Recommendations and Level of Evidence Table

Class Recommendations

Class I   There is evidence and/or agreement that a given procedure or treatment is useful and effective.

Class II   There is conflicting evidence and/or a divergence of opinion about the usefulness/efficacy of a procedure or treatment.

     IIa   The weight of evidence/opinion is in favor of usefulness/efficacy.

     IIb   The usefulness/efficacy is less well established by evidence/opinion.

Class III   There is evidence and/or general agreement that the procedure/treatment is not useful/effective and in some cases may be harmful.

Level of Evidence

A   Data derived from multiple large randomized trials.

B   Data derived from limited number of randomized trials involving small number of patients or careful analyses of nonrandomized studies or observational registries.

C   Expert consensus.

Source: Adapted from Gregoratos G, Abrams J, et al. *Circulation* 2002;106:2145–2161.

D1364906

CARDIAC EMERGENCIES

Edited by

W. Frank Peacock IV, MD, FACEP
Vice Chief
Department of Emergency Medicine
The Cleveland Clinic
Cleveland, Ohio

Brian R. Tiffany, MD, PhD, FACEP
Chairman
Department of Emergency Medicine
Chandler Regional Hospital
Medical Director
Heart Emergency Center
Arizona Heart Hospital
Phoenix, Arizona

McGraw-Hill
Medical Publishing Division

New York   Chicago   San Francisco   Lisbon   London   Madrid   Mexico City   Milan
New Delhi   San Juan   Seoul   Singapore   Sydney   Toronto

The **McGraw·Hill** Companies

Cardiac Emergencies

Copyright © 2006 by The McGraw-Hill Companies, Inc. All rights reserved. Printed in the United States of America. Except as permitted under the United States Copyright Act of 1976, no part of this publication may be reproduced or distributed in any form or by any means, or stored in a data base or retrieval system, without the prior written permission of the publisher.

1 2 3 4 5 6 7 8 9 0   DOC/DOC   0 9 8 7 6 5

ISBN: 0-07-143131-4

Notice

Medicine is an ever-changing science. As new research and clinical experience broaden our knowledge, changes in treatment and drug therapy are required. The authors and the publisher of this work have checked with sources believed to be reliable in their efforts to provide information that is complete and generally in accord with the standards accepted at the time of publication. However, in view of the possibility of human error or changes in medical sciences, neither the editors nor the publisher nor any other party who has been involved in the preparation or publication of this work warrants that the information contained herein is in every respect accurate or complete, and they disclaim all responsibility for any errors or omissions or for the results obtained from use of the information contained in this work. Readers are encouraged to confirm the information contained herein with other sources. For example and in particular, readers are advised to check the product information sheet included in the package of each drug they plan to administer to be certain that the information contained in this work is accurate and that changes have not been made in the recommended dose or in the contraindications for administration. This recommendation is of particular importance in connection with new or infrequently used drugs.

This book was set in Times by International Typesetting and Composition.
The editors were Marc Strauss and Karen G. Edmonson.
The production supervisor was Sherri Souffrance.
Project management was provided by International Typesetting and Composition.
The cover designer was Aimee Nordin.
The indexer was Susan G. Hunter.
RR Donnelley was printer and binder.

This book is printed on acid-free paper.

Cataloging-in-Publication Data for this title is on file at the Library of Congress.

This book is dedicated to my grandmother, Nanny, for teaching me the most important lessons in life; to my Mom and Dad for showing me what is real; and to my wife, Judy, and my kids, Ayla and Dakota, for putting up with me while I worked on chapters at baseball games, on camping trips, and in the back of the car while driving on vacations. W. Frank Peacock IV

To my wonderful wife, Joni, and my boys, Ben, Ryan, and Jacob, for letting this project be an enormous part of their lives too; to my parents, for their example of how to live a life; and to Blaine White, MD, for instilling in me his love of learning, and for showing me that limits are just things you place on yourself. Brian R. Tiffany

CONTENTS

CONTRIBUTORS

David Amponsah, MD [1]
Senior Staff Physician
Department of Emergency Medicine
Henry Ford Hospital
Detroit, Michigan

Ezra A. Amsterdam, MD, FACC [18]
Professor of Medicine (Cardiology)
University of California, Davis School of Medicine
Medical Director, Coronary Care Unit
University of California, Davis Medical Center
Sacramento, California

Douglas S. Ander, MD [28]
Associate Professor
Department of Emergency Medicine
Emory University School of Medicine
Atlanta, Georgia

Andra L. Blomkalns, MD, FACEP [11, 17]
Assistant Professor and Director of Residency Program
Department of Emergency Medicine
University of Cincinnati College of Medicine
Cincinnati, Ohio

Gerard X. Brogan, Jr., MD, FACEP [16]
Vice President of Emergency Services
North Shore University Hospital at Plainview
North Shore University Hospital at Syosset
Franklin Hospital Medical Center
Associate Professor of Clinical Emergency Medicine
New York University School of Medicine
New York, New York

Abhinav Chandra, MD [35]
Assistant Clinical Professor
Director, Clinical Evaluation Unit
Division of Emergency Medicine
Duke University Medical Center
Durham, North Carolina

Sean P. Collins, MD, MS [31, 33]
Assistant Professor of Emergency Medicine
Department of Emergency Medicine
University of Cincinnati College of Medicine
Cincinnati, Ohio

Thomas E. Collins, Jr., MD, FACEP [24]
Emergency Medical Services Director
Department of Emergency Medicine
Metro Health Medical Center
Medical Director, City of Cleveland
Department of Public Safety
Assistant Professor, Case Western Reserve University
   School of Medicine
Cleveland, Ohio

Deborah B. Diercks, MD, FACEP [18, 25, 26]
Assistant Professor of Emergency Medicine
University of California, Davis
Sacramento, California

Lala M. Dunbar, MD, PhD, FACEP [21]
Clinical Professor of Medicine and Emergency Medicine
Director of Medical Emergency Room
Director of Emergency Medicine Research
Louisiana State University Health Sciences Center
New Orleans, Louisiana

Charles L. Emerman, MD, FACEP [29]
Professor and Chairman of Emergency Medicine
Department of Emergency Medicine
Case Western Reserve University
Cleveland, Ohio

Gregory J. Fermann, MD, FACEP [4]
Director
Emergency Medicine
The Christ Hospital
Assistant Professor, Department of Emergency Medicine
University of Cincinnati College of Medicine
Cincinnati, Ohio

Francis M. Fesmire, MD, FACEP [9]
Director
Heart & Stroke Center
Erlanger Medical Center
Associate Professor of Medicine
University of Tennessee College
   of Medicine
Chattanooga, Tennessee

J. Christian Fox, MD, RDMS, FACEP, FAAEM [10]
Assistant Clinical Professor of Emergency Medicine
Director, Emergency Ultrasound Program
Department of Emergency Medicine
University of California, Irvine Medical Center
Irvine, California

David French, MD [8]
Department of Emergency Medicine
Carolinas Medical Center
Charlotte, North Carolina

J. Lee Garvey, MD, FACEP [8]
Department of Emergency Medicine
Carolinas Medical Center
Charlotte, North Carolina

W. Brian Gibler, MD, FACEP [17]
Professor and Chairman
Department of Emergency Medicine
University of Cincinnati College of Medicine
Cincinnati, Ohio

Eric A. Gross, MD, FACEP [36]
Assistant Program Director
Department of Emergency Medicine
Maricopa Medical Center
Phoenix, Arizona

James W. Hoekstra, MD, FACEP [15]
Professor and Chairman
Department of Emergency Medicine
Wake Forest University School of Medicine
Winston-Salem, North Carolina

Judd E. Hollander, MD, FACEP [7]
Professor
Clinical Research Director
Department of Emergency Medicine
Hospital of the University of Pennsylvania
Philadelphia, Pennsylvania

J. Douglas Kirk, MD, FACEP [18]
Associate Professor of Emergency Medicine
University of California, Davis School of Medicine
Medical Director, Chest Pain Evaluation Unit
University of California, Davis Medical Center
Sacramento, California

Jason Knight, MD [20]
Department of Emergency Medicine
Maricopa Medical Center
Phoenix, Arizona

Kenneth C. Jackimczyk, MD, FACEP [39]
Vice Chairman
Attending Physician
Department of Emergency Medicine
Maricopa Medical Center
Phoenix, Arizona

Raymond E. Jackson, MD [39]
Codirector of Clinical Research
Department of Emergency Medicine
William Beaumont Hospital
Clinical Associate Professor of Emergency Medicine
Department of Emergency Medicine
Wayne State University School of Medicine
Detroit, Michigan

Michael C. Kontos, MD, FACC [19]
Assistant Professor of Internal Medicine (Cardiology)
Virginia Commonwealth University Medical Center
Richmond, Virginia

Evan C. Leibner, MD, FACEP [37]
Chandler Emergency Medical Group
Chandler Regional Hospital
Chandler, Arizona

Phillip D. Levy, MD [34]
Assistant Residency Director
Detroit Receiving Hospital
Assistant Professor of Emergency Medicine
Wayne State University School of Medicine
Detroit, Michigan

Laszlo Littmann, MD [8]
Department of Internal Medicine
Carolinas Medical Center
Charlotte, North Carolina

Sharon E. Mace, MD, FACEP, FAPP [40, 41, 42, 43]
Director, Pediatric Education and
　Quality Improvement
Director, Observation Unit
The Cleveland Clinic Foundation
Associate Professor, Department of
　Emergency Medicine
Ohio State University School of Medicine
Cleveland, Ohio

Chadwick Miller, MD [15]
Assistant Residency Director
Department of Emergency Medicine
Wake Forest University School of Medicine
Winston-Salem, North Carolina

Donald A. Moffa, MD, FACEP [22]
Director of Education
Department of Emergency Medicine
The Cleveland Clinic
Cleveland, Ohio

Richard M. Nowak, MD, FACEP [1]
Senior Staff
Department of Emergency Medicine
Henry Ford Hospital
Detroit, Michigan

Brian S. Oliver, MD [39]
Department of Emergency Medicine
Maricopa Medical Center
Phoenix, Arizona

Brian P. O'Neil, MD, FACEP [5, 6]
Research Director
William Beaumont Hospitals
Professor of Emergency Medicine
Wayne State University
Detroit, Michigan

Joseph P. Ornato, MD, FACP, FACC, FACEP [19]
Professor and Chairman
Department of Emergency Medicine
Virginia Commonwealth University
　Medical Center
Richmond, Virginia

Ronny M. Otero, MD [35]
Senior Staff, Department of Emergency Medicine
Henry Ford Hospital
Detroit, Michigan

W. Frank Peacock IV, MD, FACEP [30]
Vice Chief
Department of Emergency Medicine
The Cleveland Clinic
Cleveland, Ohio

Sridevi Pitta, MD [23]
Department of Internal Medicine
Wayne State University School
　of Medicine
Detroit Receiving Hospital
Detroit, Michigan

Charles V. Pollack, Jr., MA, MD [12]
Chairman
Department of Emergency Medicine
Pennsylvania Hospital
Associate Professor of Emergency Medicine
University of Pennsylvania School
　of Medicine
Philadelphia, Pennsylvania

David J. Robinson, MD [13]
Assistant Professor
Research Director and Vice Chairman
Department of Emergency Medicine
University of Texas Health Science Center
　at Houston
Memorial Hermann Hospital
Houston, Texas

Michael A. Ross, MD, FACEP [5]
Chest Pain Center Medical Director
Emergency Center Observation Director
William Beaumont Hospitals
Clinical Associate Professor
Department of Emergency Medicine
Wayne State University
Detroit, Michigan

John Sarko, MD [20]
Department of Emergency Medicine
Maricopa Medical Center
Phoenix, Arizona

Assaad J. Sayah, MD, FACEP [14]
Tufts University School of Medicine
Caritas Good Samaritan Medical Center
Brockton, Massachussetts

Chong Meng Seet, MD [27]
Consultant Physician
Emergency Department
National University Hospital
Republic of Singapore

Steve D. Slauson, MD [36]
Department of Emergency Medicine
Maricopa Medical Center
Phoenix, Arizona

Alan B. Storrow, MD [27]
Associate Professor
Department of Emergency Medicine
University of Cincinnati College of Medicine
Cincinnati, Ohio

Richard L. Summers, MD, FACEP [32]
Professor of Emergency Medicine
Assistant Professor of Physiology and Biophysics
Department of Emergency Medicine
University of Mississippi
Jackson, Mississippi

James L. Tatum, MD [19]
Professor
Department of Radiology
Virginia Commonwealth University Medical Center
Richmond, Virginia

Brian R. Tiffany, MD, PhD, FACEP [2]
Chairman
Department of Emergency Medicine
Chandler Regional Hospital
Medical Director
Heart Emergency Center
Arizona Heart Hospital
Phoenix, Arizona

Robert Wahl, MD, FACEP [23]
Program Director
Department of Emergency Medicine
Detroit Receiving Hospital
Associate Professor of Emergency Medicine
Wayne State University School of Medicine
Detroit, Michigan

Daniel J. Walters, MD, PharmD [21]
Emergency Physician
Charity Hospital
Department of Emergency Medicine
Louisiana State University Health Sciences Center
New Orleans, Louisiana

James Edward Weber, DO, FACEP [3, 38]
Assistant Professor
Department of Emergency Medicine
University of Michigan Medical School
Ann Arbor, Michigan

Robert D. Welch, MD, MS, FACEP [34]
Department of Emergency Medicine
Detroit Receiving Hospital
Associate Professor of Emergency Medicine
Wayne State University School of Medicine
Detroit, Michigan

Joseph Wood, MD, JD, RDMS, FACEP, FAAEM [10]
Assistant Professor
Mayo Clinic Medical School
Mayo Clinic Hospital
Scottsdale, Arizona

Robert J. Zalenski, MD [23]
Department of Medicine
Urgent Care Section
John D. Dingell Veterans Hospital
Brooks F. Bock Endowed Professor
Department of Emergency Medicine
Wayne State University
Detroit, Michigan

Alexander M. Zlidenny, MD, RDMS [10]
Director of Emergency Ultrasound
California Emergency Physicians
Providence Holy Cross Medical Center
Mission Hills, California

FOREWORD

CARDIOVASCULAR DISEASE is now the world's leading cause of morbidity and mortality. In adult men worldwide, nearly 12% suffer from coronary heart disease or stroke. Compare that to the approximately 7% affected with HIV/AIDS, 5% with unipolar depressive disorders, and about 5% with road traffic injuries. Statistics are nearly as alarming for adult women worldwide: just over 10% with coronary heart disease or stroke, compared to about 8% with unipolar depressive disorders, and 7% with HIV/AIDS.[1]

Deaths from coronary heart disease worldwide are staggering. In sheer numbers, the leading countries in terms of deaths from coronary heart disease are the Russian Federation, China, and India. Croatia, Kazakhstan, Belarus, Ukraine, and Romania all experienced increases in death rates from 1988 to 1998 of 20–62%.[1] Increases in life expectancy, genetics, and lifestyle are the major factors affecting mortality rates. Emphasis on prevention and improved diagnosis and treatment has led to decreases in mortality rates in the United States, Australia, the Scandinavian countries, and many countries of Western Europe.

In 1893, Einthoven developed the electrocardiogram, and transmitted an ECG over 1.5 km by telephone cable. He received the Nobel Prize in 1924 for these accomplishments. The first right heart catheterization documented with radiographs in a human was performed by Forssman in 1929. The benefits of aspirin were described in 1948 by Lawrence Craven, and the first report of human defibrillation was published by Paul Zoll in 1956. The first coronary PTCA was performed by Andreas Gruentzig in 1977 in Switzerland. Despite many decades of steady advancements in cardiac diagnostics and treatment, we are still learning how to apply these advances in a timely and effective fashion to the patients we care for every day.

The Emergency Department is now the translational environment for the application of the skills of diagnosis, resuscitation, and stabilization that were developed over 50 years ago. The scope of Emergency Medicine includes all those aspects of cardiac care from the prehospital phase to the catheterization laboratory and coronary care unit. Continued stresses on hospital resources will be expected to further shift care for low-probability acute coronary events and dysrhythmias to the Emergency Department. Effective patient care will mean successful integration of knowledge and tasks between emergency physicians and cardiologists. The breadth and depth of this text represents the successful translation and integration of knowledge that is now a must for all contemporary emergency physicians.

Judith Tintinalli, MD, MS
Professor and Chair
Department of Emergency Medicine
University of North Carolina at Chapel Hill
Chapel Hill, North Carolina

IN THE EARLY 1990s, the Medical College of Virginia (now Virginia Commonwealth University Health System) had a medicine emergency room (ER). While the medicine ER was staffed by internists and IM residents, there was a clear demarcation between ER and inpatient services, and an overriding philosophy was that we (cardiologists) accepted admissions from the ER but did not assume their care until they physically arrived in the CCU. It was "us versus them." Challenges of the early fibrinolytic protocols confounded by the growing "Rule-out MI" population mandated that acute care cardiology assume a more active presence in the ER. One of the tenets of our original systematic chest pain protocol was "vertical integration." This term was later co-opted by the business re-engineering community, but from our perspective was intended to convey the seamless care for cardiac patients from arrival, and as they transitioned from the ground-floor ER to the fourth-floor CCU.

---

1. MacKay J, Mensah GA. *The Atlas of Heart Disease and Stroke.* The World Health Organization, Geneva, Switzerland, 2004.

For this vision to become a reality, Cardiology had to maintain an active presence and functional relationship with the ER.

We use the term *emergency room* correctly because at the time there was a medicine ER run by the Department of Medicine (along with a surgical ER, a pediatrics ER, and an obstetrics/gynecology ER). Several years later these individual departmental ERs gave way to a true Department of Emergency Medicine, staffed by EM physicians with a fledgling EM residency program. The ED-Cardiology integration had to be redefined, but the history of the strong interdependence carried significant weight, especially at the nursing level. Definitions inherent in the chest pain protocols had over the years become a common language between ED and CCU nursing and physicians, and an active joint clinical research program had provided resources that bolstered this relationship. Despite some growing pains, the strong interaction between EM and Cardiology was reforged around important quality and performance programs.

Through this process we learned the importance of devising systems to drive quality, to disseminate new guidelines, and to facilitate implementation of these processes into acute cardiac care. Most important is the concept that accountability for both processes of care and outcomes in acute cardiac patients lies jointly in the hands of EM and Cardiology. We firmly believe that this model of shared governance, including education, communication, and facilitation, is vital to the delivery of optimal acute cardiac care. It is the growing relationship between EM and Cardiology as seen in the codevelopment of clinical practice guidelines, and in projects such as this book, that will ultimately result in the key changes needed to improve ACS care.

Robert L. Jesse, MD, PhD
National Program Director for Cardiology
Veterans Health Administration
Professor, Internal Medicine/Cardiology
Director, Acute Cardiac Care Program
Virginia Commonwealth University Health System
Richmond, Virginia

Charlotte S. Roberts, RN, ACNP
On behalf of the Acute Cardiac Team
Virginia Commonwealth University Health System
Richmond, Virginia

EVOLUTION IS THE SCIENCE of change, and no more appropriate word describes how the specialty of emergency medicine has arrived at a place where this textbook could be published. This book represents the work of dozens of emergency physicians and cardiologists who are at the forefront of shaping current practice, and it rests on the foundation work of the thousands of physicians from many different specialties who went before us. It has been an honor to be entrusted with this project on behalf of our colleagues.

When we were young residents, there were no "old" emergency docs. The specialty was too new. But there were young, aggressive, and sometimes arrogant physicians who were willing to take on the status quo and to create a new specialty from nothing. While we could both mention dozens of colleagues and mentors who have broken the trail that the rest of us may now follow, we here single out two individuals for special recognition.

No individual has been more dedicated to the cause of establishing emergency medicine as a legitimate specialty, complete with its own literature, a healthy, rapidly evolving research base, and its own TV show, than Judy Tintinalli. Her text, the *Emergency Medicine Study Guide*, was one of the first to break ground in this new territory, and it has become the defining text of emergency medicine. Judy's efforts continue today. Without her mentorship, guidance, leadership, prodding, and sometimes a good hard poke, this book would not have happened.

No discussion of resuscitation research in emergency medicine can go far without talking about Blaine White. Blaine was one of the first to do meaningful basic science research in emergency medicine, doing pioneering resuscitation work and blazing a trail with research fellowship training and federal grant funding that dozens of emergency medicine researchers follow today with great success. His example of the value of collaboration and his refusal to allow his area of expertise to be limited by the label "emergency physician" (or for that matter, the label "physician") have inspired a generation of academic emergency physicians. Many of the contributors to this book can trace their emergency medicine "genealogies" straight to Blaine.

We offer this text as another step in the evolution of emergency medicine, to begin to define a new area of expertise, emergency cardiology. It is unique in that it is a shared vision between emergency physicians and cardiologists, working to attain the common goal of improved patient care. Besides, we are now becoming old emergency physicians who will someday require the services of our younger brethren. We want them to know what they are doing.

W. Frank Peacock IV, MD, FACEP

Brian R. Tiffany, MD, PhD, FACEP

1

Algorithms for the Management of Cardiovascular Emergencies

David Amponsah
Richard M. Nowak

GUIDELINES FOR THE MANAGEMENT OF PATIENTS WITH ST-SEGMENT ELEVATION MYOCARDIAL INFARCTION/NEW LEFT BUNDLE BRANCH BLOCK

ST-segment elevation myocardial infarction (STEMI) is defined as greater than or equal to 1 mm ST-segment elevation in two or more contiguous limb leads, or greater than or equal to 2 mm ST-segment elevation in the precordial leads.[1] Right ventricular (RV) infarction is associated with occlusion of the proximal segment of the right coronary artery. The ECG sign of RV infarction is demonstration of ST-elevation of more than 1 mm in lead V4R with an upright T-wave in that lead.[2]

ECG diagnosis of acute MI (AMI) can be masked in the setting of spontaneous or pacing-induced left bundle branch block (LBBB). The finding of a new LBBB in a patient with acute chest pain is highly suggestive of an AMI. Sgarbossa has devised some rules to assist in the recognition of an AMI in the setting of a LBBB. An ST-segment elevation of at least 1 mm that is concordant with (in the same direction as) the QRS-complex or ST-segment depression of at least 1 mm in lead V_1, V_2, or V_3 is a specific marker of infarction, even with no other observed ECG changes. The sole presence of ST-segment elevation of greater than or equal to 5 mm that is discordant with (in the opposite direction from) the QRS-complex indicates a moderate-to-high probability of MI.[3] These rules, in addition to a clinical history of ischemic-type chest discomfort, clinical examination, and serum cardiac markers, will assist in confirming the diagnosis of AMI in the setting of a LBBB.

INITIAL RECOGNITION AND EMERGENCY DEPARTMENT MANAGEMENT

1. An AMI protocol should be established in the ED to identify patients with STEMI or new LBBB by ECG within 10 min of arrival.

2. Early diagnosis of STEMI/LBBB will help assure a door-to-needle time for fibrinolytic therapy within 30 min in eligible patients. Similarly, primary percutaneous transluminal coronary angioplasty (PTCA) can be achieved in 90 ± 30 min.

3. Patients diagnosed with STEMI/LBBB should receive supplemental oxygen, intravenous (IV) access, and continuous ECG monitoring.

4. Early consultation with a cardiologist should be made to assure timely definitive intervention, particularly involving primary PTCA.

5. Figure 1-1 illustrates an algorithm for the initial assessment and evaluation of the patient with acute chest pain.

Pharmacotherapy

Aspirin and Other Platelet-Active Drugs

- A dose of 162–325 mg of nonenteric aspirin should be administered as soon as possible.

- Aspirin may be chewed for more rapid absorption, particularly in patients who are not on a daily regimen.

- Aspirin should be avoided in those with known hypersensitivity and used cautiously in those with blood dyscrasias or severe hepatic disease.

- Clopidogrel is indicated in patients who have a hypersensitivity to aspirin. Clopidogrel is preferable to ticlopidine due to its less severe or lower incidence of adverse effects.[4,5] The daily dose of clopidogrel is 75 mg PO.

- Clopidogrel is normally added to aspirin in patients undergoing percutaneous coronary intervention (PCI), especially stenting. The recommended loading dose is 300 mg orally.

β-Adrenoceptor Blocking Agents

- β-blockers should be given IV to patients with STEMI who can be treated within 12 hours of onset of infarction, irrespective of administration of concomitant thrombolytic therapy or primary PTCA.

- IV metoprolol should be given slowly in 5 mg IVP increments, repeated every 5 min to a total initial dose of 15 mg. Alternatively, IV atenolol may be given slowly in 5 mg IV push increments, repeated in 5 min to a total dose of 10 mg.

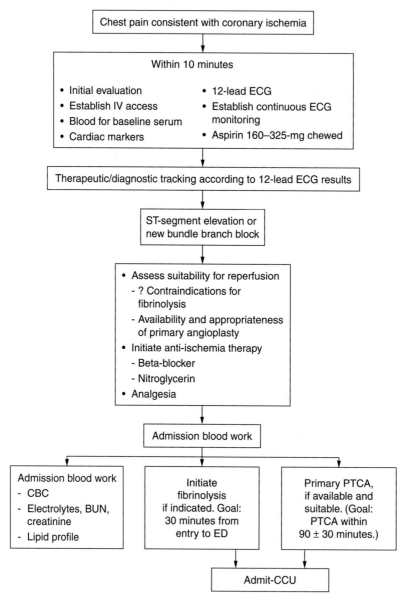

Fig. 1-1. Approach to patient with suspected acute coronary syndrome.

- Relative contraindications to β-blockers include:

  HR <60 bpm
  Systolic arterial pressure <100 mmHg
  Moderate left ventricular (LV) failure
  Signs of peripheral hypoperfusion
  PR interval >0.24 s (see Fig. 1-3)
  Second- or third-degree atrioventricular (AV) block
  Severe chronic obstructive pulmonary disease
  History of asthma
  Severe peripheral vascular disease
  Insulin-dependent diabetes mellitus

Nitroglycerin

- Patients with ischemic type chest discomfort should receive sublingual nitroglycerin (NTG) (0.4 mg tablet), unless the initial systolic blood pressure is less than 90 mmHg.
- IV NTG is indicated in patients with AMI and congestive heart failure (CHF), large anterior infarction, persistent ischemia or hypertension.
- IV NTG therapy can be initiated at 10–20 mg/min, with an increase in dosage by 5–10 µg every 5–10 min while carefully monitoring hemodynamic and clinical responses.
- Titration end points are control of clinical symptoms or decrease in mean arterial pressure of 10% in normotensive patients, or 30% in hypertensive patients (but never a systolic pressure <90 mgHg), and an increase in heart rate (HR) greater than 10 bpm (but not exceeding 110 bpm).
- Doses greater than 200 µg/min are associated with an increased risk of hypotension.
- Long-acting oral nitrate preparations should be avoided in the early management of STEMI.
- Sublingual or transdermal NTG can be used, but IV infusion of NTG allows for more precise minute-to-minute control of the agent.
- NTG should be avoided in the presence of marked bradycardia (<50 bpm) or tachycardia (>110 bpm) and used with extreme caution, if at all, in patients with suspected RV infarction.

Morphine Sulphate

- Effective analgesia (e.g., IV morphine) should be administered promptly at the time of diagnosis and should not be delayed on the premise; to do so will obscure ability to evaluate the results of antiischemic therapy.
- Morphine sulphate can be administered IV at a rate of 2–4 mg. This may be repeated every 5 min, with close monitoring of vital signs.
- Morphine-induced respiratory depression can be reversed with 0.4 mg of naloxone IV at up to 3-min intervals to a maximum of 3 doses.

Atropine

The following recommendations are applicable from early AMI to 6 or 8 hours afterward:

- Sinus bradycardia with evidence of low cardiac output and peripheral hypoperfusion or frequent premature ventricular contractions (PVCs) at onset of symptoms of AMI.
- Acute inferior MI with type 1 second- or third-degree AV block associated with symptoms of hypotension, ischemic discomfort, or ventricular arrhythmias.
- Sustained bradycardia and hypotension after administration of NTG.
- For nausea and vomiting associated with administration of morphine.
- Ventricular asystole.
- Recommended dose of atropine for bradycardia is 0.5–1.0 mg IV, repeated if needed every 3–5 min to a total dose of no more than 2.5 mg (0.03–0.04 mg/kg).
- Pacing is the treatment of choice for symptomatic bradycardia not responding promptly to atropine administration.

Anticoagulants

- Unfractionated heparin (IV) is recommended for patients undergoing PTCA or reperfusion therapy with alteplase/reteplase/anistreplase and not streptokinase.
- Recommended dose of unfractionated heparin is bolus 60 U/kg IV followed by an infusion rate of 12 U/kg/hour (with a maximum of 4000 U bolus and 1000 U/hour infusion for patients weighing >70 kg), adjusted to maintain aPTT at 1.5–2.0 times control (50–70 s) for 48 hours.
- There are no current guidelines recommending the use of low molecular weight heparin for treatment of STEMI.

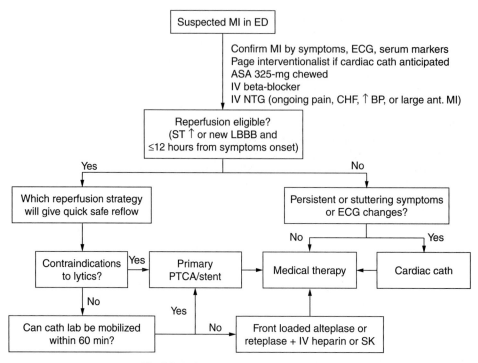

Fig. 1-2. Patient management in suspected MI.

Thrombolytic Therapy

See Fig. 1-2.

- Before thrombolytic agents are administered it is important to rule out any contraindications which may result in significant bleeding including intracranial hemorrhage. A list of potential absolute and relative contraindications is shown in Table 1-1.
- Recognition that acute coronary thrombosis is primary to the pathogenesis of STEMI led to the consideration of plasminogen activators as a preferred therapeutic approach to achieving rapid thrombolysis.
- Table 1-2 shows some of the comparative features of the Food and Drug Administration (FDA)-approved thrombolytic agents.

Fibrinolytic Dosing

- Alteplase 15 mg bolus IV, followed by 0.75 mg/kg infusion (up to 50 mg) over 30 min, followed by 0.50 mg/kg (up to 35 mg) over the next 60 min.

- Reteplase 10 U bolus over 2 min; repeat 10 U bolus after 30 min (total dose 20 U).
- Anistreplase 30 mg IV infusion over 5 min.
- Streptokinase (SK) 1.5 MU infused over 30–60 min (note: no heparin infusion when administering SK).

A newer fibrinolytic agent, tenecteplase, recently approved by the FDA for treatment of patients with AMI, has been shown to be as safe and effective as alteplase (t-PA) based on the results of the Assessment of Safety and Efficacy of a New Thrombolytic agent (ASSENT-2) trial.[6] This agent is also administered with unfractionated heparin. Dosing protocol for tenecteplase (IV bolus to be administered over 5 s) is shown in Table 1-3.

GUIDELINES FOR THE MANAGEMENT OF PATIENTS WITH SUPRAVENTRICULAR ARRHYTHMIAS

In these guidelines, supraventricular tachycardia (SVT) is used to describe reentrant arrhythmias involving the AV junction (atrioventricular nodal reciprocating

Table 1-1. Contraindications and Cautions for Fibrinolytic Use in Myocardial Infarction[*]

Absolute contraindications
- Previous hemorrhagic stroke at any time: other strokes or cerebrovascular events within 1 year
- Known intracranial neoplasm
- Active internal bleeding (does not include menses)
- Suspected aortic dissection

Cautions/relative contraindications
- Severe uncontrolled hypertension on presentation (blood pressure >180/110 mmHg)[†]
- History of prior cerebrovascular accident or known intracerebral pathology not covered in contraindications
- Current use of anticoagulants in therapeutic doses (INR[‡] ≥ 2–3); known bleeding diathesis
- Recent trauma (within 2–4 weeks), including head trauma
- Noncompressible vascular punctures
- Recent (within 2–4 weeks) internal bleeding
- For streptokinase/anistreplase: prior exposure (especially within 5 days to 2 years) or prior allergic reaction
- Pregnancy
- Active peptic ulcer
- History of chronic hypertension

[*]Viewed as advisory for clinical decision making and may not be all-inclusive or definitive.
[†]Could be an absolute contraindication in low-risk patients with myocardial infarction.
[‡]INR indicates International Normalized Ratio.

tachycardia [AVNRT]), atrium (atrial tachycardia [AT]), or AV-reciprocating rhythms (atrioventricular-reciprocating tachycardia [AVRT]). A number of predisposing factors may be responsible for patients presenting with a history suggestive of an arrhythmia without ECG documentation. Table 1-4 presents a list of possible causes.

General Evaluation of Patients with Documented Arrhythmia

- A 12-lead ECG should be done during tachycardia, but should not delay immediate therapy to terminate the arrhythmia if the patient is hemodynamically unstable.

Table 1-2. Comparison of Approved Fibrinolytic Agents

	Streptokinase	**Anistreplase**	**Alteplase**	**Reteplase**
Dose	1.5 MU in 30–60 min	30 mg in 5 min	100 mg in 90 min	2–10 U doses 30 min apart
Bolus administration	No	Yes	No	Yes
Antigenic	Yes	Yes	No	No
Allergic reactions (hypotension most common)	Yes	Yes	No	No
Systemic fibrinogen depletion	Marked	Marked	Mild	Moderate
90-min patency rates (%)	~50	~65	~75	~75
TIMI[*] grade 3 flow (%)	32	43	54	60
Mortality rate in most recent comparative trials (%)	7.3	10.5	7.2	7.5
Cost per dose (US)	$294	$2116	$2196	$2196

[*]TIMI (thrombolysis in myocardial infarction study) grade 3 flow rate indicates normal flow.

Table 1-3. Dosing Protocol for Tenecteplase

FT WT(kg)	TNK Dose(mg)
<60	30
60–69	35
70–79	40
80–89	45
>90	50

Source: Adapted from reference 4.

- If ventricular activation (QRS) is <120 ms, then the tachycardia is almost always supraventricular in origin.
- AVNRT is the most common mechanism if no atrial activity or P waves are apparent, with a regular RR interval.
- AVRT is most likely if a P-wave is present in the ST-segment and separated from the QRS by 70 ms.
- If the RP interval (Fig. 1-3) is longer than the PR interval, the most typical diagnosis is atypical

Table 1-4. Predisposing or Precipitating Factors for Patients with Palpitations

Noncardiac causes
Nicotine, alcohol, caffeine
Physical or mental stress
Hyperthyroidism
Premenstrual or menstrual
Electrolyte disturbance
Certain drugs (antiarrhythmic, antidepressant, antibiotic
    drugs; stimulants; antihistamines; appetite suppressants)
Anemia
Anxiety or hypovolemia
Fever, infection
Lack of sleep

Cardiac causes
Coronary artery disease; old myocardial infarction,
    especially for ventricular tachycardias
Congestive heart failure
Cardiomyopathy
Valvular disease
Congenital heart disease
Other conditions that may cause myocardial scarring
    (i.e., sarcoidosis, tuberculosis)
Primary electrical disorders (i.e., long QT syndrome,
    Brugada syndrome)
Accessory pathways

AVNRT, permanent form of junctional-reciprocating tachycardia (PJRT) (i.e., AVRT via a slowly conducting accessory pathway), or AT.

- Figure 1-4 illustrates a differential diagnosis for narrow QRS-complex tachycardia.
- It is important to differentiate between SVT and ventricular tachycardia (VT) when the QRS is wide (i.e., >120 ms).
- Stable vital signs during tachycardias cannot be used as criteria for distinguishing between SVT and VT.
- IV diltiazem or verapamil, which may be used for the treatment of SVT, may on the other hand precipitate hemodynamic collapse for the patient with VT.
- Wide QRS tachycardia may represent SVT with bundle branch block (BBB) or aberration, SVT with AV conduction over an accessory pathway, or VT. In the absence of a specific diagnosis of SVT, patients should be treated as having VT if the QRS is wide (>120 ms). Figure 1-5 illustrates a differential diagnosis for wide QRS-complex tachycardia (>120 ms).

Acute Management of Patients with Hemodynamically Stable and Regular Tachycardia

- Acute treatment should be initiated on the basis of the underlying mechanism when a definitive diagnosis is made based on ECG and clinical criteria. Figure 1-6 outlines the acute management of hemodynamically stable regular tachycardia.

Acute Management of Narrow QRS-Complex Tachycardia

- In regular narrow QRS-complex tachycardia, vagal maneuvers (i.e., Valsalva, carotid massage) may be initiated to terminate the arrhythmia or to modify AV conduction.
- IV antiarrhythmic drugs should be used to terminate the arrhythmia in hemodynamically stable patients.
- Adenosine is the drug of choice for terminating hemodynamically stable regular narrow QRS-complex tachycardia.

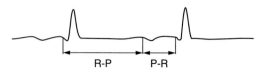

Fig. 1-3. ECG intervals.

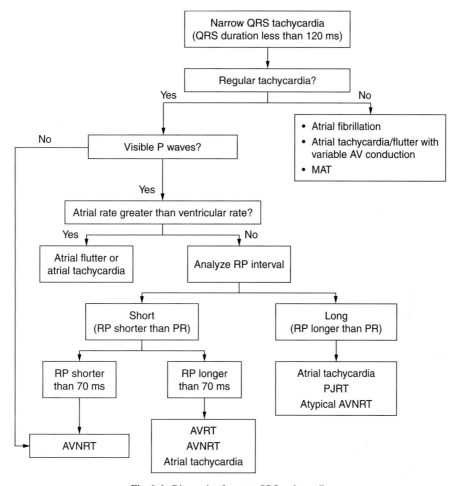

Fig. 1-4. Diagnosis of narrow QRS tachycardia.

- Adenosine should be given by rapid IVP with a flush at an initial dose of 6 mg, followed after 1–2 min if no response, with a 12 mg rapid IVP.
- Adenosine should be avoided in patients with bronchial asthma. It should also be used with caution in patients with severe coronary artery disease and may produce atrial fibrillation (AF), which may result in rapid ventricular rates for patients with preexcitation.
- Nondihydropyridine calcium-channel antagonists (e.g., diltiazem/verapamil) are also effective in terminating SVT in hemodynamically stable patients.
- IV diltiazem can be given at a dose of 20 mg (0.25 mg/kg) IV over 2 min.

- Verapamil can be used as an alternative to diltiazem at a dose of 5–10 mg IV over 2 min. Verapamil may not be used in patients with heart failure (HF) due to systolic dysfunction and associated hypotension.
- IV metoprolol can be given at dose of 2.5–5 mg over 2 min; this may be repeated every 5 min up to 3 doses.
- IV propranolol can be given at an initial dose of 0.5–1.0 mg over 1 min. This may be repeated every 5 min up to 3 doses.
- Rapid therapeutic effect for SVT can also be achieved using dc synchronized cardioversion, starting with 100–200 J, increasing energy levels to achieve desired effect. Atrial flutter can be controlled with energy levels, starting as low as 25–50 J.

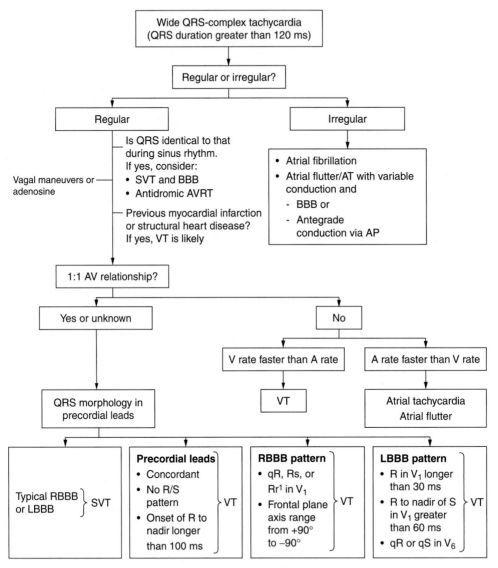

Fig. 1-5. Diagnosis of wide QRS complex tachycardia.

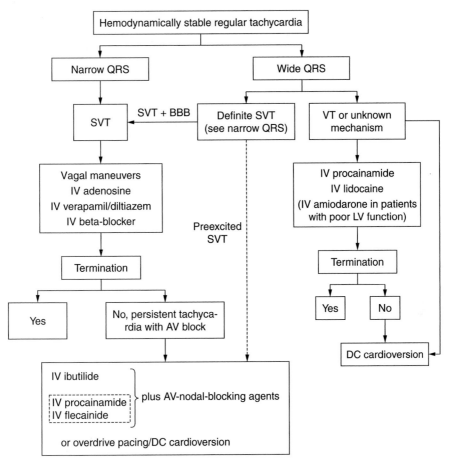

Fig. 1-6. Treatment of hemodynamically stable regular tachycardia.

Acute Management of Wide QRS-Complex Tachycardia

- If a wide QRS-complex tachycardia is definitely determined to be supraventricular in origin in a hemodynamically stable patient, then treatment should be as described for narrow complex.

- Amiodarone is the preferred drug for wide QRS-complex tachycardia, particularly for patients with impaired LV function or signs of HF.

- The initial dose of amiodarone is 150 mg IV over 10 min, followed by an infusion of 1 mg/min for 6 hours, after which 0.5 mg/min is infused as maintenance.

- IV procainamide may be given at a dose of 20–30 mg/min IV by continued infusion until the arrhythmia is suppressed, patient becomes hypotensive or QRS widens 50% above baseline, or a maximum dose of 17 mg/kg is administered. Once arrhythmia is suppressed, procainamide may be infused at a continuous rate of 1–4 mg/min.

- IV lidocaine can be given as an alternative to amiodarone at an initial bolus of 1.0–1.5 mg/kg followed by additional dose of 0.5–0.75 mg/kg every 5–10 min to a total cumulative dose of 3 mg/kg. Maintenance infusion may be started at 2 mg/min, titrating up to 4 mg/min.

- DC cardioversion is recommended for termination of irregular wide QRS-complex tachycardia (i.e., pre-excited AF), starting at 200 J.
- It is important to stress that the most effective and rapid means of terminating any hemodynamically unstable narrow or wide QRS-complex tachycardia is dc cardioversion.

ATRIAL FLUTTER

- Atrial flutter is characterized by an organized atrial rhythm with a rate typically between 250 and 350 bpm.
- Acute therapy for atrial flutter depends on the clinical presentation or the patient's hemodynamic status.
- Atrial flutter can be usually reverted to sinus rhythm with cardioversion, with energies <50 J using monophasic shocks and with less energy using biphasic shocks.
- AV nodal blocking agents are effective for rate control for atrial flutter. IV diltiazem can successfully be used for rate control. IV β-blockers may have similar effects as the calcium-channel blockers for rate control. IV verapamil should be used with caution, since it may result in symptomatic hypotension.
- IV diltiazem can be given at an initial dose of 20 mg (0.25 mg/kg) IV over 2 min as a bolus. The bolus

can be repeated after 15 min at 25 mg (0.35 mg/kg) if the rate is not adequately controlled. A maintenance dose of 5–15 mg/hour can be administered for further rate control.

- IV verapamil can be given at a dose of 5–10 mg IV over 2 min.
- Metoprolol 2.5–5 mg IV bolus over 2 min can be used, up to 3 doses for rate control.
- Esmolol at a bolus dose of 0.5 mg/kg IV can be given over 1 min followed by a maintenance dose of 0.05 mg/kg/min IV. If no therapeutic effect is observed after 5 min, the maintenance dose can be increased to 0.1 mg/kg/min IV after a second bolus of 0.5 mg/kg IV.
- IV ibutilide is especially effective for patients with atrial flutter but should not be used in patients with known LV dysfunction with ejection fraction (EF) <30% due to increased risk of polymorphic VT. The recommended dose is 0.01 mg/kg up to 1 mg IV over 10 min. Dose may be repeated only once after 10 min if no response is seen. It should also be avoided in patients with prolonged QT or those with underlying sinus node disease.
- Patients with atrial flutter of >48 hours duration should be anticoagulated prior to any mode of cardioversion. Figure 1-7 illustrates the proposed management of atrial flutter.

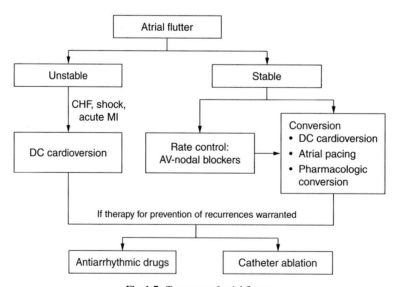

Fig. 1-7. Treatment of atrial flutter.

ATRIAL FIBRILLATION

- AF is a supraventricular tachyarrhythmia characterized by uncoordinated atrial activation with consequent deterioration of atrial mechanical function.

- Regular RR intervals are possible in the presence of AV block or interference due to ventricular or junctional tachycardia.

- A rapid irregular, sustained wide QRS-complex strongly suggests AF with conduction over an accessory pathway or AF with underlying BBB.

- Extremely rapid rates (over 200 bpm) suggest the presence of an accessory pathway.

- Table 1-5 includes a list of pharmacologic agents recommended for the management of acute AF, to achieve control of ventricular response in the emergency setting.

- IV ibutilide is effective for acute conversion of AF. The dose is similar to that for atrial flutter at 0.01 mg/kg up to 1 mg IV over 10 min. It may be repeated after 10 min, if unsuccessful.

- If a rapid ventricular response is associated with symptomatic hypotension, angina, or CHF, prompt dc synchronized cardioversion should be considered with an initial energy of 200 J or more.

APPENDIX

The following algorithms (Figs. 1-8 to 1-12) from the Advanced Cardiac Life Support (ACLS) manual have been included for easy reference.

1. Ventricular fibrillation (VF)/pulseless ventricular tachycardia (VT)
2. Pulseless electrical activity (PEA)
3. Asystole
4. Tachycardia algorithms
    a. Stable wide complex tachycardias
    b. Narrow-complex supraventricular tachycardias
5. Bradycardias: atrioventricular blocks and emergency pacing

Table 1-5. Intravenous Pharmacologic Agents for Heart Rate Control in Patients with Atrial Fibrillation

Drug[a]	Loading Dose	Onset	Maintenance Dose	Major Side Effects	Class Recommendation[b]
Diltiazem	0.25 mg/kg IV over 2 min	2–7 min	5–15 mg/h infusion	Hypotension, heart block, HF[c]	I[d]
Esmolol[d]	0.5 mg/kg over 1 min	5 min	0.05–0.2 mg/kg/min	Hypotension, heart block, bradycardia, asthma, HF	I
Metoprolol[e]	2.5–5 mg IV bolus over 2 min; up to 3 doses	5 min	NA	Hypotension, heart block, bradycardia, asthma, HF	I[d]
Propranolol[e]	0.15 mg/kg IV	5 min	NA	Hypotension, heart block, bradycardia, asthma, HF	I[d]
Verapamil	0.075–0.15 mg/kg IV over 2 min	3–5 min	NA	Hypotension, heart block, HF	I[d]
Digoxin	0.25 mg IV each 2 h, up to 1.5 mg	2 h	0.125–0.25 mg daily	Digitalis toxicity, heart block, bradycardia	IIb[f]

[a]Drugs are listed alphabetically within each class of recommendation.
[b]See class table (p. i) for class recommendations and level of evidence definitions.
[c]HF indicates heart failure.
[d]Type I in congestive HF.
[e]Only representative members of the type of β-adrenergic antagonist drugs are included in the table, but other, similar agents could be used for this indication in appropriate doses.
[f]Type IIb in congestive HF.

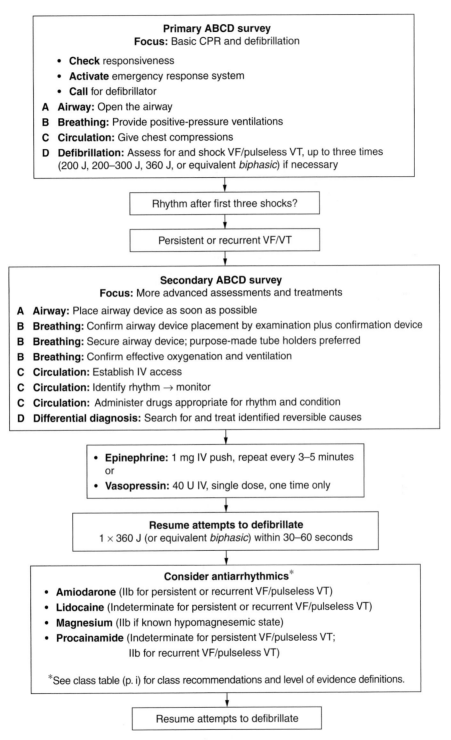

Primary ABCD survey
Focus: Basic CPR and defibrillation

- **Check** responsiveness
- **Activate** emergency response system
- **Call** for defibrillator

A **Airway:** Open the airway
B **Breathing:** Provide positive-pressure ventilations
C **Circulation:** Give chest compressions
D **Defibrillation:** Assess for and shock VF/pulseless VT, up to three times (200 J, 200–300 J, 360 J, or equivalent *biphasic*) if necessary

Rhythm after first three shocks?

Persistent or recurrent VF/VT

Secondary ABCD survey
Focus: More advanced assessments and treatments

A **Airway:** Place airway device as soon as possible
B **Breathing:** Confirm airway device placement by examination plus confirmation device
B **Breathing:** Secure airway device; purpose-made tube holders preferred
B **Breathing:** Confirm effective oxygenation and ventilation
C **Circulation:** Establish IV access
C **Circulation:** Identify rhythm → monitor
C **Circulation:** Administer drugs appropriate for rhythm and condition
D **Differential diagnosis:** Search for and treat identified reversible causes

- **Epinephrine:** 1 mg IV push, repeat every 3–5 minutes
  or
- **Vasopressin:** 40 U IV, single dose, one time only

Resume attempts to defibrillate
1 × 360 J (or equivalent *biphasic*) within 30–60 seconds

Consider antiarrhythmics[*]
- **Amiodarone** (IIb for persistent or recurrent VF/pulseless VT)
- **Lidocaine** (Indeterminate for persistent or recurrent VF/pulseless VT)
- **Magnesium** (IIb if known hypomagnesemic state)
- **Procainamide** (Indeterminate for persistent VF/pulseless VT; IIb for recurrent VF/pulseless VT)

[*]See class table (p. i) for class recommendations and level of evidence definitions.

Resume attempts to defibrillate

Fig. 1-8. Treatment of VF/VT: antiarrhythmics for persistent or recurrent VF/VT.

Pulseless electrical activity
(**PEA** = rhythm on monitor, without detectable pulse)

↓

Primary ABCD survey
Focus: Basic CPR and defibrillation

- **Check** responsiveness
- **Activate** emergency response system
- **Call** for defibrillator

A **Airway:** Open the airway
B **Breathing:** Provide positive-pressure ventilations
C **Circulation:** Give chest compressions
D **Defibrillation:** Assess for and shock VF/pulseless VT

↓

Secondary ABCD survey
Focus: More advanced assessments and treatments

A **Airway:** Place airway device as soon as possible
B **Breathing:** Confirm airway device placement by examination plus confirmation device
B **Breathing:** Secure airway device; purpose-made tube holders preferred
B **Breathing:** Confirm effective oxygenation and ventilation
C **Circulation:** Establish IV access
C **Circulation:** Identify rhythm → monitor
C **Circulation:** Administer drugs appropriate for rhythm and condition
C **Circulation:** Assess for occult blood flow (*pseudo-EMD*)
D **Differential diagnosis:** Search for and treat identified reversible causes

↓

Review for most frequent causes

- Hypovolemia
- Hypoxia
- Hydrogen ion (acidosis)
- Hyperkalemia/hypokalemia
- Hypothermia

- Tablets (drug OD, accidents)
- Tamponade, cardiac
- Tension pneumothorax
- Thrombosis, coronary (ACS)
- Thrombosis, pulmonary (embolism)

↓

Epinephrine 1 mg IV push,
repeat every 3–5 minutes

↓

Atropine 1 mg IV (if PEA rate is **slow**),
repeat every 3–5 minutes as needed, to a total
dose of 0.04 mg/kg

Fig. 1-9. Pulseless electrical activity algorithm.

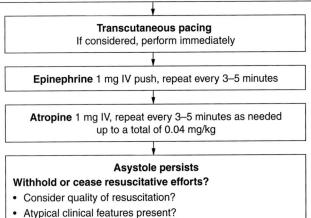

Asystole: The silent heart algorithm

↓

Primary ABCD survey

Focus: Basic CPR and defibrillation

Rapid scene survey: Is there any evidence that personnel should **not** attempt resuscitation (e.g., DNR order and signs of death)?

- **Check** responsiveness
- **Activate** emergency response system
- **Call** for defibrillator

A Airway: Open the airway

B Breathing: Provide positive-pressure ventilations

C Circulation: Give chest compressions

C Confirm: True asystole

D Defibrillation: Assess for VF/pulseless VT; shock if indicated

↓

Secondary ABCD survey

Focus: More advanced assessments and treatments

A Airway: Place airway device as soon as possible

B Breathing: Confirm airway device placement by examination plus confirmation device

B Breathing: Secure airway device; purpose-made tube holders preferred

B Breathing: Confirm effective oxygenation and ventilation

C Circulation: Confirm true asystole

C Circulation: Establish IV access

C Circulation: Identify rhythm → monitor

C Circulation: Give medications appropriate for rhythm and condition

C Circulation: Assess for occult blood flow (*pseudo-EMD*)

D Differential diagnosis: Search for and treat identified reversible causes

↓

Transcutaneous pacing
If considered, perform immediately

↓

Epinephrine 1 mg IV push, repeat every 3–5 minutes

↓

Atropine 1 mg IV, repeat every 3–5 minutes as needed
up to a total of 0.04 mg/kg

↓

Asystole persists
Withhold or cease resuscitative efforts?

- Consider quality of resuscitation?
- Atypical clinical features present?
- Support for cease-efforts protocols in place?

Fig. 1-10. Asystole: the silent heart algorithm.

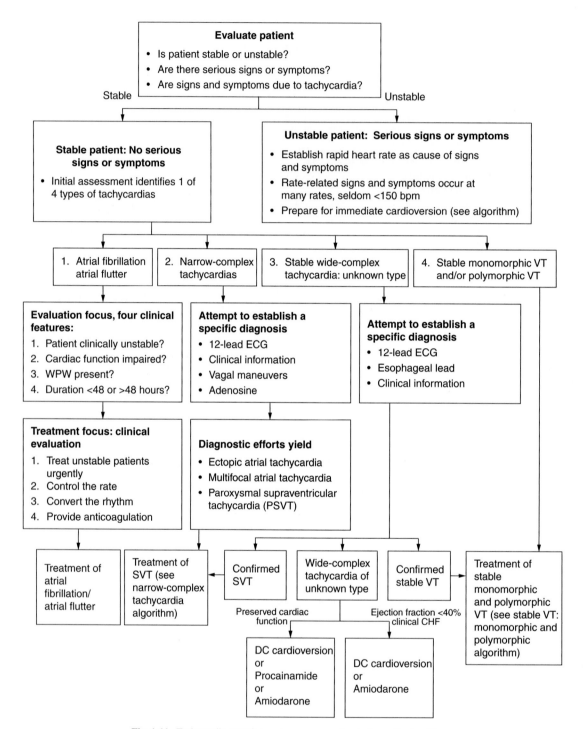

Fig. 1-11. Tachycardia overview and narrow-complex tachycardia algorithms.

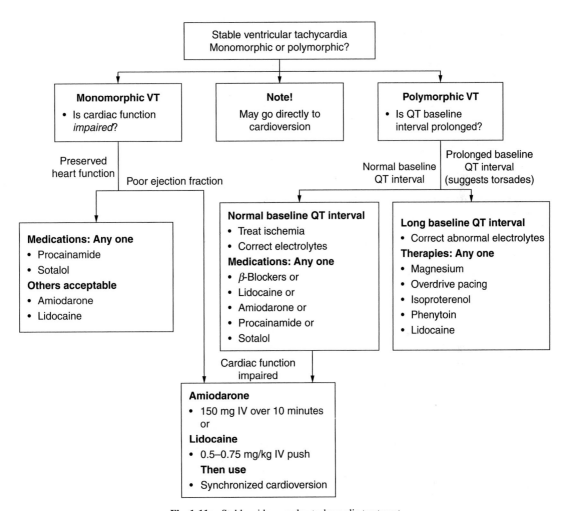

Fig. 1-11a. Stable wide-complex tachycardia treatment.

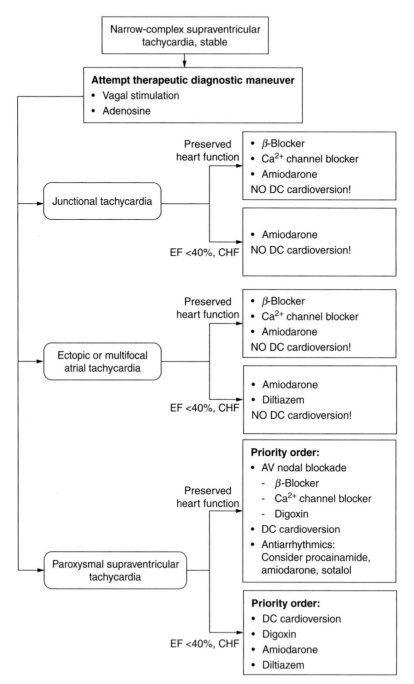

Fig. 1-11b. Narrow-complex supraventricular tachycardia treatment.

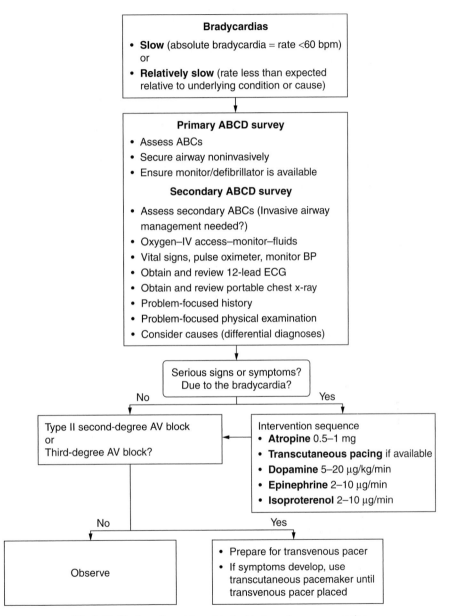

Fig. 1-12. Bradycardias: atrioventricular blocks and emergency pacing.

REFERENCES

1. ACC/AHA Guidelines for the Management of Patients with Acute Myocardial Infarction: 1999 update: A Report of the American College of Cardiology/American Heart Association Task Force on Practice Guidelines (Committee on Management of Acute Myocardial Infarction). Available at: www.acc.org.
2. Zimetbaum PJ, Josephson ME. Use of the electrocardiogram in acute myocardial infarction. *N Engl J Med* 2003;348:933–940.
3. Sgarbossa EB, Pinski SL, Barbagelata A, et al. Electrocardiographic diagnoses of evolving acute myocardial infarction in the presence of left bundle branch block. *N Engl J Med* 1996;334:481–487.
4. Quinn MJ, Fitzgerald DJ, Ticlodipine and clopidogrel. *Circulation* 1999;100(15):1667–1672.
5. Spinier SA, Hilleman DE, Cheng JWM, et al. New recommendations from the 1999 American College of Cardiology/ American Heart Association Acute Myocardial Infarction Guidelines. *Ann Pharmacother* 2001;35:589–617.
6. Angeja BG, Alexander JH, Chin R, Li X, et al. Safety of the weight-adjusted dosing regimen of tenecteplase in the ASSENT—Trial. *Am J Cardiol* 2001;88:1240–1245.

INFORMATION RESOURCES

1. ACC/AHA/ESC 2003 Guidelines for the Management of Patients with Supraventricular Arrhythmias: A Report of the American College of Cardiology/American Heart Association Task Force on Practice Guidelines. American College of Cardiology. Available at: www.acc.org/clinical/guidelines/ arrhythmias/sva_index.pdf.
2. ACC/AHA/ESC 2001 Guidelines for the Management of Patients with Atrial Fibrillation: A Report of the American College of Cardiology/American Heart Association Task Force on Practice Guidelines and the European Society of Cardiology Committee for Practice and Policy Conferences. American College of Cardiology. Available at: www.acc.org.

2

Cardiac Arrest

Brian R. Tiffany

HIGH YIELD FACTS

- Risk factors for sudden cardiac death (SCD) are the same as those for coronary artery disease.
- ECG findings such as unifocal or multifocal premature ventricular contractions (PVCs) have little value in identifying a population of patients at high risk for SCD.
- Circulatory adjuncts such as interposed abdominal compression and active compression-decompression cardiopulmonary resuscitation (CPR) appear to improve cardiac output and may improve outcomes in cardiac arrest.
- Early defibrillation is the only intervention that has been demonstrated to improve survival in cardiac arrest due to ventricular tachycardia (VT) or ventricular fibrillation (VF).
- Among antiarrhythmic agents used for VT/VF arrest, only amiodarone has been shown to improve survival to hospitalization, and no drug intervention, including epinephrine, has demonstrated a benefit on survival to discharge.

INTRODUCTION

Nontraumatic cardiac arrest is the terminal event of a number of different pathways leading to death (Table 2-1). Sudden unexpected death, defined as *death within 24 hours of symptom onset in a previously asymptomatic individual*, accounts for about one-third of all nontraumatic deaths. Of these, 75% are due to primary cardiac causes. SCD is defined as *natural death due to cardiac causes, heralded by abrupt loss of consciousness within 1 hour of the onset of acute symptoms. Preexisting heart disease may or may not have been known to be present, but the time and mode of death are unexpected.* This chapter will focus on the characteristics and treatment of cardiac arrest from primary cardiac causes.

EPIDEMIOLOGY

There are an estimated 250,000–400,000 SCDs annually in the United States, representing 50% of all cardiovascular deaths.[1] This translates into an annual incidence of 0.1–0.2% in an unselected adult (35 years and older) population. The incidence under 35 is 1 in 100,000 per year. Several high-risk subgroups with a 10-fold or greater incidence can be identified, allowing for intervention to reduce morbidity and mortality.

Heredity

Since SCD is largely a function of underlying coronary artery disease, the same risk factors operate nonspecifically for SCD. Family history is the strongest predictor of CAD, so it is no surprise that familial clusters of SCD are reported in the literature. There are also specific hereditary syndromes such as the congenital long-QT syndrome, Brugada syndrome, and hypertrophic cardiomyopathy that convey a high risk of SCD.[2]

Gender

In the Framingham study, 89% of SCD occurred in men.[3] Other studies of prehospital cardiac arrest have shown a preponderance of men ranging from 75 to 89%. When stratified by age, the male preponderance is 6:1 in the 40–64-year-old population, then declining to roughly 2:1 in the older population.

Electrocardiographic Findings

The ECG is surprisingly unhelpful in identifying a high-risk population for SCD. Seventy-five percent of SCD victims have a prior myocardial infarction. Postinfarction Q-waves are predictive of both an increased risk of SCD and all causes of cardiac mortality. However, the proportion of patients with death due to SCD is not

Table 2-1. Mechanisms of Cardiac Arrest

Etiology	Inciting Event	Underlying Cause(s)
Cardiac	Lethal dysarrhythmia	Coronary ischemia
		Cardiomyopathy
		Toxic ingestions
	PEA	Electrolyte abnormalities
		Ventricular rupture
		Valvular failure
Respiratory	Hypoxia	Hypoventilation
		Airway obstruction
		Pulmonary dysfunction
		Asphyxiation
Circulatory	Lack of venous return	Hypovolemia
		Pulmonary embolus
		Tension pneumothorax
	Vascular collapse	Sepsis
		Toxic ingestions
Metabolic	Lethal dysarrhythmia	Hyperkalemia
		Hypokalemia
		Hypomagnesemia
		Hypocalcemia
Environmental	Lethal dysarrhythmia	Lightning
		Electrocution
		Hypothermia

increased. The proportion of cardiac deaths due to SCD is not increased in patients with electrocardiographic left ventricular hypertrophy and nonspecific ST-T wave abnormalities. Among conduction abnormalities, only the presence of intraventricular conduction delays have been shown to mark an increased proportion of SCDs.[4]

The presence of unifocal PVCs in the absence of known coronary disease in patients under the age of 30 conveys no additional risk of SCD. As age increases over 30, the presence of PVCs indicates an increasing risk of coronary disease and SCD. Multifocal PVCs, PVCs > 10/hour, bigeminy, salvos of three or more complexes, and R-on-T complexes all mark a higher risk group.[5] Interestingly, three major trials of antiarrhythmics in these high-risk groups.[6–8] have failed to show a benefit of antiarrhythmic therapy; in fact both two of these trials had higher mortalities in the treatment groups.

Left Ventricular Dysfunction

Patients with left ventricular ejection fraction (LVEF) <30% are in the highest risk group for SCD. Patients with >10 PVCs/hour and LVEF <30% have a 1-year mortality in excess of 40% and an increased proportion of SCD.[9] The absolute risk of SCD increases with decreasing LVEF. Particularly relevant to emergency medical practice is the finding that unexplained syncope in a patients with functional class III or IV congestive heart failure (CHF) is associated with a 45% 1-year mortality.[10]

Time Dependence

Risk of SCD changes with time after the appearance of a risk factor. SCD frequency is highest in the first 6–18 months after a major cardiac event such as new onset CHF, out-of-hospital cardiac arrest, or recent acute myocardial infarction.

MECHANISMS

Eighty percent of SCDs are associated with athero-sclerotic disease. A number of mechanisms appear to operate in the setting of atherosclerosis which predispose to lethal dysrrhythmia.

Fixed lesions

Steady-state reductions in blood flow create a local environment where small fluctuations in electrolytes or in the metabolic state of the myocardium can quickly lead to tachydysrrhythmia. These fixed lesions can also result in local ischemia and electrical instability during periods of increased myocardial oxygen demand, likely the mechanism behind SCD during intense physical activity. Young athletes with undetected vascular anomalies such as myocardial bridging may have functional coronary flow limitations and suffer SCD by this same mechanism.

Vasospasm

Coronary artery spasm can significantly reduce blood flow in both normal vessels and those with preexisting disease. Since vasospasm is by nature a transient event, the at-risk myocardium is subjected to the hazards of both ischemia and reperfusion. Underlying etiologies include local inflammation, neurogenic modulation, toxic ingestions such as cocaine and methamphetamines, and humoral factors generated during platelet activation.

Endothelial damage

Endothelial damage, most commonly from a ruptured atherosclerotic plaque, is the most common inciting mechanism for SCD. The "active" plaque can produce occlusive or partially occlusive thrombus, acutely reducing coronary blood flow, and leading to ischemia. Platelet-derived factors play a complex role. Some platelet-derived factors produce vasospasm while others are vasodilators. Prostacyclin has been shown experimentally to protect against VF, as do thromboxane synthetase inhibitors (which theoretically shunts prostaglandin H2 toward prostacyclin production). Inhibitors of cyclooxygenase reduce prostacyclin production and experimentally enhance VF induction. Clinical evidence supporting this role for prostacyclin is the finding from the Aspirin-Myocardial Infarction Study[11] that aspirin, while reducing the incidence of reinfarction, may actually increase the absolute number of SCDs in post-MI patients.

It is also clear from indirect evidence that far more than mechanical obstruction to blood flow is involved in producing SCD. In one study, 95% of patients with SCD had either plaque fissuring, coronary thrombi, or both. However, only 18% had more than a 75% occlusion, and 44% had more than half the cross-sectional area occluded by thrombus.[12] The low rate of AMI in survivors of out-of-hospital SCD[13] also supports this view.

ELECTROPHYSIOLOGIC EFFECTS OF ISCHEMIA AND REPERFUSION

After the onset of ischemia aerobic metabolism ceases within seconds and cell revert to anaerobic metabolism, which is less efficient and does not produce adequate adenosine triphosphate to maintain the resting membrane potential. As the membrane potential falls in a given cell, excitability is reduced, upstroke velocity slows, and repolarization is slower. Once the potential reaches −60 mV, the cell is no longer excitable and cannot contribute to conduction. Since the depth of tissue hypoxia varies across the ischemic area, these changes occur at different rates in adjacent tissue resulting in a heterogeneous environment for conduction.

During reperfusion, as myocardial tissue recovers its membrane potentials, it passes again through the vulnerable zone of intermediate resting membrane potentials. In addition, continued myocardial Ca^{2+} influx due to membrane damage, the presence of superoxide radicals, and neurophysiologically induced after-potentials all contribute to arrhythmogenesis.

Local reentry is the primary mechanism underlying VT and VF. The conditions necessary for this to occur, slow conduction allowing for heterogeneity of depolarization/repolarization, and unidirectional block, are both present during ischemia and reperfusion. As would be expected from these mechanisms, there is a highly vulnerable period during the first 30 min of ischemia that abates as the resting membrane potential in ischemia myocardium falls below the excitability threshold. Continued vulnerability to lethal arrhythmias is present due to both the ischemic penumbra around the infarct zone and reperfusion.

Experimentally, several factors influence the arrhythmogenic state of ischemic myocardium. Tissue that has healed after ischemic injury maintains an increased dispersion of refractory periods, so acute ischemic injury after a healed MI is more arrhythmogenic than the same extent of ischemia in normal tissue.[14] Chronic left ventricular pressure overload, hypokalemia, and elevated adrenergic tone all increase the likelihood of arrythmogenesis from a given ischemic insult.

MANAGEMENT

Management of the suspected cardiac arrest patient can be divided into three phases: (1) initial assessment and basic life support, (2) advanced life support, and (3) postarrest care. The skill and equipment requirements increase as the patient moves through each phase.

Initial Assessment and Basic Life Support

Initial assessment consists of a few elementary diagnostic maneuvers and interventions, all of which can be performed by trained laypersons.

The first action when an unexpected collapse is encountered must be to establish the presence of a life-threatening situation. This is done by establishing the patient's level of consciousness, response to voice and touch stimuli, the presence of respiratory efforts and their quality, and the palpation for major artery pulsations at the carotid or femoral levels. If a life-threatening situation exists, the rescuer's next priority is to summon help by activating the medical rescue system.

Respiratory efforts can continue for a minute or more after cessation of circulation. Absence of respiratory efforts, or the presence of stridor with respiratory efforts, suggests a primary respiratory cause and should lead the rescuer to immediately to attempt to ventilate the patient, to search for oropharyngeal foreign bodies, and to consider attempting the Heimlich maneuver. The absence of a femoral or carotid pulse is the primary diagnostic criterion of cardiac arrest in this phase of resuscitation. Absent pulses should lead immediately to the initiation of chest compressions and ventilatory efforts.

The use of the precordial thump or "thumpversion" is controversial. The technique is to deliver one or two closed-fist blows to the upper portion of the lower third of the sternum. Each blow delivers the equivalent of a 5–10 J electrical discharge and has been shown to successfully convert VF back to an organized rhythm in a small percentage of patients. There is a corresponding theoretical risk of converting VT into VF. In 5000 patients, the largest prospective trial of precordial thump use to date, Caldwell demonstrated reversion in 5 cases of VF, 11 cases of VT, 2 cases of asystole, and 2 cases of undefined cardiovascular collapse. No cases of VT to VF conversion were found.[15] The take-home message is that thumpversion has a small but definite likelihood of working and is unlikely to cause harm, and therefore should be considered part of the initial approach to the pulseless patient. It should not be used in a conscious patient with a tachyarrhythmia. A related technique is "cough-version" in the conscious patient, which has some success at converting VT; again, there appears to be no downside risk of attempting this technique.[15]

Chest Compressions

There is, prima facie, a need to replace the lost pumping mechanism of the heart and generate forward blood flow during resuscitation. Since it was first described in 1960, closed chest cardiac massage has been the mainstay of conventional CPR.[16] Although the practice of closed chest massage is essentially unchanged from its initial description, our understanding of the physiology of circulation during cardiac arrest and resuscitation has changed dramatically in recent years.

Three different pump mechanisms are capable of moving blood during CPR. The first is the cardiac pump. Direct compression of a heart with competent valves results in forward flow as blood is forced out of the ventricles against closed mitral and tricuspid valves through the aortic and pulmonic valves. Passive filling of the ventricles occur during relaxation. This is similar to the pumping mechanism of the normally beating heart. The second mechanism is the thoracic pump. Compression of the chest causes a rise in intrathoracic pressure, forcing blood through the pulmonary vasculature, through the heart, and into the periphery. The heart acts as a passive conduit, with more or less complete incompetence of its valves.[17,18] The third mechanism is the abdominal pump. Compression of the abdomen forces blood from the abdominal aorta into the periphery against a closed aortic valve. Blood in the IVC is forced in the right atrium and ventricle where resistance is much lower than in the peripheral venous system.

The cardiac pump is the only mechanism operating during open chest cardiac massage. Intuitively, one would expect that closed chest massage would also compress the heart between the sternum and the spine and thus function by means of the cardiac pump. However, echocardiographic studies have shown that the heart valves do not open and close during CPR, and animal studies have shown that the pressure gradient across the heart is minimal, even when there is a substantial extrathoracic AV pressure gradient and measurable carotid blood flow. The thoracic pump is thus the primary circulatory mechanism during standard CPR.

A number of modifications to traditional CPR have been developed in an effort to take advantage of our understanding of the pump mechanisms, most notably interposed abdominal compressions (IAC-CPR), simultaneous compression/ventilation (SCV-CPR), and active compression-decompression (ACD-CPR). Collectively, these modified approaches are referred to as circulatory adjuncts.

In IAC-CPR, abdominal compressions by a second rescuer alternate with standard chest compressions. The hands are placed halfway between the xiphoid process and the umbilicus with the hands stacked as in standard chest compressions, and the heel of the hand is maintained in the midline over the aorta and inferior vena cava with the fingers off the abdomen as much as possible. The abdomen is compressed 1.5–2 in., or about the same depth as properly performed chest compressions. Pressures of 110 mmHg can be achieved using this technique,[19] and human trials show roughly double the forward flow achieved with standard chest compressions, or about 2 L/min in an average adult.[20] Manual abdominal compressions sufficient to produce aortic pressures at this level can be tolerated without pain by conscious adults,[21] and appear to be safe. In-hospital cardiac arrest studies have demonstrated significant improvement in outcome measures when compared with standard CPR.[20,22] The only real contraindications to IAC are pregnancy and the presence of a known abdominal aortic aneurysm.

SCV-CPR attempts to take advantage of the thoracic pump mechanism by increasing peak intrathoracic pressure generated during the compression phase of CPR. Animal models suggested an improvement in carotid flow and short-term survival, but human clinical trials were disappointing, with standard CPR actually outperforming SCV-CPR in hemodynamic parameters.[23,24]

It is intuitive that improving the "priming of the pump" in the thoracic pump model would improve hemodynamics, and indeed active decompression of the chest during the relaxation phase of chest compressions improves forward flow.[25,26] Decompression is achieved using a suction cup style device such as the Cardiopump (Ambu Inc., Glostrup, Denmark) or using sticky pads such as those incorporated into the Lifestick (Datascope, Fairfield, NJ). Use of an impedance device to prevent inflow of air through the endotracheal tube during decompression further improves forward flow.[26] Active abdominal decompression has been demonstrated to improve the circulatory effectiveness of IAC. Thoracic and abdominal ACD techniques have also been combined into four-phase CPR, or phased thoracoabdominal CPR (PTACD-CPR), in which active decompression of the abdomen and compression of the chest alternates with active decompression of the chest and compression of the abdomen. Hemodynamic modeling suggests that PTACD-CPR should deliver flow rates near 4 L/min, or near normal values.[21] The Lifestick is one device attempting to achieve practically useful PTACD-CPR. It has adhesive pads which attach to the chest and abdomen on each end of a bar, allowing alternating compression/ decompression of the chest and abdomen by a single rescuer using a rocking motion.[27]

The improved understanding of the value of circulatory adjuncts has been recognized in the most recent revision of American Heart Association (AHA) Guidelines for CPR and Emergency Cardiac Care.[28] Both ACD-CPR and IAC-CPR are considered IIb interventions, allowable within the standard of care and firmly within the realm of mainstream clinical discretion.

Defibrillation

Rapid conversion to an organized and effective rhythm is the "prime directive" in resuscitation, and other interventions such as intubation, chest compressions, IV access, or delivery of resuscitative drugs must not be allowed to delay conversion attempts. When VF or a rapid VT is identified, a defibrillation should be made immediately with a shock of 200 J, followed rapidly by shocks at 300 and 360 J if the initial shock is unsuccessful. Failure of the initial shocks to successfully cardiovert to an effective rhythm is a poor prognostic sign. After failure of three shocks up to a maximum of 360 J of energy, CPR should be continued while the patient is intubated and intravenous access is obtained. It should be kept in mind that defibrillation attempts are the primary means of resuscitation and should never be unduly delayed by intubation, obtaining intravenous access, or delivery of drugs. A slavish adherence to a specific sequence of interventions, always administering the first dose of epinephrine prior to the fourth shock, will lead to unacceptable delays in defibrillation attempts and reduce the likelihood of a successful resuscitation.

Pressor Support

The use of vasopressors during CPR results in an increase in peripheral vascular resistance and a higher "diastolic" blood pressure. Since coronary perfusion during CPR is driven by the gradient between mean arterial pressure and coronary sinus pressure, vasopressor use is crucial during prolonged CPR. Epinephrine, in a 1 mg intravenous dose, is administered and followed by repeated defibrillation attempts at 360 J. Epinephrine may be repeated at 3–5 min intervals with defibrillator shocks in between. High-dose and escalating dose epinephrine regimens do not appear to improve outcomes and are no longer recommended in AHA guidelines. Vasopressin in a single 40 U IV dose is now included in the AHA guidelines as a class IIb alternative to epinephrine on the basis of limited clinical studies showing an improved rate of return of spontaneous circulation (ROSC) in out-of-hospital cardiac arrests.[29,30] Vasopressin has a longer half-life than epinephrine (about 20 min) and thus is given as a single dose. Although no human studies have addressed this issue, if resuscitation continues beyond 20 min, it is reasonable to repeat the vasopressin dose or return to epinephrine 1.0 mg IV every 3–5 min.

Antiarrhythmic Agents

For the patient who continues to have VT or VF despite defibrillation attempts after epinephrine, electrical stability of the heart *may* be improved by intravenous administration of antiarrhythmic agents during continued resuscitation. It is important to be cognizant of the fact that the drugs which have stocked our resuscitation kits for more than 20 years were brought into wide use through rationale conjecture and extrapolation from animal studies and the use of these drugs in other settings. Antiarrhythmic agents have assumed more and more of a secondary role in resuscitation from VF/VT as the discovery of their proarrhythmic effects have undermined the already shaky underpinnings of the case for their use in these patients.

Lidocaine has a long history as the primary antiarrhythmic used in CPR. It is given as an intravenous bolus, at a dose of 1.0–1.5 mg/kg, with the dose repeated in 3–5 min up to a maximum of 3.0 mg/kg. Its use is supported by extrapolation from its efficacy in suppressing postmyocardial infarction ventricular arrhythmias and a single retrospective prehospital study.[31] Other studies have suggested an increased defibrillation threshold with lidocaine use and a lower rate of ROSC.[32] The current American Heart Association Advanced Cardiac Life Support (ACLS) guidelines give lidocaine an indeterminate rating for use in VF/VT.

Intravenous amiodarone has been studied extensively in the treatment of unstable VT, but only one randomized trial in the setting of cardiac arrest has been done.[33] In this placebo-controlled trial, a single 300 mg IV dose of amiodarone improved ROSC and improved survival to hospital admission. No benefit on survival to discharge was observed. On this basis, amiodarone is classed as a IIb intervention for shock-resistant VT/VF. Storage issues and its expense have limited its acceptance in widespread clinical practice, but amiodarone remains the only antiarrhythmic agent with convincing evidence of any sort of benefit in the VF/VT arrest setting.

Magnesium sulfate may be helpful in patients with torsades de pointes,[34] and in patients known or suspected of having a hypomagnesemic state. No evidence supports its routine use in shock-resistant VT/VF, and routine use may increase postresuscitation hypotension.[35] The use of procainamide for shock-resistant VT/VF use is supported by a single retrospective study, and the need for slow infusion and its serious side effects limits its use.[36] Bretylium tosylate has limited availability and limiting side effects. It has been completely removed from the AHA ACLS guidelines.

Asystolic Arrest and Pulseless Electrical Activity

The approach to the cardiac arrest patient whose initial rhythm is asystolic or pulseless electrical activity (PEA) differs from the approach to patients with tachyarrhythmic arrests (VT/VF). The first priority here is to institute appropriate CPR, intubation, and establishing IV access. Pressor support in the form of epinepherine (1.0 mg IV every 3–5 min) should be administered to support CPR. A prompt search for reversible causes should be performed and any reasonable possibilities addressed. The "five Hs" and the "five Ts" (Table 2-2) are useful tools in thinking through this differential diagnosis.

PEA as the initial rhythm has roughly the same successful resuscitation rate as pulseless VT/VF, while asystole as an initial arrest rhythm is uncommon, and generally implies that significant time has elapsed since the arrest. The prognosis of asystole is extremely poor. If pacing is to be attempted, it should be done as early as possible in the resuscitation. Assessing survivability, determining an endpoint for the resuscitation attempt, and preparing the resuscitation team and family for ending the resuscitation efforts should become early priorities.

OUTCOMES

Return of spontaneous circulation from out-of-hospital cardiac arrest ranges from 9 to 65%, with survival to discharge ranging from 1 to 31%. In these studies, typically one-third of discharged patients have persistent neurologic deficits, and only about half return to their prearrest function.

Highly optimized prehospital care systems in urban areas with very short response times consistently generate the highest ROSC rates. ROSC and survival to hospitalization is strongly correlated with time to first defibrillation attempt,[37,38] a fact which has led to the push to put

Table 2-2. Potentially Reversible Causes of PEA

Etiology	Treatment
Hypovolemia	Fluid resuscitation
Hypoxia	Oxygenate, ventilate
Hydrogen ion (acidosis)	Sodium bicarbonate, ventilation
Hyperkalemia	Calcium, glucose, insulin
Hypothermia	Rewarming
Tablets (accidental/ intentional drug overdose)	Drug-specific antidotes, sodium bicarbonate
Tamponade	Pericardiocentesis
Tension pneumothorax	Needle decompression
Thrombosis, coronary	Fibrinolysis or mechanical revascularization
Thrombosis, pulmonary	Fibrinolysis

more automatic external defibrillators into the hands of first-responders.

Interventions other than defibrillation, as we have discussed earlier, have little evidence that they improve long-term outcomes. The Ontario Prehospital Advanced Life Support Study (OPALS) enrolled 5638 out-of-hospital cardiac arrests, testing the efficacy of the addition of advanced life support regimens (intubation and IV drug administration) to simple rapid defibrillation.[39] Survival to hospital admission improved from 10.9 to 14.6%, but survival to discharge remained unchanged, suggesting that our clinical attention, our research efforts, and our funding should be directed toward minimizing time to defibrillation rather than at drug therapy.

REFERENCES

1. Myerburg RJ, Kessler KM, Castellanos A. Sudden cardiac death: Epidemiology, transient risk, and intervention assessment. *Ann Intern Med* 1993;119:1187–1197.
2. Priori SG, Barhanin J, Hauer RNW, et al. Genetic and molecular basis of cardiac arrhythmias: Impact on clinical management. *Circulation* 1999;99:518–528.
3. Friedman M, Manwaring JH, Rosenman RH, et al. Instantaneous and sudden deaths: Clinical and pathological differentiation in coronary artery disease. *JAMA* 1973;225: 1319–1328.
4. Kannel WB, Thomas HE. Sudden coronary death: The Framingham study. *Ann NY Acad Sci* 1982;382:3–21.
5. Myerburg RJ, Kessler KM, Luceri RM, et al. Classification of ventricular arrhythmias based on parallel hierarchies of frequency and form. *Am J Cardiol* 1984;54:1355–1358.
6. The Cardiac Arrhythmia Suppression Trial II Investigators. Effect of the antiarrhythmic agent morcizine on survival after myocardial infarction. *N Engl J Med* 1992;327:227–233.
7. Echt DS, Liebson PR, Mitchell LB, et al. Mortality and morbidity in patients receiving encainide, flecainide, or placebo: The Cardiac Arrhythmia Supression Trial. *N Engl J Med* 1991;324:781–788.
8. Waldo AL, Camm AJ, deRuyter H, et al. for the SWORD Investigators. Effect of d-sotalol on mortality in patients with left ventricular dysfunction after recent and remote myocardial infarction. *Lancet* 1996;348:7–12.
9. Bigger JT. Relation between left ventricular dysfunction and arrhythmias after myocardial infarction. *Am J Cardiol* 1986;57:8B–14B.
10. Middlekauff HR, Stevenson WG, Stevenson LW, et al. Syncope in advanced heart failure: High sudden death risk regardless of syncope etiology. *J Am Coll Cardiol* 1993;21: 110–116.
11. Aspirin-Myocardial Infarcation Research Study Group. A randomized controlled tiral of aspirin in persons recovered from myocardial infarction. *JAMA* 1980;243:661–669.
12. Davies MJ, Thomas A. Thrombosis and acute coronary lesions in sudden cardiac ischemic death. *N Engl J Med* 1984;310:1137–1140.
13. Myerburger RJ, Kessler KM, Zaman L, et al. Survivors of prehospital cardiac arrest. *JAMA* 1982;247:1485–1490.
14. Furukawa T, Moroe K, Myrovitz HN, et al. Arrhythmogenic effects of graded coronary blood flow reductions superimposed on prior myocardial infarctions in dogs. *Circulation* 1991;84:368–377.
15. Caldwell G. Simple mechanical methods for cardioversion: Defence of the precordial thump and cough version. *Br Med J (Clin Res Ed)* 1985;291:627–630.
16. Kouwenhoven WB, Jude JR, Knickerbocker GG. Closed-chest cardiac massage. *JAMA* 1960;173:1064–1067.
17. Feneley MP, Maier GW, Gaynor JW, et al. Sequence of mitral valve motion and transmitral blood flow during manual cardiopulmonary resuscitation in dogs. *Circulation* 1987;76:363–375.
18. Paradis NA, Martin GB, Goetting MG, et al. Simultaneous aortic, jugular bulb, and right atrial pressures during cardiopulmonary resuscitation in humans: Insights into mechanisms. *Circulation* 1989;80:361–368.
19. Berryman CR, Phillips GM. Interposed abdominal compression-CPR in human subjects. *Ann Emerg Med* 1984;13: 226–229.
20. Ward KR, Sullivan RJ, Zelenak RR, et al. A comparison of interposed abdominal compression CPR and standard CPR by monitoring end-tidal PCO2. *Ann Emerg Med* 1989;18: 831–837.
21. Babbs CF. Interposed abdominal compressions-cardiopulmonary resuscitation: Are we missing the mark in clinical trials? *Am Heart J.* 1993;126:1035–1041.
22. Sack JB, Kesselbrenner MB, Bregman D. Survival from in-hospital cardiac arrest with interposed abdominal counterpulsation during cardiopulmonary resuscitation. *JAMA* 1994;267:379–385.
23. Martin GB, Carden DL, Nowak RM, et al. Aortic and right atrial pressures during standard and simultaneous compression and ventilation CPR in human beings. *Ann Emerg Med* 1986;15:125–130.
24. Swenson RD, Weaver WD, Niskanen RA, et al. Hemodynamics in humans during conventional and experimental methods of cardiopulmonary resuscitation. *Circulation.* 1988;78: 630–639.
25. Cohen TJ, Tucker KJ, Lurie KG, et al. Active-compression decompression CPR improves vital organ perfusion in a dog model of ventricular fibrillation. *Chest* 1994;106:1250–1259.
26. Plaisance P, Lurie KG, Payne D. Inspiratory impedance during active compression-decompression cardiopulmonary resuscitation: A randomized evaluation in patients in cardiac arrest. *Circulation* 2000;101:989–994.
27. Sterz F, Behringer W, Berzlanovich A, et al. Active compression-decompression of thorax and abdomen (Lifestick™-CPR) in patients with cardiac arrest. *Circulation* 1996;94(Suppl I):9 (abstract).

28. Cummins RO. Guidelines 2000 for cardiopulmonary resuscitation and emergency cardiovascular care: International consensus on science. *Circulation* 2000;102(Suppl 1):1–384.

29. Lindner KH, Prengel AW, Brinkmann A, et al. Vasopressin administration in refractory cardiac arrest. *Ann Intern Med* 1996;124:1061–1064.

30. Morris DC, Dereczyk BE, Grzybowski M. Vasopressin can increase coronary perfusion pressure during human cardiopulmonary resuscitation. *Acad Emerg Med* 1997;20:609–614.

31. Herlitz J, Ekstrom L, Wennerblom B, et al. Lidocaine in out-of-hospital ventricular fibrillation: Does it improve survival? *Resuscitation* 1997;33:199–205.

32. von Walraven C, Stiell IG, Wells GA, et al. for the OTAC Study Group. Do advanced cardiac life support drugs increase resuscitation rates from in-hospital cardiac arrest? *Ann Emerg Med* 1998;32:544–553.

33. Kudenchuk PJ, Cobb LA, Copass MK, et al. Amiodarone for resuscitation after out-of-hospital cardiac arrest due to ventricular fibrillation. *N Engl J Med.* 1999;341:871–878.

34. Tzivoni D, Banai S, Schuger C, et al. Treatment of torsade de pointes with magnesium sulfate. *Circulation* 1988;77: 392–397.

35. Miller B, Craddock L, Hoffenberg S, et al. Pilot study of intravenous magnesium sulfate in refractory cardiac arrest: safety data and recommendations for future studies. *Resuscitation* 1995;30:3–14.

36. Stiell IG, Wells GA, Hebert PC, et al. Association of drug therapy with survival in cardiac arrest: limited role of advanced cardiac life support drugs. *Acad Emerg Med* 1995;2:264–273.

37. Herlitz J, Bang A, Holmberg M, et al. Rhythm changes during resuscitation form ventricular fibrillation in relation to delay until defibrillation, number of shocks delivered, and survival. *Resuscitation* 1997;34:17–22.

38. White RD, Asplin BR, Bugliosi TF, et al. High discharge survival rate after out-of-hospital ventricular fibrillation with rapid defibrillation by police and paramedics. *Ann Emerg Med* 1996;28:480–485.

39. Stiell IG, Wells GA, Field B, et al. Advanced cardiac life support in out-of-hospital cardiac arrest. *N Engl J Med* 2004;351:647–656.

3

Cardiogenic Shock

James Edward Weber

HIGH YIELD FACTS

- Cardiogenic shock (CS) is the most common cause of in-hospital mortality secondary to acute myocardial infarction (AMI), resulting in approximately 70,000 deaths per year.
- The mortality rate exceeds 70% in medically managed patients. Despite early percutaneous coronary intervention (PCI) or coronary artery bypass graft (CABG), mortality rates remain high (~50%) with half of deaths occurring within the first 48 hours.
- Medical therapy is only a temporizing measure. Definitive treatment is the restoration of coronary artery patency.
- Reperfusion modalities that have been shown to reduce mortality include thrombolytic therapy, intraaortic balloon counterpulsation, and PCI.
- If reperfusion modalities are not available, the patient should be transferred to a facility that is capable of providing these services.

INTRODUCTION

Cardiogenic shock (CS) is defined as a state of decreased pump function (cardiac output) resulting in inadequate tissue perfusion despite adequate or excessive circulating volume.[1] CS most commonly occurs secondary to an AMI that affects at least 40% of the left ventricular (LV) myocardium. CS is the most common cause of AMI-related in-hospital death, accounting for approximately 70,000 deaths annually in the United States. With medical therapy alone, mortality rates range from 70 to 90%. Although early revascularization (PCI or CABG) is superior to aggressive medical therapy, mortality rates remain as high as 50%, with half of all deaths occurring within the first 48 hours.[2,3] The overall incidence of CS

in AMI is 6–8%; a rate that has remained constant for 20 years.[4,5] CS following AMI generally develops after admission to the hospital (90%), although a small number of patients are in shock at presentation.[6] The median delay from the onset of infarction to the development of shock is 8 hours.

ETIOLOGY

Etiologies and risk factors for post-AMI CS are listed in Tables 3-1 and 3-2. The greater number of risk factors that are present suggests a larger amount of vulnerable myocardium and an increased likelihood of CS. Aggressive reperfusion strategies, employed with early identification of increased risk, may prevent CS.

AMI is the most common event precipitating CS. Acute heart failure may occur with loss of systolic contractile function of at least 25% of the LV. Once more than 40% of the LV loses contractile function, clinical CS ensues. Most cases of AMI-related CS have ST-segment elevation on the initial electrocardiogram (STEMI) that, in time, will evolve Q waves in the same ECG leads. Prior LV dysfunction can affect these percentages; a relatively small AMI may cause CS in a patient with preexisting LV dysfunction. In addition, disease in non-infarct-related coronary arteries, diastolic dysfunction, or arrhythmia can amplify the negative impact and result in CS with lesser insult.

CS can develop from mechanical complications of AMI: myocardial free-wall rupture, acute ventricular septal defect (VSD), or mitral regurgitation (MR) from valvular dysfunction or chordae rupture. Less common causes of CS include myocardial depression from conditions such as sepsis or myocarditis, LV outflow obstruction (e.g., aortic stenosis), and severe regurgitation of LV output (acute aortic regurgitation or mitral valve chordae rupture).

A portion of patients presenting with decompensated heart failure (HF) may have occult CS and may be clinically indistinguishable from those with mildly decompensated HF and stable HF.[7] Central venous oximetry and serum lactate measurements may be required to detect those with occult CS.

PATHOPHYSIOLOGY

Mechanics

While CS is characterized by both systolic and diastolic dysfunction, the main mechanical defect in CS is a marked reduction in contractility. As a result, even with preserved

Table 3-1. Etiologies of Cardiogenic Shock

Acute myocardial infarction
Pump failure
Mechanical complications
    Acute mitral regurgitation secondary to papillary
      muscle rupture
    Ventricular septal defect
    Free-wall rupture
Right ventricular infarction
Severe depression of cardiac contractility
Sepsis
Myocarditis
Myocardial contusion
Prolonged bypass
Mechanical obstruction to forward blood flow
Aortic stenosis
Hypertrophic cardiomyopathy
Mitral stenosis
Left atrial myxoma
Regurgitation of left ventricular output
Chordal rupture
Acute aortic insufficiency

---

systolic pressure, less blood volume per beat is ejected from the ventricle. To compensate for the diminished stroke volume, diastolic compliance decreases, and leads to decreased diastolic filling and an increase in end-diastolic pressure. As a result of decreased contractility, the patient develops elevated LV and right ventricular (RV) filling

Table 3-2. Risk Factors for Cardiogenic Shock

Elderly
Female
Current ischemic event
    Impaired ejection fraction (EF)
    Extensive infarct (evidence of large cardiac marker
      leak)
    Proximal left anterior descending (LAD) artery
      occlusion
    Anterior MI location
    Associated with multivessel disease
Prior medical history
    Previous MI
    CHF
    Diabetes

---

pressures and low cardiac output. Ultimately, higher LV diastolic filling pressures increase myocardial oxygen demand and cause pulmonary edema. Mixed venous oxygen saturation (MVO_2) falls because of the increased tissue oxygen extraction, which is due to the low cardiac output. This, combined with the intrapulmonary shunting that is often present, contributes to substantial arterial oxygen desaturation.

RV infarction complicates up to 30% of inferior wall AMI.[8] Although hypotension is not rare with an RV infarct, shock is much less common, and accounts for only 3–4% of CS cases. The major determinate of CS with RV infarction is the presence of LV dysfunction. With decreased LV contractility, systolic septal function is impaired and RV stroke volume is reduced. With less volume coursing through the RV, LV preload is reduced and LV stroke volume is decreased, producing more arterial hypotension and further reduction in coronary perfusion pressure.

Cellular

Patients who develop CS from AMI commonly demonstrate evidence of progressive myocardial necrosis with infarct extension. Myocytes in the ischemic border zone exhibit various stages of cell death, probably from inadequate collateral blood flow. With progression, areas of focal necrosis develop throughout the heart, producing further loss of contractile function and hypotension. Tissue hypoperfusion, with subsequent cellular hypoxia, causes anaerobic glycolysis, the accumulation of lactic acid, and intracellular acidosis. In addition, apoptosis (programmed cell death) occurs with activation of inflammatory mediators, oxidative stress, and stretching of the myocytes.[9]

Ischemia remote from the infarcted zone is an important contributor to shock and is further exacerbated by hypotension. Large areas of dysfunctional but viable myocardium can also contribute to the development of CS in patients with MI. This potentially reversible dysfunction is often described as myocardial stunning or hibernating myocardium. Stunning is defined as postischemic myocyte dysfunction that persists despite restoration of normal blood flow that eventually resolves completely. The mechanism of myocardial stunning involves a combination of oxidative stress, abnormalities of calcium homeostasis, and circulating myocardial depressant factors.

Hibernating myocardium is a state of persistently impaired myocardial function at rest, which occurs because of severely reduced coronary perfusion. Hibernation appears to be an adaptive response to hypoperfusion that may minimize the potential for further ischemia or necrosis. Consideration for the presence of myocardial stunning and hibernation is vital in patients with CS because of the therapeutic implications of these conditions. Revascularization of the hibernating (and/or stunned) myocardium generally leads to improved myocardial function. Although hibernation is considered a different physiologic process than that of myocardial stunning, the conditions are difficult to distinguish in the clinical setting and they often coexist. If ischemia is severe and prolonged, myocardial cellular injury becomes irreversible and leads to myonecrosis.

Systemic Compensation

With AMI, if depressed myocardial function occurs, neurohormonal mechanisms are triggered to maintain CO and tissue perfusion. Sympathetic nervous system activation leads to increased heart rate, systemic vasoconstriction, and increased myocardial contractility. The raised heart rate and contractility increases myocardial oxygen demand, further worsening myocardial ischemia. Increased contractility is seen as hyperkinesis in the uninvolved myocardium. Absence of hyperkinesis, from fibrosis or diffuse coronary artery disease, results in end-systolic LV volume increases, and is associated with increased CS risk. Another neurohormonal reflex that occurs is activation of the renin-angiotensin aldosterone system as a result of inadequate renal perfusion pressure. Increased angiotensin II leads to peripheral vasoconstriction and aldosterone synthesis. Aldosterone causes sodium and water retention, which increases LV preload. Fluid retention and impaired LV diastolic filling triggered by tachycardia and ischemia contribute to pulmonary venous congestion and hypoxemia. The net effect of sympathetic nervous system and renin-angiotensin activation may preserve CO and maintain end-organ perfusion, but at the cost of increased systemic vascular resistance (SVR) and higher myocardial oxygen consumption (MVO_2). Once initiated, this cycle ultimately results in total organ failure and death, if uninterrupted.

PRESENTATION

Clinical signs of CS include (1) evidence of poor cardiac output with tissue hypoperfusion (hypotension, mental status changes, cool mottled skin) and (2) evidence of volume overload (dyspnea, rales). Hemodynamic criteria for CS include (1) sustained hypotension (systolic blood pressure <90 mmHg), (2) reduced cardiac index (<2.2 L/min·m²), and (3) an elevated (>18 mmHg) pulmonary

artery occlusion pressure (PAOP). CS is a true emergency that needs aggressive intervention to avert an extremely high mortality rate.[4] While usually caused by pump failure of myocardium, other processes may impair CO to produce shock (Table 3-1).

History

History can be difficult to obtain due to the severity of the clinical presentation; mental obtundation or confusion may preclude patient cooperation. Emergency medical service (EMS) personnel, family, or the medical record may offer clues to the etiology of decompensation. If not obtunded, patients commonly complain of breathlessness. When AMI has caused the presentation, the patient may report chest pain or an ischemic equivalent. Historical findings suggestive of an alternative diagnosis should be sought; these may include complaints of fever, pleuritic chest pain, injection drug use, or a history of rheumatic heart disease.

Physical Examination

Patients in shock demonstrate clinical evidence of hypoperfusion, which is manifested by cyanosis, compensatory tachycardia, low urine output, cool skin, and mottled extremities. Systemic hypotension, defined as systolic blood pressure below 90 mmHg or a decrease in mean blood pressure by 30 mmHg, ultimately develops and further propagates tissue hypoperfusion. A higher BP may reflect compensatory increases in SVR. A pulse pressure <20 mmHg may also suggest CS. Peripheral pulses are often faint and irregular if arrhythmia is present. Unless the patient has advanced to the stage of respiratory fatigue or agonal respirations, tachypnea is common. The lung examination commonly shows rales as evidence of pulmonary edema. Jugular venous distention (JVD) and a positive abdominal jugular reflex are usually present. However, with RV infarction the lung fields may be clear despite hypotension and JVD. Cool, pale extremities with skin mottling indicate poor perfusion. Peripheral edema suggests preexisting heart failure. Diaphoresis indicates a sympathetic nervous system response.

A normal cardiac point of maximal impulse (PMI) suggests an acute presentation, as compared to a chronic heart failure exacerbation, when the PMI may be laterally shifted and diffuse from cardiac remodeling and enlargement. Loud or new systolic murmurs suggest mechanical dysfunction. Acute MR can occur from either chordae tendinea rupture or papillary muscle dysfunction.

Chordae tendinea rupture exhibits a soft holosystolic murmur at the apex, radiating to the axilla, but is often obscured by rales. With papillary muscle dysfunction, the murmur is not usually completely holosystolic, starting with the first heart sound but terminating before the second. An acute VSD is associated with a new loud holosystolic left parasternal ejection murmur, often with a palpable thrill, that decreases in intensity as the intraventricular pressures equalize.

EVALUATION AND MONITORING

Electrocardiogram (ECG)

Patients who develop CS after AMI often have profoundly abnormal ECG patterns or characteristics such as persistent ST-segment elevation, associated widespread ST-segment depression, or conduction abnormalities. Increased heart rate, prolonged QRS duration, and an increased sum of ST-segment depression in all leads in patients with inferior MI are predictive of mortality at 1 year.[10] LV hypertrophy suggests chronic heart failure or hypertension. ST-segment elevation in two or more ECG leads supports the diagnosis of AMI. RV infarction complicates inferior MI and is detected by ST-segment elevation in the right precordial ECG leads (usually V_4R). RV infarction complicating inferior MI increases mortality from about 6% (in absence of RV involvement) to 31% (with RV involvement).[8]

Chest Radiography

Chest radiography findings are useful for excluding other causes of shock or chest pain. The radiologic features of LV failure include pulmonary congestion or edema manifested by the presence of Kerley B lines, increased pulmonary vascularity, alveolar infiltrates, and pleural effusion. These findings may lag the clinical appearance by hours, therefore, their absence does not exclude CS. Cardiomegaly is the end result of long-standing myocardial remodeling and its presence may not explain the acute symptoms. Obtaining prior radiographs may help. The chest radiograph can suggest alternative or confounding diagnoses, such as pneumonia, pneumothorax, aortic dissection, or pericardial effusion.

Laboratory

The levels of serum B-type natruretic peptide (BNP) and N-terminal (NT) proBNP correlate with LV end-diastolic pressure and stretch. BNP has good direct correlation with PAOPs as measured by a pulmonary artery catheter and is an excellent predictor of the clinical development of heart failure after AMI.[11] The use of either as a diagnostic for CS is undefined. Normal serum BNP levels are less than 100 pg/mL, and normal NT proBNP levels are less than 125 pg/mL or 450 pg/mL, depending on age less than or greater than 75 years, respectively.

In CS, cardiac markers of acute ischemia may be useful. AMI can be diagnosed, but not excluded, by a single measurement. Arterial blood gas (ABG) measurements help identify those at risk of CO_2 retention, quantify the presence and severity of acidosis, and determine the contribution of metabolic or respiratory components. An elevated serum lactate may identify unsuspected hypoperfusion. Measurement of routine biochemistry parameters, such as electrolytes, renal function (e.g., urea and creatinine), and liver function tests (e.g., bilirubin, aspartate aminotransferase, alanine aminotransferase, lactate dehydrogenase [LDH]), are useful for assessing proper functioning of vital organs. A complete blood count (CBC) excludes anemia, which can contribute to cardiac ischemia. Whether to obtain specific drug levels (i.e., digoxin, ethanol, or illicit drugs) is guided by the clinical presentation. Serum magnesium should be measured with arrhythmia or severe hypokalemia.

Echocardiography

Transthoracic echocardiography (TTE) is a useful technique for establishing the cause of CS, and providing information predictive of outcome. Both short- and long-term mortality appear to be associated with initial LV systolic function and MR. Interestingly, a benefit of emergency revascularization is noted regardless of the baseline LV ejection fraction or MR.[12] Echocardiography provides information on ventricular dysfunction (e.g., regional hypokinesis, akinesis, or dyskinesis) and can identify early myocardial dysfunction by visualizing a lack of compensatory hyperkinesis in uninvolved cardiac segments. With the addition of color flow Doppler, TTE can also define the mechanical causes of CS, such as papillary muscle rupture causing acute myocardial regurgitation, acute VSD, free myocardial wall rupture, or pericardial tamponade.

TTE is useful for determining other causes of decreased CO. Acute RV dilatation, tricuspid insufficiency, paradoxical systolic septal motion, and high estimated PA and RV pressures suggest pulmonary hypertension, as occurs with pulmonary embolus. Loss of RV contractility, RV dilatation, and normal estimated pulmonary pressures occur more commonly with RV infarction. Pericardial effusion, with diastolic collapse of the right atrium or right ventricle, indicates hemodynamically significant cardiac tamponade. Finally, TTE may allow for visualization of aortic root dissection, although other imaging modalities are superior (e.g., CT angiography) if dissection is suspected.

Hemodynamic Monitoring

Invasive hemodynamic monitoring (Swan-Ganz catheterization) is very useful in helping to exclude other causes of shock, e.g., volume depletion, and obstructive or septic shock. Hemodynamic assessment by pulmonary artery catheterization in AMI patients has identified four profiles based on CO and LV preload that are strong predictors of mortality, independent of reperfusion therapy (Table 3-3).[13] Patients in CS typically have low cardiac index (CI < 2.2 L/min·m²) and elevated LV end-diastolic pressure (PAOP > 18 mmHg). While the pulmonary artery catheter can provide confirmatory data and guide treatment, it is typically unavailable to most emergency physicians.[13] Recently, a randomized evaluation of patients hospitalized with decompensated HF has concluded that

therapy guided by Swan-Ganz hemodynamic monitoring is just as safe as treatment based on clinical signs alone. However, the procedure is not associated with improved clinical outcomes.[14]

Noninvasive hemodynamic monitoring shows promise. One technique uses bioimpedance to measure stroke volume and multiplies this value by heart rate to calculate cardiac output. Approved by the FDA, impedance cardiographic monitoring is reasonably accurate, useful for diagnosis, and may exclude other causes of shock, such as volume depletion or sepsis.[15] Impedance cardiographic data are collected by the application of two ECG-type electrodes to each side of the neck and thorax. The signal is then analyzed and coupled with BP and ECG data to provide real time CO, SVR, and thoracic fluid content (TFC) values.[15,16] See Chap. 32.

DIFFERENTIAL DIAGNOSIS

AMI should first be suspected in patients with CS. Dyspnea in CS is common; therefore, pulmonary embolus, emphysema exacerbation, and pneumonia should also be considered. Hypertension, peripheral vasoconstriction, and dyspnea, suggest acute pulmonary

Table 3-3. Mean Hemodynamic Values in AMI Subsets

Class	Description	Cardiac Index (L/min·m²)	Pulmonary Artery Occlusion Pressure (mmHg)	Approximate Mortality (%)	Comment
I	No congestion or peripheral hypoperfusion	2.7 (normal)	12 (normal)	2	Good prognosis
II	Isolated congestion	2.3 (low-normal)	23 (elevated)	10	Vasodilation and diuresis result in clinical improvement
III	Isolated peripheral hypoperfusion	1.9 (decreased)	12 (normal)	22	There is relative or absolute volume deficiency. CO can be improved by volume infusions that increase stroke volume using the Frank-Starling relationship
IV	Both congestion and peripheral hypoperfusion	1.7 (decreased)	27 (elevated)	55	Clinical shock is typically present

edema. While diffuse ST-T changes can be seen with acute pericarditis or myocarditis, a nondiagnostic ECG should prompt the consideration of other causes of hypotension. These include aortic dissection, pulmonary embolus, pericardial tamponade, acute valvular insufficiency, hemorrhage, or sepsis. Finally, overdose by a toxin with negative inotropic or chronotropic effects (e.g., β-blocker, calcium-channel blocker, or digitalis overdose) should be considered.

TREATMENT

Stabilization

In the prehospital setting, the EMS should consider directing the suspected CS patient to a facility with intraaortic balloon pump and 24-hour emergency cardiac revascularization capability (i.e., cardiac bypass team). Initial management focuses on airway stability and improving myocardial pump function. Therapy begins with supplemental oxygen to reduce dyspnea and hypoxic anxiety. Since hypoxia is a greater risk than hypercarbia, supplemental oxygen is not withheld due to CO_2 retention concerns. Impending or acute respiratory failure requires immediate mechanical ventilation. Failure to expectantly manage airway and ventilatory requirements may result in rapid cardiovascular collapse. Cardiac monitoring and intravenous access are necessary. Hypoxia, hypovolemia, rhythm disturbances, electrolyte abnormalities, and acid-base alterations should be corrected as soon as possible. An arterial line, although not mandatory, helps for frequent ABGs and BP monitoring. A Foley catheter may be used to monitor urine output in response to therapy. Pulmonary artery catheter and hemodynamic monitoring should be considered in all unstable patients.

Medical Therapy

Medical therapy should be considered a temporizing measure while arranging for definitive treatment to reestablish coronary patency.[5,24–26] Diagnostic and therapeutic interventions should proceed simultaneously in unstable patients. More stable patients who are alert and able to speak may provide valuable historical information. When mechanical catastrophe is present, patients are usually in extremis and emergent echocardiography may be the best diagnostic tool. In the case of myocardial free-wall rupture, death is probable unless a pseudoaneurysm forms, which may be detected as an acute pericardial effusion on echocardiography. An acute VSD is confirmed by echocardiography, or right heart

catheterization demonstrating an O_2 saturation step-up from the right atrium to the RV. Acute MR, from papillary muscle rupture or dysfunction, can complicate inferior MI. Because the murmur may be undetectable by auscultation, echocardiography is warranted. Acute MR is associated with hypotension, pulmonary edema, and a holosystolic apical murmur.

In AMI, aspirin and antithrombin therapy should be given unless there is an absolute contraindication.[5] If there is adequate blood pressure, chest pain may be relieved by cautious use of intravenous nitroglycerin or morphine. β-Blockers, and angiotensin-converting enzyme inhibitors, demonstrated to improve outcomes in AMI, should be withheld until the patient's condition is stabilized. Similarly, other vasodilators cannot be used in most cases when hypotension is present.

Initial therapy must be guided by clinical findings. Because some patients with CS develop hypotension without pulmonary congestion, a small fluid challenge (normal saline 100–250 mL) may be appropriate. If there is pulmonary congestion, crystalloid infusion should be withheld. In patients with inadequate tissue perfusion and adequate intravascular volume, initiation of inotropic and/or vasopressor drug therapy may be necessary (see Table 3-4).

While inotropic agents do not improve outcome, they can be useful as a temporizing measure while arranging interventions to restore coronary artery perfusion and LV function.[17,18] Inotropic selection is dependent on the suspected etiology of hypotension. If hemodynamics stabilize after inotropics are started, therapy for pulmonary congestion may be started (i.e., diuretics), while arranging the ICU admission.

Pure vasoconstrictors such as phenylephrine are generally contraindicated because they increase cardiac afterload without augmenting the inotropic state. Dopamine increases myocardial contractility and supports the blood pressure; however, it may increase the heart rate, thus increasing myocardial oxygen demand. Dobutamine may be preferable if the systolic blood pressure is higher than 80 mmHg and it has the advantage of not affecting myocardial oxygen demand as much as dopamine. However, the resulting tachycardia may preclude the use of this inotropic agent in some patients. Dobutamine should be avoided in patients with moderate or severe hypotension (e.g., systolic blood pressure <80 mmHg) because of the peripheral vasodilation.

Phosphodiesterase inhibitors (e.g., milrinone) augment the inotropic state, but have significant vasodilatory properties (thereby decreasing afterload) and can decrease blood pressure to a greater extent than dobutamine.

Table 3-4. Inotropic Medications Used for CS

Dopamine
Mechanism: Adrenergic and dopaminergic agonists
Dosage: 5–50 µg/kg·min continuous IV infusion
Effect: Dose dependent
    <2 µg/kg·min—renal and mesenteric vasodilation (dopaminergic)
    2.5–5 µg/kg·min—increases heart rate and contractility (β_1-adrenergic)
    5.0–10 µg/kg·min—increases heart rate and contractility (α- and β_1-adrenergic)
    >10 µg/kg·min—increases blood pressure and SVR (α-adrenergic)
Complications: Arrhythmias, extremity gangrene, and tachycardia at high doses (which increases myocardial oxygen demand, and may extend ischemia).

Dobutamine
Mechanism: β_1-adrenergic agonist, it also has α- and β_2-adrenergic effects
Dosage: Started at 2–5 µg/kg·min, it is titrated up to 20 µg/kg·min
Effect: Primarily sympathomimetic; improves myocardial contractility and augments diastolic coronary blood flow without inducing excessive tachycardia. The net effect is increased CO, lower SVR, and lower LV filling pressure, with little BP change.
Dopamine may be added to support BP if response to dobutamine is inadequate.
Complications: Arrhythmias, nausea, and headache. If there is an inadequate response to this agent alone, dopamine may be added to support BP.

Norepinephrine
Mechanism: Pure α-adrenergic agonist
Dosage: Started at 2 µg/min and titrated according to response
Effect: Sympathomimetic; used when response to first-line pressor agents is inadequate
Complications: Similar to high dose dopamine

Milrinone
Mechanism: Phosphodiesterase inhibitor
Dosage: Loading dose of 50 µg/kg IV over 10 min, followed by a maintenance infusion of 0.5 µg/kg·min.
Effect: Increases cyclic adenosine monophosphate (cAMP), it increases inotropism, CO, and causes peripheral vasodilation.
Complications: The drop in SVR may require additional therapy with pressors to maintain BP; milrinone use in CS is best guided by hemodynamic measurements from a pulmonary artery catheter.

Therefore, concomitant therapy with a vasopressor may be necessary. Therapeutic decisions in this scenario are best guided with a pulmonary artery catheter. Phosphodiesterase inhibitors increase myocardial oxygen demand and tachycardia to a lesser extent than catecholamines. However, they are associated with a greater incidence of tachyarrhythmias than dobutamine.

In an RV infarct with hypotension, intravenous fluids should be administered as a first priority. In the absence of profound hypotension, dobutamine is a mainstay of initial pharmacologic treatment.[17] With systolic pressure <70 mmHg, dopamine is preferred, either as a single agent or in combination with dobutamine. When shock persists despite use of these agents, mechanical inotropic support with an intraaortic balloon pump is required.[5,19,20]

In acute MR, hemodynamic support can be initiated with dobutamine and nitroprusside. This supports contractility and provides afterload reduction, respectively, while promoting forward systemic blood flow. The intraaortic balloon pump is also beneficial for temporary support.[5] Acute VSD is treated with dobutamine, nitroprusside, and an intraaortic balloon counter pulsation (IABP).[5]

Confirmatory evidence for these emergent conditions with two-dimensional echocardiography should be sought, concomitant with emergency consultation from the cardiac surgical team.

In patients with AMI, activation of inflammatory cytokines leads to high levels of nitric oxide synthetase, nitric oxide, and peroxynitrite, all of which serve to directly inhibit myocardial contractility, suppress mitochondrial respiration in nonischemic myocardium, reduce catecholamine responsivity, and induce systemic vasodilation. Current studies are underway evaluating the efficacy of pharmacologic strategies aimed at suppressing this pathway.

Reperfusion for Cardiogenic Shock

Thrombolytic Therapy

When used early in the course of MI, thrombolytic therapy reduces the likelihood of subsequent development of CS after the initial event. In addition, recent data suggest that patients in CS treated with thrombolytics had better outcomes than those without thrombolytics.[21,22] The lowest mortality rate was observed with the treatment of thrombolytics followed by revascularization.[21,22] These were most likely patients in CS who reperfused with thrombolytics and were revascularized afterward. Incomplete lysis in the infarct-related artery and the high frequency of multivessel disease in patients with CS may limit the efficacy of thrombolytic therapy.[22]

Intraaortic Balloon Counter Pulsation

IABP provides hemodynamic support by decreasing afterload (which lowers MVO_2) and increasing diastolic BP (which augments coronary perfusion) and should be considered in patients presenting with CS.[5,19,20] See page 348. Recent data suggest that IABP improves survival after thrombolytic therapy by augmenting diastolic perfusion pressure and unloading the LV.[21–23] IABP does not improve survival in the absence of successful revascularization or surgical correction of an acute mechanical catastrophe.[22]

Early Revascularization

In CS, early revascularization with either percutaneous transluminal coronary angioplasty (PTCA) or CABG is the most important life-saving intervention.[5,21,22,24,25] In the randomized SHOCK trial, a strategy of early revascularization resulted in 132 lives saved at 1 year per 1000 patients as compared with initial medical therapy.[22] The

greatest short-term benefit is reported in patients less than 75 years of age, those with previous MI, and those treated within 6 hours of symptom onset. Patients older than 75 years had better survival with medical management.[5,21] CABG requires extensive surgical and medical resources, and poses significant operative risk for these seriously ill patients, thereby limiting its use. However, outcome studies supports that early revascularization should be performed in most patients under 75 years of age with CS.[21,22] The best predictors of improved in-hospital survival include younger age, absence of triple vessel disease, shorter time between symptom onset and PCI, and restoration of TIMI-3 normal epicardial flow.[26] Current recommendations for early revascularization are listed in Fig. 3-1. Mechanical complications (e.g., acute VSD or MR) producing CS require temporary inotropic support with IABP, followed by early surgical repair.[5]

CS Treatment at Hospitals without Invasive Therapy

When a CS patient presents to a facility without invasive revascularization availability, emergent transfer to an institution with this capability should be considered. The method of transfer should be selected for the expediency by which it may be accomplished (i.e., ground vs. air medical). In a large CS registry, mortality rates were 77% without thrombolytic therapy or IABP, 63% with thrombolytic therapy alone, 57% with IABP alone, and 47% with thrombolytic therapy and IABP.[22] Those with IABP were more likely to receive invasive revascularization, but there was no outcome difference as long as IABP was begun within 6 hours. While further study is needed, this suggests that the best results may be obtained by thrombolytic therapy and IABP if possible, and early transfer.[5]

DISPOSITION

All with CS requiring hemodynamic monitoring, thrombolytic or inotropic therapy, or on an IABP, require ICU admission. The occasional stable patient without multiple comorbidities or a history of HF, and who does not require hemodynamic monitoring or inotropic support, is appropriate for admission to a monitored setting. Not all patients may benefit from aggressive care, particularly elderly patients with multiple comorbid conditions. The decision to perform or withhold therapies should be made in conjunction with the patient's wishes. Factors that may influence the decision to pursue aggressive therapy include advanced age and diminished functional status.

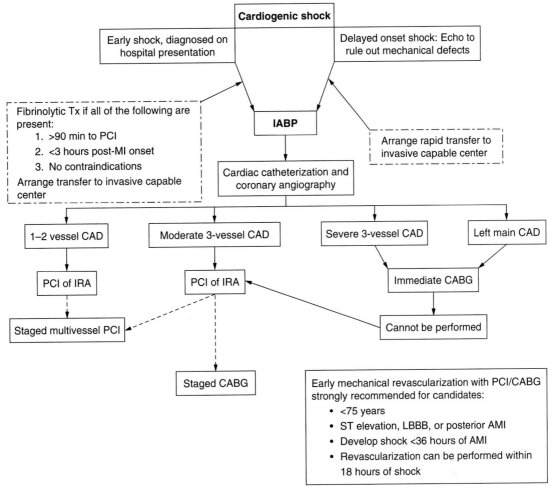

Fig. 3-1. Recommendations for initial reperfusion therapy when CS complicates AMI. Dashed lines indicate that the procedure should be performed in patients with specific indications only. IRA, infarct related artery; CAD, coronary artery disease; PCI, percutaneous coronary intervention; CABG, coronary artery bypass graffing. (Source: Reprinted from Hockman JS. Cardiogenic shock complicating acute myocardial infarction: Expanding the paradigm. *Circulation* 2003;107:2998–3002.)

REFERENCES

1. Hollenberg SM, Kavinsky CJ, Parrillo JE. Cardiogenic shock. *Ann Intern Med* 1999;131:47–59.
2. Hochman JS, Buller CE, Sleeper LA. Cardiogenic shock complicating acute myocardial infarction: Etiologies, management and outcome: Overall findings from the SHOCK Trial Registry. *J Am Coll Cardiol* 2000;36:1063–1070.
3. Webb JG, Sanborn TA, Sleeper LA, et al. Percutaneous coronary intervention for cardiogenic shock in the SHOCK Trial Registry. *Am Heart J* 2001;141;964–970.
4. Goldberg RJ, Samad NA, Yarzebski J, et al. Temporal trends in cardiogenic shock complicating acute myocardial infarction. *N Engl J Med* 1999;340:1162–1168.
5. Menon V, Hochman JS. Management of cardiogenic shock complication acute myocardial infarction. *Heart* 2002; 88:531–537.
6. Califf RM, Bengtson JR. Cardiogenic shock. *N Engl J Med* 1994;330:1724–1730.
7. Ander DS, Jaggi M, Rivers E, et al. Undetected cardiogenic shock in patients with congestive heart failure presenting to the emergency department. *Am J Cardiol* 1998;82:888–891.

8. Zehender M, Kasper W, Kauder E, et al. Right ventricular infarction as an independent predictor of prognosis after acute inferior myocardial infarction. *N Engl J Med* 1993;328:981–988.

9. Bartling B, Holtz J, Darmer D. Contribution of myocyte apoptosis to myocardial infarction? *Basic Res Cardiol* 1998;93:71–84.

10. White HD, Palmeri ST, Sleeper LA, et al. Electrocardiographic findings in cardiogenic shock, risk prediction, and the effects of emergency revascularization: Results from the SHOCK trial. *Am Heart J* 2004;148:810–817.

11. Sabatine MS, Morrow DA, de Lemos JA, et al. Multimarker approach to risk stratification in non-ST elevation acute coronary syndromes: Simultaneous assessment of troponin I, C-reactive protein, and B-type natriuretic peptide. *Circulation* 2002;105:1760–1763.

12. Picard MH, Davidoff R, Sleeper LA, et al. Echocardiographic predictors of survival and response to early revascularization in cardiogenic shock. *Circulation* 2003;107:279–284.

13. Forrester JS, Diamond GA, Swan HJC. Correlative classification of clinical and hemodynamic function after acute myocardial infarction. *Am J Cardiol* 1977;39:137–145.

14. Evaluation Study of Congestive Heart Failure and Pulmonary Artery Catheterization Effectiveness (ESCAPE): American Heart Association Scientific Sessions, 2004.

15. Shoemaker WC, Belzberg H, Wo CC, et al. Multicenter study of noninvasive monitoring systems as alternatives to invasive monitoring of acutely ill emergency patients. *Chest* 1998;114:1643–1652.

16. Peacock WF, Kies P, Albert NM, et al. Bioimpedance monitoring for detecting pulmonary fluid in heart failure: Equal to chest radiography? *Congest Heart Fail* 2000;6:86–89.

17. McGhie AI, Goldstein RA. Pathogenesis and management of acute heart failure and cardiogenic shock: Role of inotropic therapy. *Chest* 1992;102(Suppl 2):626S–632S.

18. Garber PJ, Mathieson AL, Ducas J, et al. Thrombolytic therapy in cardiogenic shock: Effect of increased aortic pressure and rapid tPA administration. *Can J Cardiol* 1995;11:30–36.

19. Anderson RD, Ohman EM, Holmes DR, et al. Use of intra-aortic balloon counterpulsation in patients presenting with cardiogenic shock: Observations from the GUSTO-1 study. *J Am Coll Cardiol* 1997;30:708–715.

20. Webb JG. Interventional management of cardiogenic shock. *Can J Cardiol* 1998;14:233–244.

21. Hochman JS, Sleeper LA, White HD, et al. One-year survival following early revascularization for cardiogenic shock. *JAMA* 2001;285:190–192.

22. Sanborn TA, Sleeper LA, Bates ER, et al. Impact of thrombolysis, intra-aortic balloon pump counterpulsation, and their combination in cardiogenic shock complicating acute myocardial infarction: A report from the SHOCK trial registry. Should we emergently revascularize occluded coronaries for cardiogenic shock? *J Am Coll Cardiol* 2000;36(Suppl A):1123–1129.

23. Kovack PJ, Rasak MA, Bates ER, et al. Thrombolysis plus aortic counterpulsation: Improved survival in patients who present to community hospitals with cardiogenic shock. *J Am Coll Cardiol* 1997;29:1454–1458.

24. Hochman JS, Sleeper LA, Webb JG, et al. Early revascularization in acute myocardial infarction complicated by cardiogenic shock. *N Engl J Med* 1999;341:625–634.

25. Sutton AGC, Finn P, Hall JA, et al. Predictors of outcome after percutaneous treatment for cardiogenic shock. *Heart* 2005;91:339–344.

26. Zeymer U, Vogt A, Zahn R, et al. Predictors of in-hospital mortality in 1333 patients with acute myocardial infarction complicated by cardiogenic shock treated with percutaneous coronary intervention. *Eur Heart J* 2004;25:322–328.

4

Basic Electrophysiology

Gregory J. Fermann

HIGH YIELD FACTS

- The process of linking impulse conduction and mechanical contraction is largely the result of the calcium ion. Pharmacologic manipulation of the calcium concentration alters cardiac inotropy and chronotropy.
- The cardiac action potential is the result of the interplay of calcium, potassium, and sodium channels. The enigmatic pacemaker current is responsible for cardiac automaticity.
- The molecular basis of cardiac activity is modulated primarily through membrane receptor-enzyme systems. The two most well-known systems are the adenylate cyclase (ADC) and phospholipase C (PLC) system.
- The genetic basis of channel and enzyme-receptor physiology is fertile ground for future research, particularly in the field of heart failure.

INTRODUCTION

The heart is actually two separate pumps. The right heart pumps blood to the lungs. The left heart pumps blood to peripheral organs. Each pump is comprised of an atrium and a ventricle. The atrium weakly pumps blood into the ventricle, which supplies the main force that propels blood to either the lungs or peripheral organs. Physiologically, the heart can be conceptualized as a pump, the rhythmic contractions of which are coordinated by highly specialized conductive fibers. The function of the heart muscle, valves, and various chambers will be addressed in other chapters. This chapter will focus on the impulse generation and propagation system of the heart. When functioning normally, the atria contract about one-sixth of a second before the ventricles, allowing extra filling of the ventricle just prior to it

sending blood to either the lungs or peripheral organs. All portions of the ventricle contract simultaneously, allowing for effective pressure generation. Unfortunately, this elegant conduction system of the heart is very susceptible to damage, particularly due to ischemic heart disease.

CONDUCTING SYSTEMS—GROSS ANATOMY

Under normal circumstances, the rhythmic impulses of the heart are generated in the sinoatrial node (SA node). The internodal pathways conduct the impulse from the SA node to the atrioventricular node (AV node). The AV node delays the impulse before conduction to the ventricles. The AV bundle, or His bundle, conducts impulses from the AV node. The AV bundle separates into two main fascicles, the left and right bundles, which then branch into a fine network of Purkinje fibers[1,2] (Fig. 4-1).

Sinoatrial Node

The SA node is a small ellipsoid strip of specialized muscle measuring 3 mm in width, 15 mm in length, and 1 mm in thickness. The SA fibers are continuous with adjacent atrial fibers such that the impulse generated proceeds immediately to the atria. The location of the SA node is in the anterosuperior wall of the atria immediately anterolateral to the ostium of the superior vena cava. The cellular properties of the SA node allow it to function as a cardiac generator in normal individuals.

Internodal Pathways

The SA node fibers fuse with the surrounding atrial muscle fibers thereby conducting action potentials to the entire atrial muscle mass. The velocity of conduction in the atrial muscle is slower than that of a specialized band of tissue called the intraatrial band. The intraatrial band (Bachmann's bundle) passes through the anterior wall of the atrium to the left atrium and conducts impulses more rapidly than surrounding atrial muscle. Likewise, three small bundles called the anterior, middle, and posterior internodal pathways conduct impulses from the SA node to the AV node more rapidly than surrounding atrial muscle.

Atrioventricular Node and Infranodal System

In order to allow the atria to deliver their contents to the ventricles, an inherent delay point in the conduction system is found at the AV node. The AV node is found in the septal wall of the right atrium, immediately posterior to the tricuspid valve. The impulse generated at the SA node reaches the AV node in about 0.04 s. The impulse leaves the AV node and appears in the AV bundle in about 0.15 s. The significant delay in this region is due to a slowed conduction velocity in junctional fibers and nodal fibers. Junctional fibers are very small fibers that connect normal atrial muscle fibers and nodal fibers. The velocity of conduction is very slow (0.02 m/s) compared with the rapid (1 m/s) conduction of the intraatrial band and internodal pathways. The slowed impulse passes through the junctional fibers to the nodal fibers. The conduction of the nodal fibers is also low (0.1 m/s). The impulse proceeds from the nodal fibers to the transitional fibers, and finally, to the AV bundle.

Purkinje System

The Purkinje fibers lead from the AV node through the AV bundle, into the ventricles. They are very large fibers and, contrary to the AV nodal fibers, transmit impulses at a very fast velocity (1.5–4.0 m/s). The transmission in the Purkinje system is about six times faster than usual cardiac muscle allowing almost immediate transmission of impulses to the entire ventricle. Purkinje fibers, like the majority of the conductive tissue, have few myofibrils and contract minimally during the course of impulse transmission.

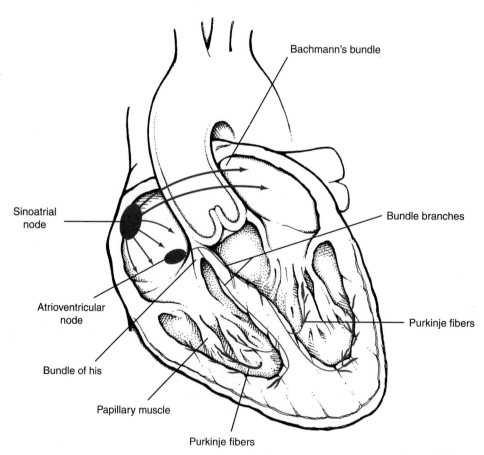

Fig. 4-1. Schematic representations of the conduction system of the heart. (Source: Redrawn with permission of Berne RM, Levy MN (eds.). *Physiology.* St. Louis, MO: Mosby, 1993.)

The Purkinje fibers originate in the AV node, form the AV bundle, which weaves between the heart valves to the ventricular septum. The AV bundle bifurcates into the left and right bundles, which lay beneath the endocardium of the right and left ventricular septum. Each branch proceeds toward the apex, the left dividing into two discreet fascicles, the anterior and posterior fascicle. After curving around the apex, the fibers proceed toward the base of the heart. The terminal Purkinje fibers penetrate into about one-third of the ventricular wall terminating in the ventricular muscle fibers.

Ventricular Muscle Impulse Transmission

After the impulse has reached the terminus of the Purkinje fibers, transmission occurs from cell to cell by the ventricular muscle fibrils. The velocity of transmission is considerably slowed (0.3–0.5 m/s) in comparison to the Purkinje system. The ventricle depolarizes from the septum to the apex to the base. The septum depolarizes from the left to the right. Ventricular myocardium depolarizes from the endocardium to the epicardium. Despite regional differences, the depolarization of the ventricle is almost simultaneous. The time from first ventricular cell contraction to the last is only 0.06 s. The ventricular muscle fiber then remains contracted for 0.3 s.

CELLULAR STRUCTURE OF CARDIAC MUSCLE

Cardiac muscle is composed of highly branched network of small cells. Each cell is surrounded by a thin cell membrane called sarcolemma. Invaginations of the sarcolemma are called T-tubules. The internal membrane system of the cardiac cell is vital for conducting the electrical impulse from the cell membrane to the contractile units located in the interior of the cell. The sarcoplasmic reticulum (SR), specialized endoplasmic reticulum, forms a membrane-bounded intracellular compartment. The tubular network of SR surrounds the myofibrils. Enlarged sacs of SR can be found close to the surface membrane where they are called sarcolemmal cisternae. Where the SR enlarges into sacs next to the T-tubule, the term lateral sac or terminal cisternae is used.

Like skeletal muscle, cardiac muscle is striated. Actin and myosin filaments form an overlapping array. The sarcomere is the basic contractile unit. The terminology used to describe the structural elements (A band, I band, Z line, and H zone) is similar to those used in skeletal muscle. Bundles of protein filaments are termed myofibrils.

Intercalated disks separate cardiac cells from one another. Intercalated disks provide minimal electric resistance to impulse propagation by allowing very permeable junction between cells that allow relatively free diffusion of ions. Electrically, cardiac cells are connected in series. Impulses are rapidly transmitted along the long axis of the myofibril while transmission occurs more slowly perpendicular to the long axis. The cellular structure of the heart can be thought of as two syncytia. Depolarization of one focus in syncytia rapidly leads to contraction of the entire unit. The atrial syncytium is separated by the ventricular syncytia by thick fibrous tissue supporting the valvular structures of the heart.

EXCITATION-CONTRACTION COUPLING

The ability of an action potential to cause myofibrils to contract is termed excitation-contraction coupling. This coupling is largely the result of the function of the T-tubule (Fig. 4-2). The action potential spreads from the cardiac muscle membrane to the interior of the cardiac muscle fiber. The calcium ion is essential in linking impulse conduction and mechanical contraction. During the plateau phase of the myocyte action potential, calcium moves inwardly across the sarcolemma and T-tubules. Opening the calcium channels is due to cyclic adenosine monophosphate (cAMP)-protein kinase-dependent phosphorylation of the calcium channel. Calcium influx from the interstitium alone is insufficient to cause myofibril contraction. The additional source of calcium is released from the intracellular calcium storage unit called the SR. The release of calcium from the SR is triggered by calcium influx from the interstitium, a process termed calcium-activated calcium release. The additional calcium release is sufficient to allow the binding of calcium to troponin C. The calcium-troponin C complex interacts with tropomyosin to unblock active sites between actin and myosin. The cross bridging of actin and myosin results in myofibril contraction, thus completing the excitation-contraction coupling sequence.

Calcium release mechanism in cardiac muscle is termed "all or nothing." Like the action potential, once the sequence of events is set in motion there is no modulation of the process until the next cycle is initiated. Mechanisms that alter cytosolic calcium concentration alter the force of myocardial contraction. Catecholamines increase intracellular movement of calcium by the cAMP-dependent protein kinase. Increasing extracellular calcium, decreasing extracellular sodium, or decreasing intracellular sodium result in increasing contractile force.

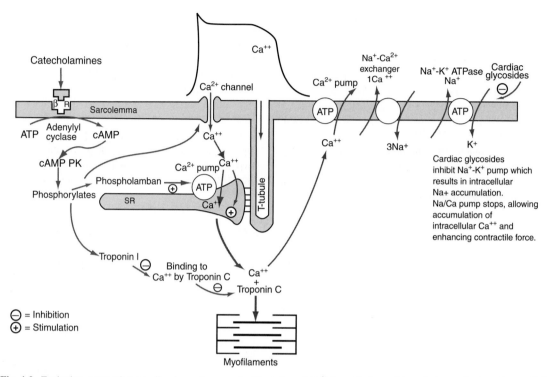

Fig. 4-2. Excitation-contraction coupling in cardiac muscle. The influx of Ca^{2+} from the interstitium during excitation triggers Ca^{2+} release from the sarcoplasmic reticulum (SR). Cytosolic Ca^{2+} activates the myofilaments in systole. Relaxation in diastolic occurs as calcium is either sequestered by SR reuptake, removed by Na-Ca exchange, or pumped outside by the Ca^{2+} pump. βR, beta-adrenergic receptor; cAMP, cyclic adenosine monophosphate; cAMP PK, cyclic AMP-dependent protein kinase.

Cardiac glycosides increase intracellular sodium by inactivating the sodium-potassium ATPase pump. Digoxin causes the accumulation of sodium intracellularly, reducing the activity of the Na^+-Ca^{2+} exchanger such that more calcium remains in the sarcoplasm and available for contraction.

Conversely, administration of calcium-channel blockers prevents calcium from entering the sarcoplasm, reducing contractile tension. At the end of the plateau phase of the action potential, the influx of calcium ions from the T-tubule and SR to the interior of the cells is shut off, and the calcium ions are rapidly pumped out of the sarcoplasm back into the SR. This process is mediated through an adenosine triphosphate (ATP)-driven calcium pump. The calcium pump is stimulated by a phosphorylated phospholamban. Phosphorylation of troponin I inhibits the binding of calcium to troponin C, allowing tropomyosin to block actin—myosin binding. Thus, diastolic relaxation occurs until this next action potential.

Calcium that enters the cell during systole must be removed during diastole. The Na^+-Ca^{2+} exchanger is largely responsible for this function but is aided to a lesser degree by a calcium pump on the sarcolemmal membrane.

CARDIAC ACTION POTENTIAL

In a resting, or nondepolarized state, the inside (cytoplasm/sarcoplasm) of each cardiac muscle cell is negatively charged in comparison to the outside (extracellular space/interstitium). In a resting, healthy, ventricular muscle cell, this relative charge difference is termed *resting membrane potential*. In atrial and ventricular muscle cells, the resting membrane potential is constant and does not change until given an adequate stimulus. If, in the presence of a stimulus, the cell is moved from its resting membrane potential to its threshold potential, a series of ion shifts, called action potential, ensues. The cells of the SA node, AV node, and

AV bundle, in contrast to atrial and ventricular myocytes, undergo spontaneous depolarization from resting potential to threshold potential. This characteristic termed *automaticity* allows them to serve as pacemakers. Membrane potentials plotted over time are useful in describing the cellular activities of the two main types of cardiac cells: nonpacemaking and pacemaking cells[3] (Fig. 4-3).

Phase Zero—Upstroke

Once a cell reaches threshold potential, rapid depolarization is caused by rapid increase in sodium (Na^+) conductance of the membrane. Sodium ions rapidly flow from the extracellular to intracellular space, forming the inwardly negative sodium current (I_{Na}). As the positively

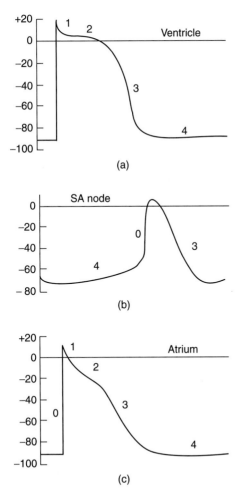

Fig. 4-3. Typical action potentials in (a) ventricle, (b) SA node, (c) atria.

charged sodium ions rush in, the membrane potential rapidly become less negative (depolarizes). The sodium ions rush in to such an extent that the membrane becomes transiently positive (+20 mV) called overshoot. The membrane potential does not quite reach the equilibrium potential (E_{Na}) of +70 mV.

Phase I—Rapid Depolarization Phase

After reaching overshoot potential, sodium channels become inactive. Potassium channels provide rapid repolarization. The type of potassium channel active in phase 1 is called the transient outward potassium current (I_{TO}).

Phase II—Plateau Phase

Two currents dominate the action potential plateau: inward calcium current (I_{Ca}) and the delayed rectifier potassium current (I_K). The calcium current, following its concentration gradient, moves from the extracellular space to the intracellular space resulting in an inwardly directed depolarizing current. However, potassium ions move in the other direction, which is outwardly directed repolarizing current. Changes in membrane potential depend on the balance of inward I_{Ca} and outward I_K currents. Often the currents are equally weighted, resulting in the relatively flat plateau phase.

Phase III—Final Repolarization

Final repolarization results when the I_{Ca} current becomes inactivated. Since only potassium conductance remains, the membrane potential moves toward potassium equilibrium potential (E_K) of –90 mV. The delayed rectifier potassium currents (I_{Ks} and I_{Kr}) close as the cell repolarizes, allowing the inward rectifier (I_{K1}) to predominate.

Phase IV—Interval Phase

In atrial and ventricular muscle cells, the resting potential remains constant during the diastolic interval. The I_{K1} remains dominant, but since the resting potential of the membrane (–75 mV) is only slightly more positive than the E_K of –90 mV, there is little driving force for movement across the channel. During this phase, the sodium-potassium ATPase (Na^+-K^+-ATPase) reestablishes ion gradients following membrane activity.

Rhythmicity and Action Potential of Pacemaker Cells

The action potential of the SA node, AV node, and His bundle differ markedly from atrial, ventricular, and Purkinje cells. Sodium channels play little role in the action potential of nonnodal cells. The upstroke (phase zero) in nodal cells results from the inward movement of calcium ions. The upstroke is less rapid with less overshoot. The plateau phase is less evident and phase III occurs more gradually. Unlike ventricular, atrial, and Purkinje tissues, the resting potential in nodal tissue is not stable. During phase IV, the resting potential of nodal cells is less negative (−55 mV) than the nonnodal counterparts (−80 to 90 mV). There is gradual depolarization to the threshold potential. The threshold potential is about −40 mV in the SA node.

The SA node is responsible for the heart's rhythmicity and under usual circumstances fires 70–80 times/min. The SA node's ability to reset other pacemaking tissues is termed overdrive suppression. However, when not stimulated from outside sources, AV nodal fibers fire at an intrinsic rate of 40–60 times/min and Purkinje fibers discharge at 15–40 times/min. Each time the SA node discharges, the impulse is conducted to the AV node and Purkinje fibers. Each of these tissues recovers, become hyperpolarized, and slowly depolarize to threshold. The SA node loses hyperpolarization and depolarizes to threshold more rapidly than any other nodal tissue. Thus, the SA node is the cardiac pacemaker because its rate of discharge is greater than any other part of the heart. If the SA node stops or slows, other pacemaking cells can takeover as the cardiac pacemaker. The usual order of succession is the SA node >60 bpm, atrial focus 40–60 bpm, AV node 40 bpm, and ventricular ectopic foci 20–40 bpm.

Refractory Periods

During the action potential of cardiac tissues, an additional stimulus will be incapable of initiating a new action potential. This timeframe is termed *the effective* or *absolute refractory period* (*ERP*). The brief time following the ERP is called the *relative refractory period* (*RRP*). During this time, only a supernormal stimulus may generate a new action potential. In ventricular muscle, the ERP is due to the inactivation of fast sodium channels and lasts from phase zero until the end of phase III. In nodal tissue, the ERP is due to the inactivation of calcium channels, and also lasts from phase zero until the end of phase III. The ERP and RRP last longer in nodal tissue than nonnodal cardiac tissue.

IONIC BASIS FOR CARDIAC ACTION POTENTIAL

General Concepts

Action potentials in cardiac tissues are caused by the movement of several different ions, through especially

adapted membrane channels.[4] Cardiac excitation relies on the function of integral membrane protein macromolecules that mediate the movement of ions across the cell membrane (Fig. 4-4). Ion channels are water-filled pores allowing for the passive movement of ion through the lipid bilayer. Ion pumps require metabolic energy from ATP to transport ions across the cell membrane. Ion exchangers use the electrochemical gradient of one ion to transport another across the membrane.

Ion channels rely on two fundamental properties. In response to appropriate stimuli, ion channels open or close, a process described as gating. When channels are open, they must choose which ion is allowed to pass, a process known as ion selectivity. Each channel is the result of genetic expression and thus is subject to mutation. These channels are often the targets of pharmacologic agents.

Gating Behavior

Ion channels can generally be classified based on their gating mechanism. If the opening or closing of the channel is influenced by membrane voltage, the pore is said to be voltage gated. The primary sodium, calcium, and many of the potassium channels are voltage gated. Ligand-gated ion channels open or close based on the availability of an appropriate substance or ligand either on the intracellular or extracellular space (Fig. 4-5). Examples of ligands include acetylcholine (Ach) and ATP which gate inwardly rectifying potassium currents.

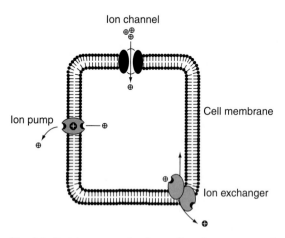

Fig. 4-4. Protein macromolecules mediate the movement of ions across the cell membrane. (Source: Redrawn with permission of Jalife J, Delmar M, Davidenko JM, et al. *Basic Cardiac Electrophysiology for the Davidenko Clinician.* Armonk, NY: Futura Publishing, 1999.

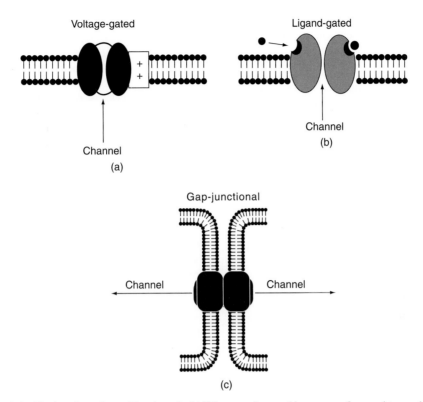

Fig. 4-5. General classification of sarcolemmal ion channels. (a) Voltage gated, opened in presence of appropriate membrane voltage; (b) ligand gated, opened in presence of appropriate molecule; hormone, peptide; (c) gap-junctional channels, allow the exchange of ions and small molecules between adjacent cells. (Source: Redrawn with permission Jalife J, Delmar M, Davidenko JM, et al. *Basic Cardiac Electrophysiology for the Clinician.* Armonk, NY: Futura Publishing, 1999.)

Ion Selectivity

Ion selectivity is a concept that is incompletely understood. Stearic hindrance is a theory that describes the conformational change in an ion channel protein that blocks large ions but allows smaller ones to pass. Since smaller ions are not universally permeable, other concepts must be at play. One such concept is that the channel must be "preconditioned" by binding that ion to specific sites on the pore. These sites are in very electrostatically sensitive areas that are ideal for repelling the other ion species.

Driving Force

When ion channels are open, a specific current will flow through them. The direction and magnitude of this current depend on the driving force for ionic movement. The driving forces depend on the difference between the membrane potential and equilibrium potential for that ion. For each ion, the driving force can be derived from the Nernst Equation: $[E]_x = -61 \log([x]_i/[x]_0)$, the $[x]_0$ is extracellular concentration of an ion and $[x]_i$ is the intracellular concentration of an ion. If the membrane potential is more positive than the equilibrium potential, cations like sodium and potassium will flow out of the cell. If it is more negative, they will flow into the cell.

Given the equilibrium potentials shown in Table 4-1, during the entire cardiac action potential, potassium currents are outward while sodium currents are inward. Inward currents depolarize the membrane while outward currents hyperpolarize or repolarize the membrane. During cardiac action potential, three ion currents predominate: sodium current, calcium current, and potassium current (Fig. 4-6).

Table 4-1. Cardiac Myocyte Intracellular and Extracellular Ion Concentrations and Ion Equilibrium Potentials

Ion	Extracellular (mM)	Intracellular (mM)	Equilibrium Potassium (mV)
K^+	4	135	−90
Na^+	145	10	+70
Ca^{2+}	2	10^{-4}	+130

Specific Currents

Sodium Current (I_{Na})

The sodium current is the major current that excites cardiac cells of the atria, ventricles, and the Purkinje system. Depolarization is caused by the rapid inward

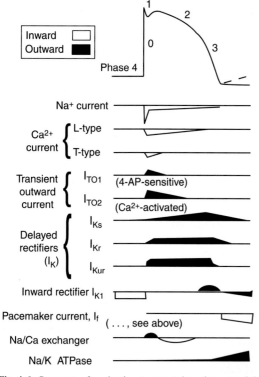

Fig. 4-6. Summary of predominant currents in action potential. Current magnitudes are not to scale. The Na^+ current is 50-fold larger than any other current. 4-Aminopyridne (4-AP) is widely used in vitro blockers of channels. The delayed rectifier has been separated on how rapidly they activate. Slowly I_{Ks}, rapidly I_{Kr}, and ultra rapidly I_{Kur}. (Source: Redrawn with permission Jalife J, Delmar M, Davidenko JM, et al. *Basic Cardiac Electrophysiology for the Clinician.* Armonk, NY: Futura Publishing, 1999.)

movement of sodium ions.[5] The magnitude of the sodium current is 50 times larger than any other current. In the nonpacemaker cell, the sodium current plays little role in the action potential. The sodium channel is regulated by norepinephrine (NE) and Ach. At the molecular level, cAMP and protein kinase A (PKA) phosphorylation of the channel exert an inhibitory effect. The sodium channel is also sensitive to such ions as cadmium and zinc. A variety of marine animals (newts, puffer fish, and snails) produce tetrodotoxin (TTX) and saxitoxin that block the I_{Na} using a guanidium ion moiety. Ion channels are often classified by their sensitivity to TTX.[1]

Calcium Current (I_{Ca})

The calcium current is a transient inward current that lacks sensitivity to TTX. The current subclassified as a transient (I_{Ca-T}) and a long-lasting (I_{Ca-L}) calcium channels have slightly different biophysical and pharmacologic properties (Table 4-2). The L-type calcium channel maintains depolarization through the plateau. The influx of calcium ions plays a crucial role in the contractile process. The calcium influx links the excitatory cascade with the contractile mechanism. In pacemaker cells, the I_{Ca-L} current is responsible for phase zero depolarization rather than the I_{Na} current as noted in the ventricular myocyte. The I_{Ca-T} is limited to the generation of pacemaker potential.

Potassium Currents

The potassium channels are a diverse group.[6] The functional roles are described in Table 4-3.

Delayed Rectifier Potassium Current

The delayed rectifier potassium current (I_K) is important in the repolarization of cardiac action potential. When the membrane potential becomes more positive than −40 mV, the delayed rectifier potassium current becomes activated. This outward current repolarizes the cell. It is also thought that the I_K current is an ionic mechanism partially responsible for initiating phase IV depolarization in pacemaking cells. Further study has revealed that there is more than one type of delayed rectifier potassium currents described (Table 4-4). These two potassium channels are described in terms of their kinetics and voltage dependence. The K_r is a rapidly activated inward rectifying current with a sensitivity to sotalol a class III antiarrhythmic. The K_s is a slowly activated current not sensitive to sotalol. During an action potential, both K_s and K_r contribute equally to the repolarization process.

Table 4-2. Biophysical and Pharmacologic Profiles of Cardiac T- and L-Type Ca Currents

	T Type	**L Type**
Activation threshold	Positive to –60 mV	Positive to –30 mV
Inactivation threshold	–90 to –60 mV	Positive to –40 mV
Conductance ($[Ca^{2+}]_0 = 5$ mM)	8.5 pS	16 pS
Pharmacologic sensitivity		
Dihydropyridines	No	Yes
Nickel	High	Low
Cadmium	Low	High

Source: Reprinted with permission of Jalife J, Delmar M, Davidenko JM, et al. *Basic Cardiac Electrophysiology for the Clinician.* Armonk, NY: Futura Publishing, 1999.

Pacemaker Current (I_f)

The pacemaker current when discovered in the 1980s displayed rather unique properties and was called I_h (h for hyperpolarization activated), I_f (f for funny), or I_q (q for queer). This channel is also referred to as hyperpolarization-activated and cyclic nucleotide-gated channels (HCN channels).[7] Unlike most other voltage-gated channels, the I_f is opened by hyperpolarization rather than by depolarization of the membrane. Although the channel has some permeability toward K ions, at normal physiologic potassium concentrations, the I_f carries sodium inwardly. Since the pacemaker channel carries an inward sodium current, the membrane slowly depolarizes toward the threshold. This "leakiness" of sodium ions allows for diastolic or phase IV depolarization of cells in the conduction system. The SA node identifies itself as the cardiac pacemaker by depolarizing most rapidly. Activation of I_f leads to steeper diastolic depolarization causing the cell to reach the threshold

more quickly. The channel is directly enhanced by cAMP and cGMP hence the name acronym HCN. Other research properties include: (a) low concentrations of cesium ions block the current, (b) extracellular chloride ions modulate the permeation of cations, (c) relative ion permeability of sodium over potassium depends on extracellular potassium concentrations.[8]

Gap-Junctional Currents

Gap-junctional channels are located in the intercalated disc which is a membrane separating the interiors of two adjacent myocardial cells. These gap-junctional channels are aqueous pores with large diameters and relatively low ionic selectivity. These channel proteins, also referred to as connexin, appear to be regulated by time- and voltage-dependent activation properties. These gap-junctional currents are essential for the rapid spread of cardiac cell excitability. At an ultrastructural level, they are slightly different than other types of ion channels.

Table 4-3. Functional Roles of Other Major Cardiac Potassium Currents

K Channel Type	**Functional Role in the Cardiac Cell**
Inward rectifier	Opens with hyperpolarization; establishes the cardiac cell resting potential.
Transient outward	Opens transiently after initial depolarization; involved in phase I repolarization.
ATP sensitive	Opens at low ATP levels in cardiac cells, such as in metabolically compromised myocardium.
Acetylcholine sensitive	Opens in the presence of Ach, such as with vagal stimulation; efflux of K causes hyperpolarization, which shortens the action potential.
Calcium activated	Opens in the presence of high levels of intracellular Ca.

Source: Reprinted with permission of Jalife J, Delmar M, Davidenko JM, et al. *Basic Cardiac Electrophysiology for the Clinician.* Armonk, NY: Futura Publishing, 1999.

Table 4-4. Properties of the Two Components of Cardiac Delayed Rectifier Current, I_K

	I_{Ks}	I_{Kr}
Activation time constants (0 mV)	400, 2500 ms	50 ms
Rectification	Slight	Marked
Conductance ($[K^+]_0 = 150$ mM)	1–3 pS	10 pS
Block by class III antiarrhythmic agent, E-4031	No	Yes
Activation by isoproterenol	Yes	No

Source: Reprinted with permission of Jalife J, Delmar M, Davidenko JM, et al. *Basic Cardiac Electrophysiology for the Clinician.* Armonk, NY: Futura Publishing, 1999.

Other Currents

The cardiac cell has background, pump, and exchanger currents. The background current is an inward current using Na+, Ca2+, and K+ as charge carriers. The Na background current may provide membrane depolarization between –50 and –20 mV. The Na-Ca exchange current is an inward current throughout the range of diastolic depolarization in pacemaker cells, providing a background, depolarizing current during diastole.[9] The sodium potassium antiporter (Na-K-ATPase) pump with a coupling ratio of 3:2 is a mechanism by which the cardiac cell can reestablish ion gradients following membrane activity. Because of the 3:2 ratio, this pump tends to cause an outward current because of the extrapositive sodium ions that are moved out of the cell.

ION CHANNEL REGULATION

The autonomic nervous system directly impacts chronotropy by stimulating the pacemaker cells of the heart. Conduction of impulses through the atria, AV nodal tissues, and the ventricles is also under autonomic control. Myocardial contractility is influenced by altering the calcium pool. The sympathetic nervous system releases NE from the nerve terminal while the parasympathetic system releases Ach. These neurotransmitters diffuse from the terminal and combine with receptor on the extracellular face of the cardiac cell membrane. The receptor-ligand complex triggers a cascade of events resulting in the alteration of ion channels and pumps.[8,10–12] The changes in gating behavior result in changes in electric and mechanical function of the heart.[13–17] Besides Ach and NE, other agents such as neuropeptides, hormones, cations, protons, and temperature influence ion channels. The exact mechanism behind ion channel

regulation is the subject of extensive research scrutiny, but several systems are well described.

Membrane Receptor and Enzyme Systems

This regulatory pathway starts at the receptor-ligand complex activating a G protein. The G protein is a membrane-bound, GTP-binding protein. The G protein combines with a membrane-bound enzyme generating a second messenger in the cytosol. The second messenger acts on a protein kinase which is usually located on an intracellular site. The protein kinase phosphorylates, or transfers a terminal phosphate group, to a target protein. The conformation change is terminated by removal of the phosphate group by a phosphatase. Using conventional terminology, neurotransmitters or hormones (first messengers) initiate a signal. The cytosolic agents (second messengers) translate the signal by causing a conformational change at the effector protein.[18,19] The two most well-known cascades are the ADC system and the PLC enzyme system (Fig. 4-7).

Adenylate Cyclase System

The ADC system is initiated by the ligand (NE) coupling with the receptor (β-adrenergic receptor) at the extracellular surface. The G protein undergoes a conformational change when it recognizes the receptor-ligand complex. The activated G protein interacts with ADC which produces cAMP. The cAMP activates PKA which phosphorylates serine and threonine residues on the target protein (Fig. 4-8).

Two vital features of any enzyme cascade are exhibited by the ADC system: amplification and signal termination. Each receptor-ligand complex can interact with several G proteins. Each G protein can activate several ADC enzymes, thus amplifying the original signal. The signal

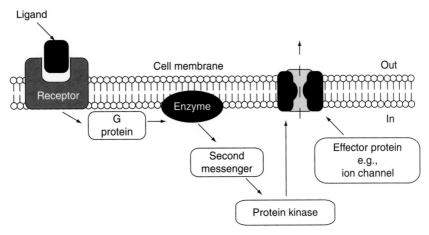

Fig. 4-7. Schematic illustration of steps in second messenger receptor-enzyme signaling pathway. (Source: Redrawn with permission Jalife J, Delmar M, Davidenko JM, et al. *Basic Cardiac Electrophysiology for the Clinician*. Armonk, NY: Futura Publishing, 1999.)

is terminated by inactivation of cAMP to AMP by the phosphodiesterase enzyme and by dephosphorylation of effector proteins by phosphatases (Fig. 4-9).

Phospholipase C System

The α-adrenergic receptor uses the more complex and less well-understood PLC system (Fig. 4-10).

Enzyme Cascade Shortcut

In enzyme shortcuts, several elements typically found in enzyme cascades are bypassed. The membrane-bound G protein regulates the ion channel directly or by another membrane intermediary. Since no cytosolic elements are involved, the process is termed membrane delimited. Direct G protein modulation may explain regulation in

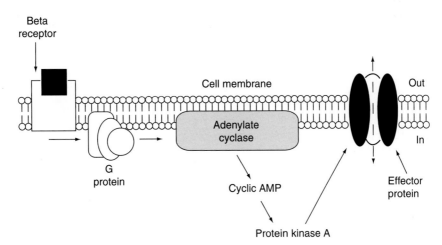

Fig. 4-8. Adenylate cyclase (ADC) signaling pathway. Coupling of a ligand (epinephrine, norepinephrine) to a β-adrenergic receptor on the extracellular surface initiates the cascade. (Source: Redrawn with permission Jalife J, Delmar M, Davidenko JM, et al. *Basic Cardiac Electrophysiology for the Clinician*. Armonk, NY: Futura Publishing, 1999.)

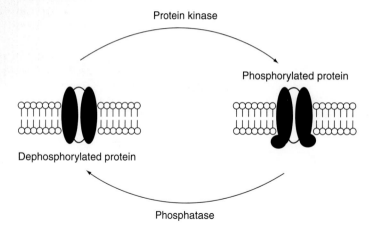

Fig. 4-9. Protein kinases phosphorylate specific residues (serine, tyrosine, threonine) on the target protein, causing a conformational change. The change to the ion channel alters the conductance. Phosphatases remove the phosphate molecule terminating the modulation effect. (Source: Redrawn with permission Jalife J, Delmar M, Davidenko JM, et al. *Basic Cardiac Electrophysiology for the Clinician.* Armonk, NY: Futura Publishing, 1999.)

rapid ion channels such as the atrial muscarinic K channel (I_{KAch}). The membrane-delimited model is also thought to exist in other channels, like I_{Ca}, and may play a role in those states where increase vagal tone overrides the ADC system (Fig. 4-11).

Proton Regulation

Since acidification of the cellular environment is a major factor in myocardial ischemia, proton-dependent effects on ion channels are important. Increasing the proton (acid) load to a cell results in membrane hyperpolarization. The proton buildup stimulates the Na^+-H^+ exchanger

to rid the cell of dangerous protons while allowing the buildup of Na^+. The buildup of intracellular Na causes the Na^+-K^+ exchanger to extrude Na^+ in exchange for K^+. The inward movement of K^+ in ischemic states hyperpolarizes the cell.

AUTONOMIC CONTROL OF THE HEART

The sympathetic stimulation through NE and epinephrine release augment myocardial contractility, shortens AV nodal conduction time, and enhances chronotropy. Stimulation of β receptors by NE activates the ADC

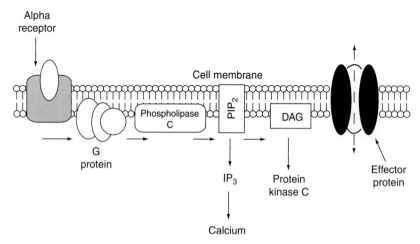

Fig. 4-10. Phospholipase C (PLC) signaling pathway. Coupling a ligand (norepinephrine) to an α-adrenergic receptor initiates the pathway. Phosphatidylinositol 4,5-diphosphate (PIP$_2$), inositol 1,4,5-triphosphate (IP$_3$), diacylglycerol (DAG). (Source: Redrawn with permission Jalife J, Delmar M, Davidenko JM, et al. *Basic Cardiac Electrophysiology for the Clinician.* Armonk, NY: Futura Publishing, 1999.)

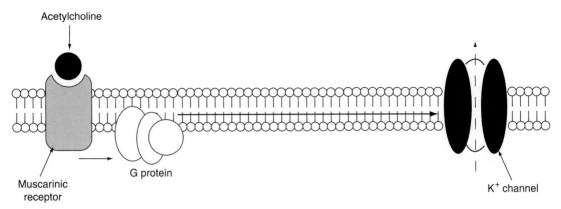

Fig. 4-11. Direct (membrane-delimited) G protein regulation of ion channels.

pathway. The effector protein is the pacemaker channel (I_f). Activating the I_f causes phase IV diastolic depolarization to become steeper. The cell reaches threshold more quickly and the heart rate increases (Fig. 4-12). Parasympathetics stimulate muscarinic receptors. Through the membrane-delimited mechanism described above, the I_{KAch} channel is activated. Opening the I_K hyperpolarizes the cell and flattens phase IV. The cells reach threshold more slowly and the heart rate decreases. Sympathetics innervate all portions of the heart and increase automaticity and strength of cardiac muscle activity. Parasympathetics innervate above the ventricles; the SA node, atria, and AV node, and serve to slow automaticity.

Future Directions

Much of the current research in electrophysiology focuses on the genetic basis of acquired and hereditary channel abnormalities—termed channelopathies. Whether inherited or acquired, channelopathies alter repolarization and lead to sudden cardiac death from ventricular arrhythmias. Unstable repolarization is magnified by prolongation of the Q-T interval. The prolonged Q-T syndrome is heritable or acquired. The inherited form is caused by discreet mutations in genes that encode ion channels. The sodium channel gene, *SCN5A*, or one of the four genes that encode the I_K channel can be affected.[18,20–22] The Brugada syndrome is characterized by ST-segment elevation in V_1 to V_3 unrelated to ischemia, electrolyte imbalance, or structural disease, with right bundle branch block morphology. The *SCN5A* gene is mutated in the Brugada syndrome leading to life-threatening ventricular arrhythmias.

The study of inherited channelopathies has led to insightful discoveries of more common diseases. Heart failure, from whatever etiology, represents an acquired form of prolonged Q-T syndrome. Selected downregulation of two potassium currents, the I_{TO} and I_{K1}, occurs at the transcriptional level.[15] In the short term, potassium downregulation decreases depolarization allowing for more time for excitation-contraction coupling.[18] In the

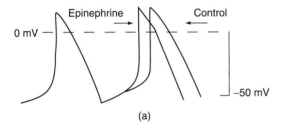

(a)

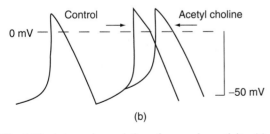

(b)

Fig. 4-12. Autonomic regulation of pacemaker activity. (a) Sympathetic stimulation, via the release of epinephrine and nor-epinephrine, increases pacemaker frequency; (b) parasympathetic stimulation, via the release of acetylcholine (Ach), inhibits pacemaker activity. (Source: Redrawn with permission Jalife J, Delmar M, Davidenko JM, et al. *Basic Cardiac Electrophysiology for the Clinician.* Armonk, NY: Futura Publishing, 1999.)

long term, downregulation predisposes individuals to disordered repolarization, delayed afterdepolarizations, and ventricular tachyarrhythmias. Upregulation of the Na^+-Ca^{2+} exchanger aggravates arrhymogenicity by altering intracellular calcium levels.[9,17]

Enzyme-receptor physiology is also altered in heart failure. Downregulation of the β_1-adrenergic receptor results in the increase in the relative cardiac β_2-adrenergic receptor expression.[10,14,16] Polymorphisms of the β_2-adrenergic receptor determines exercise capacity and outcome in the heart failure patient. Genetic expression of cardiac channels and enzyme-receptor systems is subject of aggressive ongoing research in cardiac electrophysiology. Future directions, such as gene therapy, risk stratification, and cardiac pharmacology are likely to be focused on these important enzyme-receptor systems.

REFERENCES

1. Catterall WA. Molecular properties of sodium and calcium channels. *J Bioenerg Biomembr* 1996;28:219–230.
2. Berne RM, Levy MN (eds.). *Physiology*. St. Louis, MO: Mosby, 1993.
3. Jalife J, Delmar M, Davidenko JM, et al. *Basic Cardiac Electrophysiology for the Clinician*. Armonk, NY: Futura Publishing, 1999.
4. Luo CH, Rudy Y. A dynamic model of the cardiac ventricular action potential. I. Simulations of ionic currents and concentration changes. *Circ Res* 1994;74:1071–1096.
5. Marban E, Yamagishi T, Tomaselli GF. Structure and function of voltage-gated sodium channels. *J Physiol* 1998;508(Pt 3):647–657.
6. Tristani-Firouzi M, Chen J, Mitcheson JS, et al. Molecular biology of k(+) channels and their role in cardiac arrhythmias. *Am J Med* 2001;110:50–59.
7. Kaupp UB, Seifert R. Molecular diversity of pacemaker ion channels. *Annu Rev Physiol* 2001;63:235–257.
8. Jaber M, Koch WJ, Rockman H, et al. Essential role of beta-adrenergic receptor kinase 1 in cardiac development and function. *Proc Natl Acad Sci U S A* 1996;93:12974–12979.
9. Philipson KD, Nicoll DA. Sodium-calcium exchange: A molecular perspective. *Annu Rev Physiol* 2000;62:111–133.
10. Dorn GW, II, Tepe NM, Lorenz JN, et al . Low- and high-level transgenic expression of beta2-adrenergic receptors differentially affect cardiac hypertrophy and function in Galphaq-overexpressing mice. *Proc Natl Acad Sci U S A* 1999;96:6400–6405.
11. Freeman K, Lerman I, Kranias EG, et al. Alterations in cardiac adrenergic signaling and calcium cycling differentially affect the progression of cardiomyopathy. *J Clin Invest* 2001;107:967–974.
12. Iaccarino G, Tomhave ED, Lefkowitz RJ, et al. Reciprocal in vivo regulation of myocardial g protein-coupled receptor kinase expression by beta-adrenergic receptor stimulation and blockade. *Circulation* 1998;98:1783–1789.
13. Koch WJ, Lefkowitz RJ, Rockman HA. Functional consequences of altering myocardial adrenergic receptor signaling. *Annu Rev Physiol* 2000;62:237–260.
14. Liggett SB, Wagoner LE, Craft LL, et al. The ile164 beta2-adrenergic receptor polymorphism adversely affects the outcome of congestive heart failure. *J Clin Invest* 1998;102:1534–1539.
15. Marban E. Heart failure: The electrophysiologic connection. *J Cardiovasc Electrophysiol* 1999;10:1425–1428.
16. Wagoner LE, Craft LL, Singh B, et al. Polymorphisms of the beta(2)-adrenergic receptor determine exercise capacity in patients with heart failure. *Circ Res* 2000;86:834–840.
17. Winslow RL, Rice J, Jafri S. Modeling the cellular basis of altered excitation-contraction coupling in heart failure. *Prog Biophys Mol Biol* 1998;69:497–514.
18. Marban E. Cardiac channelopathies. *Nature* 2002;415:213–218.
19. Rockman HA, Koch WJ, Lefkowitz RJ. Seven-transmembrane-spanning receptors and heart function. *Nature* 2002;415:206–212.
20. Naccarelli GV, Antzelevitch C. The Brugada syndrome: Clinical, genetic, cellular, and molecular abnormalities. *Am J Med* 2001;110:573–581.
21. Priori SG, Barhanin J, Hauer RN, et al. Genetic and molecular basis of cardiac arrhythmias; impact on clinical management. Study group on molecular basis of arrhythmias of the working group on arrhythmias of the European Society of Cardiology. *Eur Heart J* 1999;20:174–195.
22. Tan HL, Bink-Boelkens MT, Bezzina CR, et al. A sodium-channel mutation causes isolated cardiac conduction disease. *Nature* 2001;409:1043–1047.

PART II

ACUTE MYOCARDIAL INFARCTION AND ACUTE CORONARY SYNDROMES

5

Demographics and Economics of Acute Coronary Syndromes

Michael A. Ross
Brian P. O'Neil

HIGH YIELD FACTS

- About 865,000 myocardial infarctions (MIs) occur each year in the United States, with about 565,000 of these being a first time event.

- The traditional Framingham risk factors are markers of lifetime risk of coronary disease and do not have significant value in risk stratifying chest pain in the emergency department (ED).

- Women with MI are less likely to undergo invasive therapy for acute myocardial infarction (AMI), less likely to get treated with thrombolytics, receive a beta-blocker, or receive an aspirin.

- A number of studies show that chest pain observation units lower the overall cost of evaluating chest pain patients by reducing expensive admissions and reducing the incidence of "missed MI."

- Failure to diagnose MI accounts for more than one-third of malpractice dollars paid in emergency medicine.

CARDIOVASCULAR DISEASE

Cardiovascular disease (CVD) has been broadly defined as hypertension, coronary heart disease, congestive heart failure (CHF), stroke and congenital heart disease. Coronary heart disease is further subdivided into stable disease, including stable angina pectoris, and unstable disease or acute coronary syndromes (ACSs). The latter includes patients with AMI, with or without ST elevation, and unstable angina pectoris.

It is estimated that 22.6% of individuals in the United States have some form of CVD.[1] In the Framingham heart study, average rates of first major cardiovascular events were shown to rise with advancing age from 7 per 1000 at ages 35–44 to 68 per 1000 at ages 85–94. This is particularly concerning since the U.S. census has estimated that there will be 40 million Americans over 65 by 2010.

Since 1918, CVD has become the leading cause of death in the United States. In 2001, it accounted for 38.5% of all deaths, or 1 of every 2.6 deaths. There are more deaths attributable to CVD than the next five leading causes of death combined—cancer, chronic lower respiratory disease, accidents, diabetes, and influenza/pneumonia. The Center for Disease Control (CDC) has estimated that 60% of cardiovascular deaths occur either outside the hospital or in the ED. In 2001, the leading cause of cardiovascular deaths was coronary heart disease which accounted for 54% of cardiovascular deaths, followed by stroke (18%), CHF (6%), and hypertension (5%). This chapter will focus on coronary artery disease (CAD) and ACSs.[1]

CORONARY ARTERY DISEASE

It is estimated that in 2001 there were 13.2 million Americans with coronary artery disease (CAD), representing 6.4% of the population.[1] Of these individuals, 7.8 million will have experienced a MI at some time in their life. In the same year, 865,000 million of these individuals will experience a MI, with 565,000 of these being a first time event and 300,000 being recurrent. When combining coronary disease-related deaths with MI—1.2 million patients suffered either adverse event in 2001. Currently, CAD accounts for one in five deaths in the United Sates and is the leading cause of death of men and women in the United States. Annually, 340,000 people die of coronary disease either in the ED or out of the hospital. Most are due to sudden death from ventricular fibrillation. Sudden death from CAD often occurs with no preceding symptoms—with 50% of men and 64% of women having no symptoms before their sudden death.

CAD is only one manifestation of the systemic disease process of atherosclerosis. The Framingham study identified several risk factors for the development of atherosclerosis of the coronary arteries over a time frame of several years. These include age, gender, hypertension, smoking, hyperlipidemia, diabetes, and a family history of premature CAD. Each is independently associated with greater risk of developing CAD, and subsequent AMI and its complications. Framingham coronary heart disease prediction scores have been shown to perform well in a variety of ethnic groups over a 5-year period.[2]

It is important to understand that the traditional Framingham risk factors were derived to predict a patient's probability of developing CAD, or coronary atherosclerotic plaque, and its complications over several years. They were not developed, nor should they be used, to determine if a patient experiencing chest pain in the ED is suffering an ACS, or a ruptured plaque.[3] ACSs, or coronary plaque rupture, are best identified using other risk stratification methods and will be discussed elsewhere in this textbook. With this understanding, we will later evaluate the contribution of each risk factor to the disease process.

Acute Coronary Syndromes: Prevalence and Mortality

An "acute coronary syndrome" is the term used to describe the spectrum of disease processes that occur as a result of inadequate coronary perfusion, most commonly due to a ruptured coronary artery plaque. The spectrum of ACSs include AMI with electrocardiographic ST-segment elevation, or ST elevation myocardial infarction (STEMI), AMI without ST elevation (non-STEMI), and unstable angina or acute ischemia without infarction.

Data from CDC/National Center for Health Statistics (NCHS) estimate that in the year 2001 there were 928,000 patients discharged from the hospital with a primary diagnosis of AMI (795,000) or unstable angina (133,000). This number increases to 1,680,000 if patients discharged with a secondary diagnosis of AMI (959,000) or unstable angina (758,000) are included in the total case mix.[1] An analysis of the National Registry of Myocardial Infarction, or NRMI, showed that of 1,799,704 AMI patients 41.6% presented with ST-segment elevation.[4]

The diagnosis of unstable angina has undergone a significant shift in recent years due to advances in serum cardiac markers and care of more patients in same day "chest pain units." As a result of these advances, some "unstable angina" patients with positive cardiac troponin levels are now classified as a non-STEMI, while other chest pain patients are not admitted as "unstable angina" because their work up could be completed in an ED chest pain unit. Previous National Health and Nutrition Examination Survey II, (NHANES) data (1988–1994) showed that more women are diagnosed with angina than men, both in total numbers and the age-adjusted rates.[1] Data from 2001 show the prevalence of unstable angina to be 3.5% in the total population, with rates of 2.7% among males and 4.3% among females. The incidence of stable angina in that same year is estimated at 0.2% of the population, although these numbers may be lower due to changes in billing and the potential for underreporting. Approximately 20% of coronary events are preceded by a history of angina (see Table 5-1).

Demographics of Coronary Artery Disease and Acute Coronary Syndromes by Risk Groups

Age

It is well known that coronary disease is related to age. In U.S. citizens between the ages of 29 and 44, males

Table 5-1. Annual Rates Per 1000 People for New or Recurrent Angina

Group	Age 65–74	Age 75–84	Age 85 and Older
Black men	26.1	52.2	43.5
Black women	29.4	37.7	15.2
Non-Black men	44.3	56.4	42.6
Non-Black women	18.8	30.8	19.8

experience 34,000 MIs per year and females experience 10,000 infarcts per year. This increases in patients who are 45–65 years old to 250,000 for males and 88,000 for females. Finally, among patients over age 65 there are 410,000 heart attacks in males and 372,000 in females. The average age of a person having a first heart attack is 65.8 for men and 70.8 for women.[1]

Gender

With advancing age two things occur, the incidence of infarcts drastically increases, and the difference between men and women decreases. Postmenopausal women have coronary heart disease rates that are two to three times that of premenopausal women. By age 75, the prevalence of CVD is higher among women than men. Since 1985, the annual number of deaths due to CVD has been higher for women than for men (see Fig. 5-1). When considering the top 10 causes of death in women, more women die from CVD than the following 7 leading causes of death combined.[1]

Recent studies have identified gender as a predictor of poor outcomes among patients with ACSs. Unfortunately early studies of ACSs were limited to men, leading to a delay in our understanding of gender issues. Hochman published a study evaluating the sex-based differences of presentation and outcomes from the GUSTO II (Global utilization of streptokinase and t-PA for occluded coronary arteries) study which involved 3662 women and 8480 men with ACSs, that included patients with STEMI, non-STEMI, and unstable angina.[5] In this study population women tended to be older, had significantly higher rates

of diabetes, hypertension, and heart failure. Further, women had significantly lower rates of prior AMI, were less likely to smoke, and presented with ST elevation less often than men (27.2% vs. 37%, P <0.001). It was also noted that the percentage of MIs that were "non-STEMI" was higher among men than women (47.6% vs. 36.6%, P <0.001). Women were noted to have more complications and higher mortality rates in 30 days than men (6% vs. 4%, P <0.001) with similar 30-day reinfarction rates. However, after stratification and adjustment for baseline variables there was noted to be a nonsignificant trend toward increased death in women compared to men only with ST elevation AMI (odds ratio 1.27, 95% CI 0.98–1.68, P = 0.07). Among patients with unstable angina, female gender was an independent predictor of death with an odd ratio for death of 0.65 (95% CI 0.59–0.83, P = 0.003). In a study of the NRMI database, Canto et al. found that women with acute MI were more likely than men to present without chest pain (49% vs. 38%).[6] In a review of the NRMI registry, Vaccarino et al. found that of 384,878 MI patients 155,565 (40.4%) were women.[7] Overall in-hospital mortality rate was 16.7% for women and 11.5% for men. These sex-based death rates varied by age, and interestingly the mortality rate of women under age 50 was twice that of men. This gender difference in the death rates decreased with increasing age, with no significant difference noted after the age of 74. A multivariate analysis showed that the odds for death were at 11.1% greater for women than for men for every 5-year decrease in age. It was further noted that only one-third of the risk difference could be accounted for by medical history, severity of the infarction, and

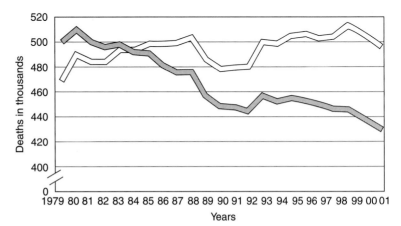

Fig. 5-1. Cardiovascular disease mortality trends for males and females in the United States: 1979–2001. (Source: CDC/NCHS, reprinted with permission from AHA.)

early management strategy. After adjustment for these factors, women still had a 7% higher risk of death for every 5 years of decreasing age (95% CI of odds ratio = 5.9–8.1).

The authors concluded that ST elevation AMI in young women had higher rates of death during hospitalization than men. In a study with an opposing viewpoint, Malacrida et al. analyzed the ISSI-3 database for major clinical events occurring from hospitalization to 35 days following discharge for 9600 women and 26,480 men that were fibrinolytic eligible AMI patients.[8] The results showed that relative to men, women had an unadjusted odds ratio for death of 1.73 (95% CI 1.61–1.86). After adjusting for the fact that women were significantly older than men the odds ratio was reduced to 1.2 (95% CI 1.11–1.29). Adjustment for other differences in baseline clinical characteristics further reduced the odds ratio to 1.14 (95% CI 1.05–1.23). The authors concluded that there is only a small independent association between female sex and mortality in patients with suspected AMI.

In a review of the AMI treatment from the Cooperative Cardiovascular Project database, Gan et al. abstracted information from 138,956 medicare beneficiaries (49% women) treated between 1994 and 1995.[9] A multivariant analysis was done to study differences between men and women with respect to the medications administered, procedures used, assignment of do not resuscite (DNR) status, and 30-day mortality. Among ideal candidates for invasive therapy, women in all age groups were less likely to undergo procedures. The difference was more pronounced among women 85 or older, with the adjusted relative risk for a procedure was 0.75 (95% CI 0.68–0.83). Women were also slightly less likely to receive thrombolytic therapy within 60 min (adjusted relative risk 0.93, 95% CI 0.9–0.96), or to receive aspirin within the first 24 hours (adjusted relative risk 0.96, 95% CI 0.95–0.97). Women were also less likely to receive beta-blockers but more likely to receive angiotensin-converting enzyme inhibitors. Women were more likely than men to have DNR orders in their records. After adjustment, women and men had similar 30-day mortality rates (hazard ratio 1.02, 95% CI 0.99–1.04). These authors concluded that compared to men, women receive somewhat less aggressive treatment during their early management of AMI. However, they noted that many of these differences were small and there was no apparent effect on mortality.

In an analysis of NRMI-2,3,4 STEMI patients with contraindications to thrombolytic therapy, Grzybowski et al. found that men were 57% more likely to receive mechanical revascularization than women.[10] Marrugat

et al. further described gender discrepancies between cardiovascular morbidity and treatment were in a 1998 study of Spanish women having their first MI. Women were found to have more comorbid conditions such as diabetes, hypertension, and angina. However after adjustment for these comorbid risk factors, their risk of death at 28 days was 1.72 times greater than for men and at 6 months it was 1.73 times greater.[11]

It is unclear why these gender differences exist and what their true magnitude is. A controversial study by Schulman et al. suggested that primary care physicians are less likely to refer patients for diagnostic cardiac catheterization who are younger, female, or Black.[12] Unfortunately, Black females have a higher age-adjusted death rate from coronary heart disease than do White females (177 per 100,000 population vs. 137 per 100,000 population), just as Black males have slightly higher rates than White males (228 per 100,000 vs. 226 per 100,000).[1] This may in part be due to the fact that as a group, Blacks show a higher prevalence of coronary disease than do Whites, whether male (41% vs. 30%) or female (40% vs. 24%).

Modifiable Risk Factors for CAD—Diabetes

Diabetes mellitus is consistently rated as one of the major risk factors for coronary disease and stroke. The CDC estimates that 49–69 million adults in the United States may have insulin resistance and one in four of them will develop type II diabetes. The data currently available from 2001 for the prevalence of physician-diagnosed diabetes in the United States were 5.5% or 11 million patients. The estimated prevalence of undiagnosed diabetes in 2001 is 2.9% of the population or nearly 6 million people.[13] It was noted that from 1994 to 2002 the prevalence of diabetes after adjusting for age increased 54% for U.S. adults, from 4.8 to 7.3%, and among American Indians and Alaskan Native adults the number increased 32.2%, from 11.5 to 15.3%. In the population of American Indians and Alaskan Natives the overall age-adjusted prevalence of diabetes was twice that of U.S. adults, with 43.5% of men and 52.4% of women between the ages of 45 and 74 having diabetes. Mokdad et al. noted that from 2001 to 2002 the prevalence of diabetes in the United States increased 8.2% overall and has increased 61% since 1990.[14]

According to the CDC/NCHS the prevalence of major coronary vascular disease, after adjusting for age, is twice that in diabetic women than nondiabetic women.[15] Further the age-adjusted hospital discharge rate for major coronary vascular disease is almost four times that for women without diabetes. Data from the CDC Diabetes Surveillance System in 2000 show the self-reported prevalence of coronary vascular conditions among diabetics aged 35–64 was 28.8%, for ages 65–74 it was 45.7%, and for those 75 and older it was 53.5%. This data from 2000 further showed that in diabetics aged 35 and older 37.2% reported some cardiovascular condition such as coronary disease or stroke. After standardizing for age, the self-reported coronary heart disease, angina, or heart attack rate was triple that for stroke (22.1% vs. 8%). Further solidifying the link between diabetes and CVD, 66–75% of people with diabetes die from some sort of heart or blood vessel disease. Death rates from heart disease among adults with diabetes are two to four times higher than rates of adults without diabetes.

Modifiable Risk Factors for CAD—Hypertension

The NHANES II (1988–1994) estimated one in five Americans and one in four adults have hypertension. The prevalence of hypertension in 2001 is 32.8% among Blacks. Specifically Black females with the highest incidence of hypertension of 44.7%, which is 35% higher than Whites and Mexicans. Not surprisingly Blacks have a corresponding increased rate of 1.3 and 1.8 times for nonfatal and fatal stroke, with a fourfold increase in the incidence of end-stage kidney disease, data from the Joint National Committee on Prevention, Detection, Evaluation and Treatment of High Blood Pressure (JNC V and VI). Of patients with hypertension, approximately one-third do not know they have it, one-third are controlled on medication, one-fourth are on medications but still uncontrolled, and one-tenth are not on medications (JNC VII).[1] The risk of developing CHF is increased two- to threefold in hypertensive patients, and hypertension is a precursor of CHF in nine-tenths of CHF patients. In the United States, hypertension is listed as a contributing cause of death in nearly 10% of deaths in the year 2000. Hypertension-associated mortality rates rose over the decade from 1991 to 2001 by 53%, with an age-adjusted rate at 36.4%. Hypertension may be contributing to 30% of deaths in Black men and 20% of deaths in Black women (JNC V and VI). The 2004 estimate for the direct and indirect costs for hypertension is $55.5 billion.

Modifiable Risk Factors for CAD—Smoking

Although heart disease is the disease process that accounts for most deaths, the leading "actual cause" of preventable

death in the United States is tobacco. In 2000, tobacco accounted for 18.1% (435,000) of U.S. deaths, followed by poor diet and inactivity (16.6%), alcohol (3.5%), microbial infections (3.1%), toxins (2.3%), motor vehicles (1.8%), and firearms (1.2%).[16] The link between smoking and coronary disease has been well documented in the Framingham studies. Of smoking-related deaths, 33.5% were cardiovascular related.[1] Thirty seven percent of nonsmokers are exposed to second hand smoke. People exposed to second hand smoke have a 30% increased risk of death from coronary heart disease, resulting in roughly 35,000 deaths per year. Fortunately tobacco use among adults has declined 40% since 1965. In 2001, 31% of Whites, 28% of Blacks, 23% of Hispanics, and 45% of Native Americans used tobacco. Smoking prevalence is greatest among those with less education (9–11 years, 35.4%) and those living below poverty incomes (33.3%). Patients coming to the ED for a smoking-related complication may present at a uniquely "teachable moment" regarding smoking cessation. As such emergency physicians should never miss this opportunity to guide patients, or family members, to smoking cessation options. The estimated costs of smoking among Americans are over 157 billion dollars annually including medical expenditures, neonatal medical expenditures related to smoking, and the decrease of productivity due to smoking.

Modifiable Risk Factors for CAD—Hyperlipidemia

After smoking, poor diet is a second leading cause cardiovascular death.[14] According to the NHANES IV from 1999 to 2000, after the age of 45 more women than men have total blood cholesterol over 200 mg/dL.[1] When broken down into subgroups with cholesterol levels over 200 mg/dL, it occurred in Black males 37.3%, Black females 46.4%, Mexican males 54.3%, Mexican females 44.7%, White males 51%, and White females 53.6%. In accordance with the American Heart Association guidelines, cholesterol screening has increased over the last 5 years from 67.3% in 1991 to almost 71% in 1999.

Trending data from NHANES I to NHANES III it is noted that the blood cholesterol dropped most dramatically among White males (163–155 mg/dL), with a slight decrease in White (166 mg/dL vs. 163 mg/dL) and Black females (174 mg/dL vs. 168 mg/dL). However, Black males had a slight increase (165 mg/dL vs. 166 mg/dL). Among American Indians aged 45–74, nearly 37.7% of the men and 37.6% of the women have total cholesterol level greater than 200 mg/dL, with 8.6% of the men and 12.7% of the women having levels greater than 240 mg/dL as higher. According to the adult treatment panel 3 (ATP3) and the National Heart Blood and Lung Institute (NHLBI), less than half of the people who meet criteria for lipid lowering treatments actually receive them. Even in high-risk patients with symptomatic coronary heart disease only half are receiving lipid lowering therapy. As troubling is the fact that patients who are prescribed lipid lowering drugs approximately only 50% are still taking these drugs 6 months later, which drops at 1 year to only 30–40% still on these medications. This unfortunate trend is compounded by the fact that on average it takes 6 months to 1 year before the benefit from the lipid lowering therapy is realized.

Using low-density lipoproteins (LDL), the "bad cholesterol," the CDC defines levels of greater than 160 mg/dL as high and greater than 190 mg/dL as very high. Using these parameters, it is noted that among non-Hispanic Whites 20.4% of men and 17% of women have LDL cholesterol of greater than 160 mg/dL. Among non-Hispanic Blacks 19.3% of men and 18.8% of women and in Mexican Americans 16.9% of men and 14% of women have high to very high LDLs. A gender trend that is reversed when compared to total cholesterol. High-density lipoproteins (HDL) or "good cholesterol levels" less than 40 mg/dL are considered low and increase the risk for heart diseases and stroke. The mean HDL level among American adults is 50.7 mg/dL. It is known those patients with low HDL cholesterol and high total cholesterol levels are at the highest risk for ACSs. It is also known that patients with low HDLs ≤ 37 mg/dL in men and ≤ 47 mg/dL in women are at high risk no matter what the total cholesterol. On the other hand, patients with high total cholesterol and higher levels of HDL (>53 mg/dL in men and >63 mg/dL in women) are at low risk for AMI. The CDC estimates each year that over $33 billion in medical costs or $9 million in lost productivity is related to the American diet.

Modifiable Risk Factors for CAD—Physical Inactivity

The third leading modifiable cause of CAD is physical activity.[14] When you look at the prevalence from 2000 to 2001 data from the Behavioral Risk Factor Surveillance System (BRFSS) study at the CDC, 54.6% of Americans over the age of 18 did not meet the physical activity recommendations. Also from the CDC/NCHS data from 1997 to 1998 it was noted that in Americans aged 18 or older 38.3% reported no physical activity, 61.7%

engaged in at least some physical activity, and 22.7% engaged in light-to-moderate physical activity at least five times per week.[1] When these subgroups are broken up by race and gender it is noted that non-Hispanic Blacks, Hispanics women, and the elderly have the least amount of activity when compared to men, the young, non-Hispanic Whites, and Asians/Pacific Island non-Hispanic adults. Further these studies show that in higher income brackets, the college educated, and those living in the West had a higher prevalence of regular physical activity. Of note, married women were more likely than women in any other marital status to engage in the least physical activity. More recent data again from the CDC/NCHS from 1997 to 2003, it is noted that in U.S. adults more than 18 years old, 31.3% engaged in regular leisure time activity. When adjusting for age, sex, results show that 34% of the non-Hispanic Whites, 26.4% of the non-Hispanic Blacks, and 21% of Hispanics engage in regular leisure time activity. The reason that this data is of such import is that the relative risk for coronary heart disease of physical inactivity ranges from 1.5 to 2.4 and for comparison this is the same increase in risk for coronary disease observed for high cholesterol, high blood pressure, and cigarette smoking.[17]

A lot of recent attention has been focused on the youth of America and for good reason. Data from the 2002 from the Youth Media Campaign Longitudinal Study of the CDC showed that 61.5% of children aged 9–13 do not participate in any organized physical activity during their nonschool hours and that 22.6% do no engage in any free time physical activity. As far as race is concerned, non-Hispanic Blacks and Hispanic children were significantly less likely than non-Hispanic White children to state involvement in organized activities, this was also true of children of parents who had lower levels of income and education. In a study published in the *New England Journal of Medicine* it was noted that parents with less education were associated with greater decline in activity for White girls of both younger and only at older ages for Black girls.[18] It is further noted that a higher body mass index (BMI) was associated with a less physical activity among girls of both races.

The U.S. Surgeon General's report of 1996 noted that physical inactivity is more prevalent among women than men, among Blacks and Hispanics than Whites, among older than younger adults, and among the less affluent than the more affluent. A study published in *JAMA* of 72,000 female nurses indicated that moderately intense physical activity such as walking was associated with substantial reduction in the total risk of ischemic stroke.[19]

The CDC estimates the annual cost for disease associated with physical inactivity at 76 billion dollars.

Modifiable Risk Factors for CAD—Overweight and Obesity

Data from NHANES IV (1999–2000) suggest that nearly 9 million children aged 6–19 are either obese (BMI greater than 30) or overweight (BMI greater than 25) with a prevalence of 15.3% in 6–11 years old and 15.5% in 12–19 years old—both increased threefold from figures in 1965. It is estimated that 10% of preschool children aged 2–5 are overweight and increase of 3% from 1995. In children aged 6–19 the incidence of overweight children was nearly doubled for non-Hispanic Blacks and Mexican Americans when compared to Whites. Data from 2001 NHANES IV suggest that one-third of American adults are obese and one-third are overweight. It estimated that each year 330,000 Americans adults die from causes related to obesity. Years of life lost are closely related to the BMI. MMWR from 2002 estimates the cost attributable to obesity-related diseases at $100 billion.[1]

Socioeconomic Status and Outcomes from Acute Coronary Syndrome

In a review of PURSUIT trial data, Rao et al. studied socioeconomic variables in patients 1 and 6 months following an acute MI.[20] They found that the use of medications and cardiac procedures proven to be beneficial to patients with AMI was lower for those in the lower income brackets. Additionally their unadjusted rate of death and AMI was higher. Parameters for income were low being under $20,000, middle being between $20,000 and $60,000, and high being over $60,000. Baseline characteristics were different with low-income patients having more chronic medical conditions and had more ST depression and CHF on presentation. For all patients, the 6 months unadjusted rates of death in succession for low, middle, and high income were 5.6%, 3.3%, and 1.6%, respectively, and for AMI were 15.8%, 14.0%, and 9.8%, respectively. The difference in the combined endpoint of death or MI was significantly different across the three income groups. The death rates in patients <65 were noted to be in succession for low, middle, and high at 3.4, 2.1, and 0.5 and for MI were noted to be 13.5%, 11.3%, and 8.1%, respectively. These differences were significant, but more so for patients under age 65. After multivariate adjustment there was no consistent pattern for disparity in the process of care; however, the strong trend for death and MI was most persistent in the low-income patients.

PROMISING RESEARCH FOR THE FUTURE

There continues to be progress in our understanding of the risk factors for CAD. Recent data presented at the 2004 European Society of Cardiology Congress from the INTERHEART Trial which is a trial of 29,000 subjects from 262 sites across 52 countries.[21] The trial included 15,152 first AMI patients, who were matched to 14,820 healthy controls by age at each site. Approximately 25% were from Europe, 25% from China, 20% from South Asia, 13% from the Middle East, 12% from South America, and 5% were from Africa. Demographic information was acquired regarding lifestyle, habits, history, psychosocial factors, use of medication, height, weight, waist to hip circumference, blood pressure, and heart rate. The presenting authors stated that most people believe that only half of global risk for heart attacks can be prevented; however, their data place the number of preventable cardiac deaths worldwide at nearly 90%. Furthermore, it is noted that the impact of these risk factors was the same in every ethnic group and in every region of the world. The authors note that the two most important risk factors for AMI were abnormal apolipoprotein B\apolipoprotien A-1 ratio and cigarette smoking. Other factors that predicted risk of AMI include diabetes, hypertension, abdominal obesity, psychosocial variables such as stress and depression, exercise, diet, and alcohol intake. Taken together current smoking and an abnormal apolipoprotein B\apolipoprotien A-1 ratio predicted 60% of global heart disease. Further this study noted the BMI was not as predictive of coronary risk as was abdominal obesity. When looked at after adjusting for age, sex, and smoking alone the odds ratio for AMI for ratio of apolipoprotein B\apolipoprotien A-1 was 3.87 with the odds ratio for AMI adjusted for all risk factors was 3.25. Of note psychosocial factors that being depression or anxiety was noted to have an odds risk ratio after adjusted for age, sex, and smoking of 2.51 and after adjustment for all factors was 2.67. This finding is rather impressive as it nearly equal to the adjusted risk of smoking at 2.95 and 2.87, respectively. The authors also calculated the population-attributable risk (PAR) for AMI in the overall population. PAR is a measure of the relative risk associated with the given factor accounting for the prevalence of the condition within the population. Using this analysis the risk for AMI after adjustment for all risks the ratio of apolipoprotein B\apolipoprotien A-1 was noted to have a PAR risk of 49.2, with the next highest risk being current smoking at 35.7. Interestingly, the next highest risk was psychosocial factors at 32.5 followed closely by abdominal obesity. The INTERHEART trial noted a clear dose effect with smoking. Patients who smoked as little as 1–5 cigarettes per day experienced a 40% increase in the risk of AMI, those who smoked 6–10 cigarettes per day had a twofold increase, and those who smoked more than 20 cigarettes had a fourfold increase in the risk of AMI. The import of this study is that it shows the risks for AMI in developing countries, which accounts for 80% of all heart disease. This is in contrast to previous data from populations from Europe and North America.

Clinical Variability of Acute Coronary Syndromes Presenting to the ED

In the ED, chest pain is the second most common chief complaint for an ED visit—accounting for 5.1% of visits.[22] According to CDC data, in 2002 there were 5,637,000 ED visits for chest pain and related symptoms. It is also the symptom most commonly associated with fatal CVDs, the leading cause of mortality in the United States. Nearly 80% of patients with AMI present to the ED. Unfortunately between 2 and 8% of patients with AMI are inadvertently discharged home.[23–26] This is because roughly 1 out of 20 patients with AMI are not at all "typical" in their presentation. It has been shown that patients with AMI who are discharged home experience twice the death rate (25%) of those admitted.[27,28] Failure to diagnose and treat AMI has consistently accounted for the greatest total dollar loss for malpractice claims against emergency physicians.[29–31]

It is traditionally described that patients with an ACS present with retrosternal chest pain that may radiate to the neck, jaw, shoulders, or down the inside of either arm. Additionally, there may be secondary symptoms such as lightheadedness, palpitations, diaphoresis, dyspnea, nausea, or vomiting. Data from the Multicenter Chest Pain Research Group demonstrated that of patients with acute MI, 59% presented with typical symptoms and 41% presented with what were called "atypical" symptoms.[32] The same study found no evidence of an ACS in the group of "chest pain" patients, 33% of patients had "typical" symptoms. It has become obvious that there is a great deal of overlap in the presenting history between patients with and without confirmed ACS. In a 2001 study, McCord et al. reported that although patients with AMI

presented within 3.9 hours of symptom onset, in 19.3% of patients the time of symptom onset could not be determined.[33] Studies of acute MI in the elderly have shown that the most common presenting chief complaint past age 70 is no longer chest pain; rather it is shortness of breath.[34] More recent studies of the NRMI registry found that 33% of patients with acute MI do not present with chest pain.[35] These chest pain free patients were more likely to be older, female, diabetic, and have a history of prior CHF. They also had longer prehospital delays (7.9 hours vs. 5.3 hours), fewer were diagnosed on admission (22% vs. 50%), fewer were treated with balloon angioplasty or thrombolytics (25% vs. 74%), and they were less likely to be treated with aspirin (60% vs. 85%) or beta-blockers (28% vs. 48%). Most dramatically, their in-hospital mortality was higher (23% vs. 9%) as was their adjusted odds ratio for inpatient death (2.21).

Understanding the conundrum of how patients with acute MI present to the ED, Graff et al. derived and validated a clinical rule to rapidly identify ED patients with acute STEMI that need a rapid (5-min) ECG.[36] The rule called for a rapid ECG on the following patients— patients older than 30 years with chest pain and patients older than 50 years with syncope, weakness, rapid heartbeat, or shortness of breath. The rule used likelihood ratios for acute MI for presenting symptoms. The rule was tested and found to identify 100% of AMI patients requiring thrombolytic therapy (STEMI patients), and 86% of AMI patients not treated with thrombolytic therapy. For MI patients who received thrombolysis, the rule decreased their time from arrival to an ECG from 10.0 to 6.3 min and their time to thrombolysis from 36.9 to 26.1 min. Although these criteria are broad, they portray the wide variety of presentation of patients with acute MI.

The initial ECG done on arrival to the ED is very useful, but also has limitations. In a study of 391,208 patients from the NRMI database, Welch et al. found that 57.0% had ST elevation diagnostic of an acute MI (STEMI); however, 35.2% had nonspecific ST changes suggestive of ischemia and 7.9% had a normal ECG on arrival to the ED.[37] In-hospital mortality rates for these three groups were 11.5%, 8.7%, and 5.7%, respectively. Understanding the limitations of an isolated initial ECG, Fesmire et al. have shown that serial ECGs increase sensitivity for acute MI from 55.4 to 68.1%.[38]

Initial cardiac markers on arrival to the ED are useful but also have limitations. This is because of the rate of release of cardiac markers from ischemic myocardium and the time from infarct onset and arrival in the ED for initial blood testing influence the sensitivity of the initial test result. The sooner a patient arrives, the less likely he/she is to have positive initial markers. In an analysis of cardiac markers studies, an increase in sensitivity for acute MI was found with serial testing for CK-MB (from 44 to 80%), myoglobin (from 49 to 90%), troponin I (from 39 to 95%), troponin T (from 44 to 93%), and a combination of CK-MB and myoglobin (from 83 to 100%).[39]

Missed Myocardial Infarction in the Emergency Department

When one considers the range of variability with which patients with MI present to the ED, it is easier to understand how patients with this serious disease might be mistakenly sent home. The incidence and rate of missed MI is best described in a 2000 study by Pope et al.[23] An analysis done on 10,689 patients presenting to 10 hospitals with symptoms suggestive of acute cardiac ischemia found that 8% were ultimately found to have AMI and 9% were found to have unstable angina. Of patients with AMI, 2.1% (1.1–3.1%, 95% CI) were mistakenly sent home from the ED, and of patients with unstable angina, 2.3% (1.3–3.2%, 95% CI) were sent home from the ED. Patients with acute cardiac ischemia or infarction were more likely to be inappropriately discharged from the ED if they were women less than 55 years old (odds ratio of 6.7), if their chief complaint was shortness of breath rather than chest pain (odds ratio of 2.7), or had a normal or nondiagnostic ECG (odds ratio of 3.3). Patients with acute MI were more likely to be discharged if they were non-White (odds ratio of 4.5) or had a normal or non-diagnostic ECG (odds ratio of 7.7). Inappropriately discharged patients with acute MI were at 90% greater risk of death at 30 days, and patients with unstable angina were at 70% greater risk of death at 30 days.

Acute MI patients with atypical presentations are identified during an extended evaluation with repeated blood tests, ECG monitoring, and physician reevaluation. In an analysis of studies reporting the rate of missed MI, there was found to be an inverse relationship between the proportion of chest pain patients who receive a complete evaluation, that is admission or observation, and the rate at which AMI is missed (see Fig. 5-2).[25] Various factors affect the physician's threshold for hospital admission decision, and thus the missed MI rate. These physician factors include: the experience of the physician as more experienced physicians admit more patients and miss less disease, the risk attitudes of the physician as physicians with low-risk personalities admit more patients and miss less disease, hospital monitored

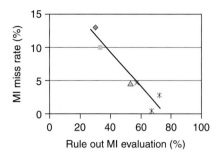

Fig. 5-2. The inverse correlation between the rate of missed MI and the percent of at-risk chest pain patients having a complete evaluation.[25]

bed capacity as physicians admit more patients when the hospital has high capacity for monitored beds and thus miss less disease, and the patients' clinical presentation as physicians are more likely to admit patients with typical presentations than atypical presentations and thus less likely to miss disease in the patient with typical signs and symptoms.[40–44] In looking at the rate of missed MI among patients with symptoms suggestive of cardiac ischemia, Graff et al. compared the rate from all prior studies, of hospitals without chest pain observation units or protocols, with EDs that had such protocols. A combination of four previous studies shows that there were 12,405 ED patients with symptoms suggestive of acute MI, among which there was a composite rate of 4.5% (4.0–5.5%, 95% CI) of missed MI. By comparison, data from a registry of EDs that had a chest pain "observation" or diagnostic protocol had a missed MI rate of 0.4% among 23,407 ED patients with symptoms suggestive of AMI.

Economic Issues Associated with Coronary Artery Disease

In the United States, approximately six billion dollars are spent annually to evaluate ED patients with chest pain.[45] Although this figure seems staggering, it is not surprising when one considers that chest pain is the second most common complaint in the ED, and historically 60–70% of chest pain patients are admitted to the hospital. Of ED chest pain patients, between 8 and 10% will be found to have MI, and between 9 and 10% will be found to have unstable angina.[23] In other words, most patients admitted to the hospital are found to have no evidence of acute cardiac ischemia. The overall average length of stay of chest pain patients is 1.9 days and their average charges are $4135.[45] Earlier studies indicated that the cost, which is often half of charges, of chest pain patients who are evaluated and discharged from the ED is $403. The cost for patients who are admitted is $2714 and those who are observed is $1210.[25] Obviously, one can decrease the overall cost of caring for an ED chest pain population by shifting more patients from admission to either discharge home or observation. Of course, this must be weighed against the risk of missing patients with acute MI. In fact, this is what was found in the chest pain evaluation registry (CHEPER) study.[25] EDs with chest pain observation units, or protocols, performed a more thorough evaluation on a greater percentage of patients through admission or observation (67% vs. 57%). In addition fewer patients were finally admitted to the hospital (47% vs. 57%), because more patients were observed. As a result it was estimated that overall costs for all chest pain patients managed in an ED with a chest pain observation unit (CPOU) was $124 lower than in an ED without a CPOU.

There have been four prospective randomized studies that specifically addressed the cost effectiveness of chest pain observation protocols. All have shown the CPOU patients had significantly lower costs compared to hospital admission (see Table 5-2). Roberts et al. randomized 165 patients to receive standard hospital care versus observation unit care.[46] The mean length of stay for observation unit patients versus hospital admission patients was 33.1 hours versus 44.8 hours and the mean total cost per patient was $1528 versus $2095. Both results were statistically significant. Interestingly, Roberts et al. also found that chest pain patients who failed observation and were admitted had higher costs than the control group, potentially because admitted patients were a "sicker" subset that

required more resources, or because the "front end" workup increases the initial cost of care and is less cost-effective if patients are not discharged (see Fig. 5-3). Gomez et al. randomized 100 patients at the University of Utah to an ED observation unit versus traditional hospital admission.[47] Those evaluated in the observation unit had shorter length of stays (15 hours vs. 55 hours) as well as lower initial ($1297 per patient vs. $5719 per patient) and 30-day costs ($1427 per patient vs. $5860 per patient). A prospective study at the Mayo Clinic by Farkouh et al. randomized 424 chest pain or unstable angina patients and found that those treated in the ED observation unit had only 62% of the costs of services provided with traditional hospitalization.[45]

A study in the United Kingdom by Goodacre et al. chose to prospectively randomize days (CPOU days vs. no CPOU days), rather than selected patients, to study the impact of the CPOU on the entire chest pain cohort.[48] Four hundred forty-two days were randomized, with 972 patients randomized into well-matched groups that had similar rates of major cardiac events (3.8% vs. 3.4%). However, ACS patients were less likely to be inappropriately discharged home on CPOU days (5.9% vs. 13.9%). Patients from CPOU days were more likely to have had a stress test during their index visit (75% vs. 29%) and 51% less likely to be hospitalized. In the 6 months following discharge, patients from the CPOU group were 35% less likely to have a return visit to the ED and 33% less likely to be readmitted to the hospital. The CPOU group had higher cost for their initial 6 hours of care (£93 vs. £73), but subsequently lower overall costs (£478 vs. £556) and better health care utility over 6 months. It is interesting to find that results concur with U.S. studies,

Table 5-2. Comparison of Cost Savings, Study Design, and Costing Method for Studies of Chest Pain Observation Units or Diagnostic Protocols[46,47,49–54]

Author/Year	Savings/patient	Study Design	Costing Method
Kerns/1993	$1,873	Contemporaneous	Charges
Hoekstra/1994	$1,160	Contemporaneous	Charges
Hoekstra/1994	$2,030	Contemporaneous	Charges
Rodriguez/1994	$1,564	Contemporaneous	Charges (mean IP)
Stomel/1999	$1,497	Contemporaneous	Costing
Mikhail/1997	$1,470	Historical	Costing
Sayre/1994	$1,449	Contemporaneous	Engineered std.
Gomez/1996	$1,165	Historical	Charges
Gomez/1996	$624	Randomized	Charges
Gaspoz/1994	$698	Contemporaneous	Costs (detailed)
Roberts/1997	$567	Randomized	Costs (detailed)

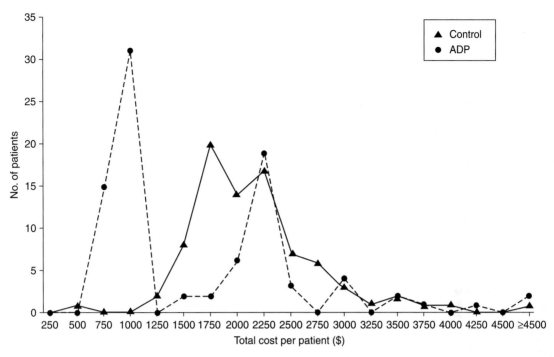

Fig. 5-3. Frequency distribution of total cost per patient of an accelerated diagnostic protocol (ADP) compared to a control group of traditionally admitted chest pain patients.[46]

COST OF MEDICAL PROCEDURES

and that these results are reproducible outside the United States. The benefits appear to be applicable to the entire chest pain cohort, not just the traditionally admitted subgroup.

During the interval from 1979 to 2001, the number of cardiac catheterizations has tripled and the number of cardiovascular operations and procedures has increased 417%. In 2001, it was estimated that nearly 1.2 million cardiac catheterizations were performed. The mean cost for diagnostic cardiac catheterization was $17,763 with a 1% in-hospital death rate. Percutaneous Translumin angioplasty (PTCA) had an average charge of $25,558 with an in-hospital death rate of 0.9%. Cardiac bypass surgery data from the NCHS 2001 estimate that 516,000 procedures were performed on 305,000 patients. The mean charges for these procedures were $60,853 with an in-hospital death rate of 2.4%. It is estimated that 571,000 PTCA procedures were preformed on 559,000 patients in 2001, which is a 266% increase from 1987 to 2001. In 2001, two-thirds of these PTCA were performed on men while 51% were performed on patients 65 and older. Data from the Health Care Costs and Utilization Project 2001 demonstrate that the primary diagnosis of coronary atherosclerosis ranked number one on the national bill at a cost of $35.1 billion, AMI ranked second at a cost of $27.7 billion, and CHF nonhypertensive was noted to be ranked fourth at a cost of $17.6 billion. Acute cerebrovascular disease was ranked eighth at a $12 billion cost and cardiac dysrhythmia was number ten at $11.4 billion. The total cost of CVD (which includes stroke), in the United States in 2004, was estimated to be $368.4 billion. This figure includes the direct costs, which includes physician, professional hospital, and nursing home costs, costs of medications, home health care, and other medical durables, plus the indirect costs of lost productivity from morbidity and mortality. For comparison data from 2003 the total cost of all cancers was $189 billion and the total cost for HIV infections in 1999 was $28.9 billion. When broken out individually estimated costs by MMWR-CDC for 2004 is heart disease alone $238.6 billion, coronary heart disease $133.2 billion, hypertensive heart disease $55.5 billion, and CHF $28.8 billion (see Figs. 5-4 to 5-6).

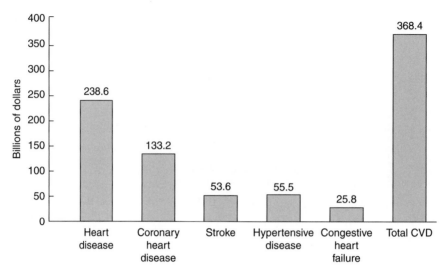

Fig. 5-4. Estimated direct and indirect costs (in billions of dollars) of cardiovascular diseases and stroke in the United States: 2004. (Source: All estimates prepared by Thomas T, NHLBI.)

COST OF LITIGATION AND THE POTENTIAL THREAT OF LITIGATION

The evaluation of the chest pain patient is a high-risk, large-volume complaint in the ED. Chest pain is high stakes because of its association with ACS. Failure to diagnose or treat AMI now accounts for the greatest total dollar loss for claims against emergency physicians. In the prethrombolytic era, such claims totaled 21% of payments and ranked sixth as the most dollars paid per case.[55] Since the thrombolytic era these claims have risen to account for up to 39% of payments and ranks second

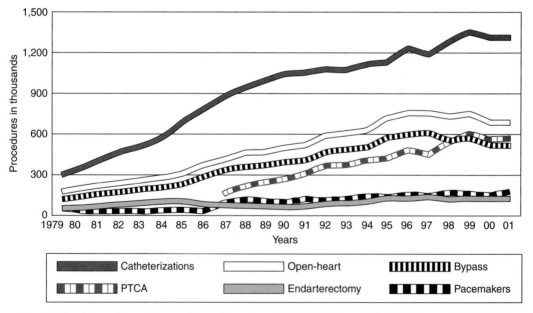

Fig. 5-5. Trends in cardiovascular operations and procedures in the United States: 1979–2001. (Source: CDC/NCHS.)

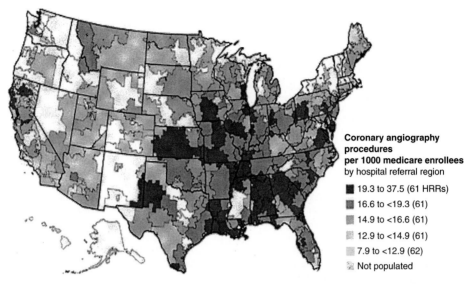

Coronary angiography procedures per 1000 medicare enrollees
by hospital referral region

- ■ 19.3 to 37.5 (61 HRRs)
- ■ 16.6 to <19.3 (61)
- ■ 14.9 to <16.6 (61)
- ▨ 12.9 to <14.9 (61)
- ▨ 7.9 to <12.9 (62)
- ▨ Not populated

Fig. 5-6. Coronary angiography procedures per 1000 medicare enrollees.

for dollar amount paid per case.[56] The nearly 50% rise in dollars per malpractice case reflects primarily the impact of thrombolytics on mortality reduction in ST elevation/Q-wave AMI. In the current health care environment emergency physicians are being pressured to admit less noncardiac chest pain without missing true coronary ischemia, all the while evaluating patients over a shorter time period in an attempt to preserve flow. The primary reasons for the failure to diagnose AMI as cited in lawsuits filed are outlined in Table 5-3.[56]

The true cost of litigation on the health system is difficult to assess even when fairly good data exist. This is because many assumptions need to be made in order to analyze the data. The very limited and nearly inaccessible data on litigation are based on closed claims, which on average take 2–4 years to close. There are no good studies that evaluate the costs of defensive medicine, i.e., the practice of ordering additional test in order to "cover themselves from litigation," in the face of a low pretest probability for disease. In fact, a poll of emergency

Table 5-3. Primary Reasons for the Failure to Diagnose Acute Myocardial Infarction

Procedure	# Files	# Files Closed	# Files Paid	% Files Paid/Closed	Indemnity	Paid File (Average)
Diagnostic, interview, evaluation	24	28	20	71.43	5,362,667	268,133
Diagnostic procedures	13	12	10	83.33	2,694,000	269,400
Physical examination	7	6	6	100.00	514,987	858,351
Medications	4	4	3	75.00	573,530	250,000
Diagnostic radiology (excluding CAT)	3	2	1	50.00	250,000	250,000

physicians attending a national meeting revealed that the risk level that most EM physicians feel comfortable sending chest pain patients home from the ED was a <1% chance of a missed diagnosis of ACS. There is no reason, particularly with the improved diagnostic and life-extending advances in cardiovascular medicine, to believe that the number or cost of litigation will decrease in the future.

REFERENCES

1. American Heart Association. *Heart Disease and Stroke Statistics—2004 Update.* Dallas, TX: American Heart Association, 2003.
2. D'Agostino RB Sr, Grundy S, Sullivan LM, et al. Validation of the Framingham coronary heart disease prediction scores: Results of a multiple ethnic groups investigation. *JAMA* 2001;286(2):180–187.
3. Jayes RL, Beshansky JR, D'Agostino RB, Selker HP. et al. Do patients' coronary risk factor reports predict acute cardiac ischemia in the emergency department? A multicenter study. *J Clin Epidemiol* 1992;45:621–626.
4. Grzybowski M, Clements EA, Parsons L, et al. Mortality benefit of immediate revascularization of acute ST-segment elevation myocardial infarction in patients with contraindications to thrombolytic therapy: A propensity analysis. *JAMA* 2003;290(14):1891–1898.
5. Hochman JS, Tamis JE, Thompson TD, et al. Sex, clinical presentations, and outcomes with acute coronary syndromes. Gusto II-b investigators. *N Engl J Med* 1999;341:226–232.
6. Canto JG, Shlipak MG, Rogers WJ, et al. Prevalence, clinical characteristics, and mortality among patients with myocardial infarction presenting without chest pain. *JAMA* 2000;283:3223–3229.
7. Vaccarino V, Parsons L, Every NR, et al. National registry of myocardial infarction 2. *N Engl J Med* 1999;341:217–225.
8. Malacrida R, Geonoi M, Maggioni P, et al. A comparison of the early outcome of acute myocardial infarction in women and men. The Third International Study of Infarcts Survival Collaborative Group. *N Engl J Med* 1999;338:8–14.
9. Gan SC, Beaver SK, Houck PM, et al. Treatment of acute myocardial infarction and thirty day mortality among men and women. *N Engl J Med* 2000;343:8–15.
10. Grzybowski M, Clements EA, Parsons L, et al. Mortality benefit of immediate revascularization of acute ST-segment elevation myocardial infarction in patients with contraindications to thrombolytic therapy: a propensity analysis. *JAMA* 2003;290:1891–1898.
11. Marrugat J, Sala J, Masiá R, et al. for the RESCATE Investigators. Mortality differences between men and women following first myocardial infarction. *JAMA* 1998;280:1405–1409.
12. Schulman KA, Berlin JA, Harless W, et al. The effect of race and sex on physicians' recommendations for cardiac catheterization. *N Engl J Med* 1999;340(8):618–626.

13. Cowie CC, Rust KF, Byrd-Holt D, et al. Prevalence of diabetes and impaired fasting glucose in adults—United States 1999–2000. *MMWR* 2003;52:833–837.
14. Mokdad AH, Ford ES, Bowman BA. Prevalence of obesity, diabetes, and obesity-related health risk factors, 2001. *JAMA* 2003;289:76–79.
15. Agency for Healthcare Research and Quality (AHRQ) and Centers for Disease Control (CDC). Major cardiovascular disease (CVD) during 1997–1999 and major CVD hospital discharge rates in 1997 among women with diabetes—United States. *MMWR* 2001;50:948–954
16. Mokdad AH, Marks JS, Stroup DF. Actual causes of death in the United States, 2000. *JAMA* 2004;291:1238–1245.
17. Pate RR, Pratt M, Blair S. Physical activity and public health. A recommendation from the Centers for Disease Control and Prevention and the American College of Sports Medicine. *JAMA* 1995;273:402–407.
18. Kimm SY, Glynn NW, Kriska AM, et al. Decline in physical activity in black girls and white girls during adolescence. *N Engl J Med* 2002;347(10):709–715.
19. Hu FB, Stampfer MJ, Colditz GA, et al. Physical activity and risk of stroke in women. *JAMA* 2000;283:2961–2967.
20. Rao SV, Kaul P, Newby K, et al. Poverty and outcome of the acute coronary syndromes. *J Am Coll Cardiol* 2003;41:1948–1954.
21. Yusuf S, Hawken S, Ounpuu S, et al. Effect of potentially modifiable risk factors associated with myocardial infarction in 52 countries (the INTERHEART study). *Lancet* 2004. Available at: *http://image.thelancet.com/extras/04art8001web.pdf.*
22. McCaig LF, Burt CW. National Hospital Ambulatory Medical Care Survey: 2002 Emergency Department Summary. *Advance Data from Vital and Health Statistics; no. 340, CDC.* Hyattsville, MD: National Center for Health Statistics, 2004.
23. Pope JH, Aufderheide TP, Ruthazer R, et al. Missed diagnoses of acute cardiac ischemia in the emergency department. *N Engl J Med* 2000;342:1163–1170.
24. Rouan GW, Hedges JR, Toltzis R, et al. Chest pain clinic to improve the follow-up of patients released from an urban university teaching hospital emergency department. *Ann Emerg Med* 1987:16;1145–1150.
25. Graff LG, Dallara J, Ross MA, et al. Impact on the Care of the Emergency Department Chest Pain Patient from the Chest Pain Evaluation Registry (CHEPER) study. *Am J Cardiol* 1997:80;563–568.
26. Pozen MW, D'Agostino RB, Selder HP, et al. A predictive instrument to improve coronary care unit admission practices in acute ischemic heart disease. *N Engl J Med* 1984:310;1273–1278.
27. Wears RL, Li S, Hernandez JD, et al. How many myocardial infarctions should we rule out? *Ann Emerg Med* 1989;18:953–963.
28. McCarthy BD, Beshansky JR, D'Agostino RB, et al. Missed diagnoses of acute myocardial infarction in the emergency department: Results from a multicenter study. *Ann Emerg Med* 1993;22:579–582.

29. Karcz A, Holbrook J, Burke MC, et al. Massachusetts emergency medicine closed malpractice claims:1988–1990. *Ann Emerg Med* 1993:22;553–559.

30. Wears RL, Li S, Hernandez JD, et al. How many myocardial infarctions should we rule out? *Ann Emerg Med* 1989;18: 953–963.

31. Rogers TT. *Risk Management in Emergency Medicine.* Dallas, TX: American College of Emergency Physicians, 1985.

32. Lee TH, Cook EH, Weisberg M, et al. Acute chest pain in the emergency room. Identification and examination of low-risk patients. *Arch Intern Med* 1985;145(1):65–69.

33. McCord J, Nowak RM, McCullough PA, et al. Ninety-minute exclusion of acute myocardial infarction by use of quantitative point of care testing of myoglobin and troponin I. *Circulation* 2001;1004:1483–1488.

34. Bayer AJ, Chanda JS, Farag RR, et al. Changing presentation of myocardial infarction with increasing age. *J Am Geriatr Soc* 1986;34: 263–266.

35. Canto JG, Shlipak MG, Rogers WJ, et al. Prevalence, clinical characteristics, and mortality among patients with myocardial infarction presenting without chest pain. *JAMA* 2000;283(24):3223–3229.

36. Graff L, Palmer A, LeMonica P, et al. Triage of patients for a rapid (5-minute) electrocardiogram: A rule based on presenting chief complaint. *Ann Emerg Med* 2000;36:554–560.

37. Welch RD, Zalenski RJ, Frederick PD. Prognostic value of a normal or nonspecific initial electrocardiogram in acute myocardial infarction. *JAMA* 2001;286:1977–1984.

38. Fesmire FM, Percy RF, Bardoner JB, et al. Usefulness of automated serial 12-lead ECG monitoring during the initial emergency department evaluation of patients with chest pain. *Ann Emerg Med* 1998;31:3–11.

39. Balk EM, Ioannidis JPA, Salem D, et al. Accuracy of biomarkers to diagnose acute cardiac ischemia in the emergency department: A meta-analysis. *Ann Emerg Med* 2001;37: 478–494.

40. Tierney WM, Fitzgerald J, McHenry R, et al. Physicians' estimates of the probability of myocardial infarction in emergency room patients with chest pain. *Med Decis Making* 1986;6:12–17.

41. Puleo PR, Meyer D, Wathern C, et al. Use of a rapid assay of subforms of creatine kinase MB to diagnose or rule out acute myocardial infarction. *N Engl J Med* 1994:331;561–566.

42. Selker HP, Beshansky JR, Griffith JL, et al. Use of the acute cardiac ischemia time insensitive predictive instrument (ACI-TIPI) to assist with triage of patients with chest pain or other symptoms suggestive of acute cardiac ischemia: A multicenter, controlled clinical trial. *Ann Intern Med* 1998;129:845–855.

43. Selker H, Griffith J, Dorey FJ, et al. How do physicians adopt when the coronary care unit is full. *JAMA* 1987:257; 1181–1185.

44. Rusnack RA, Stair TO, Hansen K, et al. Litigation against the emergency physician: Common features in cases of missed myocardial infarction. *Ann Emerg Med* 1989;18:1029–1034.

45. Farkouh ME, Smars P, Reeder GS, et al. A clinical trial of a chest pain observation unit for patients with unstable angina. *N Engl J Med* 1998;339:1882–1888.

46. Roberts RR, Zalenski RJ, Mensah EK, et al. Costs of an emergency department-based accelerated diagnostic protocol vs hospitalization in patients with chest pain: A randomized controlled trial. *JAMA* 1997;278(20):1670–1676.

47. Gomez MA, Anderson JL, Karagouris LA, et al. for the ROMIO Study Group: An emergency department-based protocol for rapidly ruling out myocardial ischemia reduces hospital time and expense: Results of a randomized study (ROMIO). *J Am Coll Cardiol* 1996;28:25–33.

48. Goodacre S, Nicholl J, Dixon S, et al. Randomised controlled trial and economic evaluation of a chest pain observation unit compared with routine care. *Br Med J* 2004;328(7434):254. Epub 2004 Jan 14. doi:10.1136/bmj.37956.664236.EE. Online access—*http://bmj.bmjjournals.com/cgi/reprint/328/7434/254.*

49. Kerns JR, Shaub TF, Fontanarosa PB. Emergency cardiac stress testing in the evaluation of emergency department patients with atypical chest pain. *Ann Emerg Med* 1999;22: 794–798.

50. Hoekstra JW, Gibler WB, Levy RC, et al. Emergency department diagnosis of acute myocardial infarction and ischemia: A cost analysis. *Acad Emerg Med* 1994;1:103–110.

51. Rodriquez S, Cowfer JP, Lyston DJ, et al. Clinical efficacy and cost effectiveness of rapid emergency department rule out myocardial infarction and non invasive cardiac evaluation in patients with acute chest pain. *J Am Coll Cardiol* 1994;23(Suppl):284A.

52. Stommel R, Grant R, Eagle KA. Lessons learned from a community hospital chest pain center. *Am J Cardiol* 1999;83:1033–1037.

53. Mikhail MG, Smith FA, Gray M, et al. Cost-effectiveness of mandatory stress testing in chest pain centre patients. *Ann Emerg Med* 1997;29:88–98.

54. Sayre MR, Bender AL, Chayan C, et al. Evaluating chest pain patients in an emergency department rapid diagnostic and treatment center is cost effective. *Acad Emerg Med* 1994;1:A45.

55. Dunn J. Chest pain. *ACEP Foresight* 1986;1:1–3.

56. Burke V, O'Neil BJ, Gawad Y. Undiagnosed myocardial infarction: Liability before and after thrombolytic therapy. *Acad Emerg Med* 1996;3(5):489.

6

Pathophysiology

Brian P. O'Neil

HIGH YIELD FACTS

- Atherosclerosis is fundamentally an inflammatory process, influenced by a host of environmental and genetic factors.
- While it is true that most acute myocardial infarctions (AMIs) arise from lesions with less than 60% stenosis, this likely reflects their predominance rather than an inherent instability in smaller plaques.
- Atherosclerotic plaque rupture is the precipitating event in acute coronary syndrome (ACS), followed by platelet adhesion, platelet aggregation, and thrombus formation.
- Currently available therapies to interrupt thrombus formation after plaque rupture include direct and indirect thrombin inhibitors, inhibitors of platelet activation, and inhibitors of platelet aggregation.
- Restenosis following angioplasty occurs through adventitial scar formation and subsequent narrowing of the arterial lumen, thrombosis, and neointimal tissue proliferation.
- Despite considerable study, a causal link between *Chlamydia pneumoniae* and atherosclerosis remains unproven.

INTRODUCTION

Patients with ACS presenting to the emergency department primarily represent the clinical manifestation of decades of atherosclerotic progression. Although modifiable risk factors have been identified and new pathogenic mechanisms are being discovered, we are still far from preventing atherosclerosis or its resulting complications. Understanding the pathophysiology behind ACS encompasses knowledge of

atherogenesis, coagulation, fibrinolysis, and the healing process. Review of current theories regarding the atheroma formation and subsequent plaque rupture will provide the foundation for all the interventions available to the emergency physician treating ACS. ACS and AMI share the same underlying pathophysiology; their clinical presentation depend on the duration of obstruction or occlusion of coronary artery circulation (see Fig. 6-1).[1]

HISTORICAL PERSPECTIVE

Atherosclerotic lesions have been identified in Egyptian mummies dating from 1580 B.C.[2] Atherosclerosis was initially described in modern times by Caleb Hillier Parry. In his book titled *Inquiry into the Symptoms and Causes of the Syncope Anginosa, Commonly Called Angina Pectoris, Illustrated by Dissections (1799)*, he noted from an autopsy that the coronary vessels had hardened and that ". . . a principle cause of the syncope anginosa is to be looked for in disordered coronary arteries."[3] In 1815, a surgeon named Joseph Hodgson published his paper on vascular disease. He stated that inflammation was the underlying cause of atherosclerosis as opposed to a natural degenerative manifestation of the aging process. He also identified that the disease process occurred in the intima, between the lumen and the media of the diseased vessels.[4] In 1841, Carl Von Rokitansky championed the *thrombogenic theory* of atherosclerosis. He proposed that the deposits observed in the inner layer of the arterial wall derived primarily from fibrin and other blood elements rather than being the result of a purulent process.[5] In 1856, Rudolf Virchow challenged Rokitansky's description of the pathogenesis of atherosclerosis by analyzing the histologic characteristics of the atherosclerotic lesions in all their stages. For the first time he used the name of "endarteritis deformans," meaning that the atheroma was a product of an inflammatory process within the intima and that the fibrous thickening evolved as a consequence of a reactive fibrosis induced by proliferating connective tissue cells within the intima.[6] Finally by 1904 the term *atherosclerosis* was coined by Marchand, who described the "gruel-like" (athere) soft contents of the plaque core covered by a hardened (sclerosis) fibrous cap.[7] In St. Petersburg, Russia, in 1908, A.I. Ignatowski observed the relationship between cholesterol-rich foods and experimental atherosclerosis.[8] This was followed by Adolf Windaus discovery that atheromatous lesions contained six times as much free cholesterol as a normal arterial wall and 20 times more esterified cholesterol.[9]

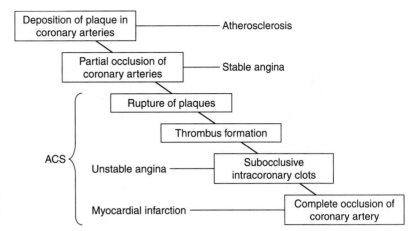

Fig. 6-1. The correlation between clinical presentation and underlying atherosclerosis.

Using cholesterol-fed rabbits to produce experimental atherosclerosis, Nikolai Anichkov demonstrated, in 1913, that it was cholesterol alone that caused these athero-sclerotic changes in the rabbit intima. By standardizing cholesterol feeding, he discovered that the amount of cholesterol uptake was directly proportional to the degree of atherosclerosis severity. Anichov's insudation theory claimed that noxious elements in the blood damaged the endothelium and formed the basis for the current *response-to-injury theory* of Ross.[10–12]

Despite over 200 years of observation and research into its pathogenesis, atherosclerotic coronary disease (ASCD) remains the primary cause of death in western civilization. Through years of research, we no longer have a static viewpoint of atherosclerosis as a "clogged pipe." Instead, it is now well recognized that atherosclerosis is a progressive and dynamic inflammatory disease. Initially dysfunction of the endothelium is accompanied by loss of protective molecules/mechanisms and expression of adhesive molecules, and procoagulants leading to development of thrombosis, smooth muscle cell (SMC) migration, and pro-liferation and atherosclerosis. Its course is marked not only by periods of quiescence and chaos, but also personalized by multiple risk factors, both fixed and modifiable. Although ASCD is an indolent chronic disease, its acute manifestations commonly present to the emergency department for evaluation and life-saving treatment.

ANATOMY OF THE ARTERY

An understanding of the normal anatomy provides the basis for describing the progression of atherosclerosis.

There are three well-defined layers of arterial anatomy, the tunica intima, media, and externa (see Fig. 6-2). The tunica intima with its endothelium has been the primary area of focus for research regarding atherogenesis. The intima is composed of three components: endothelial cells, the subendothelial space, and the basement membrane. The role of the intima in atherosclerosis is fourfold: (1) forming a semipermeable barrier, (2) sensing mechanical forces (pressure and/or flow) and secreting chemokines which change the "contractile tone" of the SMC in medial layer, (3) sensing vascular injury and producing mitogens to cause SMC, leukocytes, and platelets to migrate to the area of injury, and (4) pre-venting the coagulation of blood. The complexity of the intima can be appreciated in understanding its role in pre-serving blood in a liquid state. Heparin sulfate proteo-glycans which are embedded on the endothelial surface maintain an anticoagulant luminal surface by binding and activating antithrombin III. Further, in the early stages of thrombus formation the endothelial cell can react through thrombomodulin-mediated action by protein C and S to prevent further clotting. Protein C and S are vitamin-K-dependent glycoproteins that are involved in the inac-tivation of the coagulation cascade by modulating activated factors V and VIII. Finally, normal endothelium secretes tissue plasminogen activator, activating the fibrinolytic system to help dissolve thrombus. These compounds are all counterbalanced by the release of procoagulants including von Willebrand factor (vWF) and plasminogen activator inhibitor (PAI). It is only the uninjured endothelium with its intact pro/anticoagulative homeostasis that can sustain extended contact with blood without clotting.

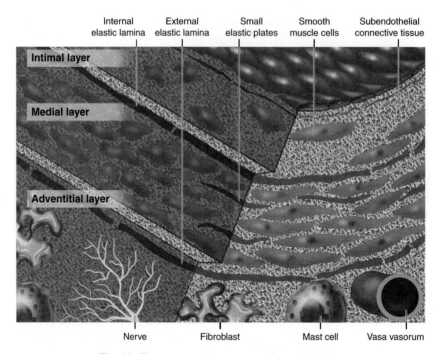

Fig. 6-2. The structure and components of normal arteries.

On the other side of the intima is the basement membrane and internal elastic membrane which separates the SMC of the media from the intima. As humans age, the intimal layer thickens and accumulates SMC and type I and III collagens secondary to presumed disruption of the basement membrane. Though a correlation with atherosclerosis is likely, this infiltration has been noted in arteries without significant atherosclerotic disease. Certain areas of the arterial tree are more prone to develop intimal thickening, especially those high pressure areas with turbulent flow and multiple branch points, i.e., coronary arteries. This has led to a theory that wall/shear stress may contribute to initial endothelial dysfunction which initiates atherosclerosis. This is further supported by the fact that arteries with few branch points (i.e., the radial and internal mammary arteries, commonly used in coronary artery bypass grafts) have an overall less atherosclerotic burden.

The tunica media is composed of SMC which are contained within layers of an elastin-rich matrix. The SMC within the media allow the artery to contract and relax in response to the modulating signals from the endothelium based on flow rates and wall stress. The elastin matrix allows the artery to stretch and recoil to absorb the kinetic energy delivered by ventricular contraction. The media, in particular the SMC, under normal conditions are relatively dormant in terms of cell replication and cytokine production. This is in sharp contrast to their enhanced activity as noted subsequent to cytokine release following endothelial injury. The enhanced activity of SMC has been regarded as a primary mechanism for the proliferation of atherosclerosis. The external elastic lamina surrounds the media and provides the border between the media and the adventitia.

The adventitia or tunica externa is the final layer of the normal artery. It is present primarily in the larger arteries and is no longer present within the arterioles. It contains the vasa vasorum, mast cells, fibroblasts, and nerve fibers in a loose pool of collagen. Understanding the role of the adventitia in atherosclerosis is still in infancy; however, research on this subject is increasing. In the setting of endothelial injury, specifically tissue hypoxia in the animal model, fibroblasts have been show to proliferate and assist in vascular remodeling. Furthermore, the fibroblasts ability to rapidly proliferate and transdifferentiate may serve a role as a stem-cell progenitor protecting the viability of the artery in response to injury.[13]

ATHEROSCLEROSIS: AN INFLAMMATORY RESPONSE

Endothelial Dysfunction

The development of atherosclerosis as proposed by Ross's *response to injury* theory initially purported that mechanical injury was the inciting event leading to endothelial *denudation*. He later proposed that endothelial denudation was an inflammatory response evoked by a huge number of stressors (atherogenic risk factors) that led to the atherosclerotic changes in the vessel wall.[12] Nowadays, the preliminary step in atherosclerosis is termed endothelial *dysfunction* and results from an interaction between genetic and environmental risk factors (especially modified lipoproteins), monocytes/ macrophages, T lymphocytes, and the normal cellular elements of the vessel wall.[14] Endothelial dysfunction refers to a loss of anticoagulant properties, an increased expression of cellular adhesion molecules (CAMs), and probable depletion of antiinflammatory endothelial nitric oxide (NO).[15]

To answer the question, "How does endothelial dysfunction start?" two main theories exist. First, it has already been noted that atherosclerosis tends to occur at branch points within the arterial tree. These areas have alterations in blood flow leading to increased wall stress, which directly allows for increased permeability of the endothelium. The effect of turbulent flow on the endothelium allows for an increased uptake of low-density lipoproteins (LDLs) and altered gene expression. Through the rabbit model evidence for increased uptake of LDLs has been identified. Following intravenous injection of LDLs, these molecules combine with surface proteoglycans (PGCs) within only 2 hours.[16] This LDL-PGC has greater vulnerability for oxidative modification from free radicals. It is these oxidized LDL (oxLDL) complexes, which are believed to play a major role in early atherogenesis. LDLs have been implicated in promoting endothelial dysfunction by increasing monocyte adhesion through the expression of CAMs and increasing monocyte and T-cell chemotaxis through cytokine production (i.e., MCP-1).[17,18] Also genetic alteration has been postulated to contribute to local endothelial cell remodeling and expression of leukocyte adhesion chemokines (including platelet-derived growth factor, transforming growth factor-beta (TGF-β), tissue plasminogen activator, and the adhesion molecules intracellular adhesion molecule-1 [ICAM-1] and vascular cell adhesion molecule [VCAM-1]).[19,20] Lastly, the known atherogenic risk factors (i.e., smoking, diabetes, hypertension, and so forth) enhance endothelial dysfunction directly through an increase in oxidative stress leading again to endothelial membrane permeability. Overall due to inherited and modifiable risk factors, the endothelium undergoes anatomic and physiologic changes leading to the second stage of atherosclerosis, monocyte, and T-cell infiltration.

Leukocyte Recruitment

After the initial insult the arterial endothelium, which normally avoids interaction with leukocytes, begins to accumulate monocytes and T lymphocytes.[21,22] The influx of leukocytes is up-regulated by the increased expression of CAMs instigated by the primary insult. Two specific types of CAMs are produced—the VCAM-1 and the ICAM-1. Of the two, VCAM-1 appears to be more specific to atherosclerotic disease due to its interaction with molecules located only in atheromas, monocytes, and T cells.[23] These molecules were initially thought to play a specific role in atherosclerosis such that serum levels were measured to identify if an association between high levels of VCAM-1 and adverse cardiovascular events could be predicted.[24,25] After contradicting research it appears that serum measurements will not provide the predictive instrument that was once hoped.[26]

Another class of CAMs identified within the intima includes the selectins. E-selection (endothelial), P-selection (platelet), and L-selection (leukocyte) have all been identified in atheromatous plaques.[27,28] However, of the three, P-selection appears to play the larger role in atherogenesis. From in vitro cultures using human aortic endothelial cells (HAECs), P-selection increases its expression on the endothelial surface in the presence of oxLDL. P-selectin's greater affinity for monocytes and lymphocytes, cell types found in atheromas, further supports its role in leukocyte recruitment during the early stages of atherosclerosis.[29]

Through recruitment by CAMs and selectins, leukocytes are able to adhere to the endothelial wall. The release of chemotaxic proteins called chemokines are required to allow leukocytes to penetrate past the initial endothelial layer into the subendothelial space.[30] The most prominent chemokine is monocyte chemoattractant protein-1 (MCP-1). MCP-1 is normally produced by both endothelial and SMC as defense against infection; however, it may also be released in the presence of oxLDL within the endothelium.[31,32] In addition to monocytes, it has recently been identified that T lymphocytes are also present within a developing plaque. Interferon-inducible protein 10 (IP-10), interferon-inducible T-cell alpha chemoattractant (I-TAC), and a monokine induced by interferon-γ (MIG) are expressed by smooth muscle cells in response to injury to attract these cells.[33]

Foam Cells

Until this stage of atherosclerosis, the endothelium appears to be functioning properly. It has correctly identified the malicious compounds, in this case oxLDLs, are present and has signaled for leukocyte assistance to eradicate the problem. However leukocytes, on arrival to the endothelium, fail to remove the oxLDLs. Instead the leukocytes express a specialized scavenger receptor to consume, engulf, and phagocytize the oxLDLs producing foam cells. The transformation of monocytes to foam cells, a cell-type specific to atherosclerosis, is the first stage of atherogenesis and represents the initial deviation from normal homeostasis. These foam cells subsequently produce substances such as cytokines, growth factors, chemokines, and proteolytic enzymes leading to athero-sclerotic plaque formation.[34] As these foam cells organize, increase in size and overall lipid content, the first visible manifestation of atherosclerosis is noted, the fatty streak. However, the role of fatty streaks as a definite precursor to arthrosclerosis has been questioned due to the identification of fatty streaks throughout the arterial tree, especially in locations where atherosclerotic pro-gression does not develop.[35] Thus, the fatty streak rep-resents a stage of atherogenesis which requires a yet unidentified modulator, possibly wall stress, to allow its progression to an actual plaque.

Stable Plaque Formation

Foam cells within the fatty streak subsequently replicate and activate SMC within the media to proliferate and migrate through the basement membrane into the suben-dothelial space. SMCs, though relatively dormant within the media, increase their rate of replication on arrival into the intima. This increased rate of cell proliferation is still only about 1% year, which underscores atherogenesis as a gradual process. As the lesion continues to expand, changes begin to occur within the wall of the artery and the plaque itself. At first the arterial lumen is not interrupted by the proliferation of cells within the plaque; instead the vessel begins to remodel outward toward the adventitia by expanding in a compensatory enlargement. Eventually as the plaque enlarges, the vessel lumen begins to diminish leading to the typical symptoms of stable angina experienced by patients under increased oxygen demand.[36] Secondly, as the plaque begins to expand it has been noted that the SMCs inside the atheroma undergo apoptosis.[37,38] This may partially

explain the role of T cells found within atheroma, which along with cytokines have been implicated in leading to death of the SMC.[39] The interaction between T cells and SMCs within the intima leads to eventual disappearance of the endothelial cells and replacement by a fibrous cap.[40] During this process the major component of the cap changes from cells to an acellular matrix. This matrix is comprised primarily of macromolecules including collagen, elastin, and PGCs.[41]

At this stage the plaque requires a change in its structure to continue growth. Analogous to tumor pathophysiology, the new atheroma generates its own microcirculation within the lesion to continue expansion. Angiogenesis provides transit for cells throughout the plaque and provides the atheroma with the oxygen and nutrients over its large surface area it requires to endure. In experimental models inhibition of angiogenesis in mice limits plaque expansion.[42] Finally, the atheromatous plaque begins to mineralize through modulation by cytokines and gamma carboxylated glutamic acid residues which sequester calcium forming a stable plaque.

The Changing Plaque

Despite the gradual nature of atherosclerotic plaque formation, angiographic studies support the viewpoint that plaque growth occurs in an intermittent fashion.[43,44] There are several explanations for the change from periods of relatively dormant growth followed by episodes of accelerated growth (see Fig. 6-3). During plaque expansion, a clinically silent event, an intraplaque hemorrhage within the atheroma's microcirculation is the catalyst for expansion. These hemorrhages promote a wave of extracellular matrix deposition and SMC prolif-eration increasing the size of the lesion.

In contrast to these intraplaque hemorrhages, external disruption of the plaque is the key mechanism leading to periods of acute thrombosis and luminal stenosis. This disruption correlates with the common symptoms of AMI and unstable angina (USA) due to decreased distal blood flow and resultant ischemia. However, not every instance of plaque rupture produces symptoms; it may simply serve to provide another episode of SMC proliferation, gradually increasing luminal stenosis. The ability to identify which lesions are more likely to produce ischemia is not yet possible. A common belief, suspected through serial angiography, is that 85% of AMIs arise from lesions with less than 60% stenosis; supposing that smaller lesions are more likely to produce symptoms than their larger counterparts.[45] In actuality, the reason smaller lesions appear to be more harmful is clarified by the fact

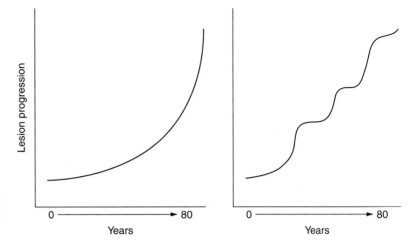

Fig. 6-3. Angiographic data demonstrates that atheroma progression is an episodic (right) rather than a linear process (left).

that low-grade stenoses are simply much more common than tight focal lesions, not that they are necessarily more dangerous or prone to rupture.[46] Therefore, during serial angiography though it appears that the smaller lesions (30–60%) cause a greater number of AMIs than their larger counterparts, this is merely a reflection of their greater overall predominance.

The Unstable Plaque

External disruption of the fibrous cap is postulated to occur by two mechanisms: (1) fracture of the "vulnerable" fibrous cap or (2) superficial erosion of the cap. The highly thrombogenic contents of the plaque core are protected from the circulation by the fibrous cap. Rupture of this cap causes exposure of the thrombogenic contents of the blood, subsequently leading to thrombosis. "Weakening" of the fibrous cap is believed to transform the stable plaque into a vulnerable form allowing for rupture. Although the clear mechanism for the initiation of degradation has not been elucidated, multiple pathways have been proposed. The first proposed mechanism is fracturing of the fibrous cap. The fibrous cap is primarily formed by collagen fibers. These fibers are produced primarily by SMCs under control of TGF-β. In a mouse model, lack of TGF-β was associated with an unstable collagen-depleted plaque phenotype.[47] Production of interferon-gamma (IFN-γ) by T cell present in the plaque, results in limitation of the production of collagen types I and III by SMC, thus leading to thinner fibrous caps.[48,49] Increased production of collagen-degrading enzymes, such as matrix metalloproteinases (MMP), also takes place in a plaque, leading to a

weaker fibrous cap. These MMPs are produced by macrophages and SMCs, and their production is enhanced by several proinflammatory mediators.[50] Therefore, both macrophages and SMCs, probably directed by T lymphocytes, contribute to the transformation to an unstable, rupture prone plaque phenotype. The second proposed mechanism of acute thrombosis, "superficial erosions" of the fibrous plaque, is poorly understood. Compared to plaque rupture, superficial erosions of the atheroma do not provide contact between the thrombus and the lipid core leading to a less pronounced reaction. In a study of 50 consecutive cases of sudden death due to coronary thrombus lesions superficial erosions were noted in 44% of patients, more often in younger patients and in women.[51,52] These unstable plaques are then susceptible to the increased wall stresses imposed by physiologic responses to emotional stress, exertion, and circadian variation (i.e., tachycardia and increased intraluminal pressure). These stressors typically rupture the unstable plaque at the junction of the atheroma and an adjacent plaque-free segment, leading to a localized clot deposition.[53]

The Platelet Plug

After years of atherosclerotic buildup, patients will begin to suffer the complications of ASCD. During periods of exercise or exertion the response of normal coronary arteries is to dilate allowing for increased supply of blood and oxygen in the face of increased demand. Initially patients with atheromatous burden in their coronary arteries will experience stable angina. Their diseased rigid arteries are unable to dilate providing a fixed supply of substrate which cannot respond to increased demand leading to typical clinical symptoms.[54] These symptoms are generally relieved by rest or coronary vasodilatory medications specifically nitroglycerin. Increases in blood pressure, heart rate, emotional stress, physical exertion as well as circadian variation not only provide for increased vascular demand, but also contribute to plaque destabilization in addition to the previously mentioned cellular pathways.[55] Transformation from stable angina to USA occurs through acute thrombosis of these ruptured atherosclerotic plaques. It is during this late phase of disease that patients present to the emergency department, where emergency physicians can act to preserve cardiac function and improve outcomes.

The first stage of acute thrombosis following plaque rupture is platelet adhesion (see Fig. 6-4). When an unstable plaque undergoes a superficial erosion or plaque rupture, its subendothelial matrix is exposed to the blood. Circulating platelets identify the area of disruption through the release of vWF from damaged endothelium and begin formation of a platelet plug. The platelet's receptor glycoprotein 1b-α, the largest of four GP Ib-IX-V polypeptides, interacts with vWF to form a tight bond which is able to overcome the shear forces present within arterial blood flow.[56,57] Additionally, platelet adhesion and subsequent activation is initiated by the collagen receptor GP VI which promotes binding of platelets to exposed collagen from the endothelial matrix.[58] While a layer of platelets is adhering to the ruptured cap, these cells undergo a series of structural changes known as platelet activation. This activation occurs through a series of second messenger systems including GMP and c-AMP which are activated by local and circulating mediators including ADP, epinephrine, and vWF.[59] Both ticlopidine and clopidogrel reduce platelet activation through inhibition of the ADP pathway.[60] Once activated, platelets not only change their physical structure to enhance thrombin binding by extending pseudopods, but also release adhesive proteins, growth factors (including PDGF, TGF-α, and TGF-β), and procoagulants (platelet factors IV and V) from their alpha granules.[61] Activated platelets also release thromboxane A_2 (TXA_2), a powerful vasoconstrictor which also results in further enhanced platelet activation.[62] Indirect antagonism of TXA_2 via irreversible binding to cyclooxygenase is the major role of aspirin in treating ACS. Lastly the platelet's membrane expresses the GP IIb/IIIa receptor, also released from alpha granules, which actively binds fibrinogen.[61]

Platelet aggregation, i.e., platelet-platelet adhesion, is the final phase in the formation of the platelet plug, a.k.a. the white clot. Fibrinogen and vWF act as ligands which bind two activated GP IIb/IIIa receptors forming a crosslink which allows the plug to expand.[63] Both compounds contain dual tripeptide RGD (arginine-glycine-aspartic acid) sequences where binding to the IIb/IIIa receptor appears to occurs.[64] Further studies have indicated that the six peptide carboxyl-terminus of the fibrinogen γ-chain as well as the RGD sequence may simply mediate interaction between fibrinogen and the IIb/IIIa receptor through yet unidentified mechanisms.[65] The interaction of these peptide chains with fibrinogen forms the target of anti-IIb/IIIa inhibitors used in clinical practice.

Coagulation Cascade and Thrombus Formation

While platelet aggregation is continuing, the extrinsic and common pathways of the coagulation cascade are also activated. The efficiency of the cascade is improved by systematic organization of the clotting factors on acidic phospholipids on the platelet membrane.[66,67] In ACS, the extrinsic pathway is primarily initiated through the release of tissue factor (TF) from the endothelial matrix.[68] TF then combines with circulating factor VIIa, usually present at low levels, forming a TF/VIIa complex.

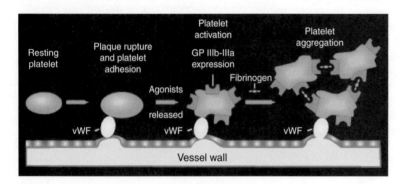

Fig. 6-4. Plaque rupture leading to platelet adhesion, activation, and aggregation.

This complex then catalyzes the conversion of factor VII into more factor VIIa, increasing the amount of available factor VIIa for binding to TF, augmenting the initial reaction.[69] The TF-VIIa enzyme then continues on to catalyze the next reaction of the extrinsic pathway, conversion of factor X to factor Xa, through two pathways. First, the enzyme works by converting factor IX to factor IXa, which then catalyzes the conversion of factor X to factor Xa. This mechanism appears to be the more kinetically favored approach as opposed to the more direct second pathway, i.e., direct activation of factor X.

Factor Xa engages in a series of reactions with factor V, calcium ions, and phospholipids derived from platelets. This composite of clotting factors and their reactions is referred to as the factor V complex or prothrombin activator. Factor V complex initiates the conversion of prothrombin (factor II) to the active form of the enzyme thrombin. Typically, in the presence of an intact endothelial layer, thrombin activates protein C, which exerts antithrombotic activity; however, as the levels of thrombin increase, thrombin exhibits procoagulative properties. This duality is known as the thrombin paradox.[70] Once formed thrombin not only catalyzes the conversion of fibrinogen (factor I) to fibrin but also serves an important role in sustaining the cascade by feedback activation of coagulation factors at several strategic sites, specifically cofactors VIII and V. Further, greater than 90% of thrombin formed during hemostasis is adsorbed to fibrin preventing the diffusion of thrombin to surrounding areas. To reverse the effects of thrombin, heparin and low-molecular weight heparin (LMWH) act in conjunction with native antithrombin III to neutralize thrombin and other activated clotting factors. Their major limitation rests in their inability to inactivate clot-bound thrombin.[71] Direct thrombin inhibitors including hirudin, originally derived from leeches, and bivalirudin, a synthetic analog, inactivate both free (fluid-phase) thrombin and fibrin-bound thrombin providing promise for potential therapies.[72]

Exposure of fibrinogen to thrombin results in proteolysis of fibrinogen to form the fibrin strands which stabilize the final clot. The first step in proteolysis is release of fibrinopeptide A from fibrinogen. The release of fibrinopeptide A enhances clot expansion by aggregating adjacent fibrin and fibrinogen molecules to be further processed into the final clot. A second peptide, fibrinopeptide B, is then cleaved by thrombin, and the ensuing fibrin monomer formed by this second proteolytic cleavage polymerizes spontaneously to form an insoluble gel. The polymerized fibrin, held together by noncovalent and electrostatic forces, is stabilized by transamidating enzyme factor XIIIa, produced by the action of thrombin on factor XIII.[73] At this stage the extent of ischemia or necrosis is dependent on the duration and extent of vessel occlusion and constriction.

ANTITHROMBOTIC MECHANISMS

Thus far we have discussed the development of atherosclerosis and plaque rupture leading to ACS. However, not every episode of plaque rupture leads to an ACS. The body has several defense mechanisms built-in to prevent intravascular thrombosis as well as limit its progression after endothelial injury.[74] First, an intact endothelium is able to release prostaglandin I_2 (PGI_2), NO, CD39, and carbon monoxide (CO) which all serve as inhibitors of the platelet adhesion.[75] NO and PGI_2 function both as direct vasodilators and through second messenger systems within the platelet to prevent adhesion and aggregation. CD39, a.k.a. ecto-ADPase, rapidly metabolizes ADP, a major agonist for platelet activation and thrombus formation.[76] Finally CO, a natural by-product of the breakdown of heme into biliverdin by heme oxygenase (HO), also inhibits SMC proliferation and platelet aggregation through second messenger systems.[77] Administration of CO, a natural platelet inhibitor, may become an innovative treatment of ACS.[78] The combination of these four molecules promotes blood fluidity in the presence of an intact endothelium.

In times of endothelial injury the body relies on three distinct anticoagulative systems to terminate clot formation. The heparin-antithrombin III (AT III) system, the protein C anticoagulant pathway, and the tissue factor pathway inhibitor (TFPI) work synergistically to regulate in vivo anticoagulation.[79–81] Defects in any of these mechanisms result in a hypercoagulable state. AT III is a glycoprotein inhibitor that neutralizes coagulation factors, especially factor Xa and thrombin.[79] Heparin, a natural endothelial PGC, serves as a site for both thrombin and AT III to bind. Following a structural alteration of the AT III molecule, catalyzed by this attachment with heparin, AT III is able to boost its anticoagulative activity by 1000 fold.[82] As opposed to its high affinity for thrombin, the interaction between the heparin: AT III complex and factor Xa plays a smaller anticoagulative role. Synthetic heparin and LMWHs act similar to their natural counterparts differentiated primarily by their respective attraction for thrombin versus factor Xa. Unfractionated heparin, owning to its larger size, preferentially reacts with thrombin to produce its anticoagulative effects; while LMWHs inhibit factor Xa. The ratio of antifactor Xa to antifactor IIa activity (Xa:IIa ratio) is commonly used to describe the efficacy of LMWHs.

TFPI is the major physiologic inhibitor of the extrinsic coagulation pathway, whose main instigator is the TF-VIIa complex.[83] TFPI is released from endothelial cells and platelets. TFPI, a tridomain protein, is hypothesized to inhibit TF-VIIa through a two-stage process. Initially TFPI binds with factor Xa inhibiting its activity directly.[81] A conformational change then occurs in the TFPI-Xa complex which later attaches to TF-VIIa inhibiting the extrinsic pathway.[84] Lastly, the protein C anticoagulant pathway is the final antithrombotic mechanism. Activated protein C (aPC) primarily inhibits factor Va and factor VIIa, the two primary cofactors of the coagulation cascade. Under normal conditions, when a clot is finished forming, i.e., the injured location is repaired, the initial stimulus for aggregation becomes depleted. Consequently, all excess thrombin flows downstream and binds with thrombomodulin on endothelial cells. This thrombin/thrombomodulin complex is able to activate circulating protein C.[85] To function effectively aPC must interact with protein S, found on the endothelial and platelet surface.[86] Then this complex is able to inactivate the target proteins, factors Va and VIIIa.[87] Resistance to the action of aPC by a specific mutation in factor Va (factor V Leiden) leads to a well-recognized hypercoagulable state.[88]

THE FIBRINOLYTIC SYSTEM

The three previous anticoagulation pathways only terminate and prevent further clot formation. It is the role of the fibrinolytic system to digest fibrin and dissolve the clot. The key enzyme for fibrinolysis is plasmin which is activated from plasminogen synthesized primarily in the liver. The entire system is initially activated by the aptly named plasminogen activators. These include tissue-type plasminogen activator (t-PA) and urokinase-type plasminogen activator (u-PA).[89] These activators are inhibited by the also aptly named plasminogen activator inhibitors (PAIs), specifically PAI-1 and PAI-2.[90] Typically, the conversion of plasminogen to plasmin by t-PA in the absence of fibrin is a slow process. Fibrin appears to provide a platform on which t-PA and plasminogen can cooperate to form plasmin. The newly formed plasmin subsequently degrades the fibrin and opens up the underlying fibrin for more plasminogen. The high affinity of plasmin for fibrin appears to help regionalize, focus the process, and promote a highly effective mechanism for clot dissolution. The combination of all these pathways is outlined in Fig. 6-5. The degradation of fibrin occurs at specific sites on the molecule leading to predictable degradation products. The most notable of these products is the D-dimer, which results from plasmin activity on crosslinked fibrin.

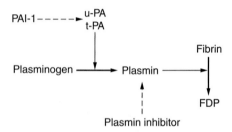

Fig. 6-5. The primary components of the fibrinolytic system.

SPECIAL CASES

Infection and Atherosclerosis

With the discovery of *Helicobacter pylori* as "the man behind the curtain" in peptic ulcer disease, there has been similar inquisition into an infectious etiology behind the stages of ASCD. Evaluation of the Framingham cohort has revealed that patients with a chronic cough tend to have an increased risk of AMI.[91] *Chlamydia pneumoniae*, cytomegalovirus (CMV), and *H. pylori* have all been associated with an increased risk of atherosclerosis.[92–94] Proving causality in this scenario is exceedingly difficult, considering the ever-present nature of atherosclerosis, respiratory pathogens, and sero-positivity for CMV in adult human populations. Of the pathogens noted, *C. pneumoniae* is the most widely studied. Despite small studies relating a positive impact from antibiotic therapy, such claims have not held up in larger studies.[95] Also, a metaanalysis reviewing 38 separate trials appears to reveal "a lack of causality" between *C. pneumoniae* and clinically manifested atherosclerosis.[93]

Restenosis Following Percutaneous Intervention

Despite the decades of buildup required for primary atherosclerosis, following balloon angioplasty (without stent) luminal narrowing recurs at 6–9 months in one-third of patients.[96] Initially the rapid rate of restenosis was attributed to SMC proliferation as a result of vessel wall injury due to mechanical manipulation. Recent trials involving serial nonstent angioplasty using intravascular ultrasound have identified that postangioplasty restenosis begins from scar formation within the adventitia which constricts the arterial lumen. This process termed "negative arterial remodeling," appears to be the main source of luminal narrowing and has renewed research efforts to further study the adventitia.[97,98] The efficacy of stents appears to be in preventing this negative remodeling by mechanically forcing the lumen to remain open. Studies show that coronary artery stenting significantly reduces the rate of target lesion revascularization (TLR), both early and long term, as compared with angioplasty alone while also improving intraluminal diameter.[99,100] However, coronary artery stenting is not a benign procedure. The presence of a metallic object within the coronary artery is inherently thrombogenic, leading to postprocedure stenosis within 2 weeks in certain patients. This had led to the development of new stents which are currently being studied including pharmacologically coated stents and biodegradable stents.[101,102] Furthermore, the metallic stent also leads to increased "neointimal tissue proliferation" along the length of the stent and is the primary cause of late stent restenosis.[103]

SUMMARY

Despite over 100 years of dedicated research in atherosclerosis and its complication a lot remains to be elucidated. We do understand now that atherosclerosis, a precursor of ACS, is an inflammatory process influenced by a list of environmental and genetic factors. Also, through research into the pathophysiology of acute thrombus formation, we have identified new treatment options for patients presenting to the emergency department having ACS. As research continues, we will be able to further outline the entire story of atherosclerosis and ACS allowing for newer and more effective treatments.

REFERENCES

1. Fuster V, Badimon L, Badimon JJ, et al. The pathogenesis of coronary artery disease and the acute coronary syndromes. *N Engl J Med* 1992;326:242–250, 310–318.
2. Ruffer MA. On arterial lesions found in Egyptian mummies. *J Pathol Bacteriol* 1911;15:453.
3. Parry CH. *An Inquiry into the Symptoms and Causes of the Syncope Anginosa, Commonly Called Angina Pectoris; Illustrated by Dissections.* London, UK: Cadell & Davis, 1799, pp. 43–44.
4. Acierno LJ. *Atherosclerosis (Arteriosclerosis). The History of Cardiology.* New York: The Parthenon Publishing Group, 1994.
5. Von Rokitansky K. *Uber einige der wichtigsten Krankheiten der Arterien*, Vienna: Meidiger, 1852.
6. Virchow R. *Phlogose und Thrombose im Gefass-system. Gesamelte Abhandlungen zur Wissenschaftligen Medicin.* Frankfurt, Medinger: Sohn und Co, 1856.
7. Marchand F. Uber Arteriosklerose (atherosklerose). Verhandlungen des 21 Kongress fur Innere Medizin. Leipzig, 1904.
8. Ignatowski AI. Ueber die Wirkung der tiershen Einwesses auf die Aorta. *Virchows Arch Pathol Anat* 1909;198:248.
9. Windaus A. Ueber der Gehalt normaler und atheromastoser Aorten an Cholesterol and Cholesterinester. *Zeitschrift Physiol Chem* 1910;67:174.
10. Anichkov N, Chalatov S. Ueber experimentelle Cholesterinsteatose: Ihre Bedeutung fur die Enstehung einiger pathologischer Proessen. *Centrbl Allg Pathol Pathol Anat* 1913;24:1–9.
11. Ross R. The pathogenesis of atherosclerosis: A perspective for the 1990s. *Nature* 1993;362:801–809.
12. Ross R. Atherosclerosis: An inflammatory disease. *N Engl J Med* 1999;340:115–126.
13. Stenmark KR, Gerasimovskaya E, Nemenoff RA, et al. Hypoxic activation of adventitial fibroblasts: Role in vascular remodeling. *Chest* 2002;122(6 suppl):3265–3345.
14. Lusis AJ. Atherosclerosis. *Nature* 2000;407:233–241.
15. Cines DB, Pollak ES, Buck CA, et al. Endothelial cells in physiology and in the pathophysiology of vascular disorders. *Blood* 1998;91:3527–3561.
16. Nievelstein PF, Fogelman AM, Mottino G, et al. Lipid accumulation in rabbit aortic intima 2 hours after bolus infusion of low density lipoprotein. A deep-etch and immunolocalization study of ultrarapidly frozen tissue. *Arterioscler Thromb* 1991;11(6):1795–1805.
17. Krieglstein CF, Granger DN. Adhesion molecules and their role in vascular disease. *Am J Hypertens* 2001;14:44S–54S.
18. Shin WS, Szuba A, Rockson SG. The role of chemokines in human cardiovascular pathology: Enhanced biological insights. *Atherosclerosis* 2002;160:91–102.
19. Tardy Y, Resnick N, Nagel T, et al. Shear stress gradients remodel endothelial monolayers in vitro via a cell proliferation-migration-loss cycle. *Arterioscler Thromb Vasc Biol* 1997;17(11):3102–3106.
20. Gimbrone MA Jr. Endothelial dysfunction, hemodynamic forces, and atherosclerosis. *Thromb Haemost* 1999;82:722–726.
21. Emeson EE, Robertson AL Jr. T lymphocytes in aortic and coronary intimas. *Am J Pathol* 1988;130:369–376.
22. Hansson G, Libby P. The role of the lymphocyte. In: Fuster V, Ross R, Topol E (eds.), *Atherosclerosis and Coronary Artery Disease.* New York; Lippincott-Raven, Vol. 1, 1996.
23. Li H, Cybulsky MI, Gimbrone MA Jr., et al. An atherogenic diet rapidly induces VCAM-1, a cytokine regulatable mononuclear leukocyte adhesion molecule, in rabbit endothelium. *Arterioscler Thromb* 1993;13:197–204.
24. Rohde LE, Lee RT, Rivero J, et al. Circulating cell adhesion molecules are correlated with ultrasound-based assessment of carotid atherosclerosis. *Arterioscler Thromb Vasc Biol* 1998;18:1765–1770.
25. Blankenberg S, Rupprecht HJ, Bickel C, et al. Circulating cell adhesion molecules and death in patients with coronary artery disease. *Circulation* 2001;104:1336–1342.
26. Malik I, Danesh J, Whincup P, et al. Soluble adhesion molecules and prediction of coronary heart disease: A prospective study and metaanalysis. *Lancet* 2001;358:971–976.

27. Blankenberg S, Barbaux S, Tiret L. Adhesion molecules and atherosclerosis. *Atherosclerosis* 2003;170(2):191–203.

28. Dong ZM, Chapman SM, Brown AA, et al. The combined role of P- and E-selections in atherosclerosis. *J Clin Invest* 19981;102(1):145–152.

29. Vora DK, Fang ZT, Liva SM, et al. Induction of P-selectin by oxidized lipoproteins: Separate effects on synthesis and surface expression. *Circ Res* 1997;80:810–818.

30. Luster AD. Chemokines—chemotactic cytokines that mediate inflammation. *N Engl J Med* 1998;338:436–445.

31. Gu L, Okada Y, Clinton S, et al. Absence of monocyte chemoattractant protein-1 reduces atherosclerosis in low-density lipoprotein-deficient mice. *Mol Cell* 1998; 2:275–281.

32. Boring L, Gosling J, Cleary M, et al. Decreased lesion formation in CCR2–/– mice reveals a role for chemokines in the initiation of atherosclerosis. *Nature* 1998;394:894–897.

33. Mach F, Sauty A, Iarossi A, et al. Differential expression of three T lymphocyte-activating CXC chemokines by human atheroma-associated cells. *J Clin Invest* 1999; 104:1041–1050.

34. Libby P. Changing concepts of atherogenesis. *J Intern Med* 2000;247:349–358.

35. Becker AE. Atherosclerose: een dynamischpathologisch concept. In: van der Werf T, Verheugt FWA (eds.), *Atherosclerose en coronaire insufficientie.* Utrecht: Interuniversitair Cardiologisch Instituut Nederland (ICIN), 1992.

36. Clarkson TB, Prichard RW, Morgan TM, et al. Remodeling of coronary arteries in human and nonhuman primates. *JAMA* 1994;271:289–294.

37. Isner JM, Kearney M, Bortman S, et al. Apoptosis in human atherosclerosis and restenosis. *Circulation* 1995;91:2703–2711.

38. Han D, Haudenschild C, Hong M, et al. Evidence for apoptosis in human atherogenesis and in a rat vascular injury model. *Am J Pathol* 1995;147:267–277.

39. Geng Y-J, Henderson L, Levesque E, et al. Fas is expressed in human atherosclerotic intima and promotes apoptosis of cytokine-primed human vascular smooth muscle cells. *Arterioscler Thromb Vasc Biol* 1997;17:2200–2208.

40. Burrig KF. The endothelium of advanced arteriosclerotic plaques in humans. *Arterioscler Thromb* 1991;11: 1678–1689.

41. Amento EP, Ehsani N, Palmer H, et al. Cytokines positively and negatively regulate interstitial collagen gene expression in human vascular smooth muscle cells. *Arteriosclerosis* 1991;11:1223–1230.

42. Moulton KS, Vakili K, Zurakowski D, et al. Inhibition of plaque neovascularization reduces macrophage accumulation and progression of advanced atherosclerosis. *Proc Natl Acad Sci U S A* 2003;100(8):4736–4741.

43. Bruschke AV, Kramer J Jr, Bal ET, et al. The dynamics of progression of coronary atherosclerosis studied in 168 medically treated patients who underwent coronary arteriography three times. *Am Heart J* 1989;117:296–305.

44. Yokoya K, Takatsu H, Suzuki T, et al. Process of progression of coronary artery lesions from mild or moderate stenosis to moderate or severe stenosis: A study based on four serial coronary arteriograms per year. *Circulation* 1999;100:903–909.

45. Hackett D, Davies G, Maseri A. Pre-existing coronary stenoses in patients with first myocardial infarction are not necessarily severe. *Eur Heart J* 1988;9:1317–1323.

46. Falk E, Shah P, Fuster V. Coronary plaque disruption. *Circulation* 1995;92:657–671.

47. Mallat Z, Gojova A, Marchiol-Fournigault C, et al. Inhibition of transforming growth factor-beta signaling accelerates atherosclerosis and induces an unstable plaque phenotype in mice. *Circ Res* 2001;89:930–934.

48. Amento EP, Ehsani N, Palmer H, et al. Cytokines and growth factors positively and negatively regulate interstitial collagen gene expression in human vascular smooth muscle cells. *Arterioscler Thromb* 1991;11:1223–1230.

49. Gupta S, Pablo AM, Jiang X, et al. IFN-gamma potentiates atherosclerosis in ApoE knock-out mice. *J Clin Invest* 1997;99:2752–2761.

50. Yanagi H, Sasaguri Y, Sugama K, et al. Production of tissue collagenase (matrix metalloproteinase 1) by human aortic smooth muscle cells in response to platelet-derived growth factor. *Atherosclerosis* 1991;91:207–216.

51. Farb A, Burke A, Tang A, et al. Coronary plaque erosion without rupture into a lipid core: A frequent cause of coronary thrombosis in sudden coronary death. *Circulation* 1996;93:1354–1363.

52. van der Wal AC, Becker AE, van der Loos CM, et al. Site of intimal rupture or erosion of thrombosed coronary atherosclerotic plaques is characterized by an inflammatory process irrespective of the dominant plaque morphology. *Circulation* 1994;89(1):36–44.

53. Malek AM, Alper SL, Izumo S. Hemodynamic shear stress and its role in atherosclerosis. *JAMA* 1999;282:2035–2042.

54. Braunwald E. Unstable angina: An etiologic approach to management. *Circulation* 1998;98:2219–2222.

55. Muller JE, Tofler GH, Stone PH. Circadian variation and triggers of onset of acute cardiovascular disease. *Circulation* 1989;79:733–743.

56. Schade AJ, Arya M, Gao S, et al. Cytoplasmic truncation of glycoprotein Ib alpha weakens its interaction with von Willebrand factor and impairs cell adhesion. *Biochemistry* 2003;42(7):2245–2251.

57. Ware J. Molecular analyses of the platelet glycoprotein Ib-IX-V receptor. *Thromb Haemost* 1998;79:466–478.

58. Andrews RK, Shen Y, Gardiner EE, et al. Platelet adhesion receptors and (patho)physiological thrombus formation. *Histol Histopathol* 2001;16(3):969–980.

59. Blockmans D, Deckmyn H, Vermylen J. Platelet activation. *Blood Rev* 1995;9:143–156.

60. Patscheke H. Platelet aggregation disorders. *Hamostaseologie* 2003;23(4):181–185.

61. Harrison P, Cramer EM. Platelet alpha-granules. *Blood Rev* 1993;7:52–62.

62. Thomas DW, Mannon RB, Mannon PJ, et al. Coagulation defects and altered hemodynamic responses in mice lacking receptors for thromboxane A_2. *J Clin Invest* 1998;102:1994–2001.

63. Kroll MH, Hellums JD, McIntire LV, et al. Platelets and shear stress. *Blood* 1996;88:1525–1541.

64. Schafer AI. Antiplatelet therapy. *Am J Med* 1996;101(2): 199–209.

65. Bennett JS. Platelet-fibrinogen interactions. *Ann N Y Acad Sci* 2001;936:340–354.

66. Jenny NS, Mann KG. Coagulation cascade: An overview. In: Loscalzo J, Schafer AI (eds.), *Thrombosis and Hemorrhage*, 2nd ed. Baltimore, MD: Williams & Wilkins, 1998, pp. 3–27.

67. Zwaal RF, Comfurius P, Beevers EM. Lipid–protein interactions in blood coagulation. *Biochim Biophys Acta* 1998;1376:433–453.

68. Osterud B. Tissue factor: A complex biological role. *Thromb Haemost* 1997;78:755–758.

69. Huang H, Norledge BV, Liu C, et al. Selective attenuation of the extrinsic limb of the tissue factor-driven coagulation protease cascade by occupancy of a novel peptidyl docking site on tissue factor. *Biochemistry* 2003;42(36): 10619–10626.

70. Griffin JH. The thrombin paradox. *Nature* 1995;378:337–338.

71. Hall RD, Pineo GF, Raskob GE. Hirudin versus heparin and low-molecular-weight heparin: And the winner is. . . *J Lab Clin Med* 1998;132:171–174.

72. Bates SM, Weitz JI. The mechanism of action of thrombin inhibitors. *J Invasive Cardiol* 2000;12(Suppl F):27F–32F.

73. Folk JE, Finlayson JS, Peyton MP. Cross-link fibrin polymerized by factor XIII: Epsilon (γ-glutamyl) lysine. *Science* 1968;160:892.

74. Schafer AI. Hypercoagulable states: Molecular genetics to clinical practice. *Lancet* 1994;344:1739–1742.

75. Vanhoutte PM, Mombouli JV. Vascular endothelium: Vasoactive mediators. *Prog Cardiovasc Dis* 1996;39: 229–238.

76. Marcus AJ, Broekman MJ, Drosopoulos JH et al. Inhibition of platelet recruitment by endothelial cell CD39/ecto-ADPase: Significance for occlusive vascular diseases. *Ital Heart J* 2001;2(11):824–830.

77. Durante W, Schafer AI. Carbon monoxide and vascular cell function. *Int J Mol Med* 1998;2:255–263.

78. Durante W. Heme oxygenase-1 in growth control and its clinical application to vascular disease. *J Cell Physiol* 2003;195(3):373–382.

79. Marcum JA, Rosenberg RD. Anticoagulantly active heparin-like molecules. In: Simionescu N, Simionescu M (eds.), *Endothelial Cell Biology in Health and Disease*. New York: Plenum Press, 1988, p. 207.

80. Esmon CT. The roles of protein C and thrombomodulin in the regulation of blood coagulation. *J Biol Chem* 1989;264:4743.

81. Rapaport SI. Inhibition of factor VIIa/tissue factor-induced blood coagulation with particular emphasis upon a factor Xa-dependent inhibitory mechanism. *Blood* 1989;73:359.

82. Craig PA, Olson ST, Shore JD. Transient kinetics of heparin-catalyzed protease inactivation by antithrombin III: Characterization of assembly, product formation and heparin dissociation in the factor Xa reaction. *J Biol Chem* 1989;264:5452.

83. Hembrough TA, Ruiz JF, Swerdlow BM, et al. Identification and characterization of a very low density lipoprotein receptor binding peptide from tissue factor pathway inhibitor that has antitumor and antiangiogenic activity. *Blood* 2004;103:3374–3380.

84. Rao LV, Rapaport SI. Studies of a mechanism inhibiting the initiation of the extrinsic pathway of coagulation. *Blood* 1987;69:645–651.

85. Esmon CT, Owen WG. Identification of an endothelial cell cofactor for thrombin-catalyzed activation of protein C. *Proc Natl Acad Sci U S A* 1981;78:2249.

86. Hackeng TM, Hessing M, van't Veer C, et al. Protein S binding to human endothelial cells is required for expression of cofactor activity for activated protein C. *J Biol Chem* 1993;268:3993.

87. Fulcher CA, Gardiner JE, Griffin JH, et al. Proteolytic inactivation of human factor VIII procoagulant protein by activated protein C and its analogy with factor V. *Blood* 1984;63:486.

88. De Stefano V, Finazzi G, Mannucci PM. Inherited thrombophilia: Pathogenesis, clinical syndromes and management. *Blood* 1996;87:3531–3544.

89. Collen D, Lijnen HR. Basic and clinical aspects of fibrinolysis and thrombolysis. *Blood* 1991;78:3114.

90. Eitzman DT, Ginsberg D. Of mice and men: The function of plasminogen activator inhibitors (PAIs) in vivo. *Adv Exp Med Biol* 1997;425:131–141.

91. Haider AW, Larson MG, O'Donnell CJ, et al. The association of chronic cough with the risk of myocardial infarction: The Framingham Heart Study. *Am J Med* 1999;106(3):279–284.

92. Adiloglu AK, Nazli C, Cicioglu-Aridogan B, et al. Gastroduodenal Helicobacter pylori infection diagnosed by Helicobacter pylori stool antigen is related to atherosclerosis. *Acta Cardiol* 2003;58(4):335–339.

93. Bloemenkamp DG, Mali WP, Visseren FL, et al. Meta-analysis of sero-epidemiologic studies of the relation between Chlamydia pneumoniae and atherosclerosis: Does study design influence results? *Am Heart J* 2003;145(3): 409–417.

94. Libby P, Egan D, Skarlatos S. Roles of infectious agents in atherosclerosis and restenosis: An assessment of the evidence and need for future research. *Circulation* 1997;96:4095–4103.

95. Kalayoglu MV, Libby P, Byrne GI, *Chlamydia pneumoniae* as an emerging risk factor in cardiovascular disease. *JAMA* 2002;288:2724–2731.

96. Nobuyoshi M, Kimura T, Nosaka H, et al. Restenosis after successful percutaneous transluminal coronary angioplasty: Serial angiographic follow-up of 229 patients. *J Am Coll Cardiol* 1988;12:616–623.

97. Mintz GS. Remodeling and restenosis: Observations from serial intravascular ultrasound studies. *Curr Interv Cardiol Rep* 2000;2(4):316–325.

98. Wilcox JN. Molecular biology: insight into the causes and prevention of restenosis after arterial intervention. *Am J Cardiol* 1993;72(13):88E–95E.

99. Kimura T, Yokoi H, Nakagawa Y, et al. Three-year follow-up after implantation of metallic coronary-artery stents. *N Engl J Med* 1996;334:561–566.

100. Debbas N, Sigwart U, Eeckhout E, et al. Intracoronary stenting for restenosis: Long-term follow-up: A single center experience. *J Invasive Cardiol* 1996;8:241–248.

101. Tamai H, Igaki K, Kyo E, et al. Initial and 6-month results of biodegradable poly-1-lactic acid coronary stents in humans *Circulation* 2000;102:399.

102. Chong PH, Cheng JW. Early experiences and clinical implications of drug-eluting stents: Part 1. *Ann Pharmacother* 2004;38:661–669.

103. Hoffmann R, Mintz GS, Dussaillant GR, et al. Patterns and mechanisms of in-stent restenosis. A serial intravascular ultrasound study. *Circulation* 1996;94:1247–1254.

7

Risk Stratification of AMI and ACS

Judd E. Hollander

HIGH YIELD FACTS

- Risk stratification aims to identify patients in one of three categories: a low-risk group that can be safely discharged, an intermediate risk group requiring further diagnostic testing, and a high-risk group requiring tailored diagnostic and therapeutic intervention.

- Traditional coronary artery disease (CAD) risk factors are poor predictors of acute coronary syndrome (ACS) in symptomatic patients.

- The electrocardiogram (ECG) is the single best tool for both identifying patients with acute myocardial infarction (AMI) and risk stratification of patients with potential ACSs.

- Cardiac markers with high negative predictive values are useful in "ruling out" ACSs in low-risk patients, while markers with high positive predictive values are useful in identifying patients who require more expensive and/or invasive evaluation.

- Single cardiac marker determinations should not be used to make admission discharge decisions.

- Provocative testing should be part of the evaluation, whether done immediately or in closely arranged followup.

INTRODUCTION

Risk stratification of patients with potential ACSs includes two overlapping diagnostic strategies: identifying patients at such low risk that they can be safely and rapidly discharged home and identifying patients at high risk requiring tailored diagnostic and therapeutic

interventions. This chapter will cover both ends of the risk stratification spectrum; however, other chapters in this book will further dictate appropriate care of patients who meet either very low- or very high-risk criteria.

HISTORY AND PHYSICAL EXAMINATION

The history and physical examination comprise the initial assessment of patients presenting with potential ACS. ACSs represent a disease spectrum from chronic stable angina to AMI. The Canadian Cardiovascular Society divides angina into four classes (Table 7-1) and unstable angina has been divided into three principal presentations by the Agency for Health Care Policy and Research Clinical Practice Guidelines (AHCPR) (Table 7-2).

The use of these classifications and definitions in the emergency department (ED) is problematic because it is often not clear whether symptoms are cardiac or noncardiac in origin. Application of the Canadian Cardiovascular Society Classification and the AHCPR guidelines is only appropriate if the patient has a diagnosis of ischemic chest pain. At ED presentation, the most immediate concern is distinguishing patients with ACS from those without ACS (e.g., patients with a noncardiac etiology for their symptoms). Approximately 5% of ED chest pain patients sustain an AMI; an additional 10% have non-AMI ACS. Thus, 85% of patients have a non-ACS etiology for their presenting symptoms. It is important to expeditiously distinguish between these two groups of patients (see Table 7-3).

The utility of clinical features for the evaluation of chest pain is quite variable (Table 7-4).[1-3] Features associated with a lower probability of AMI, such as pleuritic, positional, and sharp chest pain have poor to fair inter-physician reliability (kappa values of 0.27–0.44). High-risk features (radiation to left arm, substernal location, and history of AMI) are more reliable (kappa values of 0.74–0.89).[1] Thus, history is most reliable in "ruling in" high-risk patients but is less reliable when being used to "rule out" ACS.

Traditional cardiac risk factors are predictive of CAD in asymptomatic patients; however, in symptomatic patients (those with chest pain), cardiac risk factors are poor predictors of risk for ACS.[4] These traditional cardiac risk factors were derived from population-based longitudinal cohort studies of asymptomatic patients. In contrast, ED patients are already at increased risk because they are already symptomatic. The lack of cardiac risk factors does not identify ED patients who can be safely discharged from the ED.

Table 7-1. Canadian Cardiovascular Society Classification of Angina

Class I	Angina only occurs with strenuous, rapid, or prolonged exertion. Ordinary physical activity does not cause angina.
Class II	Slight limitation of ordinary activity. Angina occurs with climbing stairs rapidly, walking uphill, walking after meals, in cold, in wind, or under emotional stress.
Class III	Marked limitations of ordinary physical activity. Angina occurs on walking 1–2 blocks on level or climbing one flight of stairs at usual pace.
Class IV	Inability to carry on physical activity without discomfort. Anginal symptoms may be present at rest.

Source: Braunwald E, Mark DB, Jones RH, et al. *Unstable Angina: Diagnosis and Management.* Clinical Practice Guideline Number 10 (amended) AHCPR Publication No. 94-0602. Rockville, MD: Agency for Health Care Policy and Research and the National Health, Lung and Blood Institute, Public Health Service, U.S. Department of Health and Human Services, 1994.

Table 7-2. Main Presentations of Unstable Angina

Rest angina	Angina occurring at rest and usually prolonged >20 min occurring within a week of presentation.
New onset angina	Angina of at least CCSC III severity with onset within 2 months of presentation.
Increasing angina	Previously diagnosed angina that is distinctly more frequent, longer in duration, or lower in threshold (increased by at least one CCSC class to at least CCSC III severity).

Source: Braunwald E, Mark DB, Jones RH, et al. *Unstable Angina: Diagnosis and Management.* Clinical Practice Guideline Number 10 (amended) AHCPR Publication No. 94-0602. Rockville, MD: Agency for Health Care Policy and Research and the National Health, Lung and Blood Institute, Public Health Service, U.S. Department of Health and Human Services, 1994.

Table 7-3. Likelihood of Signs and Symptoms Representing ACS Secondary to CAD

Characteristic	High Likelihood (Any of the Following Features)	Intermediate Likelihood (Absence of High Likelihood Features and Any of the Following)	Low Likelihood (Absence of High or Intermediate Features, but May Have Any of the Following)
History	Typical symptoms reproducing prior angina History of prior AMI or known history of CAD	Chest or left arm discomfort as chief symptom Male sex Diabetes mellitus Multiple cardiac risk factors	Probable ischemic symptoms Recent cocaine use
Examination	Transient MR, hypotension, diaphoresis, pulmonary edema or rales	Extracardiac vascular disease	Chest discomfort reproduced by palpation
ECG	New transient ST-segment deviation (>0.05 mV) or T-wave inversions (>0.2 mV) with symptoms	Fixed Q waves Abnormal ST segments or T waves not known to new	T-wave flattening or inversion of T waves in leads with dominant R waves
Cardiac markers	Elevated cardiac TnI, TnT, or CK-MB	Normal	Normal ECG

Source: Braunwald E, Mark DB, Jones RH, et al. *Unstable Angina: Diagnosis and Management.* Clinical Practice 10 (amended) AHCPR Publication No. 94-0602. Rockville, MD: Agency for Health Care Policy and Research Health, Lung and Blood Institute, Public Health Service, U.S. Department of Health and Human Services, 1994.

Table 7-4. Likelihood Ratios for Clinical Features that Increase or Decrease Risk of AMI in Patients Presenting with Chest Pain

Clinical Feature	Likelihood Ratio (95% CI)
Increased likelihood of AMI	
Pain in chest or left arm	2.7*
Chest pain radiation	
To right shoulder	2.9 (1.4–6.0)
To left arm	2.3 (1.7–3.1)
To both left and right arm	7.1 (3.6–14.2)
Chest pain most important symptom	2.0*
History of MI	1.5–3.0†
Nausea or vomiting	1.9 (1.7–2.3)
Diaphoresis	2.0 (1.9–2.2)
Third heart sound	3.2 (1.6–6.5)
Hypotension (systolic BP <80 mmHg)	3.1 (1.8–5.2)
Pulmonary crackles	2.1 (1.4–3.1)
Decreased likelihood of AMI	
Pleuritic chest pain	0.2 (0.2–0.3)
Chest pain sharp or stabbing	0.3 (0.2–0.5)
Positional chest pain	0.3 (0.2–0.4)
Chest pain reproduced by palpation	0.2–0.4†

*Data not available to calculate confidence intervals.
†In heterogeneous studies the likelihood ratios are reported as ranges.
Source: Panju AA, Hemmelgarm BR, Guyatt GH, et al. Is this patient having a myocardial infarction? *JAMA* 1998;280: 1256–1263.

Table 7-5. Electrocardiographic Features Predictive of AMI in Acute Chest Pain Patients

Electrocardiographic Feature	Likelihood Ratio (95% CI)
New ST-segment elevation ≥1 mm	5.7–53.9*
New Q wave	5.3–24.8*
Any ST-segment elevation	11.2 (7.1–17.8)
New conduction defect	6.3 (2.5–15.7)
New ST-segment depression	3.0–5.2*
Any Q wave	3.9 (2.7–5.7)
Any ST-segment depression	3.2 (2.5–4.1)
T-wave peaking and/or inversion ≥1 mm	3.1†
New T-wave inversion	2.4–2.8*
Any conduction defect	2.7 (1.4–5.4)

*In heterogeneous studies the likelihood ratios are reported as ranges.
†Data not available to calculate confidence intervals.
Source: Panju AA, Hemmelgarm BR, Guyatt GH, et al. Is this patient having a myocardial infarction? *JAMA* 1998;280: 1256–1263.

The physical examination does not distinguish patients with ACS from patients with noncardiac symptoms. Patients with ACSs may appear deceptively well or may be in obvious distress. An S_4 is common in patients with long-standing hypertension or myocardial dysfunction. The presence of a murmur can be an ominous sign (flail leaflet of the mitral valve or a ventricular-septal defect) or it can reflect long-standing valvular heart disease. Knowledge about the patient's baseline condition may therefore be helpful.

ELECTROCARDIOGRAM

The 12-lead ECG is the single best test to immediately identify patients with AMI.[5] It is also useful for cardiovascular risk stratification of patients with potential ACSs

(Table 7-5). Although it is the best individual test, the ECG still has relatively low sensitivity for detection of AMI: it detects less than 50% of AMIs at the time of presentation.[5,6] Patients with normal or nonspecific ECGs have a 1–5% incidence of AMI and a 4–23% incidence of having unstable angina.[5–8] Patients with nondiagnostic ECGs or with ischemia that is not known to be old have a 4–7% incidence of AMI and a 21–48% incidence of unstable angina. Demonstration of new ischemia increases the risk of AMI to 25–73% and the unstable angina risk to 14–43%.[5] Right-sided lead, rV_4, should be used in the setting of inferior wall infarction to assess possible RV involvement.[7] Even among patients with ST elevation myocardial infarction (STEMI), ECG variables can further risk stratify the likelihood of 30-day mortality (Table 7-6).[9]

RISK STRATIFICATION ALGORITHMS

Several risk stratification algorithms can be used clinically at the time of initial presentation.

Goldman Risk Score

The Goldman risk score has been prospectively validated and is useful as an initial risk stratification tool.[10] The final algorithm is heavily based on electrocardiographic

Table 7-6. Multivariate Significance of the Electrocardiogram in Patients with STEMI Enrolled in GUSTO-1

Electrocardiographic Feature	Odds Ratio For 30-day Mortality (95% CI)
Sum of ST-segment deviation (19 mm vs. 8 mm)	1.53 (1.38–1.69)
Sum of ST-segment decrease (–1 mm vs. –7 mm)	0.77 (0.72–0.83)
Heart rate (84 bpm vs. 60 bpm)	1.49 (1.41–1.59)
Sum of ST-segment increase in II, III, and a VF (6 mm vs. 0 mm)	0.79 (0.71–0.89)
QRS duration (100 ms vs. 80 ms)	
Anterior infarct	1.55 (1.43–1.68)
Other location	1.08 (1.03–1.13)
Anterior infarction	
QRS duration (100 ms)	1.08 (1.03–1.13)
QRS duration (50 ms)	0.61 (0.43–0.86)
Inferior infarction	
No prior AMI	0.67 (0.50–0.90)
Prior AMI	1.41 (0.98–2.02)
Prior infarction	
Inferior infarction	2.47 (2.02–3.00)
Other location	1.17 (0.98–1.41)

Source: Hathaway WR, Peterson ED, Wagner GS, et al. Prognostic significance of the initial electrocardiogram in patients with acute myocardial infarction. *JAMA* 1998;279: 387–391.

findings and chest pain characteristics (Fig. 7-1) and does not incorporate initial cardiac marker determinations. It stratifies patients into groups with a 1–77% risk of AMI and has a sensitivity for predicting AMI of 88–91% with a specificity of 78–92%.[11] It does not identify any group with less than 1% risk; and therefore has not been able to identify patient group safe for ED discharge. This group also derived a rule to predict the need for intensive care unit admission and development of cardiovascular complications.[12] ST-segment elevation or Q waves on the ECG, other ECG findings indicating myocardial ischemia, low systolic blood pressure, pulmonary rales above the bases, or an exacerbation of known ischemic heart disease all predict complications. This algorithm has been independently validated and strict adherence to the protocol would reduce intensive care unit admission by 16%, resulting in potentially large cost savings.[13]

ACI-TIPI

The ACI-TIPI is a computer-generated method to determine the likelihood of ACS at the time of initial clinical evaluation. The acute coronary insufficiency time insensitive predictive index (ACI-TIPI) electrocardiograph incorporates age, sex, presence of chest or left arm pain, a chief symptom of chest or left arm pain, pathologic Q waves, and the presence and degree of ST-segment elevation or depression and T-wave elevation or inversion.[14] It reports the percent likelihood of "acute cardiac ischemia" on the electrocardiographic record. Four studies including 5496 patients have found that when combined with physician impression it has a sensitivity of 86–95% and a specificity of 78–92% for prediction of ACS.[11] The ACI-TIPI has not been shown to make a clinically relevant difference in diagnostic accuracy compared with physician judgment alone. It has not been widely incorporated into clinical practice.

Neural Network

The artificial neural network is a nonlinear statistical paradigm shown to be a powerful modality for the recognition of complex patterns that can maintain accuracy when some input data are missing. This is a distinct advantage for use in "real time," when some clinical information may not be readily available. It can accurately identify the presence of myocardial infarction in patients with chest pain.[15] When initial cardiac troponin I and CK-MB determinations are added to the variables used by the network, the network had a sensitivity of 95% and a specificity of 96% despite the fact that an average of 5% of the input data required by the network were missing on all patients.[15] For prediction of AMI, the neural network has better sensitivity and specificity than the Goldman risk score and ACI-TIPI score.[16] It incorporates more clinical information than either the Goldman score or ACI-TIPI (Table 7-7).

TIMI Risk Score

The thrombolysis in myocardial infarction (TIMI) risk score was derived to enhance treatment decisions by identifying patients most likely to benefit from certain therapies. The TIMI risk score for patients with unstable angina can predict at least one component of a primary end-point comprising death, new or recurrent MI, or severe recurrent ischemia requiring urgent revascularization through 14 days following index presentation. The seven TIMI risk score predictor variables are shown in Table 7-8. The total score is simply the number of these

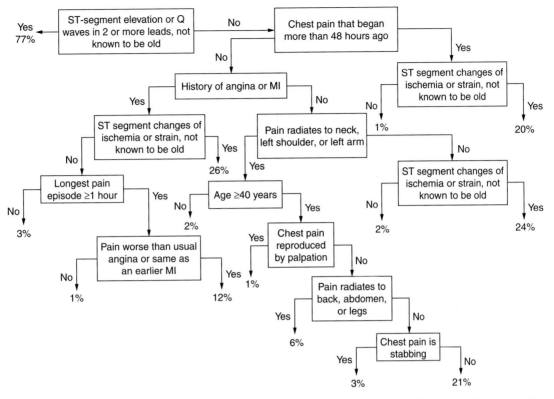

Fig. 7-1. The Goldman risk stratification algorithm for prediction of acute myocardial infarction. (Source: Lee TH, Juarez G, Cook EF, et al. Ruling out acute myocardial infarction. A prospective multicenter validation of a 12 hour strategy for patients at low risk. *N Engl J Med* 1991;324:1239–1246.)

individual risk factors. Event rates increase significantly as the TIMI risk score increases: 4.7% for a score of 0/1; 8.3% for 2; 13.2% for 3; 19.9% for 4; 26.2% for 5; and 40.9% for 6/7.[17] The TIMI risk score has also been evaluated in patients presenting to the ED with chest pain and it shows a higher 30-day risk of death, AMI, and revascularization in patients with higher scores (range 1.5–70%).[18]

A separate TIMI risk score for ST-elevation myocardial infarction exists. It is a simple integer score (Table 7-9) that showed an increased mortality with higher scores (range 1.1–30.0%).[19] Among patients not receiving reperfusion therapy, the risk score underestimated death rates.[19]

MARKERS OF MYOCARDIAL INJURY

The utility of cardiac markers is somewhat dependent on the goal of the physician in any individual patient.

Markers with high negative predictive values enhance the ability to rapidly "rule out" ACSs and can facilitate discharge from the ED (Table 7-10). Markers with high positive predictive values are ideal to mobilize more costly evaluation and treatments for patients at high risk of cardiovascular complications. More complete discussion of cardiac markers can be found in Chap. 9. In this chapter the ability of cardiac markers to help in risk stratification will be discussed.

CK-MB

Serial CK-MB mass measurements are only 36–48% sensitive when used at or shortly after presentation.[11,20] As a result, single CK-MB measurements cannot generally be used to assist in the admission/discharge decision since they do not attain adequate negative predictive values for ACS. Over reliance on serial markers will result in an unacceptable rate of missed AMI and

Table 7-7. Clinical Criteria Included in Several ED Risk Stratification Schemes

	Goldman Score	ACI-TIPI	Baxt Neural Network
Demographics	Age ≥40 years	Age Gender	Age Gender Race
Presentation characteristics	Chest pain duration ≥48 h Longest pain episode >1 h History of angina or MI Pain worse than usual angina or same as prior MI Pain radiates to neck, left shoulder, or left arm Pain radiates to back, abdomen, or legs Chest pain reproduced by palpation Chest pain is stabbing	Presence of chest or left arm pain Chief symptom of chest or left arm pain	Left anterior chest pain Left arm pain History of prior coronary angina, or CHI Pain pressing in nature Pain crushing in nature Pain radiating in nature Pain radiating in nature Shortness of breath Diaphoresis Nausea and vomiting
Past history			Hypertension Diabetes mellitus Elevated cholesterol Family history disease
Electrocardiographic criteria	ST-segment elevation or Q waves in 2 or more leads, not known to be old ST-segment changes of ischemia or strain, not known to be old	Pathologic Q waves Presence and degree of ST-segment elevation or depression T-wave elevation or inversion	Q waves [old] Q waves not known to be old ST-segment elevation [old] ST-segment elevation not known to be old T-wave inversion [old] T-wave inversion not known to be old ST-segment depression [old] ST-segment depression not known to be old Left bundle branch [old] Left bundle branch known to be old Hyperacute T waves old Hyperacute T waves not known to be old
Cardiac marker determination			Presentation CK, CK-MB, and troponins

Source: Hollander JE. Acute coronary syndrome in the emergency department: Diagnosis, risk stratification and management In: Theroux P (ed.), *Acute Coronary Syndromes: A Companion to Braunwald's Heart Disease.* Philadelphia, PA: W.B. Saunders, 2003, pp. 152–167.

Table 7-8. Elements of the TIMI Score for Unstable Angina/Non-ST-Segment Elevation MI*

Age 65 years or older
Three or more traditional risk factors for coronary artery
    disease
Prior coronary stenosis of 50% or more
ST-segment deviation on presenting electrocardiogram
Two or more anginal events in prior 24 h
Aspirin use within the 7 days prior to presentation
Elevated cardiac markers

*The presence of each of the above is assigned 1 point. The maximal possible score is 7.

cardiovascular complications. Serial CK-MB measurements over 6–9 hours have been widely employed in chest pain observation units and are considered sufficient, if negative, to safely exclude AMI allowing further diagnostic testing or ED release, depending on the clinical scenario. An alternative strategy is to examine the change in CK-MB values within 2 hours of ED presentation. A rise in CK-MB ≥1.6 ng/mL over the 2-hour period following presentation achieves a sensitivity for detection of AMI of 94%, which is better than using the 2-hour CK-MB value alone (75%).[21]

Table 7-9. Elements of the TIMI Score for ST-Segment Elevation AMI

Clinical Risk Indicators	Points
Historical	
Age >75 years	3
Age 65–74 years	2
History of diabetes, hypertension, or angina	1
Physical examination	
Systolic blood pressure	
Systolic blood pressure <100 mmHg	3
Heart rate >100 bpm	2
Killip class II–IV	2
Weight <67 kg	1
Presentation	
Anterior ST-segment elevation or left bundle branch block (LBBB)	1
Time to reperfusion >4 h	1
Total points possible	14

Source: Morrow DA, Antman EM, Parsons L, et al. Application of the TIMI risk score for ST-elevation MI in the National Registry of Myocardial Infarction 3. *JAMA* 2001;286:1356–1359.

Table 7-10. Summary of Predictive Properties of Cardiac Markers of Diagnosis of AMI

Marker	No. Studies	No. Subjects	Sensitivity (95% CI)	Specificity (95% CI)	Diagnostic Odds Ratio (95% CI)
At time of presentation					
Creatine kinase	12	3,195	37 (31–44)	87 (80–91)	3.9 (2.7–5.7)
CK-MB	19	6,425	42 (36–48)	97 (95–98)	25 (18–36)
Myoglobin	18	4,172	49 (53–55)	91 (87–94)	11 (8–15)
Troponin I	4	1,149	39 (10–78)	93 (88–97)	11 (3.4–34)
Troponin T	6	1,348	39 (26–53)	93 (90–96)	9.5 (5.7–16)
CK-MB and myoglobin	3	2,283	83 (51–96)	82 (68–90)	17 (7.6–40)
Serial markers					
Creatine kinase	2	786	69–99	68–84	12–220
CK-MB	14	11,625	79 (71–86)	96 (95–97)	140 (65–310)
Myoglobin	10	1,277	89 (80–94)	87 (80–92)	84 (44–160)
Troponin I	2	1,393	90–100	83–96	230–460
Troponin T	3	904	93 (85–97)	85 (76–91)	83 (33–210)
CK-MB and myoglobin	2	291	100	75–91	4.3–14

Source: Lau J, Ioannidis JPA, Balk EM, et al. Diagnosing acute cardiac ischemia in the Emergency Department: A systematic review of the accuracy and clinical effect of current technologies. *Ann Emerg Med* 2001;37:453–460.

Cardiac Troponins

Combined analysis of four studies assessing the predictive properties of single cardiac troponin I values at the time of presentation for AMI found a sensitivity of 39% and specificity of 93%.[11] A similar analysis of six cardiac troponin T studies found the same results.[11] Thus, the cardiac troponins have similar sensitivity and specificity for detection of AMI as CK-MB.[22–24] In patients with unselected chest pain syndromes and those with definite ACSs, elevations in cardiac troponin I and troponin T both predict cardiovascular complications independent of CK-MB and the ECG.[23,24] Minor elevations in cardiac troponin I and T can also identify patients more likely to benefit from an early invasive treatment strategy.[25] In patients admitted to chest pain observation units, cardiac troponin T has higher sensitivity for detection of myocardial necrosis and multivessel CAD than CK-MB.[26] In unselected ED patient populations with chest pain syndromes, cardiac troponin T elevations are associated with a 3.5-fold increased risk of 60-day adverse cardiovascular events.[27] Elevated values of the cardiac troponins in patients with non-ST-segment elevation AMI increase the short-term risk of death 3.1 fold (1.6% vs. 5.2%).[28] Although the cardiac troponins are useful for both diagnosis and risk stratification of patients with chest pain,[29] ACS, and AMI, cardiac maker testing in the ED will not identify most ED patients who subsequently develop adverse events.[30,31] Thus, patients with negative markers still require an evaluation and testing, as dictated by their clinical presentation.

Myoglobin

The sensitivity of myoglobin at the time of ED presentation is 49%, exceeding that of CK-MB or troponins, but the specificity is only 87%.[11] However, serial quantitative testing over 1 hour, evaluating both absolute values and a change of 40 ng/mL has 91% sensitivity and up to a 99% negative predictive value for AMI within 1 hour of ED presentation (approximately 3–4 hours after symptom onset).[32] One study has evaluated the ability of myoglobin to risk stratify ED patients with potential ACS and it found that an elevated myoglobin predicted a 3.4-fold risk of adverse cardiovascular events and identified some high-risk patients not otherwise identified by clinical characteristics, CK-MB, or troponin T.[33]

Combinations of Markers

Although both troponin T and CK-MB have approximately the same rate of detection in serum, there is benefit to using both markers to risk stratify patients. At the time of ED presentation, the use of both markers rather than either alone, increases diagnostic sensitivity more than 25%.[33] A combination of myoglobin and troponin I can achieve a diagnostic sensitivity of 97% with a 99% negative predictive value, within 90 min of ED presentation.[34] The addition of CK-MB did not improve diagnostic accuracy within this time frame, but the CK-MB and myoglobin combination had 92% sensitivity and 99% negative predictive value within this same time frame.

IMAGING MODALITIES

Cardiac imaging can detect abnormalities prior to irreversible myocardial damage.

Echocardiography

Echocardiography, when used to assess wall motion, has a sensitivity for detection of AMI of approximately 93%, but a specificity of only 53–57%.[35] Echocardiography is most useful in patients without a past history of CAD since it cannot distinguish old from new infarcts. Larger areas of infarction and more depressed left ventricular function predict a higher likelihood of cardiovascular complications and an increased mortality. The addition of echocardiography to baseline clinical variables and the initial ECG appears to have independent predictive value.[36] The predictive properties of echocardiography and myocardial perfusion imaging are similar with respect to AMI, PTCA, and presence of CAD.[37]

Rest Sestamibi Imaging

Sestamibi imaging is very useful for ED risk stratification of chest pain patients. A very high negative predictive value of resting sestamibi imaging can allow early ED discharge of low-risk patients. An abnormal sestamibi scan is associated with 50-fold increased risk of AMI; a 14.5-fold increased risk of revascularization over the next 30 days; and a 30-fold increased risk of death over the ensuing 12 months.[38] Early perfusion imaging is considerably more sensitive than initial cardiac troponin I determinations.[39]

Immediate Provocative Testing

Stress testing is common in chest pain observation units despite a paucity of evidence to show that they are cost-effective tools for risk stratification of ED chest pain patients. There are no large studies demonstrating the sensitivity and specificity for detection of CAD in this patient population and some studies in this patient population have more "false positive" than "true positive" tests.[40] Exercise treadmill or pharmacologic testing with or without nuclear imaging, as well as stress echocardiography are safe and can assist cardiovascular risk stratification in the ED.[41–43] Patients with an uneventful observation period, negative cardiac markers, and a normal stress test can be safely discharged with a referral for follow-up. There is some evidence supporting the use of immediate exercise testing in low-risk ED chest pain patients without known ventricular dysfunction and with normal or nonspecific ECGs, even prior to cardiac marker determination.[44]

Previous Diagnostic Testing for Coronary Artery Disease

Prior cardiac catheterization results are very useful for risk stratification. Patients documented to have minimal (<25%) stenosis or normal coronary arteriograms have an excellent long-term prognosis with greater than 98% free from myocardial infarction 10 years later.[45] Repeat cardiac catheterizations an average of 9 years later found that approximately 90% of patients did not develop even a single vessel CAD.[46] Recent cardiac catheterization with normal or minimally diseased vessels almost eliminates the possibility of an ACS.

EMERGENCY DEPARTMENT DISPOSITION

Patients should be risk stratified based on the likelihood that they have an ACS. The single best tool for initial risk stratification of chest pain patients is the ECG,[5] despite the fact that it will not identify all patients with AMI. Patients with STEMI should receive reperfusion therapy and be triaged to the cardiac care unit. Other patients should be further evaluated for their risk of ACS, preferably using validated tools (Goldman or TIMI score, consensus guidelines, or computerized algorithms) rather than simply clinical impression.

Patients with nonischemic etiologies of their chest pain and those with a less than 1% risk of 30-day adverse events could be released home from the ED. Patients with stable anginal patterns do not require inpatient evaluation. Patients less than 40 years old without any cardiac risk factors and without a prior cardiac history have a <1% risk of ACS and <1% risk of 30-day death, AMI, or revascularization. Likewise, patients less 40 years old with a normal ECG and no prior cardiac history also have a <1% risk of ACS or adverse 30-day cardiovascular events.[47] These groups would be considered very low risk for ACS

and are reasonable to discharge without further evaluation. Sestamibi imaging during acute chest pain can sufficiently exclude ACS such that some patients can be safely discharged from the ED without further observation or cardiac marker testing.[38]

Most patients at low risk should be treated in an ED observation unit or inpatient setting. Chest pain observation units allow brief periods of observation while obviating the need for more costly hospital admission in a large cohort of patients with nonspecific chest pain syndromes. A variety of different protocols exist, but most observation protocols incorporate frequent serial marker testing (at 1–4 hour intervals) for at least 6 hours, telemetry monitoring (with continuous single or 12-lead ECG), and some form of provocative testing for patients who "rule out" for myocardial infarction and do not have cardiovascular complications during the observation period. Patients without recurrent symptoms or cardiovascular complications with negative cardiac marker determinations are safe for release from the ED. If released without provocative testing, low-risk patients should have close follow-up arranged. Aggressive multiple marker strategies, including serial CK-MB, myoglobin, and cardiac troponin I values over 90 min for low-risk chest pain patients may also allow safe rapid release of some of these patients.[48]

Intermediate risk patients should receive serial cardiac markers and provocative testing. Elevated cardiac markers on initial determination may warrant "upgrading" of some patients originally triaged to non-ICU telemetry settings, since it increases risk of adverse events. Patients with abnormal but nondiagnostic ECGs may benefit from more intensive observation and monitoring in the cardiac care unit, when initial cardiac markers are elevated. Patients with normal or nonspecific ECGs are at low risk for complications, and therefore do not automatically warrant more than a non-ICU telemetry setting unless dictated by other clinical parameters (ECG changes, continued chest pain, or cardiovascular complications). Initial cardiac marker determinations should not be used to make admission/discharge decision. Even when a undetectable troponin I on presentation is combined with a Goldman AMI risk of <4%, there is an unacceptable rate of adverse events at 30 days (1% death, 2% AMI, and 2% revascularization).[49]

Important premorbid factors related to short- and long-term prognosis in patients with ACSs are the severity of CAD, the left ventricular function, age, and comorbid diseases. For this reason, prior invasive and noninvasive assessments of cardiac function should be taken into account when making ED disposition decisions.

REFERENCES

1. Hickan DH, Sox HC, Sox CH. Systematic bias in recording history in patients with chest pain. *J Chronic Dis* 1985; 38:91–100.

2. Gadsboll N, Hoiland-Carlsen PF, Nielsen GG, et al. Symptoms and signs of heart failure in patients with myocardial infarction: Reproducibility and relationship to chest x-ray, radionuclide ventriculography and right heart catheterization. *Eur Heart J* 1989;10:1017–1028.

3. Panju AA, Hemmelgarm BR, Guyatt GH, et al. Is this patient having a myocardial infarction. *JAMA* 1998;280:1256–1263.

4. Jayes RL, Beshansky JR, D'Agostino RB, et al. Do patients' coronary risk factor reports predict acute cardiac ischemia in the emergency department? A multicenter study. *J Clin Epidemiol* 1992;45:621–626.

5. Lee T, Cook F, Weisberg M, et al. Acute chest pain in the emergency room: Identification and examination of low risk patients. *Arch Intern Med* 1985;145:65–69.

6. Selker HP, Zalenski RJ, Antman EM, et al. An evaluation of technologies for identification of acute cardiac ischemia in the emergency department: A report from a National Heart Attack Alert Program Working Group. *Ann Emerg Med* 1997;29:13–87.

7. Hathaway WR, Peterson ED, Wagner GS, et al. Prognostic significance of the initial electrocardiogram in patients with acute myocardial infarction. *JAMA* 1998;279:387–391.

8. Slater DK, Hlatky MA, Mark DB, et al. Outcome in suspected acute myocardial infarction with normal or minimally abnormally admission electrocardiographic findings. *Am J Cardiol* 1987;60:766–770.

9. Brush JE, Brand DA, Acampora D, et al. Use of the initial electrocardiogram to predict in-hospital complications of acute myocardial infarction. *N Engl J Med* 1985;312: 1137–1141.

10. Lee TH, Juarez G, Cook EF, et al. Ruling out myocardial infarction. A prospective multicenter validation of a 12 hour strategy for patients at low risk. *N Engl J Med* 1991;324: 1239–1246.

11. Lau J, Ioannidis JPA, Balk EM, et al. Diagnosing acute cardiac ischemia in the Emergency Department: A systematic review of the accuracy and clinical effect of current technologies. *Ann Emerg Med* 2001;37:453–460.

12. Goldman L, Cook EF, Johnson PA, et al. Prediction of the need for intensive care in patients who come to emergency departments with chest pain. *N Engl J Med* 1996;334: 1498–1508.

13. Qamar A, McPherson C, Babb J, et al. The Goldman algorithm revisited: Prospective evaluation of a computer-derived algorithm versus unaided physician judgment in suspected acute myocardial infarction. *Am Heart J* 1999; 138:705–709.

14. Selker HP, Beshanski JR, Griffith JL, et al. Use of the acute cardiac ischemia time-insensitive predictive instrument (aci-tipi) to assist with triage of patients with chest pain or other symptoms suggestive of acute cardiac ischemia: a multicenter, controlled clinical trial. *Ann Intern Med* 1998; 129:845–855.

15. Baxt WG, Shofer FS, Sites FD, et al. A neural computational aid to the diagnosis of acute myocardial infarction. *Ann Emerg Med* 2002;39:366–373.

16. Baxt WG. *Neural Computational Aid to the Diagnosis of Acute Myocardial Infarction.* Atlanta, GA: Presented at Society of a Academic Emergency Medicine Annual Meeting, May, 2001.

17. Antman EM, Cohen M, Bernink PJ, et al. The TIMI risk score for unstable angina/non-ST elevation MI: A method for prognostication and therapeutic decision making. *JAMA* 2000;284:835–834.

18. Hollander JE, Pollack CV Jr., Sites FD, et al. Validation of the TIMI risk score in the emergency department chest pain patient population (abstract). *Acad Emerg Med* 2003; 10(5):42.

19. Morrow DA, Antman EM, Parsons L, et al. Application of the TIMI risk score for ST-elevation MI in the National Registry of Myocardial Infarction 3. *JAMA* 2001;286:1356–1359.

20. Gibler WB, Lewis LM, Erb RE, et al. Early detection of acute myocardial infarction in patients presenting with chest pain and nondiagnostic ECGs: Serial CK-MB sampling in the emergency department. *Ann Emerg Med* 1990;19:1359–1366.

21. Fesmire FM, Percy RF, Bardoner JB, et al. Serial creatinine kinase MB testing during emergency department evaluation of chest pain. Utility of a 2 hour delta CK-MB of +1.6 ng/ml. *Am Heart J* 1998;136:237–244.

22. Brogan GX Jr., Hollander JE, McCuskey CF, et al. Evaluation of a new assay for cardiac Troponin I vs Creatine Kinase-MB for the diagnosis of acute myocardial infarction. *Acad Emerg Med* 1997;4:6–12.

23. Green GB, Li DJ, Bessman ES, et al. The prognostic significance of troponin I and troponin T. *Acad Emerg Med* 1998;5:758–767.

24. Antman EM, Tanasijevic MJ, Thompson B, et al. Cardiac specific troponin I levels predict the risk of mortality in patients with acute coronary syndromes. *N Engl J Med* 1996;335:1342–1349.

25. Morrow DA, Cannon CP, Rifai N, et al. Ability of minor elevations of troponins I and T to predict benefit from an early invasive strategy in patients with unstable angina and non ST segment elevation myocardial infarction. *JAMA* 2001;286:2405–2412.

26. Newby LK, Kaplan AL, Granger BB, et al. Comparison of cardiac troponin T versus creatine kinase-MB for risk stratification in a chest pain evaluation unit. *Am J Cardiol* 2000;85:801–805.

27. Sayre MR, Kaufmann KH, Chen IW, et al. Measurement of cardiac troponin T is an effective method for predicting complications among Emergency Department patients with chest pain. *Ann Emerg Med* 1998;31:539–549.

28. Heidenreich PA, Alloggiamento T, Melsop K, et al. The prognostic value of troponin in patients with non-ST elevation acute coronary syndromes: A meta-analysis. *J Am Coll Cardiol* 2001;38:478–485.

29. Hamm CW, Goldmann BU, Heeschen C, et al. Emergency room triage of patients with acute chest pain by means of rapid testing for cardiac troponin T or troponin I. *N Engl J Med* 1997;337:1648–1653.
30. McErlean ES, Deluca SA, van Lente F, et al. Comparison of troponin T versus creatine kinase MB in suspected acute coronary syndromes. *Am J Cardiol* 2000;85:421–426.
31. Kontos MC, Anderson FP, Alimard R, et al. Ability of troponin I to predict cardiac events in patients admitted from the Emergency Department. *J Am Coll Cardiol* 2000;36:1818–1823.
32. Brogan GX Jr., Friedman S, McCuskey C, et al. Evaluation of a new rapid quantitative immunoassay for serum myoglobin versus CK-MB for ruling out acute myocardial infarction in the emergency department. *Ann Emerg Med* 1994;24:665–671.
33. Green GB, Beaudreau RW, Chan DW, et al. Use of troponin T and creatine kinase MB subunit levels for risk stratification of emergency department patients with possible myocardial ischemia. *Ann Emerg Med* 1998;31:19–29.
34. McCord J, Nowak RM, McCullough PA, et al. Ninety-minute exclusion of acute myocardial infarction by use of quantitative point-of-care testing of myoglobin and troponin I. *Circulation* 2001;104(13):1483–1488.
35. Selker HP, Zalenski RJ, Antman EM, et al. An evaluation of technologies for identification of acute cardiac ischemia in the emergency department: A report from a National Heart Attack Alert Program Working Group. *Ann Emerg Med* 1997;29:13–87.
36. Kontos MC, Arrowood JA, Paulsen WHJ, et al. Early echocardiography can predict cardiac events in Emergency Department patients with chest pain. *Ann Emerg Med* 1998;31:550–557.
37. Paventi S, Parafati MA, DiLuzio E, et al. Usefulness of two dimensional echocardiography and myocardial perfusion imaging for immediate evaluation of chest pain in the Emergency Department. *Resuscitation* 2001;49:47–51.
38. Tatum JL, Jesse RL, Kontos MC, et al. Comprehensive strategy for the evaluation and triage of the chest pain patient. *Ann Emerg Med* 1997;29:116–125.
39. Kontos MC, Jesse RL, Anderson FA, et al. Comparison of myocardial perfusion imaging and cardiac troponin I in patients admitted to the Emergency Department with chest pain. *Circulation* 1999;99:2073–2078.
40. Lindsay J Jr., Bonnet YD, Pinnow EE. Routine stress testing for triage of patients with chest pain. Is it worth the candle? *Ann Emerg Med* 1998;32:600–603.
41. Diercks DB, Gibler WB, Liu T, et al. Identification of patients at risk by graded exercise testing in an Emergency Department chest pain center. *Am J Cardiol* 2000;86:289–292.
42. Trippi JA, Lee KS, Kopp G, et al. Dobutamine stress tele-echocardiography for evaluation of emergency department patients with chest pain. *J Am Coll Cardiol* 1997;30:627–632.
43. Colon PJ 3rd, Guarisco JS, Murgo J, et al. Utility of stress echocardiography in the triage of patients with atypical chest pain from the emergency department. *Am J Cardiol* 1998;82:1282–1284.
44. Kirk JD, Turnipseed S, Lewis WR, et al. Evaluation of chest pain in low risk patients presenting to the emergency department: the role of immediate exercise testing. *Ann Emerg Med* 1998;32:1–7.
45. Pitts WR, Lange RA, Cigarroa JE, et al. Repeat coronary angiography in patients with chest pain and previously normal coronary angiogram. *Am J Cardiol* 1997;80:1086–1087.
46. Papanicolaou MN, Califf RM, Hlatky MA, et al. Prognostic implications of angiographically normal and insignificantly narrowed coronary arteries. *Am J Cardiol* 1986;58:1181–1187.
47. Walker NJ, Sites FD, Shofer FS, et al. Characteristics and outcomes of young adults who present to the Emergency Department with chest pain. *Acad Emerg Med* 2001;8:703–708.
48. Ng SM, Krishnaswamy P, Morissey R, et al. Ninety minute accelerated critical pathway for chest pain evaluation. *Am J Cardiol* 2001;88:611–617.
49. Limkakeng A Jr., Gibler WB, Pollack C, et al. Combination of Goldman risk and initial cardiac troponin I for Emergency Department chest pain patient risk stratification. *Acad Emerg Med* 2001;8:696–702.

8

Electrocardiography in Cardiac Ischemia

David French

J. Lee Garvey

Laszlo Littmann

HIGH YIELD FACTS

- The electrocardiogram (ECG) is a critical tool in the diagnosis of acute coronary syndromes (ACS), though its sensitivity and specificity are not perfect, and a normal ECG does not preclude the diagnosis of myocardial ischemia or infarction.

- The presence of ST-segment changes, especially ST elevation (STE) with reciprocal ST depression (STD), portends a worse prognosis for myocardial infarction (MI) than does a normal or nondiagnostic ECG.

- There are many confounding patterns for STE, and some are associated with coronary artery disease (CAD), like left ventricular hypertrophy (LVH) and left bundle branch block (LBBB). This can make the diagnosis of cardiac ischemia difficult, especially in symptomatic patients.

- Pathologic Q waves are the only truly diagnostic waveform for MI, though the delay in their appearance makes routine use for decision-making impractical.

- Inferior and posterior ischemia may not be adequately imaged with the current 12-lead ECG. The use of additional leads (V_4R, V_8, and V_9) may clarify the extent of ischemia.

- ECG changes in ischemia are dynamic, and serial ECGs improve the diagnostic sensitivity of the ECG. Serial assessment begins with reviewing previous ECGs (if available) and may include the use of prehospital ECGs and continuous ST-segment analysis.

INTRODUCTION

In 1887, the first transcutaneous tracing of human cardiac electrical activity was published by Augustus Waller, founding the field of electrocardiography. These early images were obtained by capillary electrometers, which tended to obscure details in the tracing. Willem Einthoven advanced the field in 1900 when he incorporated the use of the string galvanometer and began producing cardiac tracings in the form that they are known today. The American Heart Association described the six precordial leads in 1938 with the addition of the 6 limb lead tracings shortly thereafter. Thus, began the era of the 12-lead ECG and a revolution in the field of cardiology.[1] Since its inception, the ECG has become an essential component of the cardiac evaluation for ACS, which includes unstable angina pectoris (USAP) and acute myocardial infarction (AMI).

The benefits of the ECG in this setting are clear. It is a safe and inexpensive test, and tracings are easily accessible and quickly obtained. In combination with history, physical examination, and cardiac markers, it is an essential component of the bedside diagnosis of ACS and subsequent risk stratification.[2,3] In the era of thrombolytic drugs and mechanical revascularization of the ischemic myocardium, early identification of ACS is critical, so the ECG is a vital diagnostic tool.[4]

As with all studies, the ECG has its limitations. Perhaps the greatest limitation of the ECG is its relatively low sensitivity (and specificity) for detecting ischemic changes. Miller et al. evaluated the presenting patterns of ECGs in over 900 patients subsequently diagnosed with AMI and found normal or nondiagnostic ECGs in nearly 20% of them.[5] Further, multiple underlying ECG patterns make diagnosis of ACS difficult, including LVH, LBBB, ventricular paced rhythms (VPR), benign early repolarization (BER), and previous MIs.

Several other factors contribute to the limitations of the ECG. Successful interpretation requires training and experience, and some waveforms are difficult to interpret, leading to disagreement among clinicians and misdiagnosed ischemia. The individual 12-lead ECG provides a brief picture of cardiac electrical activity and can miss ischemic changes and arrhythmias. The cardiac tracings of the ECG represent the net electrical currents of the heart, and small ischemia-related changes may not be evident. In addition, the ECG in its current form incompletely evaluates the right ventricle and the posterior wall of the heart.[3]

ANATOMY

In order to appreciate the anatomic orientation of the ECG, consideration of lead location in relation to the cardiac chambers is necessary. The heart lies nearly horizontal in the chest cavity, with the ventricles at the anterior-inferior apex. The right atrium and ventricle are more anterior than the left chambers, resulting in an interventricular septum that is nearly parallel with the frontal plane of the body.[4]

The precordial leads (V_1–V_6) of the ECG lie in the transverse plane and progress in an orderly fashion from the right ventricle to the lateral left ventricle. Lead V_1 captures the base of the right ventricle, as well as the anterior and basal portions of the interventricular septum with assistance from lead V_2. Leads V_3 and V_4 further image the septum and anterior left ventricle, while lead V_5 covers the apex with V_6. This last lead may also capture part of the posterior wall.[6] However, the right ventricle and posterior wall of the heart are not completely imaged by these leads, and additional leads may be necessary to fully evaluate these areas for suspected ischemia.

The limb leads, which lie in the frontal plane, may be organized in the standard fashion, or according to the Cabrera orientation (Fig. 8-1), which is more anatomically appropriate. In addition, while most of the frontal leads are separated by 30° increments in the classic Einthoven triangle, there is a 60° gap between leads II and III, a location which could be occupied by –aVR. Thus, the inferior and lateral aspects of the left ventricle are suboptimally imaged, while lead aVR provides a view of the right shoulder and is essentially ignored by clinicians.[4]

THE ECG IN ISCHEMIA AND INFARCTION

Despite the limitations, the ECG provides much useful information in the evaluation for ACS. However, differentiating between the ischemic changes of angina and the changes associated with MI can be difficult, especially in the acute setting. In fact, many ECG changes associated with ischemia may be present in either condition. Traditional teaching has held that changes in the ST segment and T wave of the ECG indicate myocardial ischemia, while changes in the QRS complex are associated

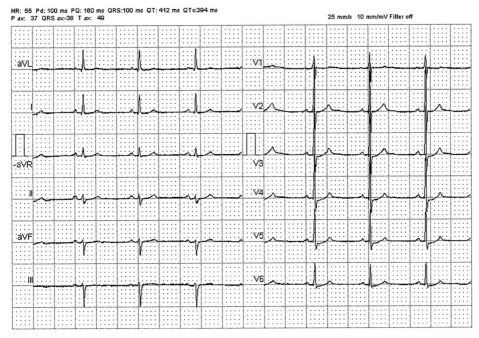

Fig. 8-1. Cabrera sequence of lead presentation. Frontal plane leads arranged sequentially following the progression around Einthoven's triangle. (aVL, I, –aVR, II, aVF, III)

with infarction and necrosis. These latter changes take time to develop on the ECG, so changes in the QRS complex play a less prominent role in the algorithms for early revascularization.

Instead, efforts have been made to describe early ischemic ECG changes that have a high likelihood of progressing to MI and necrosis. In 2000, the American College of Cardiology (ACC) published a position statement in conjunction with the European Society of Cardiology describing changes suspicious for developing ACS: ST-segment elevation at the J point ($\geq$0.2 mV in leads V_1, V_2, or V_3 or $\geq$0.1 mV in the remaining leads), STD, or T-wave changes in two or more contiguous leads. The committee acknowledged that these findings were "robust determinants" of myocardial ischemia but alone could not diagnose myocardial necrosis; the presence of pathologic Q waves was recognized as the only change truly diagnostic for an acute, recent, or resolved MI. Some ECG findings impede the use of these criteria, including Wolff-Parkinson-White (WPW) syndrome, BBB, VPR, and LVH.[7]

While these changes may not guarantee MI, some ECG patterns are very suggestive of impending necrosis. Since "time is muscle," the goal with AMI is early identification with appropriate revascularization as quickly as possible. Understandably, then the ACC definition of STE is widely used as a major criterion for the use of reperfusion therapy, since so many of these patients eventually have elevated cardiac markers indicating infarction.[8,9] Bahit et al. performed a retrospective analysis of patients from the GUSTO-IIa trial who presented with STE. Roughly 95% of patients with evolving ECG changes (including new Q waves and resolving STE) considered "evidence" for AMI had a twofold increase in CK-MB and a 3- and 11-fold increase in troponin I and T, respectively.[10] This suggests that STE, especially with dynamic ECG changes, is an appropriate indicator of impending infarction. In fact, AMIs are categorized on the basis of ST elevation myocardial infarction (STEMI) or non-ST elevation myocardial infarction (NSTEMI), with important prognostic and treatment implications.

T-Wave Changes

The T wave results from repolarization of the ventricles, and normally has a symmetric morphology with an amplitude less than 0.50 mV in the precordial leads and 1.0 mV in the limb leads. Changes in the T wave may be the earliest indication of ACS. Both hyperacute T waves and T-wave inversion can result from ischemic myocardium; however, other conditions can cause similar ECG patterns.

Hyperacute T Waves

In STEMI, hyperacute T waves present as early as a few minutes after occlusion of a coronary vessel. Hyperacute T waves are prominent, tall waves, which may be symmetric but are generally asymmetric with a wide base. They are a transient finding, usually progressing to STE within a few minutes to hours. The etiology of the hyperacute T wave is not clear, but serum markers of myocardial necrosis are not typically found to be abnormal during this period.

The differential diagnosis for prominent T waves is long. Cardiac etiologies include LVH, BER, BBB, VPR, valvular heart disease, idiopathic hypertrophic subaortic stenosis, pericarditis, and cor pulmonale. Other underlying conditions with pronounced T waves include hyperkalemia, neurologic disease, hyperthyroidism, acidosis, anemia, and some acute drug overdoses. However, there are no objective criteria defining a hyperacute T wave, and this may represent a normal variant.

The conditions most closely resembling hyperacute T waves are LVH, BER, and hyperkalemia. The former two can usually be distinguished from ischemia by the associated ECG findings. Hyperkalemia may be a bit more problematic. A clinical suspicion for electrolyte abnormalities (including a history of renal failure) provides an important diagnostic clue. The T waves of hyperkalemia are usually tall and symmetric with a narrow base, though this pattern does not absolutely differentiate it from ischemia.[11]

T-Wave Inversion

While hyperacute T waves are important to recognize, the more common T-wave abnormality associated with ACS is T-wave inversion, or coronary T waves. These T waves are usually symmetric and narrow with an isoelectric ST segment which may be bowed upward.[12] Miller et al. found that isolated T-wave inversion was present in 10.7% of patients who were subsequently diagnosed with MI and was associated with a 5% 28-day mortality, which was similar to the mortality associated with MI and normal or nondiagnostic ECGs.[5] Savonitto et al. found a similar mortality rate in their retrospective analysis of over 12,000 patients presenting with AMI, even though they had a higher incidence of isolated T-wave inversion (20% of presenting ECGs). According to their study, 32% of patients presenting with T-wave inversion were subsequently diagnosed with AMI.[2]

While abnormal T waves on an ECG may be acute, they may also be a chronic finding from a prior infarction or other processes. After reperfusion therapy, T-wave inversion can be used as an indicator of treatment efficacy. T-wave inversion noted within a few hours after thrombolytic drug treatment is a specific indicator of successful reperfusion. However, inversion noted more than 4 hours after reperfusion does not necessarily indicate successful therapy—this change can simply reflect evolving AMI.[13]

In addition, many other etiologies exist for T-wave inversion, including cardiac and noncardiac processes. T-wave inversion is a sensitive but nonspecific finding on the ECG. The list of alternative diagnoses is long and includes LVH, WPW, myocarditis, persistent juvenile T waves, pulmonary embolism, cerebrovascular accident, or central nervous system (CNS) injury. History, physical examination, and other ECG findings will help differentiate the cause of the T-wave inversion.[12,14,15]

Wellens Syndrome

Wellens syndrome is a specific pattern of T-wave inversion that is important to recognize, though it is rarely described in cardiology texts. It has primarily been identified in the emergency medicine literature. Diagnostically, it is defined as either deep, inverted, symmetric T waves or biphasic T waves in the anterior precordial leads (V_2 and V_3), though similar changes may be evident in other precordial leads (Fig. 8-2). The ST segment is usually isoelectric, and pathologic Q waves are absent in the precordial leads. The sensitivity and specificity of these ECG changes is not known. Historically, patients will complain of recent anginal symptoms, though chest pain is often absent at the time of these ECG findings.

The clinical significance of Wellens syndrome is that the ECG changes result from a critical stenosis of the proximal left anterior descending (LAD) coronary artery. The T-wave changes are a preinfarction finding, and the usual course of the syndrome is progression to a significant anterior MI. Therefore, patients presenting with Wellens syndrome should not undergo provocative (i.e., stress) testing, but rather should undergo cardiac catheterization to identify the obstruction. The T-wave changes resolve with treatment.

The differential diagnosis for the Wellens pattern is similar for other T-wave inversions. CNS-related changes most closely resemble these findings and have been characterized as "Wellenoid" in appearance. Usually, the altered T waves resulting from a neurologic cause are wide based, inverted, deep, and symmetric, but the underlying cause can be elucidated from a careful history and physical examination.[14] In the absence of neurologic findings, alternative explanations for T-wave inversion should be sought.

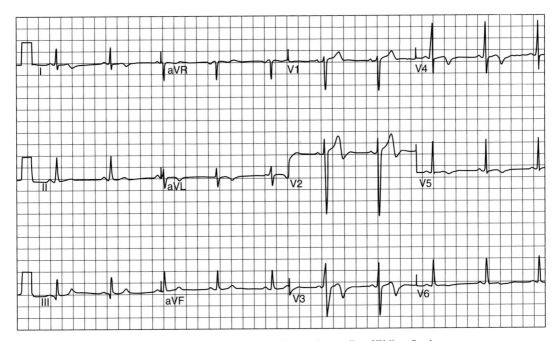

Fig. 8-2. ECG demonstrating precordial T wave abnormality of Wellens Syndrome.

ST-Segment Changes

The ST segment is measured from the J point (the *junction* of the end of the QRS complex and the start of the ST segment) to the apex of the T wave. This section of the ECG is a critical area when evaluating for ACS, primarily because it changes relatively early in the setting of ACS, resulting in either ST elevation (STE) or STD. If necrosis ensues, these findings are again categorized as STEMI or NSTEMI. It is important to remember that these changes are dynamic and eventually resolve or evolve into more permanent ECG changes, which may include Q waves and persistent T-wave inversion.

ST Elevation

STE associated with ischemia usually begins with hyperacute T waves, which rapidly evolve into STE. Pathologic STE results in myocardial necrosis in the vast majority of patients. Elevation due to ischemia is caused by a change in the electrical currents in the affected area. On the ECG, the amount of elevation is determined by the height of the J point above the isoelectric line.[7,15] Defining the site of the isoelectric line is occasionally debated. While it may be identified by the TP segment, tachycardia can obscure this interval. Other authors suggest using the PR segment.[16] Clinically significant STE has been defined either by the ACC criteria or as 100 μV of elevation in the precordial leads. Again, this finding must be present in two contiguous leads, indicating the same general anatomic location (Fig. 8-3).[7,17]

The morphology of STE in ACS is classically described as obliquely straight or convex, meaning that the tracing travels along or above an imaginary line connecting the J point and the apex of the T wave. The shape of the ST segment with convex elevation has been compared to a "tombstone." Concave elevation, in which the tracing travels below this imaginary line, is less likely to result from ACS.[12] Brady et al. found that nonconcave ST-segment elevation, defined as either convex or straight elevation, was 77% sensitive and 97% specific for AMI, and only patients with a coronary diagnosis (including USAP) had nonconcave elevation.[17] Therefore, convex and obliquely straight STEs, when present, are very useful for diagnosing ACS, but concave elevation is not absolutely incompatible with ischemia.

STE is a relatively common finding in AMI and is associated with an increased complication rate. Miller et al. demonstrated isolated STE in 20.8% of patients presenting with AMI with a 28-day mortality rate of 10.6%.[5] Savonitto et al. found a slightly lower rate for 30-day mortality and reinfarction (9.4%), which was still twice as high as the complication rate for patients with T-wave inversion alone.[2]

Resolution of STE is also an important finding, as it is an indicator of tissue reperfusion during therapy. The degree of resolution is a prognostic indicator, and the absence of resolution is indicative of treatment failure. In patients receiving thrombolytics who do not demonstrate STE resolution, rescue angioplasty may be required to reperfuse the ischemic myocardium.[13]

Other Etiologies of STE

Many nonischemic conditions can complicate the interpretation of STE on the ECG. This can occur in two ways—either through mimicking STE or through altering the ST segment and masking STE. Since identification of ischemic STE is so important, clinicians must be aware of such complicating patterns and understand how to differentiate these from ACS. This is not always done successfully. Sharkey et al. evaluated the use of thrombolytics in patients with STE and found that 11% of patients were

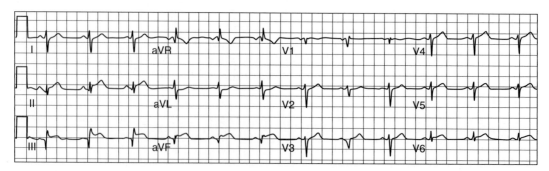

Fig. 8-3. ST segment elevation in acute inferior myocardial infarction. STE is seen in leads II, III and aVF and reciprocal STD in lead aVL.

mistakenly treated because the initial ECG was misinterpreted as diagnostic for ACS.[9] Given the frequency with which STE occurs from nonischemic causes, this is not surprising. Brady et al. retrospectively analyzed the diagnoses of patients presenting to the emergency department with STE and found that ACS was not even the most common cause of STE. LVH accounted for 25% of elevations, followed by LBBB and AMI (15% each), BER (12%), right bundle branch block (RBBB) (5%), left ventricular aneurysm (LVA) (3%), pericarditis (1%), ventricular paced rhythm (1%), and other undefined causes, including nonspecific BBBs (22%).[18] Other less common causes of STE include WPW syndrome, Prinzmetal's angina (vasospasm), hypothermia, cardiac tumors, pulmonary embolism, abdominal disorders (pancreatitis, cholecystitis, and peritonitis), and Brugada syndrome. The latter is associated with idiopathic ventricular fibrillation and presents with a RBBB pattern, downsloping STE, and inverted T waves.[4,16,19] Finally, minimal STE is a normal finding in the majority of young adults. Over 90% of males aged 16–58 years have STE of 0.1–0.3 mV in the precordial leads. This may also be evident in women, though it is less pronounced.[16] Excluding ACS in the presence of these confounding patterns requires a careful ECG analysis, a thorough history and physical examination, and a detailed knowledge of the differential diagnosis.

Left Ventricular Hypertrophy

Though LVH can cause STE, the differentiation is made by analysis of QRS voltage patterns. Two easily remembered rules are an R wave > 1.1 mV in lead aVL or a collective height of the S wave in V_1 and the R wave in either lead V_5 or V_6 >3.5 mV. A strain pattern with a downsloping STD followed by an asymmetric, discordant (in the opposite direction of the QRS) T wave is often present, as are other repolarization abnormalities causing ST-segment and T-wave changes.[11,15] It is important to remember that LVH is frequently seen in patients with CAD, and ischemia should be considered in the appropriate clinical circumstances.

Left Bundle Branch Block

LBBB is defined by (1) QRS duration > 120 ms, (2) broad, notched R waves in the lateral leads (aVL, V_5, V_6), (3) absent Q waves in the left-sided leads, and (4) prolonged R-wave peak (>60 ms) in the lateral precordial leads.[15] The ECG pattern associated with LBBB has long been recognized as a diagnostic dilemma in the setting of

ACS and has thus been extensively studied. The first problem is that LBBB is associated with an abnormal ST morphology and T-wave polarity discordant to that of the QRS. This altered morphology affects the appearance of T-wave and ST-segment changes normally associated with ACS. The second problem is that patients with BBBs frequently have concomitant CAD and are at higher risk for developing ischemia. Therefore, recognizing ACS in patients with LBBB can be difficult, though it is not an uncommon dilemma (Fig. 8-4).

Sgarbossa et al.[20] developed and validated a set of electrocardiographic criteria for the diagnosis of AMI in the setting of LBBB. They incorporated three criteria into a scoring system: (1) concordant (in the same direction as the QRS) STE of ≥1 mm (5 points), (2) discordant STE of ≥5 mm (2 points), and (3) STD of ≥1 mm in leads V_1, V_2, V_3 (3 points). They found that a score ≥3 was 36% sensitive and 96% specific for AMI. Subsequent studies have challenged the validity of this scoring system. Shapiro et al. retrospectively analyzed emergency department ECGs in 441 patients with LBBB. The specificity of the scoring system was still high at 95.9%, but the sensitivity in this study was poor (16.6%).[21] Shlipak et al. also found these criteria to have a poor sensitivity (10%) in a retrospective analysis of 83 emergency department patients but still noted a specificity of 100%.[22] Most recently, Gula et al. retrospectively evaluated 414 ECGs with LBBB in the setting of AMI and found a poor sensitivity of 6–19% for each of the individual Sgarbossa criteria and only 27% sensitivity for any ST-segment change. Equally as important, the authors noted only fair-to-moderate interobserver agreement for each of the necessary findings, with a κ of 37–52%. Concordant STE and STD in leads V_1–V_3 were the most specific findings (98.8% and 100%, respectively). The end result, according to this study, is that over half of AMIs with LBBB would be missed by these criteria. This would still be an improvement over current practice standards, in which patients with LBBB and AMI receive perfusion therapy with 10% of the frequency of patients with STEMI.[23]

With the obvious limitations of these criteria, Shlipak suggests that reperfusion therapy should be considered for all patients with LBBB and symptoms consistent with AMI, due to the low negative predictive value of Sgarbossa's scoring system.[22] Extreme caution should be used before adopting this approach, since the median age of patients with chest pain and LBBB is 74 years, which may lead to increased mortality with overaggressive thrombolysis.[4] More work must be done before ACS can be easily diagnosed in the setting of LBBB.

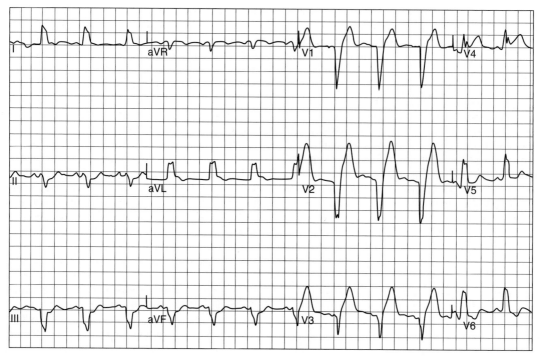

Fig. 8-4. Left bundle branch block and acute infarction. ST segment elevation concordant with the major component of the QRS complex in lead V4, V5 and aVL; ST segment elevation greater than 0.5 mV in leads V2 and V3 (discordant with QRS).

Right Bundle Branch Block

RBBB is identified by (1) QRS duration $\geq$120 ms, (2) rsR′ pattern in leads V_1 or V_2, (3) S wave $\geq$40 ms in leads I and V_6, and (4) R peak duration $\geq$50 ms in lead V_1 but normal in leads V_5 and V_6.[15] Unlike LBBB, the conduction defect in RBBB rarely obscures ischemic changes in the ST segment and T wave.[4] RBBB may itself be caused by ischemia of portions of the conducting system.

Ventricular Paced Rhythms

The difficulty in identifying ACS in a paced rhythm is similar to that associated with LBBB. In this case, repolarization forces with polarity opposite that of the QRS complex alter the morphology of the ST segment and the T wave. Sgarbossa et al. evaluated 17 patients with AMI and VPR using the same three criteria used for LBBB, though no scoring system was developed in this study. The results were similar. For the individual criteria, the sensitivity was low and ranged from 18 to 53%. The

specificity was better (82–94%), but still of marginal diagnostic utility.[24]

Left Ventricular Aneurysm

An LVA is a segment of infarcted myocardium that moves dyskinetically during systole and diastole and may be found in 3–15% of post-MI patients. The ECG from these patients reveals STE of varying morphology (usually concave) in leads associated with the location of the aneurysm. This elevation is likely caused by ischemia or wall stress within the LVA. Well-developed Q waves are frequently present.[25]

Pericarditis

While pericarditis may occur following AMI, multiple other etiologies exist. The STE seen in acute pericarditis is usually concave and diffuse, occurring in multiple anatomically disparate leads, though isolated STE has been encountered. Leads V_1 and aVR differ; STD is the norm if ST-segment changes are present in these leads. In addition, PR depression may occur, indicating atrial involvement. A similar PR pattern can be encountered with atrial infarction.[4,16,19]

Benign Early Repolarization

BER is a normal variant of the ECG and may be caused by early repolarization processes, but the exact etiology is not known. This results in an elevated, concave ST segment with a notched or slurred J point and upright, symmetric, tall T waves. The precordial leads are most likely to show this pattern; it is rarely seen in isolated limb leads. BER is not associated with underlying CAD and is found in various proportions of the population in all ages and various ethnic groups.[11,19]

Wolff-Parkinson-White

WPW syndrome results from an accessory pathway that manifests itself as a short PR interval and a delta wave at the onset of the QRS. Pinski et al.[26] analyzed six patients with WPW and STE enrolled in an acute fibrinolytic trial. AMI was subsequently diagnosed by elevated CK-MB in five of them. Though this was a very small study, the authors concluded that STE in the setting of WPW is a reasonably specific finding of AMI. Further validation of these findings is necessary.

ST Depression

Isolated STD is another important finding in the diagnosis of ACS and is thought to occur from subendocardial ischemia. The ECG shows a depressed J point with a downward sloping ST segment, though the segment may be horizontal or upward sloping. The latter is less often associated with ischemia. STD may be diffuse, but it often appears in anatomically contiguous groups of leads.[12]

As many as 48–67% of patients with STD on the presenting ECG are ultimately diagnosed with NSTEMI.[2,3] Savonitto found isolated STD in 35% of patients presenting with AMI; the 30-day mortality and reinfarction rate was 10.5% (similar to STE patients).[2] Miller found a much lower incidence of isolated STD (11.8%) but a higher 28-day mortality rate (13.1%).[5] The severity of STD is indicative of mortality and reinfarction rate during initial hospitalization for patients with NSTEMI, according to Hyde et al. In this study, patients with 0.05 mV STD had a complication rate of 2%, while

patients with 0.1 mV and ≥0.2 mV STD had higher rates (7.7% and 24%, respectively). In the long term, Hyde documented a 30% 4-year mortality rate for patients with ≥0.05 mV of STD on the presenting ECG, and the exact degree of STD continued to influence mortality.[27] Unfortunately, these patients do not receive the same benefit from thrombolytics as patients with STEMI;[4] Hyde noted that "hospital revascularization did not predict late survival" in his NSTEMI patients, though subsequent revascularization did improve long-term outcome.[27] The reasons for this are not known, and it is unclear whether these patients should be managed with aggressive interventions or more conservative management. However, the current trend is to manage these patients aggressively if they have dynamic ST-segment changes and elevated cardiac markers—indicators of AMI.

There is an exception to this principle. Patients with isolated STD in leads V_1 and V_2 may benefit from thrombolysis. This pattern can be seen with posterior MI, and since the current 12-lead does not adequately image the posterior wall of the left ventricle, STE may not be detected. STD in leads opposite the posterior segment may be the only ECG change evident.[4]

The differential diagnosis of STD includes LVH with strain pattern, hypokalemia, digitalis effect, and hyperventilation. Perhaps the most important alternative diagnosis in the patient with chest pain and STD is thoracic aortic dissection. These patients may have CK elevations, and myocardial ischemia does occur if the dissection extends to the coronary vasculature.[4,12] A chest radiograph should be reviewed in all patients to evaluate the mediastinum for aortic dissection, especially when considering the use of heparin or thrombolytics. Administration of these medications can be a critical error in patients with dissection.

Reciprocal ST Depression

STD may occur concomitantly with STE. The morphology is the same as for isolated STD and likely results from either regional ischemia or "mirroring" in which the injury current is reflected in leads 180° from the site of injury.[4] In other words, a negative electrical current depresses the ST segment in leads opposite from the leads with STE. Historically, the ECG finding of STE and STD together has been considered relatively specific for AMI; 89% of such patients were diagnosed with MI in Savonitto's study.[2] Brady et al. did not find these changes to be as useful. Initially, they determined the sensitivity to be 63% with a specificity of 34% and found that STD was present with equal frequency in STE from ischemic and nonischemic causes. Once confounding factors were controlled (LVH, BBB, VPR), the sensitivity and specificity improved significantly to 69% and 93%, respectively.[28]

Reciprocal changes are seen in approximately 75% of inferior AMIs and in 30% of anterior AMIs. They have prognostic importance, and patients with STEMI and STD have a higher morbidity and mortality.[12] Miller et al. found this pattern in 35.2% of patients presenting with AMI, which was associated with a 13.8% 28-day mortality rate.[5] Savonitto et al. had a lower incidence of STE with STD (15% of AMIs), but they, too, had a high 30-day death and reinfarction rate (12.4%). Savonitto et al. also noted that STD, both isolated and with concomitant STE, was associated with a higher incidence of three-vessel CAD. Patients with STEMI and STD also had larger infarctions, worse left ventricular ejection fractions, and more significant symptoms of congestive heart failure.[2]

QRS Complex Changes

The QRS complex results from depolarization of the ventricles and normally has a duration ≤120 ms. The Q wave, if present, is usually small (<0.5 mV) and of short duration. A pathologic Q wave is defined as having a duration ≥40 ms and appearing in two or more anatomic leads. Some consider an amplitude >25% of the height of the R wave abnormal, though this is not as reliable a finding.[15] In the setting of ACS, an abnormal Q wave is diagnostic of MI.

The appearance of Q waves is not the only QRS change that may be present in ACS. Anterior myocardial ischemia may affect the conduction system and produce BBBs (both right and left). Even in the absence of BBBs, AMI may cause widening of the QRS complex, which has prognostic significance. Brilakis et al. noted that a QRS duration ≥100 ms without BBB in 369 patients with NSTEMI was associated with increased mortality during hospitalization and at 5-year postinfarction. Five-year survival rates were 52.2% for these patients, compared to 74.3% for patients with a normal QRS duration. The reasons for this are not clear, though prolonged QRS may indicate multivessel CAD and decreased left ventricular function. This finding was not duplicated in patients with STEMI.[29]

Q wave Myocardial Infarction

While pathologic Q waves are considered diagnostic for MI, inferior Q waves may be present in 12% of young,

healthy men. In AMI, they usually appear 8–12 hours after vessel occlusion, but they have been noted as early as 1 or 2 hours after the onset of myocardial damage.[12] Some patients may not develop Q waves until 3 days after AMI, even without extension of the infarction. The development of pathologic Q waves has prognostic value, and MIs have been classified as Q wave MI (QMI) or non-Q wave MI (NQMI), replacing previous terminology of transmural and nontransmural infarctions, respectively. While QMI is associated with a larger area of infarction and increased periinfarction mortality, NQMI has a higher incidence of angina and recurrent infarction, likely due to incomplete occlusion of the coronary artery with quicker return of blood flow to ischemic segments.[30]

Since Q waves appear later than ST-segment changes, the development of Q waves in the acute setting is less practical than the STEMI criteria used for administering reperfusion therapy. Another limitation of Q waves is their permanence; Q waves without ST-segment changes preclude exact dating of the infarction. Old infarctions may further complicate the diagnosis of ACS by masking changes in an area of reinfarction. Fortunately, Q waves are rarely the only acute ECG change in AMI; they are usually accompanied by other ECG changes indicative of ischemia.[3,12]

Non-Q wave Myocardial Infarction

Some authors suggest that NSTEMI has actually replaced the category of NQMI.[12] This is not completely accurate; while most STEMI patterns result in Q waves, almost half of NQMIs present with STEMI. It is difficult to describe "classic" patterns of non-Q wave AMI, though three ECG types are frequently associated with NQMI. The first has convex STE with T-wave inversion. The second has STD ≥0.1 mV, and the third lacks obvious ST-segment changes, though nonspecific changes may be present.

Again, NQMI is usually associated with incomplete occlusion of coronary arteries. This results in less extensive infarction than in QMI and quicker return of blood flow. Resolution of coronary vasospasm and a higher degree of blood vessel collateralization may further limit infarct size. However, this incomplete occlusion leaves areas of myocardium at increased risk for recurrent events.

NQMIs comprise 37–59% of AMIs and are frequently complicated by congestive heart failure (25%) and cardiogenic shock (18%) during hospitalization. Predictors of a worse short-term outcome include previous MI or other cardiac events, diabetes, hypertension, and LVH. The in-hospital mortality rate is less than 10%, which is lower than the rate for QMI, but the long-term complication and mortality rate is equal to or greater than that for QMI.[30]

Bundle Branch Blocks

BBBs not only confound the diagnosis of STE, but the altered QRS morphology of LBBB and VPR precludes the identification of new Q waves. Further, the presence of BBB portends a worse outcome for patients with AMI. While a new BBB is highly suggestive of ACS, it is difficult or impossible to determine the acuity of this finding in many cases. In a retrospective study of nearly 300,000 patients with AMI, Go et al. found that all BBBs (acute and chronic) were associated with increased in-hospital mortality. LBBB had a 34% increase in mortality rate (odds ratio 1.34), though this could largely be explained by the fact that patients with BBB were older, had more comorbid conditions and were less likely to receive thrombolysis. RBBB was an independent predictor of mortality with a 64% increased rate (OR 1.64), even after adjustment for comorbities.[31]

Three percent of AMI patients in Miller's study presented with new LBBB. This group had the highest mortality of all ECG patterns analyzed (22.2% 28-day mortality) and the longest average length of hospital stay (12.5 days). Further, new LBBB was associated with the worst long-term outcome with a 20% 8-year survival rate.[5]

Other ECG Changes

Many other nonspecific ECG changes may be seen in AMI. The QT interval may lengthen, shorten, or remain unchanged. Inversion or amplification of U waves can occur. Ventricular arrhythmias, including premature ventricular contractions (PVCs), ventricular fibrillation (VF), and ventricular tachycardia (VT) are seen. Sinus tachycardia and atrial rhythms, such as atrial fibrillation and atrial flutter may also occur in AMI.[13,15] In fact, ACS

should be considered in all patients with unexplained, new arrhythmias.

Reperfusion can also cause arrhythmias. Accelerated idioventricular rhythms and PVCs are commonly seen, benign patterns. VF and VT may also be seen, though these are much less common and may indicate ongoing ischemia.[13]

Nondiagnostic and Normal ECGs

Unfortunately, a normal ECG does not preclude the diagnosis of ACS and was the presenting pattern in 18.5% of Miller's AMI patients, associated with a 6.0% 28-day mortality.[5] However, other studies have found that only 1% of patients discharged home with a normal ECG are subsequently diagnosed with AMI. A nondiagnostic ECG has a similarly favorable prognosis for AMI, though it does not rule out ischemia. ST changes <100 µV in two contiguous leads without pathologic Q waves, conduction abnormalities, or T-wave inversion qualify as nondiagnostic changes. Underdiagnosis is frequent in this setting, and patients with nondiagnostic ECGs account for over 50% of missed AMIs and over 60% of missed USAPs.[3]

SPECIFIC ANATOMIC PATTERNS OF ISCHEMIA

ECG changes associated with ACS require findings in two contiguous leads. The leads involved in ischemic change offer insight into the location of the at-risk myocardium and the culprit artery. To truly understand this, it is easiest to review the principal locations of ischemia with the subsequent ECG changes (Table 8-1). Remember that the right ventricle and posterior left ventricle are not adequately imaged by the current 12-lead ECG. While the following principles are generally accurate, variations in individual coronary artery anatomy, as well as

Table 8-1. Coronary Artery and ECG Lead Correlation with Anatomic Ischemia

Anatomic Location	**Occluded Artery**	**Ischemic Leads**	**Reciprocal Leads**
Anterior wall	LAD	V_2, V_3, V_4	II, III, aVF
Lateral wall	LCx	I, aVL, V_5, V_6	V_1, V_2
Inferior wall	RCA (90%), LCx	II, III, aVF	Varies
Posterior wall	LCx	V_8, V_9	V_1, V_2
Right ventricle	RCA, rarely LCx	V_1, V_4R	Varies

Abbreviations: LAD, Left anterior descending, LCx, Left circumflex, RCA, Right coronary artery.

prior coronary artery bypass surgery, prior infarction, and collateral circulation limit their specificity.[13]

Anterior Ischemia

Anterior ischemia results from occlusion of the LAD artery. ECG changes, especially STE, are noted in leads V_2, V_3, and V_4, though they are most prominent in leads V_2 or V_3. When the interventricular septum is affected, BBBs, especially RBBB or bifascicular blocks, may develop. Atrioventricular (AV) blocks may also be seen with septal ischemia and infarction. Leads I, aVL, V_5, and V_6 can show ischemic changes if the lateral wall of the ventricle is involved.

With STE, reciprocal STD can be seen in the inferior leads (II, III, and aVF), especially in the setting of proximal LAD occlusion, which indicates a larger infarction and worse prognosis. If STE is seen in leads I and aVL with anterior ischemia and reciprocal changes, the lesion is proximal to the origin of the first diagonal branch. This finding has been termed an anterolateral or "high lateral" pattern. Distal LAD occlusion usually does not cause such diffuse ST changes or inferior reciprocal STD, though STE may be present in the inferior leads if the LAD "wraps around" the apex of the heart.

Lateral Ischemia

The ECG is not as sensitive a tool for the diagnosis of lateral ischemia; STE in the lateral leads (I, aVL, V_5, and V_6) is present in less than half of AMI patients. Occlusion of the left circumflex (LCx) artery is responsible for ECG changes that occur with isolated ischemia in this area. The LCx supplies a relatively small myocardial area, which explains the inconsistent presence of ECG findings. In fact, one-third of patients may have a normal ECG, and another third will have STD, especially in leads V_1 and V_2. A more common finding is lateral ischemia associated with ECG changes elsewhere, such as anterolateral or inferolateral ischemia. The former is related to LAD occlusion, while the latter is caused by right coronary artery (RCA) occlusion.

Posterior Ischemia

Isolated posterior ischemia is a rare finding. Usually, ischemic changes occur in concert with ischemia in other anatomic distributions. For instance, occlusion of the RCA (and its posterior descending branch) will cause inferior and posterior ischemia, while LCx lesions will affect the lateral and posterior walls. With inferior ischemia, posterior involvement indicates a larger infarct and worse prognosis.

Since the 12-lead ECG does not adequately image electrical activity in the posterior wall of the heart, ischemic changes are mirrored in the anterior leads (V_1, V_2, and occasionally V_3). Instead of STE in these leads, STD with a tall R wave and an upright T wave is very suggestive of posterior ACS and infarction. Using the additional leads of V_8 and V_9 is more effective than evaluating the anterior leads and will clarify the ST changes and the diagnosis of posterior ischemia.

Inferior Ischemia

The majority of inferior ischemia is caused by occlusion of the RCA, though the LCx artery may be the culprit in 10–20% of cases. ECG changes are evident in leads II, III, and aVF. Greater STE in lead III than lead II with reciprocal STD in leads I and aVL suggests that the RCA is the source of the ischemia (sensitivity 90%, specificity 71%). Reciprocal changes in the precordial leads (V_1–V_3) indicate that the LCx is occluded, especially when STE is noted in the lateral leads (sensitivity 83%, specificity 96%). The absence of STD in leads V_1 and V_2 effectively rules out LCx involvement. Additional leads may assist with identification of the culprit artery. STE in leads V_8 and V_9 with STD in lead V_4R is more often seen with LCx occlusion. In some cases of STE, the ischemic changes extend to V_5 and V_6, indicating a significant degree of affected myocardium and a worse prognosis. This may occur with both RCA and LCx occlusion.

Conduction abnormalities are fairly common with inferior ischemia and may occur up to a few days after injury. Sinus bradycardia and AV blocks, including complete AV block with a narrow complex escape rhythm, may develop. This usually occurs early in the course of ischemia. Early presentations are generally self-limited and resolve within 24 hours; atropine is effective therapy for associated hemodynamic instability. When AV blocks occur later in the course, they can be more resistant to medications and may require a temporary or permanent pacemaker.

Right Ventricular Ischemia

Ischemic changes in leads V_1 and V_2, especially STE, are specific for RCA occlusion proximal to the right ventricular (RV) branch with resulting RV ischemia. Usually this occurs in association with inferior ischemia, and RV infarction occurs in 25–40% of inferior AMIs. Posterior infarction may be present as well, which can alter the appearance of STE in the precordial leads. ECG changes may extend as far laterally as lead V_5, indicating anterior involvement. Rarely, RV ischemia may be seen with lateral ischemia and occlusion of the LCx artery. Again, the right ventricle is not adequately imaged by the current 12-lead ECG, and the addition of a right-sided lead (V_4R) will increase the sensitivity of the ECG for ischemic changes, though this elevation can be short-lived, often resolving within 12 hours of infarction. RV infarction may be complicated by complete AV block and hypotension requiring pacing and/or preload support with intravenous fluids.[4,8,12,13]

TECHNOLOGIC ADVANCES

A major limitation of the 12-lead ECG is its static nature in the face of dynamic waveform changes seen with ACS; the ECG typically records only a 10-s period of electrical activity. While up to half of all patients with AMI present to the emergency department with normal or nondiagnostic ECGs, 20% of these patients will develop waveform changes consistent with ACS early in their hospitalization. In order to increase the sensitivity of the ECG for detecting ischemia, obtaining serial ECGs is an important process in the evaluation of ACS. This begins by comparing the presenting ECG with a prior ECG, if readily available.[12,32]

If no diagnostic ECG changes are evident on the initial tracing, serial ECGs may identify evolution of ST-segment changes. Patients with progressive STE may qualify for thrombolytics or other revascularization procedures. Even without STE, other ECG changes, like STD, may prompt the clinician to admit the patient for further cardiac testing.

ST-Segment Monitoring

While the traditional method of evaluating serial ECGs is to obtain 12-lead tracings at various time intervals, it is not the most efficient technique. Monitoring of the ST segment is a variation on the theme of serial ECGs. This technique relies on continuous computer monitoring of the ST segment with tracings obtained every 30–60 s. Alarms sound when ST changes (elevation or depression) are detected. This may be especially helpful in the setting of confounding patterns, like LBBB and LVH.[32]

Fesmire et al. in a prospective observational study, demonstrated that serial ECGs with ST-segment monitoring increased the diagnostic sensitivity (68.1% vs. 55.4% for AMI) and specificity (99.4% vs. 97.1% for ACS) when compared with the initial 12-lead ECG. In

this study, serial ECGs found ischemic changes in 16.2% more patients ultimately diagnosed with AMI than did the single ECG.[33] Serial ECGs are also important for risk stratification, with dynamic ST changes associated with a higher rate of cardiac mortality.[34]

Overall, there are limited data on the use of ST segment (STS) monitoring with serial ECGs. The Agency for Healthcare Research and Quality (AHRQ) released a technology review in 2001 that found insufficient data to form "a conclusion about the utility of this technology."[35] Despite this lack of endorsement, serial ECGs with STS monitoring have become a central component of various chest pain evaluation protocols.[36,37]

The primary limitations of ST-segment monitoring are false positives related to movement artifact. This usually occurs with body positional change, though lead misplacement, heart rate change, and transient arrhythmia may also affect the STS monitoring. Finally, some patients have acute changes in the voltage of the QRS complex and ST segment, altering the ST morphology and triggering alarms.[38]

Prehospital 12-Lead ECG

Serial ECG monitoring can begin before the patient arrives in the emergency department. Since the mid-1980s, 12-lead monitors have become increasingly prevalent in EMS systems. Critics have suggested that obtaining a 12-lead ECG in the prehospital setting delays transport to the hospital for definitive treatment and that paramedics should not be interpreting these ECGs. Kudenchuk et al. demonstrated that prehospital ECGs increased the sensitivity for detecting ACS,[39] while the AHRQ technology report acknowledged that transport times were not increased by obtaining a 12-lead ECG.[35] Most importantly, obtaining prehospital ECGs can reduce the time to thrombolytic administration by at least 20 min in some studies and more in others. With cellular communications readily available in many areas, prehospital ECGs can be obtained and transmitted to the receiving hospital for physician interpretation, though several studies have indicated that trained paramedics are greater than 90% accurate at detecting ECG changes consistent with probable infarction.[40] Barring financial limitations, this technology should be considered for all EMS agencies, especially in areas with longer transport times.

Neural Networks

Another technique for improving ECG sensitivity for ACS changes uses of computer interpretation of the ECG.

Artificial neural networks involve "training" a computer to recognize ischemic changes with a method of continuously reevaluating diagnostic criteria to improve sensitivity, essentially allowing the computer system to learn from its mistakes. This is especially useful for less experienced clinicians, though Heden et al. demonstrated an improved sensitivity for AMI detection when compared with a trained cardiologist.[41,42] Currently, there are little data on outcomes to support the routine use of this technology.[3]

15-Lead ECG

As previously discussed, the current 12-lead ECG has limitations and may miss changes associated with both posterior and RV ischemia. There is some thought that 15-lead ECGs should be standard, adding leads V_8 and V_9 for posterior changes, as well as lead V_4R to detect right-sided ischemia. To obtain a 15-lead ECG, the standard 12 leads are placed in the usual positions. Leads V_8 and V_9 are placed on the posterior thorax at the level of the anterior 5th intercostal space, with V_8 at the midscapular line and V_9 along the left paraspinal border. V_4R is attached to the right side of the chest, mirroring the position of V_4.[12] Despite the theoretical benefits of 15-lead ECG, two studies by Brady et al. and Zalenski et al. failed to demonstrate a clinically significant difference in the detection of ischemic changes in these areas. Clinicians did feel that the 15-lead ECG provided a more complete anatomic picture when ischemia was present, but the use of additional leads was not critical during routine ECG evaluation. While the use of additional leads may provide useful information in the setting of inferior and lateral ischemia,[43,44] further studies are needed to confirm this benefit.

CONCLUSIONS

The 12-lead ECG is a critical component of the early diagnosis of ACS, despite its imperfect sensitivity and specificity. With a goal of shortening the time to definitive treatment, ischemic changes in the ST segment have become a critical component of the criteria for reperfusion strategy. Specifically, STE must be recognized expeditiously to use revascularization therapies quickly and appropriately. This is not always easy due to multiple confounding patterns for STE; a thorough understanding of the differential diagnosis of STE is essential.

Several ECG patterns are associated with ACS and impending infarction. While some ST and T-wave changes may not qualify for reperfusion therapy, their importance and prognostic value should be recognized. The only truly diagnostic finding for MI is the pathologic Q wave. Unfortunately, these usually present several hours into the tissue necrosis and are less practical as a criteria for thrombolytic therapy.

Finally, a normal initial ECG does not rule out ACS, and the use of serial ECGs increases the sensitivity for detecting ischemic changes. This can begin with prehospital ECGs, which have been shown to shorten the time to thrombolytic administration. Serial ECGs with ST-segment monitoring are gaining popularity in the diagnosis of ACS. While these technologic advances are helpful in detecting ischemia, they are best used in conjunction with a thorough history and physical examination, serum markers of cardiac necrosis, and clinical acumen for detecting ACS.

REFERENCES

1. Fisch C. Centennial of the string galvanometer and the electrocardiogram. *J Am Coll Cardiol* 2000;36:1737–1745.
2. Savonitto S, Ardissino D, Granger CB, et al. Prognostic value of the admission electrocardiogram in acute coronary syndromes. *JAMA* 1999;281:707–713.
3. Pope JH, Selker HP. Diagnosis of acute cardiac ischemia. *Emerg Med Clin N Am* 2003;21:27–59.
4. Sgarbossa EB, Birnbaum Y, Parrillo JE. Electrocardiographic diagnosis of acute myocardial infarction: Current concepts for the clinician. *Am Heart J* 2001;141:507–517.
5. Miller WL, Sgura FA, Kopecky SL, et al. Characteristics of presenting electrocardiograms of acute myocardial infarction from a community-based population predict short-and long-term mortality. *Am J Cardiol* 2001;87:1045–1050.
6. Anderson ST, Pahlm O, Selvester RH, et al. Panoramic display of the orderly sequenced 12-lead EKG. *J Electrocardiol* 1994;27:347–352.
7. Thygesen T, Alpert JS, et al. Myocardial infarction redefined—A consensus document of the Joint European Society of Cardiology/American College of Cardiology Committee for the redefinition of myocardial infarction. *J Am Coll Cardiol* 2000;36:959–969.
8. Horacek BM, Wagner GS. Electrocardiographic ST-segment changes during acute myocardial ischemia. *Cardiac Electrophysiol Rev* 2002;6:196–203.
9. Sharkey SW, Berger CR, Brunette DD, et al. Impact of the electrocardiogram on the delivery of thrombolytic therapy for acute myocardial infarction. *Am J Cardiol* 1994;73:550–553.
10. Bahit MC, Criger DA, Ohman EM, et al. Thresholds for the electrocardiographic change range of biochemical markers of acute myocardial infarction (GUSTO-IIa data). *Am J Cardiol* 2002;90:233–237.

11. Somers MP, Brady WJ, Perron AP, et al. The prominent T wave: Electrocardiographic differential diagnosis. *Am J Emerg Med* 2002;20:243–251.

12. Brady WJ, Aufderheide TP, Chan T, et al. Electrocardiographic diagnosis of acute myocardial infarction. *Emerg Med Clin N Am* 2001;19:295–320.

13. Zimetbaum PJ, Josephson ME. Use of the electrocardiogram in acute myocardial infarction. *N Engl J Med* 2003;348:933–940.

14. Rhinehardt J, Brady WJ, Perron AD, et al. Electrocardiographic manifestations of Wellens' syndrome. *Am J Emerg Med* 2002;20:638–643.

15. Surawicz B, Knilans TK. *Chou's Electrocardiography in Clinical Practice.* Philadelphia, PA: W.B. Saunders, 2001.

16. Wang K, Asinger RW, Marriott HJL. ST-segment elevation in conditions other than acute myocardial infarction. *N Engl J Med* 2003;349:2128–2135.

17. Brady WJ, Syverud SA, Beagle C, et al. Electrocardiographic ST-segment elevation: The diagnosis of acute myocardial infarction by morphologic analysis of the ST segment. *Acad Emerg Med* 2001;8:961–967.

18. Brady WJ, Perron AD, Martin ML, et al. Cause of ST segment abnormality in ED chest pain patients. *Am J Emerg Med* 2001;19:25–28.

19. Brady WJ. Benign early repolarization: Electrocardiographic manifestations and differentiation from other ST segment elevation syndromes. *Am J Emerg Med* 1998;16:592–597.

20. Sgarbossa EB, Pinski SL, Barbagelata A, et al. Electrocardiographic diagnosis of evolving acute myocardial infarction in the presence of left bundle-branch block. *N Engl J Med* 1996;334:481–487.

21. Shapiro NI, Fisher J, Zimmer GD, et al. Validation of electrocardiographic criteria for diagnosing acute myocardial infarction in the presence of left bundle branch block [abstract]. *Acad Emerg Med* 1998;5:508–509.

22. Shlipak MG, Lyons WL, Go AS, et al. Should the electrocardiogram be used to guide therapy for patients with left bundle-branch block and suspected myocardial infarction? *JAMA* 1999;281:714–719.

23. Gula LJ, Dick A, Massel D. Diagnosing acute myocardial infarction in the setting of left bundle branch block: Prevalence and observer variability from a large community study. *Coronary Artery Dis* 2003;14:387–393.

24. Sgarbossa EB, Pinski SL, Gates KB, et al. Early electrocardiographic diagnosis of acute myocardial infarction in the presence of ventricular paced rhythm. *Am J Cardiol* 1996;77:423–424.

25. Engel J, Brady WJ, Mattu A, et al. Electrocardiographic ST segment elevation: Left ventricular aneurysm. *Am J Emerg Med* 2002;20:238–242.

26. Pinski SL, Sgarbossa EB, Wagner GS, et al. Electrocardiographic manifestations of acute myocardial infarction in patients with Wolff-Parkinson-White syndrome [abstract]. *PACE* 1995;18:1739.

27. Hyde TA, French JK, Wong CK, et al. Four-year survival of patients with acute coronary syndromes without ST-segment elevation and prognostic significance of 0.5-mm ST-segment depression. *Am J Cardiol* 1999;84:379–385.

28. Brady WJ, Perron AD, Syverud SA, et al. Reciprocal ST segment depression: Impact on the electrocardiographic diagnosis of ST segment elevation acute myocardial infarction. *Am J Emerg Med* 2002;20:35–38.

29. Brilakis ES, Mavrogiorgos NC, Kopecky SL, et al. Usefulness of QRS duration in the absence of bundle branch block as an early predictor of survival in non-ST elevation acute myocardial infarction. *Am J Cardiol* 2002;89:1013–1018.

30. Liebson PR, Klein LW. The non-Q wave myocardial infarction revisited: 10 years later. *Prog Cardiovas Dis* 1997;39:399–444.

31. Go AS, Barron HV, Rundle AC, et al. Bundle-branch block and in-hospital mortality in acute myocardial infarction. *Ann Intern Med* 1998;129:690–697.

32. Velez J, Brady WJ, Perron AD, et al. Serial electrocardiography. *Am J Emerg Med* 2002;20:43–49.

33. Fesmire FM, Percy RF, Bardoner JB, et al. Usefulness of automated serial 12-lead ECG monitoring during the initial emergency department evaluation of patients with chest pain. *Ann Emerg Med* 1998;31:3–11.

34. Jernberg T, Lindahl B, Wallentin L. ST-segment monitoring with continuous 12-lead ECG improves early risk stratification in patients with chest pain and ECG nondiagnostic of acute myocardial infarction. *J Am Coll Cardiol* 1999;34:1413–1419.

35. Lau J, Ioannidis JPA, Balk EM, et al. for the Agency for Healthcare Research and Quality: Evaluation of technologies for identifying acute cardiac ischemia in emergency departments. *Evid Rep Technol Assess* 2001;26:1–15.

36. Fesmire FM, Hughes AD, Fody EP, et al. The Erlanger chest pain evaluation protocol: A one-year experience with serial 12-lead ECG monitoring, two-hour delta serum marker measurements, and selective nuclear stress testing to identify and exclude acute coronary syndromes. *Ann Emerg Med* 2002;40:584–594.

37. Zalenski RJ, McCarren M, Roberts R, et al. An evaluation of a chest pain diagnostic protocol to exclude acute cardiac ischemia in the emergency department. *Arch Intern Med* 1997;157:1085–1091.

38. Drew BJ, Wung SF, Adams MG, et al. Bedside diagnosis of myocardial ischemia with ST-segment monitoring technology: Measurement issues for real-time clinical decision-making and trial designs. *J Electrocardiol* 1998;30(Suppl):157–165.

39. Kudenchuk PJ, Maynard C, Cobb LA, et al. Utility of the prehospital electrocardiogram in diagnosing acute coronary syndromes: The myocardial infarction triage and intervention (MITI) project. *J Am Coll Cardiol* 1998;32:17–27.

40. Ferguson JD, Brady WJ, Perron AD, et al. The prehospital 12-lead electrocardiogram: Impact on management of the out-of-hospital acute coronary syndrome patient. *Am J Emerg Med* 2003;21:136–142.

41. Cross SS, Harrison RF, Kennedy RL. Introduction to neural networks. *Lancet* 1995;346:1075–1079.
42. Heden B, Ohlin H, Rittner R, et al. Acute myocardial infarction detected in the 12-lead ECG by artificial neural networks. *Circulation* 1997;96:1798–1802.
43. Zalenski RJ, Rydman RJ, Sloan EP, et al. Value of posterior and right ventricular leads in comparison to the standard 12-lead electrocardiogram in evaluation of ST-segment elevation in suspected acute myocardial infarction. *Am J Cardiol* 1997;79:1579–1585.
44. Brady WJ, Hwang V, Sullivan R, et al. A comparison of 12- and 15-lead ECGs in ED chest pain patients: Impact on diagnosis, therapy, and disposition. *Am J Emerg Med* 2000;18:239–243.

9

Diagnosis
Serum Markers

Francis M. Fesmire

HIGH YIELD FACTS

- Troponins are highly sensitive to myocardial injury, and are therefore elevated in a number of nonacute coronary syndrome (non-ACS) diseases where myocardial oxygen delivery may not be adequate to meet demand.

- No single marker measurement has sufficient power to reliably identify or exclude acute myocardial infarction (AMI) within 6 hours of symptom onset.

- Serial multi-marker testing and the usage of delta marker strategies improve the testing offers increased sensitivity for AMI.

- It is important to recognize that "not AMI" does not equate to "not ACS," and evaluation strategies must be designed not only to detect AMI, but to risk stratify patients.

INTRODUCTION

Overview

The last 25 years have seen an explosion in research and development in cardiac markers for detection of AMI. In the 1980s, creatine kinase (CK)-MB enzyme activity supplanted lactate dehydrogenase (LDH) isoforms and total CK as the gold standard in the detection of myocardial necrosis. The mid-1990s led to the usage of cardiac-specific troponins (I and T) for the risk stratification of patients with ACS, though CK-MB mass was considered to be the proven marker for diagnosis of AMI. Now in the 2000s, AMI has been redefined with recommendations that the troponins be the definitive marker of myocardial necrosis. In addition to markers of necrosis, there are a whole host of new markers on the horizon, markers of ischemia, markers of inflammation, markers of failure, all of which may be useful in conjunction with markers

of necrosis in the overall risk stratification of patients with ACS.

In the following sections, we will first discuss World Health Organization (WHO) and European Society of Cardiology (ESC)/American College of Cardiology (ACC) definitions of AMI. We then will discuss the most common markers of myocardial necrosis, followed by a discussion of clinical decision making in the usage of individual markers, combination of markers (i.e., multimarker approach), and delta marker measurements for identification and exclusion of AMI. We will conclude with a brief discussion of point-of-care testing and new markers on the horizon that may prove to be useful in the evaluation and management of patients with suspected ACS. Finally, it must be emphasized that the majority of studies and recommendations discussed in this chapter are based on usage of WHO or modified WHO diagnostic criteria and may be outdated when applied against a 99th percentile troponin cutoff as the gold standard for diagnosing AMI.

AMI Definition

WHO Criteria

The WHO criteria developed in the 1970s defined AMI based on two of the following three criteria: typical ischemic chest discomfort (typically greater than 20 min), increase in total CK to two times upper limit of normal, or new Q waves on 12-lead electrocardiogram (ECG)[1,2] (Table 9-1). With the advent of the troponins, a population of patients with ACS was discovered who were CK-MB negative, but troponin positive. These patients were found to be at higher risk for adverse outcome with the recommendations that troponins were useful in the risk stratification of ACS patients.[3,4] The National Academy of Clinical Biochemistry published a consensus report in 1999 recommending the usage of two decision limits for the troponin assay: a low abnormal value identifying high-risk non-AMI ACS patients, and a higher value suggestive of AMI as defined by WHO criteria.[5]

ESC/ACC Criteria

Studies on the pathophysiology of AMI and troponin positive unstable angina have established a common pathway that is initiated by plaque rupture, thrombus formation, and subsequent myocardial necrosis. The extent of necrosis is influenced by a host of factors including degree of occlusion, degree of cholesterol embolism, and presence of collateral flow. As a result of this common pathway, the ESC and ACC published in

Table 9-1. WHO Diagnostic Criteria for Acute
Myocardial Infarction (One of following)

1. Definite ECG[*], or
2. Symptoms[†] typical or atypical or inadequately
   described, together with probable ECG[‡] and abnormal
   enzymes[§], or
3. Symptoms typical[†] and abnormal enzymes[§] with
   ischemic or noncodable ECG or ECG not available, or
4. Fatal case, whether sudden or not, with naked-eye
   appearance of fresh myocardial infarction and/or recent
   coronary occlusion found at necropsy.

[*]Definite ECG: (a) the development in serial records of a
diagnostic Q wave and/or (b) the evolution of an injury current
that lasts more than 1 day.
[†]Duration of more than 20 min.
[‡]Probable ECG: evolution of major ST elevation, major ST
depression, and/or major T-wave inversion.
[§]Abnormal enzymes: if at least one reading is more than twice
the upper limit of normal.
Source: Adapted from reference 2.

2000 new recommendations for the redefinition of
myocardial infarction.[6] This new definition of AMI
requires a typical rise and fall of biochemical markers of
myocardial necrosis with at least one of the following:
ischemic symptoms, development of pathologic Q waves
on the ECG, ECG changes indicative of ischemia, or
coronary artery intervention (Table 9-2). Furthermore,
the committee recommends that cardiac troponin I and

Table 9-2. ESC/ACC Diagnostic Criteria for Acute
Myocardial Infarction (One of following criteria)

Typical rise and gradual fall (troponin[*]) or more rapid
rise and fall (CK-MB[*]) of biochemical markers of
myocardial necrosis with at least one of the following:
   Ischemic symptoms
   Development of pathologic Q waves on the ECG
   ECG changes indicative of ischemia
   Coronary artery intervention
Pathologic findings of AMI

[*]An increased value for cardiac troponin or CK-MB should be
defined as one that exceeds the 99th percentile in a reference
control group. In most situations, elevated values for biomarkers
should be recorded from two successive blood samples to
diagnose MI. Cardiac troponins are the preferred biomarkers for
myocardial damage.
Source: Adapted from reference 6.

troponin T become the preferred markers of necrosis with
a cutoff level at the 99th percentile of the reference population. Despite these recommendations, few researchers
and clinicians have incorporated these recommendations
into actual practice. It currently is estimated that usage of
this new definition of AMI will result in an increase in
number of patients given a diagnosis of AMI by 25–200%
depending on the actual cutoff value used.[7–9]

COMMON MARKERS OF MYOCARDIAL NECROSIS

Overview

There has been much controversy in recent years
regarding which is the best marker of myocardial
necrosis. The ideal marker of myocardial necrosis should
appear in the plasma in the first hour of symptom onset,
be highly specific for cardiac necrosis, easily measured
by standard laboratory devices, and remain elevated for
days following the event. In the 1970s patients were
routinely admitted for 48–72 hours for rule out of AMI
with serial LDH isoenzymes and total CK measurements.
By the 1980s CK-MB activity was used to identify and
exclude myocardial infarction within 24 hours of presentation. In the early 1990s physicians were routinely
using CK-MB mass to identify AMI within 12 hours of
symptom. Now with frequent usage of multimarker and
delta approach, physicians are frequently ruling out AMI
within 3–6 hours of symptom onset.

The most common markers of myocardial necrosis are
CK-MB mass, myoglobin, and troponins. These markers
are proteins found within the myocytes of cardiac cells
that are released when myocytes are irreversibly injured.
Myoglobin and CK-MB are the first to be released from
the cytosol of the damaged cells (myoglobin sooner due
to its lower molecular weight). The troponin complex is
tightly bound to the fibers of the myocyte and has a
delayed release, though there is a small amount present
in the cytosol that has an early release. As a result of
these differences, the markers of necrosis each have
unique release and clearance properties. Figure 9-1 is a
typical graph of the release and clearance properties of
the common markers of myocardial necrosis following
AMI. Below, we discuss the common markers in more
detail.

Troponins

The troponins are regulatory proteins found in skeletal
and cardiac muscle. The troponin complex is made from

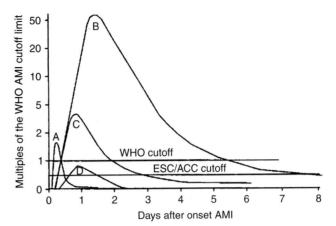

Fig. 9-1. Timing of release of common cardiac markers of necrosis. Peaks A, B, and C, respectively demonstrate release of myoglobin, troponin, and CK-MB in AMI as defined by WHO diagnostic criteria. Peak D demonstrates troponin release in troponin positive/CK-MB negative ACS now defined as AMI by ESC/ACC diagnostic criteria. (Source: Modified with permission from reference 5.)

three subunits that include troponin I, troponin T, and troponin C. The troponin C complex is identical in skeletal and cardiac muscle whereas the troponin T and troponin I complex are unique in skeletal and cardiac muscle. Thus, existing troponin assays are specific for the cardiac forms with essentially no cross-reactivity with skeletal proteins. When myocytes sustain irreversible damage, an early release of troponin is seen from the cytosolic fraction (3–6% of total). Troponin is cleared rapidly from the serum; however, there is a continued delayed release from the troponin complex that is structurally bound to the fibers of the myocyte, which accounts for its slower rise and persistent elevation as compared to CK-MB. In patients with transmural AMI, the troponins appear in the serum relatively early in symptom onset, peak at 24–36 hours, and remain elevated for 4–10 days. The first generation troponin assays were not able to detect myocardial necrosis reliably until approximately 8–12 hours after symptom onset. Newer generation troponins are now detecting myocardial necrosis in the initial hours of symptom onset.

Initial studies on cardiac troponin revealed a subset of ACS patients who were troponin positive but CK-MB negative. These patients had higher risk of adverse outcome as compared to troponin negative unstable angina patients but lower risk of adverse outcome as compared to patients with positive CK-MB and troponin.[3,4,10] In a recent study, Rao et al.[10] retrospectively analyzed 1852 patients from three previous prospective reports. Patients were grouped into one of four categories based on marker status: troponin negative/CK-MB negative; troponin negative/CK-MB positive; troponin positive/CK-MB negative; and troponin positive/CK-MB positive. The adjusted odds of death or MI occurring at 24 hours and 30 days was assessed by baseline marker status. The highest odds of 24-hour and 30-day adverse outcome occurred in patients with both markers positive. Intermediate risk was observed for patients who were troponin positive and CK-MB negative with lowest rate of risk seen in patients who were troponin negative and CK-MB negative. Current ACC/ESC recommendations would now classify these troponin positive/CK-MB negative patients as non-ST-segment elevation AMI although clearly there is a direct association between peak troponin value and increasing risk of adverse outcome.

As discussed earlier, the new ACC/ESC definition recommends usage of the 99th percentile as compared to a reference population for the definition of AMI. They furthermore recommend that the assay should have an imprecision (coefficient of variation) of ≤10% at this cutoff value. Unfortunately, few commercial assays meet this requirement. Also, unlike troponin T which has only one commercially assay available, there are dozens of commercially available troponin I assays. As there currently is no standardization in measurement of troponin I assays, further confusion results from the fact that there is up to a 100-fold difference in measurement of a fixed troponin sample among the different troponin I assays. Apple et al.[11] have attempted to minimize this confusion as well as to facilitate usage of the new ACC/ESC definition by publishing the lowest cutoff value above the 99th percentile for the commonly available troponin assays in which the imprecision is ≤10%. For the Roche Elecsys 3rd generation troponin T assay, the lowest cutoff value meeting these criteria is 0.035 ng/mL. Table 9-3 lists the lowest cutoff value with ≤10% imprecision above the 99th percentile for the most common commercially available troponin assays.

Further confusion results in determining how to implement these guidelines in the real world setting in which many nonischemic conditions exist that result in elevated troponins. Cardiomyopathy, congestive heart failure, hypertensive crisis, hypothyroidism, implantable defibrillators, myocarditis, pacing, renal failure, sepsis, shock, subarachnoid hemorrhage, and tachyarrhythmias are just a sample of the multitude of non-ACS diseases that have been associated with elevated troponin levels. Undoubtedly, many of these conditions result from myocardial oxygen supply not meeting oxygen demand with subsequent myocardial necrosis. The patient presenting with pulmonary edema, nondiagnostic ECG, and isolated elevated troponin presents a particular diagnostic dilemma frequently encountered in the real world setting. That is, did the patient have a myocardial infarction that caused the pulmonary edema, or did the pulmonary edema result in hypoxic injury to the heart with resultant myocardial necrosis? Irrespective of which came first, in

this condition and all other cardiac-related conditions, the higher the troponin elevation, the worse the prognosis.

CK-MB

CK, which is responsible for converting creatine phosphate and adenosine diphosphate to creatine and adenosine triphosphate, is composed of combinations of two possible subunits (M, muscle; B, brain). CK-BB is found in brain and kidney tissue. CK-MM is the predominate CK isoenzyme in both cardiac and skeletal muscle. However, CK-MB comprises approximately 25% of cardiac CK as compared to 0–3% of skeletal muscle CK. Initial assays used enzymatic activity to measure CK-MB whereas current assays are almost exclusively mass assays as measured by immunologic methods. CK is always present in circulation due to normal tissue turnover with significant individual variation depending on age, sex, weight, or race. In order to increase the specificity of the CK-MB assay, it is commonly recommended to use a CK-MB mass/total CK index of 2.5–3.0 in order to differentiate skeletal from myocardial damage. In patients with transmural AMI, CK-MB appears in the first hours of

Table 9-3. Recommended Cutoff Values for Current Commercial Assays for AMI Using ESC/ACC Criteria for Redefinition of AMI

	Generation	99th Percentile (ng/mL)	Recommended Cutoff (ng/mL)[*]
Troponin I assays			
Abott Axsym	1st	0.5	0.8
Bayer Immuno 1	1st	0.1	0.35
Bayer ACS: 180	1st	0.1	0.35
Bayer Centaur	1st	0.1	0.35
Beckman-Coulter Access	2nd	0.04	0.06
Biosite Triage	2nd	0.19	0.5
Dade Behring Dimension RxL	2nd	0.07	0.14
Dade Behring Stratus CS	2nd	0.07	0.07
Dade Behring Opus	1st	0.1	0.3
DPC Immulite	1st	0.2	0.6
i-STAT	1st	0.08	0.1
Ortho Vitros Eci	1st	0.08	0.12
Tosoh AIA	2nd	0.06	0.06
Troponin T Assay			
Roche Elecys	3rd	0.01	0.035

[*]Lowest cutoff value above 99% in which the assay imprecision is ≤10%.
Source: Modified with permission from reference 11.

symptom onset, reaches abnormal levels by 6–10 hours, peaks at 18–24 hours, and returns to baseline by 36–72 hours. As CK-MB is cleared from the plasma faster than CK-MM, patients with a delayed presentation may have a CK index suggesting skeletal muscle injury.

Measurements of CK-MB isoforms have increased the early sensitivity of CK-MB measurements. When CK-MB2 is released, MB2 is converted to MB1 by irreversible enzymatic cleavage. Normally the isoforms CK-MB1 and CK-MB2 exist in the plasma in equal concentrations. With myocardial injury, there is an increase in the ratio of MB2/MB1 within the initial hours of symptom onset. Studies have demonstrated an increased early sensitivity of CK-MB isoforms over CK-MB mass in the early detection of AMI. However, due to the technical expertise required to perform this assay, as well as to the availability of new generation troponin assays, it is doubtful this assay will ever be widespread in use.

Myoglobin

Myoglobin is a small protein abundant in the cytosol of all striated muscle cells. As a result, myoglobin is not a cardiac-specific marker. Due to its small size, myoglobin is released rapidly after myocardial cell necrosis and may appear as an abnormal level as early as 1 hour after symptom onset. Due to its rapid renal clearance, myoglobin may return to normal values as early as 6–8 hours after symptom onset. Due to its rapid clearance and lack of cardiospecificity, myoglobin should never be used as the sole marker of myocardial necrosis. Its best

usage appears to be for its ability to exclude AMI when used in conjunction with CK-MB and troponins.

Clinical Decision Making

Bayes' Theorem

As with any disease condition, the appropriate usage of laboratory test results requires an assessment of pretest probability. In the Erlanger Chest Pain Evaluation Protocol, chest pain patients with suspected ACS were risk stratified into four categories: category 1, ACS with clinical and ECG criteria for emergency reperfusion therapy; category 2, probable ACS with absence of clinical and ECG criteria for emergency reperfusion therapy; category 3, possible ACS; and category 4, probable non-ACS chest pain but presence of preexisting disease or significant risk factors for coronary artery disease warranting a screening evaluation. Reported rates of AMI for category 1 through 4 chest pain patients were approximately 95%, 50%, 10%, and 2%, respectively. Bayes' theorem states pretest odds of disease × likelihood ratio = posttest odds of a disease. Using the formula odds of a disease = probability of a disease/(1 − probability of a disease) converts the pretest odds of AMI into 19, 01, 0.11, and 0.02, respectively for category 1 through 4 patients, respectively. Traditional teaching is that a positive likelihood ratio ≥10 or negative likelihood ratio ≤0.1 should result in a change in clinical decision making.[12] Table 9-4 demonstrates the posttest odds and posttest probability for AMI after applying a hypothetical

Table 9-4. Utility of a Hypothetical Diagnostic Marker Test with Positive Likelihood Ratio[*] (+LR) = 10 for Identification of AMI and Negative Likelihood Ratio[†] (−LR) = 0.1 for Exclusion of AMI

		Identification of AMI (+LR = 10)	Exclusion of AMI (−LR = 0.1)
Erlanger CP Category (Prevalence AMI[‡])	Pretest Odds AMI	Posttest Odds[§] AMI (Probability[¶] %)	Posttest Odds AMI (Probability %)
1 (95%)	19	190 (99.5%)	1.9 (66%)
2 (50%)	1	10 (91%)	0.1 (9.1%)
3 (10%)	0.11	1.1 (53%)	0.01 (1.1%)
4 (2%)	0.02	0.2 (17%)	0.002 (0.2%)

[*]+LR = sensitivity/(1 − specificity).
[†]−LR = (1 − sensitivity)/specificity.
[‡]Prevalence AMI = pretest probability AMI.
[§]Odds of AMI = probability of a AMI/(1 − probability of AMI).
[¶]Probability of AMI = odds of AMI/(1 + odds of AMI).

cardiac marker test with a positive likelihood ratio = 10 and negative likelihood ratio = 0.1. As can be seen, the posttest probability for AMI of a positive test ranges from 17 to 99.5% depending on the chest pain category. Likewise, the posttest probability for AMI in patients with a negative test ranges from 0.2 to 66% depending on the chest pain category. In order to have a posttest probability of AMI of ≤0.5% (posttest odds = 0.005) for category 1 through category 4 patients would require a cardiac marker test with a negative likelihood ratio of 0.0003, 0.005, 0.05, and 0.25, respectively in order to exclude myocardial infarction with a miss rate of 1 in 200. Likewise, in order to have a posttest probability of AMI of ≥50% (posttest odds = 1) would require no serum marker testing for category 1 and 2 patients, and a cardiac marker test with positive likelihood ratio of 9.1 and 50 for category 3 and 4 patients, respectively. There are multiple websites on the Internet readily found with search engines that allows one to calculate the posttest probability using pretest probability and likelihood ratios. Figure 9-2 is a nomogram for converting pretest probabilities (left vertical axis) into posttest probabilities (right vertical axis) from likelihood ratio data.

Single Marker Usage

Table 9-5 is a summary of the relationship of reported sensitivities, specificities, positive likelihood ratios, and negative likelihood ratios for AMI of the common serum markers of necrosis in relationship to time of symptom

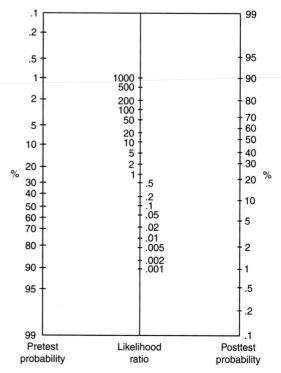

Fig. 9-2. Likelihood ratio nomogram: extension of a straight line, connecting the pretest probability (left vertical axis) with the likelihood ratio for a diagnostic test, determines the posttest probability (right vertical axis). (Source: Modified with permission from http://eduserv.hscer.washington.edu/physdx/glossary/likratio.html.)

Table 9-5. Relationship of Reported Sensitivities (Positive Likelihood Ratio) and Specificities (Negative Likelihood Ratio) for Acute Myocardial Infarction of Common Serum Markers in Relationship to Time of Symptom Onset

	CK-MB Mass		Myoglobin		Troponin T		Troponin I	
Time (h)	Sens (+LR)	Spec (−LR)	Sens (+LR)	Spec (−LR)	Sens (+LR)	Spec (−LR)	Sens (+LR)	Spec (−LR)
2	16% (19.8)	99% (0.85)	26% (2.1)	87% (0.84)	11% (6.6)	98% (0.91)	16% (4.9)	97% (0.87)
4	39% (32.8)	99% (0.61)	43% (4.0)	89% (0.64)	36% (6.2)	98% (0.68)	36% (6.2)	94% (0.68)
6	66% (4)	100% (0.34)	79% (7.4)	89% (0.24)	62% (15.8)	96% (0.40)	58% (10.1)	95% (0.45)
10	90% (226)	99.6% (0.10)	87% (8.8)	90% (0.15)	87% (24.0)	96% (0.14)	92% (17.1)	95% (0.08)
14	91% (82.3)	99% (0.10)	62% (5.3)	88% (0.43)	85% (21.8)	96% (0.16)	91% (11.6)	92% (0.10)
18	96% (239)	99.6% (0.04)	58% (5.1)	89% (0.48)	79% (18.3)	96% (0.22)	96% (14.5)	93% (0.05)
22	96% (106)	99% (0.04)	43% (4.9)	91% (0.63)	86% (15.9)	95% (0.15)	90% (15.5)	94% (0.11)

Abbreviations: Sens = sensitivity; Spec = specificity; +LR = positive likelihood ratio; −LR = negative likelihood ratio.
Source: Modified with permission from reference 13.

onset in the Diagnostic Cooperative Study.[13] An ideal single marker of cardiac necrosis should have a positive likelihood ≥10 and a negative likelihood ratio ≤0.01. No markers in the Diagnostic Cooperative Study fulfill this criterion within 6 hours of symptom onset. CK-MB mass and troponin I fulfill this criterion by 10 hours, and, myoglobin and troponin T never fulfill this criterion. As a result of these and similar findings in other studies, the 2000 clinical policy of the American College of Emergency Physicians[14] states as an Evidence-based Standard: "No single determination of one serum biochemical marker of myocardial necrosis reliably identifies or reliably excludes AMI less than 6 hours of symptom onset." The policy further recommends as a Guideline to perform repeat serum marker testing at 6–10 hours from symptom onset for CK-MB mass and subforms and 8–12 hours for the troponins prior to making an exclusionary diagnosis of non-AMI chest pain. A footnote cautions that if time of symptom onset is unknown, unreliable, or more consistent with preinfarctional angina, then time of symptom onset should be referenced to time of ED presentation. In order to increase the early sensitivity of AMI detection, the National Academy of Clinical Biochemistry recommends that one obtain an early marker of myocardial necrosis (e.g., myoglobin) in conjunction with a later definitive marker (e.g., troponin).[5]

It is important to recognize that the above recommendations for myoglobin, CK-MB mass, and troponins derive mainly from studies with first generation immunoassays using WHO or modified WHO diagnostic criteria. Clearly new CK-MB and troponin assays with analytical sensitivities <0.1 ng/mL are allowing the earlier detection of myocardial necrosis so that it is no longer clear which is the best early marker of myocardial necrosis. By default, due to the ESC/ACC redefinition of AMI, troponins are the best definitive marker of myocardial necrosis.

Multimarker Strategy

Due to the varying kinetics of release and clearance of the individual markers of necrosis, researchers and physicians have been employing measurements of combinations of the various individual markers of necrosis in order to maximize sensitivity. In the CHECKMATE Study, Newby et al. report on the use of the serial measurement of CK-MB, myoglobin, and troponin I in the risk stratification exclusion of 30-day AMI and death in 1005 patients.[15] The authors compared the strategy of CK-MB in conjunction with troponin I to the strategy of using all three markers in combination. The multimarker strategy of using all three markers identified more patients with 30-day death or AMI as compared to the strategy of using only CK-MB and troponin I. However, the sensitivity of the three-marker strategy for a 30-day outcome was only 23.9% with a specificity less than 50% thus limiting the usefulness of the multimarker approach for directing therapy. In a prospective observational study of 817 patients (65 AMI patients), McCord et al. report on a strategy of using a combination of myoglobin in conjunction with CK-MB or troponin I at baseline, 90 min, and 3 hours for the early exclusion of myocardial infarction (Table 9-6).[16] At baseline, the combination of myoglobin in conjunction with troponin I had a sensitivity of 85%, which increased in sensitivity to 97% at 90 min and outperformed all other marker combinations. The 3-hour blood draw resulted in a slight decrease in specificity without any increase in sensitivity. The authors conclude that serial measurements of myoglobin and troponin I at baseline and 90 min allow the early exclusion of AMI. As the specificity of the combination of myoglobin in conjunction with troponin I is 60% at 90 min, it is important to realize that one cannot diagnose AMI with this combination, but only exclude AMI. Patients with negative results can be entered into an unstable angina evaluation pathway if clinically indicated (e.g., early stress testing). Patients with positive results require additional testing to confirm or exclude the diagnosis of AMI.

Delta Marker Measurements

A different approach to identifying AMI with serum markers is to rely on time changes (delta changes) in the serum marker level as opposed to relying on exceeding a threshold value of normalcy. As assays are becoming ever more sensitive and precise, this approach has the potential to reliably identify and exclude AMI relatively soon after symptom onset while the absolute value of the cardiac markers are in the normal range. Also, by focusing on time changes of the markers, as opposed to absolute values, the noise resulting from patients who may normally have elevated cardiac markers (e.g., renal failure, cardiomyopathy) is eliminated. Fesmire et al. performed baseline and 2-hour CK-MB testing in 710 chest pain patients (113 AMI; CK-MB gold standard; mean time from symptom onset until presentation 108 min) with a normal baseline CK-MB.[17] A 2-hour delta change of +1.6 ng/mL was 92% sensitive and 95% specific; as compared to a sensitivity of 75% and specificity of 96% for an abnormal 2-hour absolute value of CK-MB. The authors

Table 9-6. Sensitivity, Specificity, Positive Likelihood Ratio (+LR), and Negative Likelihood Ratio (–LR) for Biochemical Marker Testing Alone and in Combination at Baseline and 90 Min after ED Presentation

	Time 0[*]				Time 0, 90 min			
	Sensitivity (%)	Specificity (%)	+LR	–LR	Sensitivity (%)	Specificity (%)	+LR	–LR
CK-MB	75	85	4.9	0.29	83	83	4.9	0.20
Myo	71	76	2.9	0.39	85	73	3.1	0.21
cTnI	65	88	5.2	0.40	77	79	3.7	0.29
CK-MB + Myo	83	70	2.8	0.24	92	68	2.8	0.11
CK-MB + cTnI[†]	80	76	3.3	0.26	89	68	2.8	0.16
Myo + cTnI	85	67	2.5	0.23	97	60	2.4	0.05
CK-MB + Myo + cTnI[†]	88	63	2.4	0.19	97	56	2.2	0.05

[*]Time 0 = time of ED presentation. Mean time from symptom onset until presentation was 3.9 hours for AMI patients."
[†]Personal communication from McCord J.
Abbreviations: myo = myoglobin; cTnI = troponin I.
Source: Modified with permission from reference 16.

conclude that a delta CK-MB ≥ +1.5 ng/mL reliably identifies (positive likelihood ratio 19.6) and reliably excludes (negative likelihood ratio 0.08) when combined with clinical judgment.

The time changes in serum marker value have also been applied to myoglobin testing with various strategies proposed being doubling of myoglobin at baseline, rise of +40 ng/mL in 1 hour, or 50% change in myoglobin value at either 1 or 2 hours.[18–20] In a recent study, Ng et al. report on the findings in 1285 ED patients with suspected AMI presenting at a veterans hospital who underwent serial testing of CK-MB, myoglobin, and troponin I at baseline, 30, 60, and 90 min.[21] In order to increase the specificity of myoglobin, the authors defined an abnormal myoglobin as a rise ≥25% above the baseline value (delta myoglobin). The best combination of markers in this study was a positive delta myoglobin in conjunction with an abnormal troponin I. By 90 min, this combination had a sensitivity for AMI of 94% and specificity of 94%. However, only 29% of the patients in this study presented within 6 hours of symptom onset and 98% of the population were males thus limiting extrapolation of these data to the typical emergency department setting.

Fesmire et al. have also demonstrated the use of a rise of CK-MB ≥ +1.5 ng/mL or rise of troponin I ≥ +0.2 ng/mL when incorporated in a comprehensive chest pain evaluation protocol which includes continuous 12-lead ECG monitoring in conjunction with selective nuclear stress testing for the early identification and exclusion of AMI.[22] In a follow-up study, the authors report the use of delta CK-MB versus delta myoglobin when using a low cutoff value of troponin as the gold standard.[23] Interestingly, this study found that the delta CK-MB significantly outperformed delta myoglobin at 2 hours. The authors suggest that the rapid clearance of myoglobin from the serum in patients with positive troponin I microinfarcts (previously classified as unstable angina) is the cause of the finding and suggest that myoglobin may no longer be the best early marker of myocardial necrosis using new ACC/ESC definition. Finally, a small pilot study using a third generation troponin I assay with a analytical sensitivity of 0.03 ng/mL (99% percentile 0.07 ng/mL with imprecision <10% at 0.06 ng/mL) found that a 2-hour delta troponin I ≥ +0.02 ng/mL outperformed all other markers tested for detection of 30-day adverse outcome and suggest that rapid serial testing with new generation troponin assays may be sufficient for the identification and exclusion of AMI.[24]

POINT-OF-CARE TESTING

The ACC and American Heart Association recommend that cardiac marker results should be available within 60 min and preferably within 30 min.[25] There are multiple quantitative point-of-care systems available with turn around times of less than 20 min. Point-of-care testing can eliminate delays associated with transportation and processing in a central laboratory. The advantages of improved time must be weighed against the increased cost and need for stringent quality control and training of emergency department personal. At the present time studies are lacking that demonstrate improved outcome with point-of-care testing, and thus no definite recommendations can be made. If point-of-care testing is not used, systems should be in place to ensure prompt notification of the physician of any abnormal marker tests.

MARKERS ON THE HORIZON

Overview

A whole host of markers are on the horizon that may be of value in the evaluation of chest pain patients. It is important for the physician to realize that markers of necrosis are used to identify and exclude AMI, but not to identify or exclude non-AMI ACS. Once AMI is excluded, physicians must make the clinical decision of whether or not to evaluate the patients for unstable angina or other potentially life-threatening nonischemic causes of chest pain (e.g., pulmonary embolism, aortic dissection).

Ischemia Markers

In February of 2003, the FDA approved the albumin cobalt binding assay as the first marker of ischemia. Under physiologic conditions, cobalt is bound tightly to the N-terminus of albumin. Free radicals produced during ischemia decrease the ability of albumin to bind to cobalt. The albumin cobalt binding assay measures this change in cobalt binding. Preliminary evidence suggests that this test when used in conjunction with troponin and the ECG has a high negative predictive value for ACS. Bhagavan et al. report a sensitivity of 88% and specificity of 94% of this assay in 167 emergency department chest pain patients (25 AMI patients; 50 unstable angina patients) for ACS.[26] Wu et al. in a retrospective study using strict application of the ESC/ACC guidelines for detection of AMI found that the combination of troponin I and the cobalt albumin assay had a sensitivity for AMI of 65% at presentation, 87% at 1–6 hours, and 92.9% at 6–12 hours with a negative predictive value of 85%, 96%, and 96%, respectively at these three time intervals.[27] Specificity of this combination of assays was 75%, 59%, and 48%, respectively for the three time intervals, thus limiting the usefulness of the combination of troponin I and cobalt albumin binding assay beyond the initial triage of chest pain patients. Future research will be required to determine which subsets of troponin negative patients will benefit the

most from this assay. Other potential markers of ischemia currently being investigated are free fatty acids, pregnancy-associated plasma protein-A, glycogen phosphorylase isoenzyme BB, and sphingosine-1-phosphate.

Inflammation Markers

In addition to ischemia markers, there are also a numerous markers of inflammation that are rapidly becoming available. Current research suggests that inflammation in coronary artery plaques plays a central role in the pathway that leads to fissuring, rupture, and subsequent thrombosis. Markers of inflammation such as C-reactive protein, acute-phase proteins, fibrinogen, and various cytokines all appear to be useful in the risk stratification of patients with ACS. C-reactive protein and fibrinogen are the most studied of these inflammatory markers. C-reactive protein is a sensitive acute-phase protein whose levels increase in response to inflammation, infection, and tissue damage. Fibrinogen also increases in response to inflammation as well as having a key role in response to elevation. Both of these markers have been shown to be independent predictors of short-term risk of new cardiac events and C-reactive protein has also been demonstrated to be predictive of long-term mortality in ACS patients.[28] As specificity of these markers is poor, these tests should be used as prognostic markers that may be useful in guiding long-term therapy.

Heart Failure Markers

The B-natriuretic peptide assay, which is discussed in more detail elsewhere in Chap. 27, may also prove to be useful in the evaluation of ACS patients. B-type natriuretic peptide (BNP) and the N-terminal fragment of its prohormone (N-proBNP) are released from the heart in response to increased wall stress. These peptides facilitate diagnosis of heart failure and help guide therapy. Studies have consistently shown that higher BNP levels in congestive heart failure correlate with greater severity of heart failure and worse clinical prognosis. Preliminary studies have indicated that BNP levels rise in response to cardiac ischemia and thus may provide additional information in the identification and risk stratification of patients with ACS.

CONCLUSIONS

In conclusion, the last 25 years have seen a marked evolution in usage of cardiac markers to identify and exclude AMI. We have gone from measurement of LDH isoenzymes over 48–72 hours of inpatient observation to rapid protocols using multimarker and delta strategies to exclude AMI within 2 hours of emergency department presentation. Clearly, there is no one right strategy for the identification and exclusion of AMI. The cardiac markers used and time frames of marker measurements must be individualized among the various institutions. One must take into account the analytical sensitivity and precision of the individual assays, the nature of the patient population, and the comfort level of the physicians practicing at the institution when establishing a cardiac marker protocol. This should be done as a collaborative effort among emergency physicians, cardiologists, clinical pathologists, and hospital administration. It is also important to recognize that "not AMI" does not equate to "not ACS." Once AMI has been excluded, it is important that clinical judgment be used to decide which patients may be safely discharged from the emergency department and which patients require further evaluation for unstable angina or other potentially noncardiac life-threatening causes of chest pain. Future studies are needed to elucidate which combination of injury markers, ischemia markers, inflammation markers, and failure markers will provide the best approach for the evaluation and treatment of patients with ACS.

REFERENCES

1. World Health Organization: Report of the Joint International Society and Federation of Cardiology/World Health Organization Task Force on Standardization of Clinical Nomenclature. Nomenclature and criteria for diagnosis of ischemic heart disease. *Circulation* 1979;59:607–609.
2. Turnstall-Pedroe, Kuulasmaa K, Amouyel P, et al. Myocardial infarction and coronary deaths in the World Health Organization MONICA Project: Registration procedures, event rates, and case-fatality rates in 38 populations from 21 countries in four continents. *Circulation* 1994;90:583–612.
3. Antman EM, Tanasijevic MJ, Thompson B, et al. Cardiospecific troponin I levels to predict the risk of mortality in patients with acute coronary syndromes. *N Eng J Med* 1996;26:301–312.
4. Ohman EM, Armstrong PW, Christenson RH, et al. Cardiac troponin T levels for risk stratification in acute myocardial ischemia. *N Engl J Med* 1996;335:1333–1341.
5. Wu AHB, Apple FS, Gibler WB, et al. National Academy of Clinical Biochemistry Standards of Laboratory Practice: Recommendations for the use of cardiac markers in coronary artery disease. *Clin Chem* 1999;45:1104–1121.
6. The Joint European Society of Cardiology/American College of Cardiology Committee: Myocardial infarction redefined—A consensus document of the Joint European Society of Cardiology/American College of Cardiology

Committee for the redefinition of myocardial infarction. *J Am Coll Cardiol* 2000;36:959–969.
7. Newby LK, Alpert JS, Ohman EM, et al. Changing the diagnosis of acute myocardial infarction: Implications for practice and clinical investigations. *Am Heart J* 2002; 144:957–980.
8. Ferguson JL, Beckett GJ, Walker SW, et al. Myocardial infarction redefined: The new ACC/ESC definition, based on cardiac troponin, increases the apparent incidence of infarction. *Heart* 2002;88:343–347.
9. Kontos MC, Fritz LM, Anderson FP, et al. Impact of the troponin standard on the prevalence of acute myocardial infarction. *Am Heart J* 2003;2003:446–452.
10. Rao SV, Ohman EM, Granger CB, et al. Prognostic value of isolated troponin elevation across the spectrum of chest pain syndromes. *Am J Cardiol* 2003;91:936–940.
11. Apple FS, Wu AHB, Jaffe AS. European Society of Cardiology and American College of Cardiology guidelines for redefinition of myocardial infarction: How to use existing assays clinically and for clinical trials. *Am Heart J* 2002;144:981–986.
12. Gallagher EJ. Clinical utility of likelihood ratios. *Ann Emerg Med* 1998;31:391–397.
13. Zimmerman J, Fromm R, Meyer D, et al. Diagnostic Marker Cooperative Study for the diagnosis of myocardial infarction. *Circulation* 1999;99:1671–1677.
14. American College of Emergency Physicians: Clinical Policy: Critical issues in the evaluation and management of adult patients presenting with suspected acute myocardial infarction or unstable angina. *Ann Emerg Med* 2000;35:521–544.
15. Newby LK, Storrow AB, Gibler WB, et al. Bedside multimarker testing for risk stratification in chest pain units: The chest pain evaluation by creatine kinase-MB, myoglobin, and troponin I (CHECKMATE) study. *Circulation* 2001; 103:1832–1837.
16. McCord J, Nowak RM, McCullough PA, et al. Ninety-minute exclusion of acute myocardial infarction by use of quantitative point-of-care testing of myoglobin and troponin I. *Circulation* 2001;104:1483–1488.
17. Fesmire FM. Delta CK-MB outperforms delta Troponin I at 2 hours during the initial ED evaluation of chest pain. *Am J Emerg Med* 2000;18:1–8.
18. Tucker JF, Collins RA, Anderson AJ, et al. Value of serial myoglobin levels in the early diagnosis of patients admitted for acute myocardial infarction. *Ann Emerg Med* 1994;24: 704–708.
19. Davis CP, Barrett K, Torre P, et al. Serial myoglobin levels for patients with possible myocardial infarction. *Acad Emerg Med* 1996;3:590–597.
20. Brogan GX, Friedman S, McCuskey C, et al. Evaluation of a new rapid quantitative immunoassay for serum myoglobin versus CK-MB for ruling out acute myocardial infarction in the emergency department. *Ann Emerg Med* 1994;24:665–671.
21. Ng SM, Krishnaswamy P, Morissey R, et al. Ninety-minute accelerated critical pathway for chest pain evaluation. *Am J Cardiol* 2001;88:611–617.

22. Fesmire FM, Hughes AD, Fody EP, et al. The Erlanger Chest Pain Evaluation Protocol: A one-year experience with serial 12-lead ECG monitoring, two-hour delta serum marker measurements, and selective nuclear stress testing to identify and exclude acute coronary syndromes. *Ann Emerg Med* 2002;40:584–594.

23. Fesmire FM, Christenson RH, Fody EP, et al. Delta CK-MB outperforms myoglobin at 2-hours during the ED identification and exclusion of troponin positive non-ST segment elevation acute coronary syndromes. *Ann Emerg Med* 2004;in press.

24. Fesmire FM, Fesmire CE. Improved identification of acute coronary syndromes with second generation cardiac troponin I assay: Utility of 2-hour delta cTnI $\geq +0.02$ ng/ml. *J Emerg Med* 2002;22:147–152.

25. Braunwald E, Antman EM, Beasley JW, et al. ACC/AHA 2002 guideline update for the management of patients with unstable angina and non-ST-segment elevation myocardial infarction: A report of the American College of Cardiology/American Heart Association Task Force on Practice Guidelines (Committee on the Management of Patients with Unstable Angina). 2002. Available at: *http://www.acc.org/clinical/guidelines/unstable/ unstable.pdf.*

26. Bhagavan NV, Lai EM, Rios PA, et al. Evaluation of human serum albumin cobalt binding assay for the assessment of myocardial ischemia and myocardial infarction. *Clin Chem* 2003;49:581–585.

27. Wu AH, Morris DL, Fletcher DR, et al. Analysis of the albumin cobalt binding (ACB) test as an adjunct to cardiac troponin for the early detection of acute myocardial infarction. *Cardiovasc Toxicol* 2001;1:147–151.

28. Lidahl B, Toss H, Siegbahn A, et al. Markers of myocardial damage and inflammation in relation to long-term mortality in unstable coronary artery disease. *N Engl J Med* 2000; 343:1139–1147.

10

Cardiac Ultrasound

Alexander M. Zlidenny
J. Christian Fox
Joseph Wood

CARDIAC ULTRASOUND

Cardiovascular illness may be the most challenging disease process for EPs in daily practice. Cardiac ultrasound performed by EPs can provide valuable information into a patient's cardiac structure, contractility, and hemodynamic status. Cardiac ultrasound was first described in the Emergency Medicine literature in the 1980s as a diagnostic tool for identifying pericardial effusions.[1] Since then many more applications have been identified as EPs have gained the knowledge and skills to incorporate cardiac ultrasound into their treatment algorithms.

The scope of cardiac ultrasound that can be performed by the EPs varies, depending on their level of training and expertise. For most, the primary focus for EPs performing bedside echocardiography should be detecting the presence of a pericardial effusion. This should be viewed as a simple, dichotomous question. Is the heart beating in a sac of fluid? Keeping the determination simple will avoid overdiagnosis and will shorten the time required to perform the ultrasound examination. As physician experience increases, they will develop a sense of what a normal cardiac contraction looks like on the ultrasound screen. Recognizing global hypocontractility can be very helpful in evaluating a patient presenting with undifferentiated shock. Patients with shock secondary to acute volume loss will usually have a hyperdynamic heart, while cardiogenic shock is manifest by global hypokinesis.

This chapter will describe the methods for obtaining and interpreting bedside echocardiograms in the ED.

HIGH YIELD FACTS

- Cardiac ultrasound is best performed with a curved phased array probe. Lower frequencies (2.5–3.5 MHz) provide the best image quality, especially when scanning in the subcostal window. Using an ultrasound probe with a small footprint will allow imaging between ribs.

- Although there are many cardiac ultrasound windows recognized by echocardiographers, emergency physicians (EPs) tend to use only the four main windows of subcostal, parasternal long (PSL) axis, parasternal short (PSS) axis, and the apical four chamber view.

- The incidence of pericardial effusions in dyspneic emergency department (ED) patients has been reported to be as high as 13.6%[23]; however, Beck's triad (hypotension, muffled heart sounds, and jugular venous distention) for predicting its presence, is present in less than 40% of patients with pericardial tamponade.[2]

- Differentiating epicardial fat pads from pericardial effusion can be challenging. Epicardial fat will have areas of echogenicity that moves with the heart's contractile activity as compared to a pericardial effusion, which should be completely anechoic and not move with systole. Pericardial effusions may also have echogenic areas if there are loculations or old clotted blood.

- In acute cardiac ischemia, regional wall motion abnormalities occur in just a few seconds, well before any ECG changes.[7,8] Consequently, the sensitivity of echocardiography is reported to 93–100% for diagnosing acute myocardial infarction (AMI).[9–12] However, if the infarct is very small, involving <20% of the myocardial wall, a wall motion abnormality may be undetectable.[12] Interpretation of wall motion abnormality is also confounded by prior MI; therefore, its specificity for predicting acute ischemia is low (69–87%).[12,13]

- In patients presenting to the ED in cardiac arrest, survival to hospital admission is unlikely if there is no cardiac activity detectable by bedside ultrasound.[30] The presence of cardiac activity predicted survival to hospital admission in 27%, whereas only 3% with cardiac standstill survived to admission.[31]

The questions addressed by the ultrasound interrogation should be appropriate to the skill level of the clinician, and should address realistic potential diagnoses. In a young patient presenting with penetrating chest trauma, it may be adequate to ascertain the presence of pericardial fluid. With the acquisition of greater skill, the EP may begin to use the screening echocardiogram to assess wall motion.

ANATOMY

The heart sits in the thoracic cavity at an oblique angle, with the apex pointing toward the left hip. In general, deoxygenated blood returns to the right side of the heart and is pumped to the body by the left side of the heart. The atrio-ventricular septum separates the heart into its left and right sides. The heart is surrounded by lung tissue and the thoracic rib cage, which interferes with obtaining proper cardiac ultrasound windows. Finally, the left lobe of the liver lies just inferior to the heart and provides a good acoustic window.

Systemic blood returns to the heart via the inferior and superior vena cava, and then passes through into the right atrium. Blood from the right atrium enters the right ventricle through the tricuspid valve. It then travels to the pulmonary circulation via the pulmonary arteries and back to the left atrium via the pulmonary veins as oxygenated blood. Blood in the left atrium enters the left ventricle through the mitral valve, which has anterior and posterior leaflets. It is then pumped to the systemic circulation through the aortic valve and the thoracic aorta, via its ascending and descending portions. The heart is surrounded by visceral pericardium, which is in contact with the surrounding parietal pericardium. Between these pericardial layers lies a potential space for fluid to accumulate, forming pericardial effusions.

CARDIAC ULTRASOUND TECHNIQUE

Cardiac ultrasound is best performed with a curved phased array probe. Lower frequencies (2.5–3.5 MHz) provide the best image quality, especially when scanning in the subcostal window. Using an ultrasound probe with a small footprint will provide the best results when viewing the heart in the parasternal windows (Fig. 10-1). The smaller probe footprint will allow the sonographer to scan between the ribs, thus avoiding rib shadow artifact.

In all emergency ultrasound applications the probe indicator, the side of transducer that corresponds to the left side of the monitor, should be pointed either toward the patient's right or cephalad. The only exception to this rule is the PSL axis view of the heart. It is important that

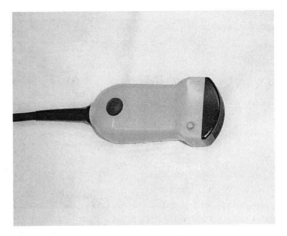

Fig. 10-1. Small footprint curved probe.

sonographers closely inspect the direction of the probe indicator each time they scan a patient (Fig. 10-2). Reversing the indicator is the most common error made by novice sonographers and will cause unnecessary confusion when viewing the cardiac ultrasound images.

Traditionally, cardiac ultrasound is performed with the sonographer standing on the right side of the supine patient, although the chaotic nature of the ED may not always allow this. ED cardiac sonographers should be prepared to perform examinations and interpret images while scanning from either side of the patient, and while using either the right or left hand to manipulate the probe. Most ED patients are lying supine during examinations. Placing patients in the left lateral decubitus position will increase the likelihood of performing a quality examination, especially when viewing from the cardiac apical window (Fig. 10-3). The left lateral decubitus position pushes the heart anteriorly and closer to the ultrasound probe during the examination.

CARDIAC ULTRASOUND WINDOWS

There are at least 11 cardiac ultrasound windows recognized by echocardiographers. In the ED, however, physicians have limited time and therefore tend to use only four main windows in performing cardiac ultrasound. The cardiac windows that are easiest to obtain while providing the most information to EPs are: subcostal, PSL axis, PSS axis, and the apical four-chamber view.

Subcostal View

The most important cardiac ultrasound window of the heart that should be mastered by EPs is the subcostal

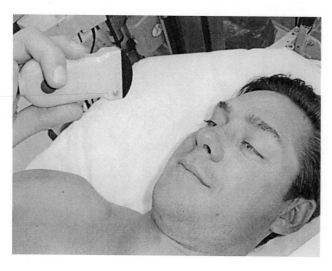

Fig. 10-2. Carefully examine probe for indicator.

view. Some patients may have anatomic and physiologic variances making it difficult to obtain a useful subcostal view. This includes the obese patient and those that have significant epigastric tenderness.

The best method to obtain the subcostal view of the heart is to start by placing the ultrasound probe at the patient's right subcostal margin (Fig. 10-4). As a general rule, the probe should be kept in the transverse plane with the indicator aimed toward the patient's right hip. The probe should be directed toward the patient's left shoulder and advanced in a sweeping motion toward the patient's subxiphoid region, using the left lobe of the liver

as a window for viewing all four chambers of the heart (Figs. 10-5 and 10-6). Once in the subxiphoid area, care should be taken to keep the ultrasound probe as flat as possible with relation to the patient's anterior chest. It is best for sonographers to place their hand on top of the ultrasound probe, with the cable exiting under the hand (Fig. 10-7). The best subcostal views are gained by using copious amounts of gel and pushing down relatively hard (toward the spine) on the ultrasound probe.

All four chambers of the heart will be visualized using the subcostal (also known as subxiphoid) approach. The sonographer should tilt the probe "up and down" as well

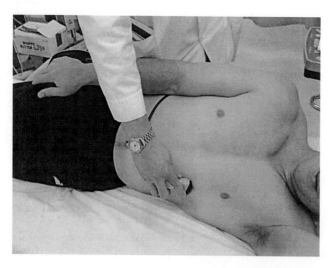

Fig. 10-3. Patient in left lateral decubitus position.

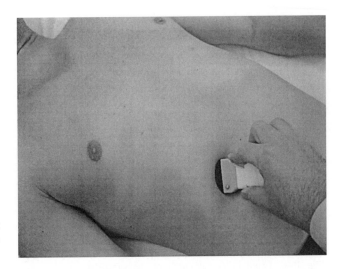

Fig. 10-4. To perform a subcostal view of the heart start by placing the ultrasound probe at the patient's right subcostal margin.

as "right to left" in order to obtain the best window. The most anterior chamber of the heart is the right ventricle and will appear just posterior to the left lobe of the liver on the ultrasound image (Fig. 10-8). The left ventricle will appear just posterior to the right ventricle, while the right and left atria will be visualized on the left side of the screen in relation to the ventricles. The mitral and tricuspid valves may also be visualized in this view, as well as the interventricular septum. The sonographer may need to increase the depth of image in order to visualize all four chambers. The most anterior portion of the cardiac image is the best area to visualize a pericardial effusion. Overall cardiac function can also be estimated accurately using this window.

Parasternal Long Axis View

The PSL axis view of the heart is very useful in patients in whom the subcostal view is difficult to obtain. The PSL view is limited in those with various hyperinflated lung diseases (e.g., chronic obstructive pulmonary disease [COPD]), and in those with chest wall tenderness. This is the best view to visualize the heart valves, but is inferior to the subcostal view at diagnosing pericardial effusions.

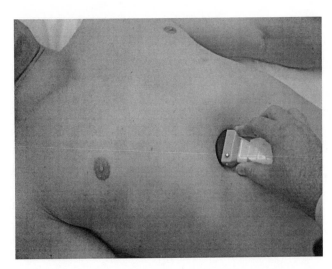

Fig. 10-5. Probe with indicator toward right hip advanced to subxiphoid position.

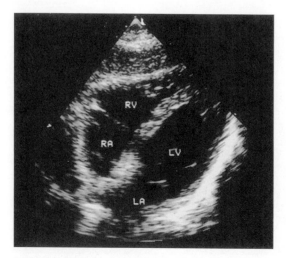

Fig. 10-6. Two-dimensional image of the subcostal four chamber plane. (Source: Extracted from Hurst's Cardiology, Chap. 13, p. 358, Fig. 13-19B.)

Obtaining a PSL window involves first imaging where the heart lies in its long axis under the chest wall. In Fig. 10-9, we have placed a hand over the chest to demonstrate how the heart lies in its longest axis. The fingernails are pointed in the direction of the apex, while the carpal bones are overlying the great vessels. Because the marker on the probe should correspond to the left side of the ultrasound monitor, and because this marker is aimed in the direction of the apex (or fingernails), we therefore expect to see the apex toward the left side of the monitor. Furthermore, the right side of the monitor corresponds to the great vessels including the aortic outflow tract. This is done by placing the ultrasound probe between the ribs just to the left of the sternum in the third or fourth intercostal space with the indicator toward the patient's left elbow. The sonographer may have to adjust the angle of the probe to obtain the best window. The probe should be held "like a pencil" with the base of the sonographer's hand against the patient's chest for best control (Fig. 10-10).

The PSL axis view visualizes the heart in its long axis, with the apex appearing on the left side of the screen (Fig. 10-11). In the near field of the image will be the right ventricle and the tricuspid valve, while the left atrium and ventricle will be visualized in the far field (Fig. 10-12). The anterior and posterior leaflets of the mitral valve may also be examined in the far field. It will be possible to view the aortic outflow tract and the aortic valve in the middle field of the image. In some cases, the descending thoracic aorta may be visualized posterior to the left ventricle.

Parasternal Short Axis View

The PSS axis view should be obtained after finding the PSL axis view and then rotating the probe 90° clockwise

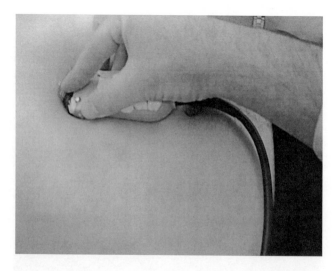

Fig. 10-7. Cable exiting under hand.

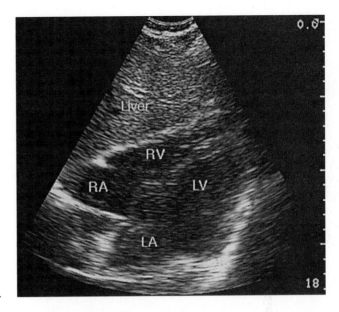

Fig. 10-8. Normal subcostal view of the heart.

(Fig. 10-13). The probe remains just left of the sternum in the third or fourth intercostal space, with the indicator toward the patient's right elbow. The PSS axis view is the best way to visualize the aortic and mitral valves (Fig. 10-14).

At the level of the aortic valve, the right ventricle will be seen in the near field and the left atrium in the far field. The right atrium may be visualized on the left side of the image in the middle field, while the pulmonary artery and valve may be seen on the right side of the middle field. The aortic valve can be identified in the middle of the image by the so-called "Mercedes Benz sign" (Fig. 10-15).

The inferior view of the PSS axis allows for visualization of the right and left ventricles at the level of the mitral valve (Fig. 10-16). A characteristic "fish mouth"

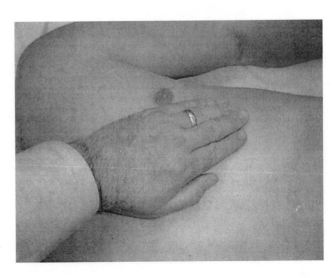

Fig. 10-9. Hand overlying long axis of heart with fingernails over the apex.

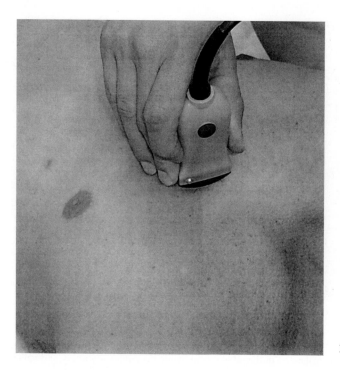

Fig. 10-10. Probe held for parasternal long (PSL) view.

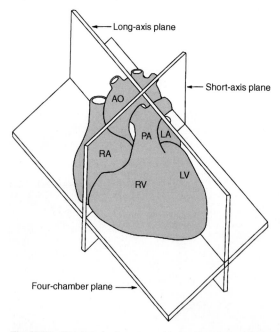

Fig. 10-11. The three basic tomographic imaging planes used in cardiac ultrasound. (Source: Extracted from Hurst's Cardiology, Chap. 13, p. 351, Fig. 13-12.)

view of the mitral valve can be seen by viewing the anterior and posterior leaflets down toward the left ventricle.

Apical Four Chamber View

The apical four chamber view is the best cardiac window for comparing chamber sizes. It is a coronal view of all four chambers that is also helpful for estimating overall function (Fig. 10-17). The apical four chamber view should be obtained by placing the ultrasound probe 2–3 cm inferior to the patient's left nipple with the indicator toward the patient's right hip. Placing patients in the left lateral decubitus position will provide the best results (Fig. 10-18).

The heart will appear with the apex aiming upward and the right side of the heart on the left side of the screen (Fig. 10-19). The mitral and tricuspid valves can be visualized, as well as the septal wall running vertically top-to-bottom in the image. Slight alterations in technique while obtaining the apical four-chamber view may yield a five-chamber view that includes the aortic valve in the middle of the image (Fig. 10-20). Patients with chest tenderness, pulmonary diseases, COPD, and/or large breasts will make obtaining the apical four-chamber view very challenging.

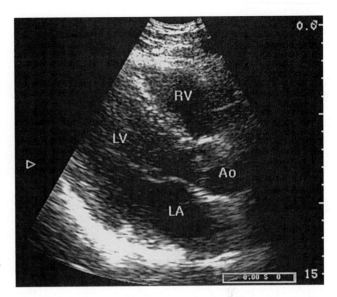

Fig. 10-12. Normal parasternal long axis (PSL) view of the heart.

INDICATIONS

Chest Trauma

Patients with blunt or penetrating chest trauma may suffer significant injuries readily diagnosed by bedside cardiac ultrasound. These include pericardial tamponade, cardiac rupture, and cardiac contusion. Cardiac windows should be viewed as part of the focused assessment for sonography in trauma (FAST) examination early in the course of trauma resuscitation and diagnosis.

Traumatic chest injuries may be life threatening. Cardiac ultrasound can provide rapid and efficient diagnosis. This is beneficial because the physical examination findings of Beck's triad (hypotension, muffled heart sounds, and jugular venous distention) are present in less than 40% of patients with pericardial tamponade.[2] The visualization of a pericardial effusion causing diastolic collapse of the right ventricle is the most accurate evidence of pericardial tamponade[3] (Fig. 10-21). Once the diagnosis of tamponade is made, immediate pericardiocentesis or surgical pericardial window is needed. The success of bedside ultrasound in diagnosing pericardial tamponade caused by penetrating chest trauma is well documented.[4] Cardiac ultrasound has also been shown to diagnose cardiac rupture after blunt chest trauma.[5]

Blunt chest trauma may also result in hemodynamic instability via direct cardiac contusion. Historically, the diagnosis of cardiac contusion has been inaccurate using

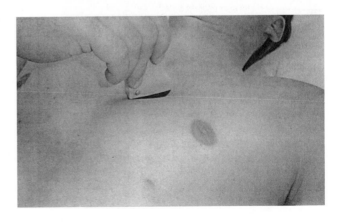

Fig. 10-13. Parasternal short (PSS) probe placement.

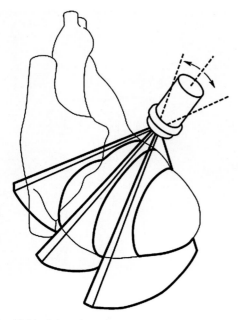

Fig. 10-14. Orientation of various short axis sector beams through the left ventricle obtained by angling the transducer in the parasternal position. (Source: Extracted from Hurst's Cardiology, Chap. 13, p. 355, Fig. 13-16a.)

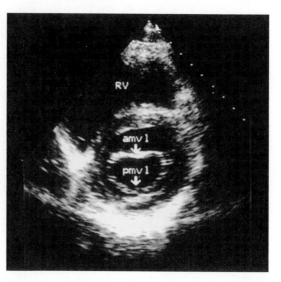

Fig. 10-16. Visualization of the right and left ventricles at the level of the mitral valve. (Source: Extracted from Hurst's Cardiology, Chap. 13, p. 355, Fig. 13-16C.)

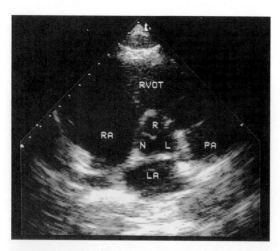

Fig. 10-15. Short axis plane through the base of the heart demonstrating the "Mercedes Benz" sign. (Source: Extracted from Hurst's Cardiology, Chap. 13, p. 355, Fig. 13-16B.)

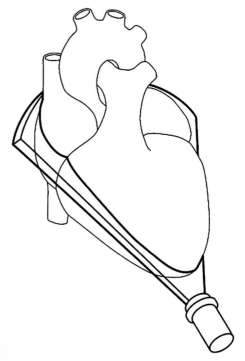

Fig. 10-17. Orientation of the sector beam and transducer position for the apical four chamber plane. (Source: Extracted from Hurst's Cardiology, Chap. 13, p. 356, Fig. 13-17A.)

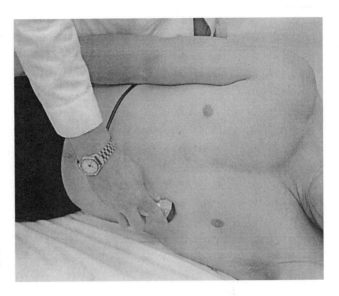

Fig. 10-18. Apical probe placement inferior to left nipple with indicator toward patient's right hip, while patient lies in left lateral decubitus position.

chest X-ray, ECG, and cardiac markers. Cardiac ultrasound can improve the diagnostic accuracy of cardiac contusion.[6] Cardiac contusion is diagnosed by noting segmental wall motion abnormalities and right ventricular (RV) dilation on cardiac ultrasound.

CHEST PAIN

The differential diagnosis for patients presenting to the ED with acute chest pain is large, and includes acute coronary syndrome (ACS), pulmonary embolus, thoracic aortic dissection, esophageal rupture, pneumothorax, costochondritis, gastroesopahgeal reflux disease (GERD), myocarditis, and pericarditis. Many of the most serious diagnoses can be differentiated with cardiac ultrasound findings, such as wall motion abnormalities, right heart dilatation, and pericardial effusions.

Acute Coronary Syndrome

Considering that the initial ECG is nondiagnostic in about 50% of ED patients ultimately diagnosed with an

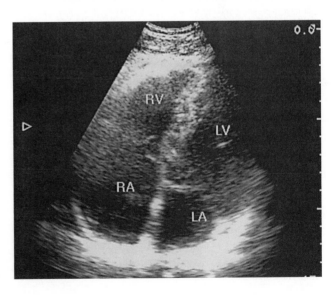

Fig. 10-19. Apical four chamber view.

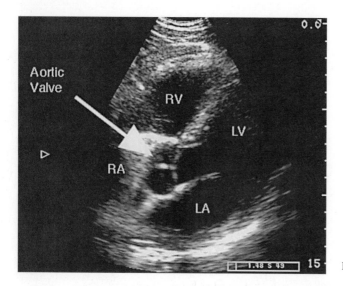

Fig. 10-20. Apical five chamber view.

AMI, accurate diagnosis of ACS can be difficult. For many years, cardiologists have used echocardiography to evaluate left ventricular function and wall motion abnormalities as a marker for AMI. Other findings associated with AMI include mitral regurgitation, left ventricular rupture, and left ventricular thrombus.

In patients with induced cardiac ischemia, early studies found regional wall motion abnormalities occur just a few seconds into the event, well before any ECG changes.[7,8] Consequently, the sensitivity of echocardiography is reported to be 93–100% for diagnosing AMI.[9–12] However, a limitation of cardiac ultrasound in

the context of ACS is when the infarct is very small, involving <20% of the myocardial wall, as there may not be a detectable wall motion abnormality.[12] Alternatively, the specificity is low (69–87%) because of the confounder of a prior MI.[12,13] In the setting of a previous MI, regional wall motion abnormalities may be difficult to differentiate from the acute event.

Bedside cardiac ultrasound can be accurate in establishing left ventricular function and ejection fraction (EF) in ED patients.[14,15] Emergency physicians, with only limited cardiac ultrasound training, were able to accurately assess left ventricular function in the ED

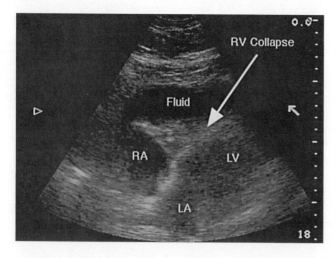

Fig. 10-21. Pericardial tamponade with RV collapse.

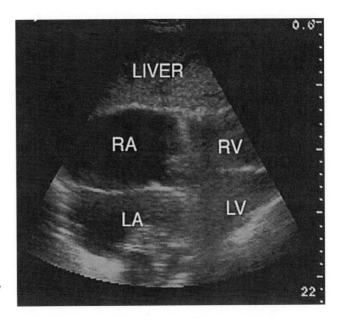

Fig. 10-22. Right-sided heart dilatation due to pulmonary embolism.

setting. Some researchers have since proposed combining ECG, cardiac markers, and bedside ultrasound results to predict adverse events after AMI.[16,17] Patients with significant wall motion abnormalities had increased adverse events post-MI, including congestive heart failure (CHF) and lethal arrhythmias. Cardiac ultrasound has also been proposed as an adjunct diagnostic tool for ED chest pain units.[18] This has the potential to decrease the number of hospital admissions and lower healthcare costs.

ED cardiac ultrasound can provide quick and noninvasive information in the diagnosis of ACS. EPs should look for regional wall motion abnormalities and decreased left ventricular function as evidence for ACS. Broad use of high quality bedside cardiac ultrasound could also increase ACS diagnostic accuracy and predict adverse events post-MI.

Pulmonary Embolism

The gold standard for pulmonary embolism (PE) diagnosis is a pulmonary arteriogram, although lower extremity Doppler ultrasound, serum D-dimer measurement, computed tomography, and ventilation/perfusion scans are more widely used in the ED setting. Cardiac ultrasound may aid in making the difficult diagnosis of PE by visualizing mitral regurgitation, RV dilatation, or RV thrombus (Fig. 10-22).

Bedside cardiac ultrasound has been found to be insensitive but very specific for diagnosing PE in the ED setting.[19] Jackson and colleagues reported a 41% sensitivity

and 91% specificity for cardiac ultrasound in diagnosing PE.[19] A separate study of in-patients found a sensitivity of 59% and specificity of 77%.[20] Cardiac ultrasound may be beneficial as a screening tool for patients that are at risk for PE, but not for definitive diagnosis.

There have also been studies reporting the benefits of cardiac ultrasound in guiding thrombolytic therapy. In a study by Konstantinides et al., patients with a known PE and evidence of right heart strain on cardiac ultrasound, received either heparin or thrombolytic therapy.[21] They found decreased mortality with thrombolytics, as compared to those who received heparin alone. In another study, Goldhaber et al. reported that patients with PE and RV hypokinesis on cardiac ultrasound had twice the mortality rate as those with a normal ultrasound.[22]

Cardiac ultrasound may be a tool to select which patients with pulmonary embolus may benefit from thrombolytic therapy. Future strategies may combine the use of cardiac ultrasound with bedside lower extremity Doppler and D-dimer tests as a rapid and noninvasive screening tool to diagnose PE in the ED.

UNEXPLAINED DYSPNEA

Nontrauma patients presenting to the ED with shortness of breath must be evaluated for an assortment of medical diagnoses that include pneumonia, CHF, arrhythmia, pneumothorax, severe anemia, pleural effusion, and PE.

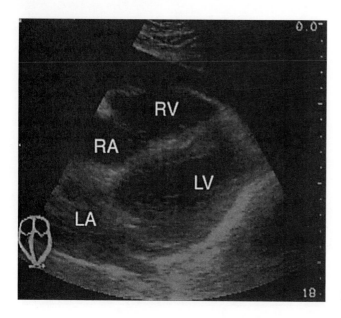

Fig. 10-23. Pericardial effusion.

A cardiac ultrasound should be performed looking for evidence of pericardial effusion once all other etiologies have been ruled out. Patients with chronic renal failure, cancer, CHF, pericarditis, lupus, and many other medical problems are at high risk for pericardial effusions.

The incidence of pericardial effusions in dyspneic ED patients has been reported to be as high as 13.6%.[23] Most of these have been misdiagnosed without the use of bedside ultrasound. Emergency physician performed cardiac ultrasound has been shown to be very accurate for the detection of pericardial effusion. In a prospective study using a gold standard of cardiologist confirmation of ultrasound results, Mandavia et al. reported sensitivity and specificity of ED ultrasound for diagnosing pericardial effusions were 96% and 98%, respectively.[24]

A pericardial effusion appears as an anechoic stripe of fluid surrounding the heart (Fig. 10-23). This fluid accumulates in the potential pericardial space, between the visceral and parietal pericardial layers. Patients may normally have 10–50 cc of serous fluid in this space. However, the acute accumulation of greater than 50–100 cc may cause tamponade and hemodynamic compromise. Nontraumatic (chronic) effusions may develop over weeks to months and will stretch the pericardium over time. In this fashion, the pericardial space can contain up to 1000 cc of fluid before there is actual tamponade.

The subcostal view of the heart is the initial window of choice when evaluating for the presence of a pericardial effusion. If present an effusion is best seen in the space anterior to the heart and closest to the ultrasound probe. Quite commonly it is difficult for the EP to discern pericardial effusions from epicardial fat (Fig. 10-24). A study by Blaivas et al. tested 5 attendings and 17 residents on previously validated cardiac ultrasound clips.[25] The physicians in the study were able to accurately discern epicardial fat pads from pericardial effusions in only 30% of patients, although the investigators used cases that were very difficult to interpret.

Epicardial fat pads are very common, particularly if obese.[25] The PSL axis view of the heart should be used, in conjunction with the subcostal view, especially in patients when there is a question of a pericardial effusion versus epicardial fat. Sonographically, epicardial fat will have areas of echogenicity and will move together with the heart's contractile activity. Conversely, pericardial effusions should be completely anechoic and not move with the heart. Pericardial effusions may also have echogenic areas if there are loculations or old clotted blood. EPs must be very diligent in discerning these two entities or risk performing unnecessary invasive procedures.

UNEXPLAINED HYPOTENSION

There are numerous etiologies for unexplained hypotension in the ED. Bedside ultrasound may have its greatest utility in differentiating the causes of acute hypotension. Immediate bedside ultrasound can diagnose an impending problem and guide definitive treatment.

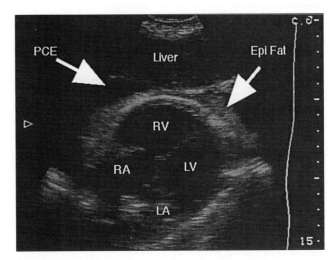

Fig. 10-24. Epicardial fat pad and pericardial effusion.

In 2001, Rose et al. proposed a bedside ultrasound algorithm for patients with unexplained hypotension.[26] This protocol calls for the emergency sonographer to perform a FAST examination, and include both cardiac windows and the abdominal aorta. The strategy behind using these windows is to look for pericardial effusion/tamponade, abdominal aortic aneurysm (AAA), or free fluid in the abdomen, which may signify intraabdominal solid organ injury. They termed this algorithm the undifferentiated hypotensive patient (UHP) ultrasound protocol. They reported three cases where their ultrasound findings diagnosed pericardial tamponade, an AAA, and a splenic injury by the detection of free fluid in the abdomen.[26] Each of the patients was reported to have swift and successful definitive treatment based on ED bedside ultrasound findings. Anecdotally, many centers have employed this ultrasound protocol in their daily practice with similar life-saving results.

Estimating cardiac function with bedside ultrasound may also contribute to the determination of the causes of hypotension, as well as guide the course of treatment. Many have examined the use of ED cardiac ultrasound in determining left ventricular function.[14,15,27] In a study by Moore et al., emergency physicians received focused training for determining EF. Comparison of emergency physician versus primary cardiologist estimate of EF yielded a Pearson's correlation coefficient $R = 0.86$, which compared favorably with interobserver correlation between cardiologists ($R = 0.84$).[14] Randazzo and col-

leagues also reported an 83.3% agreement between emergency physicians and cardiologists in estimating high central venous pressure (CVP) by measuring IVC size using bedside cardiac ultrasound.[15]

Cardiac ultrasound findings for left ventricular function and CVP offer promise as a noninvasive tool for differentiating septic from cardiogenic shock, as well as estimating the patient's volume status. Hyperdynamic cardiac function indicates a normal response to sepsis and the need for increased IV fluids, whereas depressed cardiac function indicates cardiogenic shock and the need for inotropic agents. Based on previous studies of early goal-directed therapy for septic shock, cardiac ultrasound may be used in the future in place of the pulmonary artery catheter during the "golden hours" of critical care resuscitation.[28]

CARDIAC ARREST

Cardiac ultrasound may be useful in ED cardiac arrest patients, with multiple studies showing that it predicts outcomes.[30,31] In a study by Blaivas and Fox of 136 patients presenting to the ED in cardiac arrest, no patient survived to hospital admission if there was no cardiac activity (i.e., cardiac standstill) detectable by bedside ultrasound.[30] Another study showed that the presence of cardiac activity predicted survival to hospital admission (27%), whereas only 3% with cardiac standstill survived to admission.[31] Immediate cardiac ultrasound on cardiac arrest patients may guide treatment interventions and help emergency physicians decide when to end resuscitation efforts. It may also provide evidence for an unsuspected and treatable diagnosis.

Patients with pulseless electrical activity (PEA) have several possible etiologies that include pericardial tamponade, severe hypovolemia, and severe hypocontractility. These entities may be diagnosed quickly and noninvasively at the bedside using cardiac ultrasound. Findings may guide interventions such as the need for pericardiocentesis, increased IV fluids, or inotropic agents, which restore systemic perfusion. Bedside cardiac ultrasound may also be able to unmask cardiac activity not seen on cardiac monitors.[29] A case has been reported of a patient presenting to the ED in asystole but having unorganized cardiac activity on bedside ultrasound signifying ventricular fibrillation. The patient underwent defibrillation in the ED and was converted to sinus rhythm.

PROCEDURE GUIDANCE

Cardiac ultrasound may be used as a real-time adjunct for procedures, such as pericardiocentesis, transvenous pacemaker insertion, and external pacemaker capture. The use of cardiac ultrasound makes the procedures safer and more effective.

Pacemaker Placement

Cardiac ultrasound is useful for guidance during transvenous and external pacemaker placement. Pacemakers are commonly placed for third degree heart block, type II second degree heart block, and severe bradycardia. Cardiac ultrasound is used to confirm successful external pacing by viewing ventricular contractions associated with pacer spikes on the cardiac monitor. During transvenous pacemaker placement, the pacer wire may be visualized entering into the right ventricle. Animal and human studies have shown success in using ultrasound-guided external pacing.[32,33] Traditional blind techniques for transvenous pacemaker placement are successful on the first attempt 10% of the time.[34] Two separate case series had a 100% success rate in floating ultrasound-guided transvenous pacemakers in the ED.[35,36] Ultrasound guidance may be considered for all patients undergoing ED pacemaker placement.

Pericardiocentesis

Pericardiocentesis is performed to drain a pericardial effusion using a blind needle insertion technique or by surgical pericardiotomy. Traditionally, emergency

physicians are taught to perform pericardiocentesis using the subxiphoid approach. This approach is fraught with complications, most notably lacerations of the liver, diaphragmatic perforation, pneumothorax, and ventricular perforation. Instead, the ideal needle entry site should be at the point at which the largest fluid accumulation is closest to the body surface. This is typically found in the parasternal region using a transthoracic needle approach. One study using cardiac ultrasound found the most commonly chosen point of entry was located on the chest wall (86%). Subcostal entries accounted for only 12%, and the major complication rate was low at 2%, whereas blind needle insertion techniques have been reported to have up to 19% mortality and 50% complication rates.[37–41] A study of 41 patients undergoing 46 ultrasound-guided pericardiocenteses had a 100% success rate with only 5% complications and no deaths.[42] Ultrasound-guided pericardiocentesis has been shown to be safer and more effective than traditional techniques.

Ultrasound-guided pericardiocentesis is performed by placing the patient in a semireclining position, so as to allow the fluid to collect as anterior to the heart as possible. Once the optimal needle trajectory has been ascertained, instruct the patient not to move from that position to prevent fluid from shifting away from the needle entry site. Special needles or catheters are not necessary. A pericardiocentesis kit may be assembled from standard equipment available in most EDs. Entering through the chest wall via the parasternal route, a straight needle trajectory will essentially avoid vital structures and have a much shorter path to the effusion. Furthermore, we are aided by the fact that ultrasound scatters when it encounters air-filled spaces thereby avoiding lung tissue. Most often the needle entry point of choice is located between the 5th and 6th or between the 6th and 7th intercostals spaces. Additionally, it is recommended to stay 5 cm lateral to the sternal border to avoid puncturing the internal thoracic artery. Keep in mind the neurovascular bundle courses just inferior to each rib so enter just superior to the rib margin.

The angle at which the ultrasound beam best avoids important structures and approximates the largest fluid collection is the same angle at which the needle should be inserted. This angle is created by the operator and may require several echogenic windows before the optimal trajectory is envisioned in the sonographer's mind. Once the fluid space has been identified, and the optimal needle trajectory determined, the point is marked on the skin with an indelible pen. Make sure to maintain the patient in the same position to minimize translocation of the fluid collection after the mark has been made. Apply gentle aspiration as the sheathed needle is advanced while aiming for the fluid space. Once fluid is aspirated, gently insert the needle 2 mm further. Advance the sheath over the needle, and remove the steel core. The catheter should continue to drain the pericardial fluid.

REFERENCES

1. Mayron R, Gaudio FE, Plummer D, et al. Echocardiography performed by emergency physicians: Impact on diagnosis and therapy. *Ann Emerg Med* 1988;17(2):150–154.
2. Carrel R, Shaffer MA, Franaszek JB. Emergency diagnosis, resuscitation, and treatment of acute penetrating cardiac trauma. *Ann Emerg Med* 1982;11(9):504–517.
3. Armstrong WF, Schilt BF, Helper DJ, et al. Diastolic collapse of the right ventricle with cardiac tamponade: An ecocardiographic study. *Circulation* 1982;65(7):1491–1496.
4. Plummer D, Brunette D, Asinger R, et al. Emergency department echocardiography improves outcome in penetrating cardiac injury. *Ann Emerg Med* 1992;21(6): 709–712.
5. Schiavone WA, Ghumrawi BK, Catalano DR, et al. The use of echocardiography in the emergency management of non-penetrating traumatic cardiac rupture. *Ann Emerg Med* 1991;20(11):1248–1250.
6. Kaye P, O'Sullivan I. Myocardial contusion: Emergency investigation and diagnosis. *Emerg Med J* 2002;19(1):8–10.
7. Kerber RE, Abboud FM. Echocardiographic detection of regional myocardial infarction. *Circulation* 1973;47(5): 997–1005.
8. Weiss JL, Bulkley BH, Hutchins GM, et al. Two dimensional echocardiography recognition of myocardial injury in man: Comparison with post-mortem studies. *Circulation* 1981;63(2):401–408.
9. Heger JJ, Weyman AE, Wann LS, et al. Cross-sectional echocardiography in acute myocardial infarction: Detection and localization of regional left ventricular asynergy. *Circulation* 1979;60(3):531–538.
10. Gibson RS, Bishop HL, Stamm RB, et al. Value of early two dimensional echocardiography in patients with acute myocardial infarction. *Am J Cardiol* 1982;49(5):1110–1119.
11. Sabia P, Abbott RD, Afrookteh A, et al. Importance of two-dimensional echocardiographic assessment of left ventricular systolic function in patients presenting to the emergency room with cardiac-related symptoms. *Circulation* 1991; 84(4):1615–1624.
12. Kontos MC, Arrowood JA, Paulsen WH, et al. Early echocardiography can predict cardiac events in emergency department patients with chest pain. *Ann Emerg Med* 1998;31(5)550–557.
13. Sasaki HS, Charuzi Y, Beeder C, et al. Utility of echocardiography for the early assessment of patients with non-diagnostic chest pain. *Am Heart J* 1986;112:494–497.
14. Moore CL, Rose GA, Tayal VS, et al. Determination of left ventricular function by emergency physician echocardiography of hypotensive patients. *Acad Emerg Med* 2002;9(3):186–193.
15. Randazzo MR, Snoey ER, Levitt MA, et al. Accuracy of emergency physician assessment of left ventricular ejection fraction and central venous pressure using echocardiography. *Acad Emerg Med* 2003;10(9):973–977.
16. Levitt MA, Jan BA. The effect of real time 2-D echocardiography on medical decision-making in the emergency department. *J Emerg Med* 2002;22(3):229–233.
17. Mohler ER 3RD, Ryan T, Segar DS, et al. Clinical utility of troponin T levels and echocardiography in the emergency department. *Am Heart J* 1988;135(2 pt 1):253–260.
18. Lateef F, Gibler WB. Provocative testing for chest pain. *Am J Emerg Med* 2000;18(7):793–801.
19. Jackson RE, Rudoni RR, Hauser AM, et al. Prospective evaluation of two-dimensional transthoracic echocardiography in emergency department patients with suspected pulmonary embolism. *Acad Emerg Med* 2000;7(9):994–998.
20. Steiner P, Lund GK, Debatin JF, et al. Acute pulmonary embolism: Value of transthoracic and transesophageal echocardiography in comparison with helical CT. *Am J Roentgenol* 1996;167(4):931–936.
21. Konstantinides S, Geibel A, Olshewski M, et al. Association between thrombolytic treatment and the prognosis of hemodynamically stable patients with major pulmonary embolism. *Circulation* 1997;96(3):882–888.
22. Goldhaber SZ, Visani L, DeRosa M for ICOPER. Acute pulmonary embolism: Clinical outcomes in the International Cooperative Pulmonary Embolism Registry (ICOPER). *Lancet* 1999;353(9162):1386–1389.
23. Blaivas M. Incidence of pericardial effusion in patients presenting to the emergency department with unexplained dyspnea. *Acad Emerg Med* 2001;8(12):1143–1146.
24. Mandavia DP, Heffner RJ, Mahaney K, et al. Bedside echocardiography by emergency physicians. *Ann Emerg Med* 2001;38(4):377–382.
25. Blaivas M, DeBehnke D, Phelan MB. Potential errors in the diagnosis of pericardial effusion on trauma ultrasound for penetrating injuries. *Acad Emerg Med* 2000;7(11):1261–1266.
26. Rose JS, Bair AE, Mandavia DP, et al. The UHP ultrasound protocol: A novel approach to the empiric evaluation of the undifferentiated hypotensive patient. *Am J Emerg Med* 2001;19(4):299–302.
27. Rich S, Sheikh A, Gallastegui J, et al. Determination of left ventricular ejection fraction by visual estimation during real-time two-dimensional echocardiography. *Am Heart J* 1982;104:603–606.
28. Rivers E, Nguyen B, Havstad S, et al. Early goal-directed therapy in the treatment of severe sepsis and septic shock. *N Engl J Med* 2001;345(19):1368–1377.
29. Amaya SC, Langsam A. Ultrasound detection of ventricular fibrillation disguised as asystole. *Ann Emerg Med* 1999;33(3): 344–346.

30. Blaivas M, Fox JC. Poutcome in cardiac arrest patients found to have cardiac standstill on the bedside emergency department echocardiogram. *Acad Emerg Med* 2001;8(6):616–621.

31. Salen P, O'Connor R, Sierzenski P, et al. Can cardiac sonography and capnography be used independently and in combination to predict resuscitation outcomes? *Acad Emerg Med* 2001;8(6):610–615.

32. Holger JS, Minnigan HJ, Lamon RP, et al. The utility of ultrasound to determine ventricular capture in external cardiac pacing. *Am J Emerg Med* 2001;19(2):134–136.

33. Ettin D, Cook T. Using ultrasound to determine external pacer capture. *J Emerg Med* 1999;17(6):1007–1009.

34. Syverud S, Dalsey W, Hedges J, et al. Radiologic assessment of transvenous pacemaker placement during CPR. *Ann Emerg Med* 1986;15(2):131–137.

35. Aguilera PA, Durham BA, Riley DA. Emergency transvenous cardiac pacing placement using ultrasound guidance. *Ann Emerg Med* 2000;36(3):224–227.

36. Macedo W, Sturman K, Kim JM, et al. Ultrasonographic guidance of trasnvenous pacemaker insertion in the emergency department: A report of three cases. *J Emerg Med* 1999; 17(3):491–496.

37. Morin JE, Hollomby D, Gonda A, et al. Management of uremic pericarditis: A report of 11 patients with cardiac tamponade and a review of the literature. *Ann Thrac Surg* 1976;22(6):588–592.

38. Krikorian JG, Hancock EW. Pericardiocentesis. *Am J Med* 1978;65(5):808–814.

39. Kwasnik EM, Koster JK, Lazarus JM, et al. Conservative management of uremic pericardial effusions. *J Thorac Cardiovasc Surg* 1978;76(5):629–632.

40. Wong B, Murphy J, Chang CJ, et al. The risk of pericardiocentesis. *Am J Cardiol* 1979;44(6):1110–1114.

41. Guberman BA, Fowler NO, Engel PJ, et al. Cardiac tamponade in medical patients. *Circulation* 1981;64(3): 633–640.

42. Salem K, Mulji A, Lonn E. Echocardiographically guided pericardiocentesis-the gold standard for the management of pericardial effusion and cardiac tamponade. *Can J Cardiol* 1999;15(11):1251–1255.

11

Basic MI Therapy

Andra L. Blomkalns

HIGH YIELD FACTS

- Institutions should aim to obtain an EKG as soon as possible, within 10 minutes, in all patients suspected of having an acute MI.
- Oxygen should be administered to patients with O_2 saturation <90%.
- Chest pain response to nitroglycerin treatment has no place in the diagnosis of acute coronary syndrome (ACS).
- Patients with right ventricular infarctions are often very preload dependent and may have a profound hypotensive response to nitroglycerin.
- Aspirin is the most beneficial immediate treatment for AMI and should be administered promptly to every chest pain patient without an aspirin sensitivity contraindication.
- Beta-blockers reduce myocardial oxygen demand, lower the 7-day mortality from AMI, and should be considered in all patients with cardiac ischemia.
- Angiotensin converting enzyme (ACE) inhibitors should be considered in AMI patients with persistent hypertension, anterior wall infarcts, pulmonary congestion, or left ventricular ejection fraction (LVEF) <40%.

Cardiovascular disease (CVD) accounts for 38.5% of all deaths or 1 in every 2.6 deaths in the United States in 2001. It is the leading cause of mortality in this country.[1] CVD claims more lives each year than the next five leading causes of death combined. Hence, the importance of timely identification of symptoms of possible ischemia, appropriate triage and risk stratification, and initial basic treatment are all key components in the evaluation of a patient presenting with chest discomfort. It is this "basic" treatment that can be started on nearly every patient with chest discomfort before a definitive diagnosis is made. This chapter will serve to summarize these therapies and the evidence for their use.

Guidelines for the management of patients with AMI were updated in 1999.[2] In this document and others from the American College of Cardiology (ACC) and the American Heart Association (AHA), recommendations and indications for specific procedures, therapies, or intervention are classified by the strength of the consensus group's recommendation and the level of evidence supporting that recommendation. (See class table [p. i].)

These designations help the clinician rank the various therapies based on the consensus opinion of experts in the field. These designations will be included as appropriate for each of the therapies discussed. The assessing and treating physician should consider all these initial therapies and institute them as soon as possible.

OXYGEN

Oxygen is perhaps the most widely used drug in medicine. Nearly all patients transported by emergency medical services (EMS) arrive with an oxygen mask. At many institutions, oxygen is started on every patient with chest discomfort, even before placing the patient on a monitor or obtaining an ECG. Intuitively, it would seem that an acute myocardial event is associated with an oxygen debt to the myocardium and the rest of the body. A logical assumption might be that supplemental oxygen would help pay that debt. The true evidence in support for oxygen is much less pervasive.

Recommendations for the use of oxygen are according to the guidelines as follows:

Class I: Supplemental oxygen should be administered to patients with arterial oxygen saturation less than 90%.

Class IIa: It is reasonable to administer supplemental oxygen to all patient with uncomplicated STEMI during the first 6 hours.

There has been some evidence to support the potential limitation of myocardial injury through the use of oxygen, suggesting that patients may be modestly hypoxemic due to shunting and the potential for cardiogenic pulmonary edema.[3–5] These data do not suggest, however, that this therapy should be instituted on all patients presenting with chest discomfort. The IIa recommendation for patients with diagnosed myocardial infarction in the first 6 hours of treatment is less supported by evidence, but generally thought to be effective. Beyond 6 hours, oxygen is thought to be less effective.

The clinician should also be aware that the use of oxygen is not without expense or complication. Excessive oxygen may harm patients with chronic obstructive pulmonary disease (COPD). In high flow amounts, oxygen causes peripheral vasoconstriction. The damage caused by oxygen free radicals is not yet completely understood or known.

For now, it seems that oxygen is best reserved for use in those patients who meet the following criteria:

1. Overt pulmonary edema on examination or chest radiograph.
2. Arterial oxygen saturation less than 90%.
3. Patients with AMI in the first 6 hours.

NITROGLYCERIN

Nitroglycerin is another frequently used medication in the care of patients with chest discomfort. Nearly all patients with chest pain considered to be of possible cardiac origin receive at least one sublingual nitroglycerin. Many attributes of nitroglycerin make it unique. For one, it comes in many forms: sublingual tablets, long-acting pills, spray, paste, and intravenous. Secondly, patients themselves often titrate their own doses at home before arriving in the care of a physician. It is often the failure of nitroglycerin to relieve a patient's symptoms that prompts the evaluation. Lastly, some clinicians have gone as far to use the effect of nitroglycerin on a patient's symptoms for diagnosis.

Nitroglycerin acts to relieve myocardial ischemic pain through dilatation of the vascular smooth muscle. It dilates not only the coronary vessels, but also the peripheral arteries and veins. The result can be beneficial if nitroglycerin is used judiciously and appropriately. A common and serious complication of nitroglycerin is hypotension, which further risks the ischemic myocardium. This is a particular concern in those patients who have a suspected right ventricular infraction. These patients are preload dependent and extremely sensitive to this drug and may become significantly hypotensive with even small doses.

Sublingual or transdermal nitroglycerin is a good starting place for patients in the evaluation phase. Once a patient is determined to have ACS, nitroglycerin can be best used intravenously and titrated according to the patient's pain.

Recommendations for the use of intravenous nitroglycerin are as follows[2]:

Class I: For the first 48 hours in patients with AMI and congestive hear failure (CHF), large anterior infarction, persistent ischemia, or hypertension. Use may be continued for those patients with recurrent angina or pulmonary congestion.

Class IIb: For the first 48 hours in all patients with acute MI who do not have hypotension, bradycardia, or tachycardia. Continued use is acceptable in those patients with a large or complicated infarction.

Class III: Patients with a systolic pressure <90 mmHg or with severe bradycardia <50 bpm.

Long-acting nitrates are generally contraindicated in the management of AMI. Their absorption is unpredictable with a potentially unstable patient with variable perfusion. The long half-life of such formulations is difficult to counter if the patient should become hypotensive. These medications are most adequately used in the outpatient setting for the management of chronic stable angina.

Nitroglycerin has little or no place in the diagnosis of ACS. Some clinicians feel that pain that is not improved or relieved by nitroglycerin must not be cardiac in origin. Conversely, some others maintain that a positive response to nitroglycerin portends a cardiac etiology. Both of these allegations are met with numerous examples and studies contradicting these beliefs.[6]

The appropriate and inappropriate uses of nitroglycerin are outlined below:

1. Intravenous nitroglycerin should be used in patients with large infarctions, persistent ischemia, pulmonary congestion, or hypertension.
2. Transdermal or sublingual nitroglycerin can be judiciously used in patients with chest pain consistent with possible AMI.
3. Nitroglycerin should not be used in patients with right ventricular infarctions or those who are hypotensive or bradycardic.[7]

ASPIRIN

Aspirin is an integral part in the early management of all patients with suspected AMI. It is perhaps the most beneficial immediate treatment that can be administered to the patient with myocardial ischemia and can be given promptly and with confidence to all suspected patients without aspirin sensitivity contraindications. It is widely available, inexpensive, and easy to administer. The recommendation for the use of aspirin in this population is clear and well supported.[2]

> Class I: A dose of 160–325 mg should be given on day 1 and continued indefinitely thereafter.
> Class IIb: Other antiplatelet agents such as clopidogrel may be substituted in the patient who has a true aspirin allergy or if the patient is unresponsive to aspirin.

The pivotal trial making aspirin the mainstay of initial AMI treatment was the Second International Study of Infarct Survival (ISIS-2).[8] In this trial, administration of aspirin resulted in a mortality reduction of 23%. In addition to reducing mortality, it also reduces coronary reocclusion and recurrent ischemic events.[9] This medication acts by almost immediately and totally inhibiting endogenous thromboxane A2 production.

Recommendations for aspirin include the following:

1. Aspirin (160–325 mg) should be given to all patients suspected of having acute coronary ischemia.
2. Rectal aspirin suppositories should be used in patients with severe nausea or vomiting.
3. In patients with true aspirin allergy, other antiplatelet agents such as clopidogrel should be considered.

BETA-BLOCKERS

Beta-blockers should be considered in all patients with ischemia. There is overwhelming evidence for the use of these agents both early in the patient's course and later after an event. A large metaanalysis of patients in the prethrombolytic era showed a 14% relative risk reduction in 7-day mortality.[10] Intravenous formulations should be considered in patients with ongoing pain, hypertension, or tachycardia and can be continued orally after control. These agents decrease cardiac work and myocardial oxygen demand. Slowing of the heart rate increases the duration of diastole, thereby increasing coronary and collateral blood flow. Administration should target a heart rate of about 60–70 bpm. Beta-blockers should not be given in patients with AV block, history of severe asthma or COPD, or severe LV dysfunction. If concerns exist about beta-blocker reaction, short-acting agents such as metoprolol or esmolol in small doses can be used.

The guideline recommendations for beta-blockers are as follows[11]:

> Class I: An oral beta-blocker should be administered promptly to those patients without a contraindication and is not contingent whether a patient receives concomitant fibrinolytic therapy or performance of primary PCI.
> Class IIa: It is reasonable to administer intravenous beta-blockers promptly to ST elevation myocardial infarction (STEMI) patients without contraindications, especially if tachycardia or hypertension is present.

When beta-blockers are truly contraindicated, a nondihydropyridine calcium-channel blocker, such as diltiazem, may be used in the absence of severe LV dysfunction. The immediate release form of nifedipine is contraindicated due to its reflex sympathetic activation, tachycardia, and sudden hypotension.

INHIBITORS OF THE RENIN-ANGIOTENSIN-ALDOSTERONE SYSTEM

Inhibitors of the renin-angiotensin-aldosterone system include ACE inhibitors and angiotensin receptor blockers (ARB). In the ED, ACE inhibitors should generally be considered in the acute phase of treatment if the patient is persistently hypertensive despite treatment with other previously administered agents such as nitroglycerin and beta-blockers.

In addition, guideline recommendations for the use of this class of medications include[11]:

> Class I: An ACE inhibitor should be administered orally within the first 24 hours in patients with anterior infarction, pulmonary congestion, or a LVEF less than 40%. And ARB should be administered to patients who cannot tolerate ACE inhibitors. This applies for patients with the absence of hypotension or known contraindications to this class of medications.

Class IIa: An ACE inhibitor administered orally within the first 24 hours can be useful in STEMI patients without anterior infarction, pulmonary congestion, or an LVEF less than 40%.

Of note, due to the risk of hypotension, intravenous administration of ACE inhibitors in the first 24 hours is a class III recommendation and should not occur.

A large number of randomized trials have established the benefit for the early use of ACE inhibitors. The majority of the trials support starting this medication in the first 24 hours, after other therapies have occurred and the blood pressure has been stabilized. The use of ARBs is not as well supported by clinical trial evidence, yet these agents appear to be particularly useful in patients with a depressed LVEF or signs of clinical heart failure who are intolerant of ACE inhibition.[11]

OTHER ADJUCTIVE MEASURES

Patients with AMI are by definition "unstable" and should be treated with significant care and appropriate monitoring. Other recommendations for the treatment of patients with acute ischemia include[11,12]:

1. Bed rest with continuous ECG monitoring. Patients with potential acute ischemia should not be allowed to ambulate without monitoring and supervision. Continuous monitoring serves to theoretically assist in the detection of arrhythmias.

2. Intravenous morphine sulfate when symptoms are not relieved with nitroglycerin. Initial doses of 2–4 mg seem most appropriate. This can be titrated and repeated as needed for further pain. Respiratory depression can ensue rapidly in the unstable patient.

3. Hyperglycemia should be aggressively monitored and treated. This can be achieved through insulin infusion.

4. Magnesium and other electrolyte deficits should be corrected. Electrolyte disturbances are more common in patients previously on diuretic therapy.

In summary, the overall care and choice of therapy in these patients should be governed by assessment of risk and severity of symptoms. The initial goal for all these patients is alleviate their symptoms, thereby reducing myocardial ischemia. Frequent assessment, continuous monitoring, and judicious use of appropriate therapies give the patient the best chance for a good outcome.

Hospital-based protocols may assist in providing consistent treatment. Checklists may prompt therapies that might otherwise have been omitted. Easily accessible lists of common contraindications can help reduce medical error. Successful patient treatment relies on the timely collaboration of physicians, nurses, and other caregivers.

REFERENCES

1. Association AH. *2002 Heart and Stroke Statitical Update*. Dallas, TX: American Heart Association, 2002.
2. Ryan TJ, Antman EM, Brooks NH, et al. 1999 update: ACC/AHA guidelines for the management of patients with acute myocardial infarction. A report of the American College of Cardiology/American Heart Association Task Force on Practice Guidelines (Committee on Management of Acute Myocardial Infarction). *J Am Coll Cardiol* 1999;34(3):890–911.
3. Fillmore SJ, Shapiro M, Killip T. Arterial oxygen tension in acute myocardial infarction. Serial analysis of clinical state and blood gas changes. *Am Heart J* 1970;79(5): 620–629.
4. Madias JE, Madias NE, Hood WB, Jr. Precordial ST-segment mapping. 2. Effects of oxygen inhalation on ischemic injury in patients with acute myocardial infarction. *Circulation* 1976;53(3):411–417.
5. Maroko PR, Radvany P, Braunwald E, et al. Reduction of infarct size by oxygen inhalation following acute coronary occlusion. *Circulation* 1975;52(3):360–368.
6. Constant J. The diagnosis of nonanginal chest pain. *Keio J Med* 1990;39(3):187–192.
7. Come PC, Pitt B. Nitroglycerin-induced severe hypotension and bradycardia in patients with acute myocardial infarction. *Circulation* 1976;54(4):624–628.
8. Randomized trial of intravenous streptokinase, oral aspirin, both, or neither among 17,187 cases of suspected acute myocardial infarction: ISIS-2. (Second International Study of Infarct Survival) Collaborative Group. *J Am Coll Cardiol* 1988;12(6 Suppl A):3A–13A.
9. Roux S, Christeller S, Ludin E. Effects of aspirin on coronary reocclusion and recurrent ischemia after thrombolysis: A meta-analysis. *J Am Coll Cardiol* 1992;19(3): 671–677.
10. Hennekens CH. Beta blockers. In: Hennekens CH (ed.), *Clinical Trials in Cardiovascular Disease: A Companion to Braunwald's Heart Disease*. Philadelphia, PA: W.B. Saunders, 1999, pp. 79–94.
11. Antman EM, Anbe DT, Armstrong PW, et al. ACC/AHA guidelines for the management of patients with ST-elevation myocardial infarction—executive summary. A report of the American College of Cardiology/American Heart Association Task Force on Practice Guidelines (Writing Committee to revise the 1999 guidelines for the management of patients

with acute myocardial infarction). *J Am Coll Cardiol* 2004;44(3):671–719.

12. Braunwald E, Antman EM, Beasley JW, et al. ACC/AHA 2002 guideline update for the management of patients with unstable angina and non-ST-segment elevation myocardial infarction—summary article: a report of the American College of Cardiology/American Heart Association task force on practice guidelines (Committee on the Management of Patients With Unstable Angina). *J Am Coll Cardiol* 2002;40(7): 1366–1374.

12

Nonaspirin Antiplatelet Agents for Acute Coronary Syndromes

Charles V. Pollack, Jr.

HIGH YIELD FACTS

- Platelet activation and aggregation are provoked by plaque rupture in the coronary arteries, and are at the root of thrombus formation and ischemic complications of acute coronary syndrome (ACS).
- There are multiple pharmacologic modalities via which platelet activity can be attenuated, and the benefit of antiplatelet therapy is typically magnified when used in conjunction with invasive management of ACS.
- Higher-risk ACS patients generally derive greater benefit from antiplatelet therapy.

INTRODUCTION

Only over several decades has the pivotal role of the platelet in acute thrombosis come fully to be appreciated. Thanks to this understanding, bolstered now by countless recent and ongoing randomized clinical trials, antithrombotic therapy with antiplatelet agents is now routine in cardiology and emergency medicine practice. Because of the multiple mechanisms via which platelet activation and aggregation can be interrupted, antiplatelet therapy is likely to remain a mainstay of therapy in ACS. Interference with platelet function may of course precipitate certain adverse events—particularly bleeding—as well, and therefore appropriate use of antiplatelet agents must always be guided by good clinical risk stratification and by an objective assessment of the likely risk: benefit ratio of therapy in each individual patient.

Antiplatelet therapy for ACS at this writing consists of the following choices: aspirin, adenosine diphosphate (ADP) receptor antagonists (the thienopyridines, clopidogrel, and ticlopidine), and glycoprotein (GP)

IIb/IIIa receptor antagonists (the chimeric *large molecule* antibody abciximab, and the *small molecules* eptifibatide and tirofiban). Aspirin will not be addressed in this chapter. A clear understanding of the remaining agents requires at least a cursory review of the role of platelets in acute thrombosis, which in the coronary artery in the setting of typical ACS is now often termed *atherothrombosis*.

Atherothrombosis can be defined as superimposed thrombus formation in the setting of preexisting athero-sclerotic plaque (see Fig. 12-1).[1] Platelets, which control bleeding and hemostasis, normally circulate in an inactivated state, but become activated in the presence of vascular injury. Proteins in the blood and vessel wall are released when an atherosclerotic plaque ruptures, inducing platelets to convert to an activated state. Activated platelets bind to collagen within the newly exposed arterial subendothelial matrix at the base of the plaque, inducing a conformational change in the platelet cell as well as degranulation of a variety of platelet granules. This leads to release of chemoattractant agents that recruit more platelets to the area.[2] A variety of mediators found in abundance in this matrix are known to induce the activated state in platelets; these include collagen, von Willebrand's factor, thromboxane A_2, thrombin, ADP, and epinephrine, among many others. ADP also binds to surface receptors on neighboring platelets, further amplifying the cyclical process of platelet activation, degranulation, and aggregation.[3]

The ultimate result of platelet activation is elaboration of GP IIb/IIIa receptors on the platelet surface. Once activated, these receptors bind fibrinogen, resulting in three-dimensional cross-linking among neighboring platelets and subsequent thrombus formation.[4] Activation of cyclooxygenase in platelets results in the elaboration of thromboxane A_2, which further activates neighboring platelets and helps generate a relatively more fibrinolytic-resistant aggregate. Products of the coagulation pathway, also stimulated by tissue factor from within the ruptured plaque,[5] act to convert prothrombin to thrombin, which in turn converts fibrinogen to fibrin and further stabilizes the platelet aggregate into a luminal clot. The clot may trigger an acute vascular event in situ if it is of sufficient size with respect to the vessel lumen, or it may be the source of platelet-aggregate emboli that can cause downstream ischemia or frank infarction.[6]

Interference with ADP receptors (via use of thienopyridines) and with thromboxane A_2 receptors (with aspirin) primarily reduce platelet activation, although these approaches may also attenuate platelet aggregation through a less well-understood mechanism. GP IIb/IIIa receptor antagonists exert a beneficial effect in ACS by

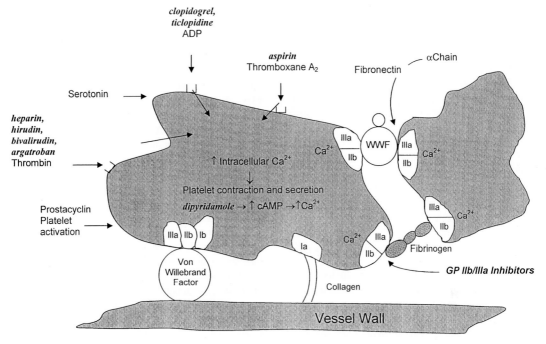

Fig. 12-1. Platelet activation and aggregation at a site of coronary atherothrombosis. Platelet interactions with agonists and antagonists of platelet aggregation, the vessel wall, other platelets, and adhesive macromolecules. Agents in italics prevent the formation, or inhibit the function, of the adjacent agonists of platelet aggregation. (Source: Adapted with permission from Almony GT, Lefkovits J, Topol EJ. Antiplatelet and anticoagulant use after myocardial infarction. *Clin Cardiol* 1996;19:357–365.)

occupying the platelet surface integrin GP IIb/IIIa receptors, preventing the binding of fibrinogen to platelets and therefore limiting platelet-to-platelet linkages and platelet aggregation.

ADP RECEPTOR ANTAGONISTS: TICLOPIDINE AND CLOPIDOGREL

Inhibition of platelet ADP receptors results in reductions in both platelet activation and platelet aggregation.[7] It may also manifest a secondary inhibitory effect by preventing degranulation of activated platelets.[2] There are two ADP receptor antagonists approved for clinical use in the United States. They are both thienopyridines and share numerous chemical characteristics. Ticlopidine was developed first, followed by clopidogrel, which differs from the former by the addition of a carboxymethyl side group. This structural change may account for clopidogrel's milder side effect profile and more rapid induction of antiplatelet activity (see below).[8] Both agents have been studied in clinical trials of patients with atherothrombosis. Both agents are recommended in PCI guidelines (class I), for AMI patients allergic or unresponsive to aspirin therapy (class IIb),[9] and for patients with unstable angina (UA) or non-ST elevation myocardial infarction (NSTEMI) who are unable to take aspirin due to hypersensitivity or major gastrointestinal (GI) intolerance (class Ib).[10]

ADP receptor antagonists are potentially indicated in the ED, but the use of ticlopidine in the acute care setting is limited by at least four important issues:

1. The slow onset of action of ticlopidine (5 days to full therapeutic effect), compared with the prompt activity after a loading dose of clopidogrel.[11,12]

2. Ticlopidine's association with significant neutropenia in about 1% of patients, mandating frequent and close monitoring of white blood cell counts, at least during the first months of therapy.[13]

3. A high frequency of adverse GI effects prompting discontinuation of ticlopidine.[14]

4. Ticlopidine's much greater association (0.2% incidence, more than 100 times that with clopidogrel) with thrombotic thrombocytopenic purpura (TTP).[15]

The most common adverse effects associated with clopidogrel are rash and GI upset; clopidogrel has been only very rarely associated with TTP and no specific laboratory monitoring is required during its use. A single 300 mg loading dose of clopidogrel provides significantly greater inhibition of ADP-induced platelet aggregation on the first day of treatment than either ticlopidine 500 mg/day or clopidogrel 75 mg/day.[16] Use of either drug is contraindicated in patients with active bleeding and both should be used only with caution in patients with a significant risk of bleeding complications.

COMBINATION ANTIPLATELET THERAPY

The synergistic effect of combination antiplatelet therapy using aspirin and a thienopyridine is important in the management of ACS. Early studies showed that more complete antiplatelet inhibition is achieved by simultaneously targeting multiple sites of platelet activation.[17,18] Cadroy and colleagues assessed the antithrombotic effects of the combination of aspirin and clopidogrel, with or without a 300 mg loading dose, versus aspirin alone in a model of arterial thrombosis. A beneficial antithrombotic effect was found 6 hours after administration of the aspirin and clopidogrel combination without a loading dose, and it was significantly superior to the effect of aspirin alone. The antithrombotic effects when a loading dose of clopidogrel was used were evident within 90 min and achieved a level at 6 hours similar to that on day 10. The clopidogrel and aspirin combination at day 10 was significantly more potent than aspirin alone.[19]

The combination of ticlopidine and aspirin was established early as the regimen of choice in coronary artery stenting.[20,21] Generally, aspirin therapy is given indefinitely, while the duration of therapy with ticlopidine is usually 2–4 weeks. Clopidogrel has recently replaced ticlopidine in this setting because of its similar efficacy, more rapid onset of activity, and more acceptable safety profile.[22] There are relatively few data on combination therapy with ADP receptor antagonists and GP IIb/IIIa receptor antagonists for patients with ACS in which the ADP agent is administered first. Data from the Tirofiban And Reopro Give similar Efficacy outcomes Trial (TARGET), however, indicate that a loading dose of clopidogrel prior to PCI with adjunctive abciximab or tirofiban given after the clopidogrel is associated with improved outcomes at 30 days.[23,24]

Clinical trials have demonstrated that ADP receptor antagonists are effective in the secondary prevention of atherosclerotic disease. In the Clopidogrel vs. Aspirin in Patients at Risk of Ischemic Events (CAPRIE) protocol, 19,185 patients with a recent acute arterial thrombotic episode (ischemic stroke within 1 week to 6 months; MI ≤35 days old; or atherosclerotic peripheral arterial disease) were randomized in double-blinded fashion to either aspirin 325 mg/day or clopidogrel 75 mg/day. The mean follow-up interval was nearly 2 years. Clopidogrel was associated with a relative risk reduction of 8.7% in the composite endpoint of ischemic stroke, MI, or vascular death. It was concluded that in a patient population similar to that in CAPRIE treated for 1 year, clopidogrel would prevent 24 major clinical events per 1000 patients, compared to 19 major events prevented with aspirin alone. The occurrence of adverse events between clopidogrel and aspirin was similar.[25]

The largest and most definitive study of the effects of an ADP receptor antagonist in ACS is the Clopidogrel in Unstable angina to prevent Recurrent Events (CURE) trial. CURE was a multicenter, randomized, prospective study to evaluate the combination of clopidogrel and aspirin versus aspirin alone in patients with non-ST-segment elevation (NSTE) ACS. The 12,562 patients were eligible for inclusion if they presented within 24 hours of experiencing chest pain and had either diagnostic ECG changes or positive cardiac markers. Clopidogrel 300 mg or placebo was administered as a loading dose as soon as treatment was allocated. This was followed by clopidogrel 75 mg/day (or placebo) and aspirin 75–325 mg/day. In addition, most patients received "best medical" therapy including a heparin agent, beta-blockers, calcium-channel antagonists, ACE inhibitors, and lipid-lowering agents; only a small minority of patients, however, received IIb/IIIa receptor blockers, and only 21% were managed interventionally. Treatment continued for a minimum of 3 months and varying periods up to 1 year.[26] The primary study endpoint was a composite of death, reinfarction, or stroke. At 12-month follow-up, 11.4% of patients randomized to placebo versus 9.3% of patients on clopidogrel reached the primary endpoint. This represents a statistically significant 20% risk reduction, driven largely by a reduction in the incidence of MI (5.2% vs. 6.7%). Major bleeding but not life-threatening bleeding was modestly but significantly increased (3.7% vs. 2.7% in placebo).[26]

Aggressive treatment and intervention for UA and NSTEMI in the ED remains a relatively new phenomenon, unlike the ED management of patients with ST-segment elevation events; that the full and irreversible therapeutic benefit of clopidogrel administered in a loading dose (300 mg bolus) is evident within 2 hours makes use of this drug consistent with an early treatment approach. A potential concern pertinent to administering clopidogrel for ACS in the ED is that at least 10–15% of these patients typically go to coronary artery by-pass grafting (CABG) during the index hospitalization,[27,28] and irreversibly inhibited platelets may create problems for, or cause delays in, surgical management. This is highlighted in the 2002 update to the 2000 ACC/AHA NSTE ACS guidelines,[10] which state that in patients taking clopidogrel in whom CABG is planned, if possible the drug should be withheld for at least 5 days, and preferably for 7 days. The timing of a clopidogrel loading dose, therefore, should be related to the intended management strategy (interventional vs. medical) and anticipated time to intervention, if any, in the individual institution, in a protocol developed jointly by emergency physicians, cardiologists, and cardiac surgeons.[29]

Late vascular occlusive sequelae postcoronary intervention are other examples of platelet-mediated events that can result in acute thrombotic events. The CLopidogrel ASpirin Stent International Cooperative Study (CLASSICS) showed that the combination of clopidogrel and aspirin is superior in safety to the combination of ticlopidine and aspirin in 1020 postcoronary stent patients started on one of three 28-day antiplatelet regimens: a 300 mg loading dose of clopidogrel followed by the combination of aspirin and clopidogrel; aspirin and clopidogrel without a loading dose; or ticlopidine and aspirin. The primary combined endpoint of major peripheral or bleeding complications, neutropenia, thrombocytopenia, or early discontinuation of therapy was reached in 9.1% of the ticlopidine-treated patients and only 4.6% in the combined clopidogrel-treated patients. The use of a 300-mg loading dose of clopidogrel was not associated with an increased risk of bleeding and was well tolerated.[30]

To evaluate the benefit of long-term clopidogrel after PCI and to determine the benefit of initiating clopidogrel with a preprocedure loading dose, the Clopidogrel for the Reduction of Events During Observation (CREDO) trial was conducted among 2116 patients who were to undergo elective PCI or were deemed at high likelihood of undergoing PCI.[31] Patients were randomly assigned to receive a 300-mg clopidogrel loading dose or placebo, 3–24 hours before PCI. All patients then received clopidogrel, 75 mg/day, through day 28. From day 29 through 12 months, patients in the loading-dose group received clopidogrel, 75 mg/day, and those in the control group received placebo, all in addition to aspirin. Both groups received aspirin throughout the study. At 1 year, long-term clopidogrel therapy was associated with a 26.9% relative reduction in the combined risk of death, MI, or stroke. Clopidogrel pretreatment did not significantly reduce the combined risk of death, MI, or urgent target vessel revascularization at 28 days, and risk of major bleeding at 1 year increased, but not significantly.[31] These data should also be considered in the decision of when to initiate clopidogrel therapy in ACS patients.

GP IIB/IIIA RECEPTOR INHIBITION THERAPY

Platelet receptor GP IIb/IIIa has been identified as the final and obligatory common pathway to platelet aggregation, regardless of the activation stimulus. GP IIb/IIIa expressed on the surface of platelets on platelet activation mediates platelet aggregation by binding to fibrinogen, which forms bridges between platelets, thus linking them together into aggregates. There are approximately 80,000 copies of GP IIb/IIIa on the surface of each activated platelet.[32] Several lines of evidence point to the platelet receptor GP IIb/IIIa as the final common pathway to platelet aggregation and, therefore, a rational therapeutic target for the prevention of arterial thrombotic events in ACS. For example, patients with Glanzmann's thrombasthenia, a condition in which platelet aggregation is disrupted, have been shown to have defective GP IIb/IIIa receptors. In addition, the platelets of these patients fail to aggregate in the presence of known platelet agonists.[33] These insights have resulted in significant research efforts to develop drug therapies that inhibit platelet receptor GP IIb/IIIa to prevent platelet aggregation and arterial thrombosis.

To date, three agents with activity at the GP IIb/IIIa receptor have been approved by the U.S. Food and Drug Administration for clinical use: the chimeric antibody abciximab, which establishes a relatively long-term and noncompetitive blockade at the receptor, and two smaller molecules, eptifibatide and tirofiban, which exert a reversible and competitive interference with fibrinogen binding. Animal data demonstrate that ADP-induced platelet aggregation is completely prevented when at least 80% of GP IIb/IIIa receptors are blocked, although there is significant heterogeneity in the extent of GP IIb/IIIa receptor blockade and platelet inhibition induced by these agents. Some 40–70% of patients achieve >90% platelet inhibition after an initial bolus.[34–36]

These concerns notwithstanding, multiple studies have confirmed the efficacy of these agents in reducing the composite risk of death, MI, or urgent revascularization at 30 days, when used in conjunction with percutaneous coronary intervention, and these effects appear to be both additive to aspirin and clopidogrel, and persistent over time.[37-42] The benefits of GP IIb/IIIa receptor blockade are clearly greater in higher-risk, ACS patients, than in lower-risk or elective PCI patients.[43] Furthermore, prolonged infusion of abciximab without intervention may have negative outcomes, as demonstrated in the Global Utilization of STrategies to Open occluded arteries (GUSTO IV-ACS) trial.[44] This trial studied 7800 patients with chest pain syndrome plus ST-segment depression or an elevated troponin level, and who received aspirin and heparin but did not undergo early intervention. Treatment of these patients with abciximab produced no benefit in death or MI at 30 days, and was actually associated with a 14% increase in death or MI at 48 hours.[44] Likewise, studies of long-term oral GP IIb/IIIa inhibitors have been routinely disappointing.[45,46]

The three currently approved drugs have different chemical structures and perform differently in clinical use. The use of abciximab results in persistent receptor occupancy despite its short half-life; platelet aggregation gradually returns to normal 24–48 hours after discontinuation of the drug. Although it is an antibody, it is not completely specific to the GP IIb/IIIa receptor. Eptifibatide and tirofiban establish receptor occupancy that is in general in equilibrium with plasma levels. They have half-lives of 2–3 hours and are highly specific for the GP IIb/IIIa receptor. Platelet aggregation returns to normal in 4–8 hours after discontinuation of a small molecule GP IIb/IIIa inhibitor. Because the various agents have not been compared directly with each other, their *relative* efficacy is not known.

Abciximab has been studied primarily in trials of interventional management, in which it has been consistently associated with a significant reduction in the rate of MI and the need for urgent revascularization. The C7e3 AntiPlatelet Therapy in Unstable REfractory Angina (CAPTURE) trial enrolled patients with refractory UA.[47] After angiographic identification of a culprit lesion suitable for angioplasty, patients were randomized to receive either abciximab or placebo administered for 20–24 hours before angioplasty and for 1 hour thereafter. The rate of the composite of death, MI, or urgent revascularization in 30 days was significantly reduced with abciximab. The difference did not persist at 6-month follow-up. Because of its longer duration of action, abciximab is not optimal for use in patients likely to need CABG; a small molecule GP IIb/IIIa antagonist is preferred in this setting. Abciximab is approved for the treatment of NSTE ACS as an adjunct to PCI, or when PCI is planned within 24 hours.

The Platelet Receptor Inhibition in ischemic Syndrome Management in Patients Limited by Unstable Signs and Symptoms (PRISM-PLUS) trial enrolled 1915 patients with clinical NSTE ACS and the presence of either ischemic ST-segment changes or creatine kinase (CK) and CK-MB elevation. Patients were randomized to receive tirofiban alone, unfractionated heparin (UFH) alone, or the combination for a period of 48–108 hours.[28] The tirofiban-alone arm was dropped during the trial because of an excess mortality rate. The combination of tirofiban and UFH compared with UFH alone reduced the primary composite endpoint of death, MI, or refractory ischemia at 7 days, 30 days, and 6 months, respectively. Computer-analyzed cine-angiography also confirmed that patients who received tirofiban exhibited a significantly lower thrombus load.[48] Tirofiban has been approved for the treatment of patients with NSTE ACS, in conjunction with heparin, in patients who are managed medically as well as those undergoing PCI.

Eptifibatide was studied in the Platelet glycoprotein IIb/IIIa in Unstable angina: Receptor Suppression Using Integrilin Therapy (PURSUIT) trial of 10,948 patients who had chest pain syndrome and ST-segment changes or CK-MB elevation.[27] Eptifibatide or placebo was added to standard management until hospital discharge or for 72 hours, although patients found to have normal coronary arteries could receive shorter infusions. The primary outcome rate of the double composite of death or nonfatal MI at 30 days was significantly reduced with eptifibatide. A substantial treatment effect was seen as early as 96 hours, and was maintained at 6-month follow-up. Eptifibatide has been approved for the treatment of patients with NSTE ACS who are treated medically or with PCI.

The aggregate effects of the GP IIb/IIIa class are clearly positive in the NSTE ACS population. A metaanalysis of the effects of GP IIb/IIIa antagonists in all six large randomized placebo-controlled trials was performed by Boersma et al.[49] A small but significant reduction in the odds of death or MI in the active treatment arm (11.8% vs. 10.8%) was observed. The effect was more pronounced in patients who underwent PCI. Major bleeding complications were increased in the GP IIb/IIIa antagonist-treated group compared to those who received placebo, although the incidence of intracranial bleeding was not increased.

The major adverse effect seen with intravenous administration of the GP IIb/IIIa receptor antagonists is an increased risk of bleeding, which is typically mucocutaneous or involves access sites used for interventions.[10] Major bleeding rates for GP IIb/IIIa receptor antagonists were as much as two to three times greater than for placebo in early trials, although substantial responsibility for that extent of bleeding is likely attributable to higher heparin doses than are currently used in conjunction with GP IIb/IIIa agents.[10] Analysis of safety data is further confounded by the use of different definitions of significant bleeding and CABG-related bleeding among the various trials. For example, in the PRISM-PLUS trial,[28] major bleeding by TIMI criteria occurred in 1.4% of patients who received tirofiban versus 0.8% of patients who received heparin only, and in PURSUIT,[27] non-CABG patients showed a 3.0% "major bleeding" rate if they received eptifibatide and 1.3% with placebo. No trials have shown an increased risk of intracranial bleeding associated with GP IIb/IIIa therapy. Given current data, the optimal employment of GP IIb/IIIa receptor blockade is for high-risk NSTE ACS patients being managed invasively. There is clearly a role for small-molecule agents (eptifibatide and tirofiban) in high-risk patients who cannot or will not be taken to intervention.[10]

SUMMARY

Antiplatelet therapy has been demonstrated as beneficial in both ACS and in routine coronary interventions, with both acute and long-term efficacy. Optimal benefit from these drugs is obtained in the context of higher-risk patients undergoing invasive management. Currently available antiplatelet modalities include antiactivation and antiaggregation agents, and an understanding of platelet biology is important in optimizing their use.

REFERENCES

1. Montalescot G. Value of antiplatelet therapy in preventing thrombotic events in generalized vascular disease. *Clin Cardiol* 2000;23(Suppl VI):VI-18–VI-22.
2. Coller BS. Platelets in cardiovascular thrombosis and thrombolysis. In: Fozzard HA, Jennings RB, Haber E, Katz AM (eds.), *The Heart and Cardiovascular System*, 2nd ed. New York: Raven Press, 1991, pp. 219–233.
3. Libby P. Multiple mechanisms of thrombosis complicating atherosclerotic plaques. *Clin Cardiol* 2000;23(Suppl VI): VI-3–VI-7.
4. Califf RM, Simoons ML. Use of glycoprotein IIb/IIIa inhibitors in coronary syndromes: State of the art. *Am Heart J* 1998;135:S31–S55.
5. Schafer AI. Coagulation cascade: An overview. In: Loscalzo J, Schafer AI (eds.), *Thrombosis and Hemorrhage*. Boston, MA: Blackwell Scientific, 1994, pp. 3–12.
6. Ambrose JA, Weinrauch M. Thrombosis in ischemic heart disease. *Arch Intern Med* 1996;156:1382–1394.
7. Humbert M, Nurden P, Bihour C, et al. Ultrastructural studies of platelet aggregates from human subjects receiving

8. Van de Graaff E, Steinhubl SR. Antiplatelet medications and their indications in preventing and treating coronary thrombosis. *Ann Med* 2000;32:561–571.
9. Ryan TJ, Antman EM, Brooks NH, et al. 1999 Update. ACC/AHA guidelines for the management of patients with acute myocardial infarction: Executive summary and recommendations. *Circulation* 1999;100:1016–1030.
10. Braunwald E, Antman EM, Beasley JW, et al. ACC/AHA guidelines for the management of patients with unstable angina and non-ST-segment elevation myocardial infarction: A report of the American College of Cardiology/American Heart Association Task Force on Practice Guidelines (Committee on the Management of Patients with Unstable Angina). *J Am Coll Cardiol* 2000;36:970–1062. Updated on March 15, 2002, at *www.americanheart.org* and *http://www.acc.org*.
11. Savcic M, Hauert J, Bachmann F, et al. Clopidogrel loading dose regimens: Kinetic profile of pharmacodynamic response in healthy subjects. *Semin Thromb Hemost* 1999;25(Suppl 2): 15–19.
12. Helft G, Osende JI, Worthley SG, et al. Acute antithrombotic effect of a front-loaded regimen of clopidogrel in patients with atherosclerosis on aspirin. *Arterioscler Thromb Vasc Biol* 2000;20:2316–2321.
13. Gill S, Majumdar S, Brown NE, et al. Ticlodipine-associated pancytopenia: Implications of an acetylsalicylate acid alternative. *Can J Cardiol* 1997;13:909–913.
14. Package insert, Ticlopidine hydrochloride, Roche Laboratories.
15. Bennet C, Weinberg P, Rozenberg-Ben-Dror K, et al. Thrombotic thrombocytopenic purpura associated with ticlopidine: A review of 60 cases. *Ann Intern Med* 1998; 128:541–544.
16. Darius H, Rupprecht H-J, Kress P, et al. Accelerated inhibition of platelet activity by clopidogrel loading dose in patients following coronary stent implantation. *Eur Heart J* 1999;20(Abstr Suppl):252.
17. Harker LA, Marzec UM, Kelly AB, et al. Clopidogrel inhibition of stent, graft, and vascular thrombogenesis with antithrombotic enhancement by aspirin in nonhuman primates. *Circulation* 1998;98:2461–2469.
18. Herbert J-M, Dol F, Bernat A, et al. The antiaggregating and antithrombotic activity of clopidogrel is potentiated by aspirin in several experimental models in the rabbit. *Thromb Haemost* 1998;80:512–518.
19. Cadroy Y, Bossavy J-P, Thalamas C, et al. Early potent antithrombotic effect with combined aspirin and a loading dose of clopidogrel on experimental arterial thrombogenesis in humans. *Circulation* 2000;101:2823–2828.
20. Cutlip DE, Leon MB, Ho KK, et al. Acute and nine-month clinical outcomes after "suboptimal" coronary stenting: Results from the STent Anti-thrombotic Registry Study (STARS) registry. *J Am Coll Cardiol* 1999;34:698–706.
21. Bertrand ME, Legrand V, Boland J, et al. Randomized multicenter comparison of conventional anticoagulation versus

clopidogrel and from a patient with an inherited defect of an ADP-dependent pathway of platelet activation. *Arterioscler Thromb Vasc Biol* 1996;16:1532–1543.

antiplatelet therapy in unplanned and elective coronary stenting. The Full Anticoagulation versus Aspirin and Ticlopidine (FANTASTIC) Study. *Circulation* 1998;98:1597–1603.

22. Moore SA, Steinhubl SR. Clopidogrel and coronary stenting: What is the next question? *J Thromb Thrombolysis* 2000;10:121–126.

23. Moliterno DJ, Topol EJ. A direct comparison of tirofiban and Abciximab during percutaneous coronary revascularization and stent placement: Rationale and design of the TARGET study. *Am Heart J* 2000;140:722–726.

24. Topol EJ, Moliterno DJ, Herrmann HC, et al. Comparison of two platelet glycoprotein IIb/IIIa inhibitors, tirofiban and abciximab, for the prevention of ischemic events with percutaneous coronary revascularization. *N Engl J Med* 2001;344:1888–1894.

25. CAPRIE Steering Committee: A randomized, blinded trial of clopidogrel versus aspirin in patients at risk of ischaemic events (CAPRIE). *Lancet* 1996;348:1329–1339.

26. The Clopidogrel in unstable Angina to Prevent Recurrent Events Trial Investigators: Effects of clopidogrel in addition to aspirin in patients with acute coronary syndromes without ST-segment elevation. *N Engl J Med* 2001;345:494–502.

27. PURSUIT Trial Investigators: Inhibition of platelet glycoprotein IIb/IIIa with eptifibatide in patients with acute coronary syndromes. *N Engl J Med* 1998;339:436–443.

28. Platelet Receptor Inhibition in Ischemic Syndrome Management in Patients Limited by Unstable Signs and Symptoms (PRISM-PLUS) Study Investigators: Inhibition of the platelet glycoprotein IIb/IIIa receptor with tirofiban in unstable angina and non-Q-wave myocardial infarction. [published erratum appears in *N Engl J Med* 1998;339:415]. *N Engl J Med* 1998;338:1488–1497.

29. Pollack CV, Roe MT, Peterson ED. 2002 update to the ACC/AHA guidelines for the management of patients with unstable angina and non-ST-segment elevation myocardial infarction: Implications for emergency department practice. *Ann Emerg Med* 2003;41:355–369.

30. Bertrand ME, Rupprecht H-J, Urban P, et al. CLASSICS Investigators: Double-blind study of the safety of clopidogrel with and without a loading dose in combination with aspirin compared with ticlopidine in combination with aspirin after coronary stenting: The Clopidogrel Aspirin Stent International Cooperative Study (CLASSICS). *Circulation* 2000;102:624–629.

31. Steinhubl SR. Early and sustained dual oral antiplatelet therapy following percutaneous coronary intervention: a randomized clinical trial. *JAMA* 2002;288:2411–2420.

32. Wagner CL, Mascelli MA, Neblock DS, et al. Analysis of GPIIb/IIIa receptor number by quantification of 7E3 binding to human platelets. *Blood* 1996;88:907–914.

33. Phillips DR, Scarborough RM. Clinical pharmacology of eptifibatide. *Am J Cardol* 1997;80(Suppl 4A):11B–20B.

34. Coller B, Folts J, Smith S, et al. Abolition of in vivo platelet thrombus formation in primates with monoclonal antibodies to the GPIIb/IIIa receptor: Correlation with bleeding time, platelet aggregation, and blockade of GPIIb/IIIa receptors. *Circulation* 1989;80:1766–1774.

35. Kereiakes D, Broderick T, Roth E, et al. Time course, magnitude, and consistency of platelet inhibition by abciximab, tirofiban, or eptifibatide in patients with unstable angina pectoris undergoing percutaneous coronary intervention. *Am J Cardiol* 1999;84:391–395.

36. Kini AS, Richard M, Suleman J, et al. Effectiveness of tirofiban, eptifibatide, and abciximab in minimizing myocardial necrosis during percutaneous coronary intervention (TEAM pilot study). *Am J Cardiol* 2002;90:526–529.

37. The EPIC Investigators: Use of a monoclonal antibody directed against the platelet glycoprotein IIb/IIIa receptors in high-risk coronary angioplasty. *N Engl J Med* 1994;330:956–961.

38. The EPILOG Investigators: Platelet glycoprotein IIb/IIIa receptor blockade and low-dose heparin during percutaneous coronary revascularization. *N Engl J Med* 1997;336:1689–1696.

39. de Bono DP, Simoons ML, Tijssen J, et al. Effect of early intravenous heparin on coronary patency, infarct size, and bleeding complications after alteplase Thrombolysis: Results of a randomized, double-blind European Cooperative Study Group trial. *Br Heart J* 1992;67:122–128.

40. The IMPACT-II Investigators: Randomised placebo-controlled trial of the effect of eptifibatide on complications of percutaneous coronary intervention. *Lancet* 1997;349:1422–1428.

41. Topol EJ, Lincoff AM, Kereiakes DJ, et al. Multi-year follow-up of abciximab in three randomized, placebo-controlled trials of percutaneous coronary revascularization. *Am J Med* 2002;113:1–6.

42. Bonz AW, Lengenfelder B, Strotmann J, et al. Effect of additional temporary glycoprotein IIb/IIIa inhibition on troponin release in elective percutaneous coronary interventions after pretreatment with aspirin and clopidogrel. *J Am Coll Cardiol* 2002;40:662–668.

43. Patrano C, Collar B, Dalen JE, et al. Platelet active drugs: The relationships among dose, effectiveness, and side effects. *Chest* 2001;119:39S–63S.

44. GUSTO IV-ACS Investigators: Effect of glycoprotein IIb/IIIa receptor blocker abciximab on outcome in patients with acute coronary syndromes without early coronary revascularization: The GUSTO IV-ACS randomized trial. *Lancet* 2001;357:1915–1924.

45. Second SYMPHONY Investigators: Randomized trial of aspirin, sibrafiban, or both for secondary prevention after acute coronary syndromes. *Circulation* 2001;103:1727–1733.

46. Chew DP, Bhatt DL, Sapp S, Topol EJ. Increased mortality with oral platelet glycoprotein IIb/IIIa antagonists: A meta-analysis of phase III multicenter randomized trials. *Circulation* 2001;103:201–206.

47. Randomised placebo-controlled trial of abciximab before and during coronary intervention in refractory unstable angina: The CAPTURE Study [erratum appears in *Lancet* 1997;350:744]. *Lancet* 1997;349:1429–1435.

48. Zhao XQ, Theroux P, Snapinn SM, et al. Intracoronary thrombus and platelet glycoprotein IIb/IIIa receptor blockade with tirofiban in unstable angina or non–Q-wave myocardial infarction: Angiographic results from the PRISM-PLUS trial. *Circulation* 1999;100:1609–1615.

49. Boersma E, Harrington RA, Moliterno DJ, et al. Platelet glycoprotein IIb/IIIa inhibitors in acute coronary syndromes: A metaanalysis of all major randomized clinical trials. *Lancet* 2002;359:189–198.

13

Thrombolytics

David J. Robinson

HIGH YIELD FACTS

- Although percutaneous coronary intervention (PCI) in the cardiac catheterization lab may represent the most effective therapy for acute myocardial infarction (AMI), it is not uniformly available on a 24/7 basis. Therefore, thrombolytics will continue to be important interventions for the acute care physician and their patients.
- Time to thrombolytics is more determinant of outcomes in ST-segment elevation myocardial infarction (STEMI), than the choice of which agent is used.
- In contradistinction to first generation thrombolytics (streptokinase [SK]) third generation thrombolytics (tenecteplase [TNK] and reteplase [rPA]) have improved outcomes when used with some form of heparin.

INTRODUCTION

Thrombolytic development over the last 50 years resulted first from the discovery of SK as a beneficial fibrinolytic for clots in the lung. Interests in thrombolysis for AMI have lead to research initially with the "naturally" existing thrombolytic SK, the related anisoylated compound anistreplase, and the direct acting family of thrombolytics beginning with alteplase. Enhancements in the core structure of alteplase have yielded a "third" generation of thrombolytics, rPA, and TNK. Both claim clinical and technological advancements over alteplase through ease of administration, reduced side effects, and improved characteristics[1] (Table 13-1). Aside from the known applications for AMI, acute ischemic stroke, and massive pulmonary embolism, fibrinolytics are now being used or tested for occluded catheter clearance, peripheral arterial occlusion, deep venous thrombosis, and several nonvascular conditions including acute congestive heart failure, sepsis, lung abscesses, empyema, and others.

RATIONALE

Platelet activation and coagulation normally do not occur in intact blood vessels. The pathogenesis of AMI involves coronary endothelial insult with resultant disruption of atherosclerotic plaque.[2] Disruption of coronary plaque and the exposure of tissue factor causes release of coagulation factors that activate the clotting cascade. Acceleration of the clotting cascade results in the production of factor X, enhancing fibrinogenesis. Plaque rupture also exposes subendothelial proteins where platelets are attracted, adhered, and aggregated. Here, fibrin serves to crosslink the platelet aggregate to form a platelet-rich thrombus. This process results in an expanding coronary thrombus at the site of endothelial disruption that rapidly causes further vessel stenosis, resulting in low flow perfusion to target myocardium, myocardial ischemia, and infarction. Lysis of the culprit thrombus with resultant restoration of coronary flow could reverse myocardial ischemia and reduce the permanent damage resulting from necrosis.

PATHOPHYSIOLOGY OF THROMBOLYTICS

The fibrinolytic system dissolves intravascular clots through the enzymatic digestion of fibrin by activated plasmin. The inactive precursor plasminogen is converted to plasmin by cleavage of a single peptide bond.[3] Plasmin is a relatively nonspecific protease; it digests fibrin clots and other plasma proteins, including several coagulation factors. Both circulating plasminogen and tissue plasminogen activator (tPA) are released from endothelial cells, as a response to fibrin production or hypoxia, and then bind to fibrin. Fibrin-bound plasminogen is converted to plasmin by tPA, which dissolves the thrombus. The fibrinolytic system digests exposed fibrin, while fibrin in wounds persists to maintain hemostasis. Although the desired therapy is thrombolysis of only the culprit coronary vessel, any exogenous fibrinolysis can cause bleeding at any site, especially in areas of recent vascular trauma (e.g., surgery, gastrointestinal [GI] bleeding, cardiovascular accident [CVA]).

OBJECTIVES OF THROMBOLYSIS FOR STEMI

Reperfusing the infarct-related artery (IRA) after AMI is the primary objective of all fibrinolytics. The advantages of thrombolytics in the acute care setting are their rapid availability, well-documented efficacy, and their proven outcome benefits in AMI. However, the limitations of potentially severe hemorrhage, failed reperfusion in up to

Table 13-1. Clinical Features of Thrombolytic Agents

Features	SK	tPA	rPA	TNK
Half-life (min)	25	5	13–16	20
Method of administration	1 h IV	1.5 h IV	2 IV boluses	1 IV bolus
Dose	1.5 mU	15 mg bolus, up to 85 mg/90 min	10 + 10 MU	45–55 mg/kg
Action	Indirect	Direct	Direct	Direct
Fibrin specificity	NA	++	+	+++
TIMI grade 3 flow at 90 min (%)	35	50–60	50–63	50–64
Major hemorrhage % (range)	0.3–4.7	0.4–5.94	0.95–4.7	4.66
ICH (%)	0.25–0.54	0.62–0.94	0.77–0.91	0.93
Antigenicity (%)	2.5	0.20	NA	0.10
Lives saved/1000	2.5	3.5	3–3.5%	3.5
Cost ($US, approximate)	290	2200	2200	2200

40% of patients, and early target vessel reocclusion, have driven the medical community toward PCI such as balloon dilatation or stenting.[4] Despite the apparent superiority of PCI, most hospitals are not equipped to provide 24-hour immediate PCI, leaving fibrinolysis as a viable strategy for AMI.

From 1990 to 1999, the National Registry for Myocardial Infarction (NRMI) reported a decrease in patients receiving primary thrombolytic therapy for STEMI from 34.3 to 20.8% while the use of primary PCI rose significantly from 2.4 to 7.3%.[5] For hospitals with active cardiac intervention labs, the use of thrombolytics dropped from 59.1% in 1994 to 47.9% in 1999 while the use of PCI doubled from 11.8 to 24.4%. These data still support the widespread use of fibrinolytics as a primary strategy for AMI management.

OUTCOMES TRIALS FOR THROMBOLYTICS

Thrombolytic clinical trials are divided into three major categories: monotherapy, combination therapy using the glycoprotein (GP) IIb/IIIa inhibitors, and pharmacoinvasive therapy (PHI) (Table 13-2). Other adjunctive therapies are listed separately.

Monotherapy

Indirect Acting Thrombolytics: Streptokinase and Anistreplase

Streptokinase

Streptokinase, a bacterial protein secreted by the group C β-hemolytic streptococci, was first reported as a thrombolyic for AMI in the 1950s. Since it does not possess any protease activity, it must first bind to plasminogen, forming a complex that converts plasminogen to plasmin. The circulating half-life is short (Table 13-1) requiring a drug infusion. Since SK has little fibrin specificity, it indiscriminately converts clot bound and circulating plasminogen to plasmin. The resultant free plasmin is rapidly inactivated by alpha-2-antiplasmin until the capacity of this inhibitor is exhausted. Once exhausted, the remaining plasmin generated from SK administration continues to degrade circulating fibrinogen, providing a sustained thrombolysis and anticoagulation. Regeneration and repletion of clotting factors occur by hepatic synthesis over 24–48 hours. The risk of serious bleeding after SK administration generally occurs during the postadministrative systemic "depletion" state noted.

SK is administered as a 1.5 mU infusion over 60 min. Patency (Thrombolysis In Myocardial Infarction [TIMI] 2 or 3 flow) is reported in 60% of patients at 90 min, and up to 80–90% of patients at 24 hours (Table 13-1). TIMI 3 flow was reported in only 35% of patients from the Global Utilization of STrategies to Open occluded arteries (GUSTO-IIB) subtrial.[6] When administered within 1 hour of symptom onset, the Gruppo Italiano per lo Studio della Sopravvivenza nell'Infarto miocardico (GISSI-2)[7] trial reported a 47% reduction in mortality with the use of SK in AMI. Major side effects of SK include bleeding, allergic reactions, and hypotension. Hemorrhage occurs in up to 10% of patients not undergoing invasive procedures and nearly 20% of those who do. Serious bleeding averages 2%, while intracranial hemorrhage (ICH) averages 0.5% (Table 13-1). Concerns for allergic reactions and anaphylaxis have contributed to the hesitancy for its use in

Table 13-2. Outcome Trials for Thrombolytics

Therapy	Trial Name	Agents	30-Day Mortality (%)	ICH (%)	Non-ICH Bleeding (%)	Ischemia/ Reocclusion (%)	Reinfarction (%)	Revascularization/ Urgent PCI (%)	TIMI 2/3 at 90 min
Monotherapy									
41,021	GUSTO I	Streptokinase	7.4	0.51	5.8		4.0		
		Alteplase	6.3	0.70	5.1		4.0		
324	RAPID-II	Reteplase	4.1*	1.20	12.4	9.0		13.6	59.9
		Alteplase	8.4	1.90	9.7	7.0		26.5	45.2
15,059	GUSTO III	Reteplase	7.5	0.90	6.9		4.2		83.4
		Alteplase	7.2	0.87	6.8		4.2		73.3
16,949	ASSENT-2	Tenecteplase	6.2	0.93	4.7	19.4†	4.1		
		Alteplase	6.2	0.93	5.9	19.5	3.8		
Combination									
16,648	GUSTO V§	Reteplase	5.9	0.60	1.8*	12.8	3.5	11.6‡	
		1/2 Reteplase + abciximab	5.6	0.60	3.5	11.3	2.3	8.3	
6095	ASSENT-3	Tenecteplase + enoxaparin 1/2	5.4	0.88	3.0	4.6	2.7	11.9	
		Tenecteplase + abciximab	6.6	0.94	4.3	3.2	2.2	9.1	
		Tenecteplase + UFH	6.0	0.93	2.2	6.5	4.2	14.4	
Pharmacoinvasive									
212	GRACIA-2	Tenecteplase + PCI	3.0	1.0		7.0	2.0		
		PCI	6.0	0		6.0	1.0		
395	PAMI	alteplase + PCI	2.6 (NS)	2			5.1		
		PCI	5.6	0			12.0*		

*Thirty-five-day mortality.
†Listed as recurrent angina.
‡At 24 h.
§Seven-day PCI and coronary artery by-pass grafting (CABG) rates lower, hemorrhage rates higher.

the United States, but its reported rates for allergy (2–5%) and anaphylaxis (<0.3%) are quite low. Hypotension is another adverse effect, occurring in up to 50% of patients receiving SK. SK should not be used up to 2 years after initial administration.

Anistreplase

Anisoylated plasminogen-streptokinase activator compound (APSAC, anistreplase) is a complex similar to SK. Once activated, APSAC converts and degrades through a several step process into SK and plasminogen. Hydrolysis of the anisoyl group enhances catalysis of plasminogen to plasmin. The gradual hydrolysis of APSAC to its active complex extends the circulating half-life to 90 min, allowing single bolus administration over SK alone. Patency rates from APSAC are reported better than SK, but are lower than the DNA recombinant direct acting thrombolytics. Adverse reactions such as bleeding, hypotension, and allergic reactions including anaphylaxis occur in APSAC with similar frequency to that of SK. Given the lower patency rates, greater fibrin specificity, and risks of antigenic reactions, SK, and anistreplase have largely been abandoned for the direct acting thrombolytics in North America.

Direct Acting Thrombolytics: Alteplase, Reteplase, Tenecteplase

The direct acting thrombolytics are all derived from recombinant or mutagenic forms of tPA. As a class, they do not carry the antigenic risk of SK or anistreplase (Table 13-1). The mechanism of action of all direct acting fibrinolytics is to enzymatically cleave single chain plasminogen molecules to double chain plasmin at the arginine 560-valine 561 site, exposing plasmin to degradation (lysis). Although the third generation thrombolytics share similarities in mechanism of action, subtle differences in function are reported in trials that distinguish each of the products.

Alteplase (tPA)

Alteplase was the first reported direct acting thrombolytic to demonstrate clinical efficacy.[8] The GUSTO-I trial[9] compared four thrombolytic strategies with SK or tPA (Table 13-2). In this trial, tPA had a significantly lower 30-day mortality (6.3%) than SK and IV heparin (7.4%), SK and subcutaneous heparin (7.2%), or SK, tPA, and heparin (7.0%, Table 13-2). A 14% relative mortality reduction was reported with tPA to SKs 1% at 30 days. Significantly more

hemorrhagic strokes occurred in the tPA arm than in SK. Angiographic substudies of the GUSTO trial[10] suggested that one explanation for tPAs success was its ability to more rapidly open (90 min) occluded coronary arteries as compared to SK (Table 13-1). This substudy reported that the tPA arm resulted in an 81% 90-min coronary artery patency versus 56% and 61% for the two SK arms. Aside from the conclusion that tPA resulted in lower mortality rates than SK, the presumption that early and complete patency was an important predictor of myocardial salvage was introduced. Future trials examining early and rapid artery patency after administration of therapy have now become an important metric in pharmacologic and pharmacoinvasive trials. Alteplase is administered as a bolus and infusion (Table 13-1).

Reteplase

Reteplase, a deletion mutation of wild-type tPA, was the first bolus thrombolytic published to show benefits in AMI. In 1995, the International Joint Efficacy Comparison of Thrombolytics (INJECT) trial[11] compared this double bolus third generation thrombolytic to SK. The primary outcome of this equivalency trial was 35-day mortality. Results from this trial yielded no difference in mortality at the primary outcome or at 6 months, and no difference in stroke rates, suggesting that a double bolus thrombolytic was equivalent to SK in outcome. RAPID-II compared 90-min coronary artery patency rates to that of the accelerated tPA protocol. The RAPID-II investigators reported that administering rPA produced statistically higher TIMI 2 or 3 patency rates at 60 and 90 min than PA with no differences in mortality, bleeding, or strokes.[12] The need for additional coronary interventions was significantly reduced in the rPA group (13.6%) than in the tPA cohort (26.5%, $P <$ 0.01). The authors concluded that rPA as a double bolus achieves both higher and more rapid rates of coronary reperfusion than tPA. A larger trial, GUSTO-III (Table 13-2), compared standard dose rPA to accelerated tPA. No difference in 30-day mortality rates, ICH, or strokes were reported suggesting similarity in efficacy and safety.[13]

Tenecteplase (TNK-PA, (TNK))

Tenecteplase is a modified form of tPA, developed through recombinant DNA technology. It differs from native tPA by three amino acid substitutions. The resulting TNK has notable properties of a long half-life necessitating only a single weight-based bolus for clinical thrombolysis in AMI, and increased fibrin specificity compared to the wild-type human tPA or rPA.

The ASsement of the Safety and Efficacy of a New Thrombolytic Agent (ASSENT-2) trial showed similar 30-day mortality rates between TNK (6.18%) and tPA (6.15%), and similar ICH rates (Table 13-2), but TNK had significantly lower noncerebral bleed rates (26.43%) than tPA (28.95%, $P = 0.0002$).[14] TIMI 10B reported 90-min TIMI grade 3 flow from 54 to 66%, and 90-min TIMI 2/3 flow ranging from 77 to 88% versus tPA's 82%.[15] Comparison of bleeding complications and angiographic outcomes resulted in the recommendation of a tiered weight-based regime to provide an optimal single bolus weight-adjusted dose of 0.5–0.6 mg/kg.

Combination Therapy

Administration of exogenous fibrinolysis results in a paradoxical increase in thrombosis through several proposed mechanisms. First, acute thrombolysis releases clot-bound fibrin into the bloodstream stimulating further platelet aggregation and thrombosis. Second, small released thrombi from thrombolysis may embolize and then travel to the microvasculature establishing secondary "downstream" clots. Third, primary clot lysis exposes the initial insult of the ruptured vulnerable plaque to thrombogenic factors that can again cause thrombosis. Active fibrinolysis enhances the expressions of these factors. One example is plasminogen activator inhibitor (PAI)-1, an inhibitor of fibrinolysis found especially on platelets. The resulting prothrombus state results IRA patency failure, reocclusion, or the need for urgent mechanical revascularization procedures in up to 60% of postthrombolytic patients.

Platelet aggregation during fibrinolysis may limit fibrinolysis success and reduce the clinical outcomes. Stimulation of the GP IIb/IIIa receptor on the platelet represents the final common pathway to platelet aggregation. GP IIb/IIIa receptor inhibitors designed to block the final pathway were first studied in acute coronary syndromes to counter impending ST-segment AMI and prevent or reduce the risk of coronary restenosis after PCI. Their success in reducing target artery ischemic complications led to trials evaluating a full or reduced dose combination of fibrinolytic and GP IIb/IIIa inhibitor in the management of STEMI. Trials evaluating the addition of GP IIb/IIIa blockade to fibrinolytic therapy weighed the benefits from lower reinfarctions, IRA reocclusion, and recurrent ischemia requiring urgent PCI, with the risk of severe or life-threatening bleeding.

Early trials with alteplase and abciximab or eptifibatide reported significantly lower IRA reocclusion rates or the need for urgent PCI, but also significantly increased bleeding complications. Further trials testing half dose thrombolytics with full dose GP IIb/IIIa inhibitors resulted in improved reperfusion results with no change in bleeding complications compared to fibrinolytic monotherapy. GUSTO-V,[16] the largest combination therapy trial to date, compared full dose rPA to half dose rPA and full dose abciximab in 16,648 patients presenting with acute STEMI within 6 hours of onset. All patients received IV heparin. Thirty-day mortality was unchanged in the two groups (Table 13-2), but the secondary endpoints of reocclusion, reinfarction, and need for emergent revascularization was significantly reduced in the combination group. Although the incidence of ICH was similar between the groups, non-ICH bleeding was twice as high in the combination group (Table 13-2).

ASSENT-3 randomized full dose TNK and enoxaparin, half dose TNK with low dose IV heparin and abciximab, or full dose TNK with standard IV heparin (control group).[17] The 30-day mortality was unchanged between the three arms; however, significantly lower refractory ischemia, reinfarction, and need for urgent PCI rates were reported in the TNK and abciximab groups. The ICH rates were similar between groups although major bleeding rates were significantly higher in the abciximab and enoxaparin groups (Table 13-2).

In both trials, however, significantly higher rates of ICH were detected in the subgroup of patients over 75 years old, suggesting that alternative reperfusion strategies such as PCI (if available) may be more suitable in the elderly population. In view of the bleeding complications without the mortality benefits, combination therapy with GP IIb/IIIa inhibition is not recommended at this time for first-line therapy in STEMI.

Pharmacoinvasive Therapy

The controversy of which management strategy, pharmacologic (primary fibrinolysis followed by rescue angioplasty) or mechanical (PCI including angioplasty, stenting, or bypass) remains unresolved as limitations in interventional cardiac catheter (ICC) lab availability or technical delays in ICC lab transfer continue to plague North American hospitals. Less than 25% of North American, and fewer than 10% of European, hospitals are equipped to perform rapid primary PCI. The NRMI-2 registry[5] of STEMI patients reported no differences in in-hospital mortality between the PCI and thrombolytic-treated groups, with an overall mean time to PCI of 111 min. Mortality rates after PCI performed between 151 and 180 min was 1.6 times higher than if PCI was completed prior to 60 min, suggesting that the problem with PCI is in its timing. Since there are no reported STEMI registries to date that demonstrate that 90-min "time to PCI" are consistently achievable, alternative strategies for STEMI management are used.

Physicians managing the STEMI patient must weigh the unknown time delay that can occur while waiting for an available intervention suite versus the increased risk of bleeding complications that may occur from thrombolytic management. Stone et al. reported that patients undergoing PCI had significantly better outcomes if their TIMI patency grades were higher before the PCI procedure.[18] Pre-PCI patency was shown to be an independent predictor of mortality outcome, suggesting that strategies to improve coronary patency before PCI could improve outcomes. Trials beginning in the 1980s considered combining thrombolysis followed by PCI. The strategy, called "facilitated PCI," is now called pharmacomechanical, or PHI therapy as they employ the patency benefits of early fibrinolysis with the long-term benefits of PCI.

GUSTO-IV pilot Strategies for Patency Enhancement in the Emergency Department (SPEED) randomized patients to half dose rPA with or without abciximab followed by immediate (<90 min) or no PCI.[19] The PHI arm had significantly lower ischemic events than those who only received thrombolysis. The PHI strategy also resulted in lower death, reinfarction, and need for urgent PCI than those in the fibrinolysis-only group. Pre-PCI TIMI 3 grade flow was higher in the PHI arm than any other trial at that time. Preliminary results published from the Grupo de Análisis de la Cardiopatía Isquémica Aguda[20] (GRACIA-2) trial comparing PCI <3 hours versus TNK and enoxaparin at 3–12 hours reported that the preintervention TIMI 3 flow significantly increased from 14% in the PCI group to 59% in the PHI group (Table 13-2). The primary outcomes of death, reinfarction, and recurrent ischemia were no different between groups. Bleeding complications including ICH were similar in this pilot study ($N = 212$). Dauerman and Sobel in reviewing the Pravastatin in Acute Coronary Treatment (PACT), SPEED, and TIMI 10B/14B trials, noted that early fibrinolysis followed by PCI resulted in earlier high-grade coronary patency, decreased rates of reinfarction, and need for urgent PCI, and in the TIMI trials, reduced death and recurrent AMI[21] (Table 13-1).

Despite the apparent benefits of PHI, the trials are small and there are limited long-term data available. Ongoing trials to assess the benefits of early reperfusion followed by directed PCI are in progress, including a PHI trial employing prehospital fibrinolysis Pre-hospital Administration of Thrombolytic therapy with urgent Culprit Artery Revascularization (PATCAR).

Adjunctive Therapy for Thrombolytics

Thrombosis and fibrinolysis represent two sides of a homeostatic process where clot is continuously generated and then dissolved. An acute insult that occurs when a vulnerable plaque ruptures in a coronary artery alters the homeostatic balance temporarily in favor of thrombosis. From the 1990s, further studies identified several limitations of fibrinolytic monotherapy. Alone, fibrinolytic agents attack only the fibrin-rich components of clot and do not dissolve platelets or disable many of the other stimuli that enhance or propagate clot formation. Recent AMI trials to test adjunctive therapies with fibrinolysis have significantly reduced the rebound thrombosis phenomenon after acute thrombolysis. As a result, today's clinical best practice guidelines for AMI pharmacotherapy, though continually changing, requires a recipe of multiple antithrombotic and antiplatelet agents in addition to fibrinolytics.

Using fibrinolytic therapy or PHI as a cornerstone for reperfusion success, a number of trials were designed to improve clinical outcomes through stabilizing clot, disabling platelets, or blocking factors responsible for fibrinogenesis.

Aspirin

The largest trial assessing the efficacy of aspirin for AMI was the second International Study of Infarct Survival (ISIS-2) results published in 1988.[22] The mortality benefit from aspirin therapy taken immediately and for 1 month after AMI significantly reduced mortality. A metaanalysis of nine randomized control trials reported that the absolute reduction in nonfatal reinfarction was reduced from 2.2 to 1.2% when aspirin in doses ranging from 75 to 150 mg/day were administered on the day of AMI.[23] With doses greater than 160 mg, a near total inhibition of thromboxane A_2 production is expected, with rapid clinical antithrombotic benefit. Higher doses did not result in greater benefits. There were no statistical increases in ICH, strokes, or bleeds requiring transfusions. Results from the metaanalysis indicated that aspirin therapy during the acute AMI phase resulted in 1 life saved for 41 AMI treated. With few exceptions, aspirin therapy is considered first-line treatment for AMI. An initial dose of 160–325 mg is recommended to be given promptly by the American College of Cardiology (ACC) and the American Heart Association (AHA) guidelines.[24] A daily maintenance dose is then recommended indefinitely.

Thienopyridines

The thienopyridines, ticlopidine, and clopidogrel, represent a different class of antiplatelet compounds that blocks the adenosine diphosphate (ADP) arm of fibrinogen's membrane GP receptor, GP IIb/IIIa. By blocking the ADP stimulus of the GP IIb/IIIa receptor, the thienopyridines act as an inhibitor of platelet activation and aggregation. The thienopyridines act at site different from aspirin. Like aspirin, they do not act as antithrombotics nor do they possess thrombolytic activity.

Clopidogrel in Unstable angina to prevent Recurrent Events (CURE), a large trial comparing aspirin and clopidogrel versus aspirin for acute coronary syndromes, showed that the former reduced mortality rates from cardiovascular causes from 11.4 to 9.3%.[25] Side effects included reversible neutropenia, thrombotic thrombocytopenic purpura (TTP), and significantly higher bleeding rates. The antiplatelet benefits from the thienopyridines generally occur later than aspirin.

Unfractionated Heparin (UFH)

GUSTO-I and III trials reported that UFH improved the outcomes of accelerated tPA or bolus rPA strategies. UFH was also shown to reduce ischemic complications such as restenosis, recurrent ischemia, and infarction, when given concomitantly with alteplase. Early GUSTO results reported that IV UFH provided no additional benefits to SK, over aspirin, or subcutaneous (SQ) heparin, while increasing the bleeding risk. The non-fibrin-specific thrombolytics (e.g., SK) show little benefit from the addition of UFH, whereas fibrin selective thrombolytics (tPA, rPA, TNK) do benefit from adjunctive UFH therapy. The ACC/AHA guidelines recommend the use of IV UFH as an adjunct for STEMI patients receiving alteplase (class IIa), but does not recommended UFH for use with the non-fibrin-specific thrombolytics (SK, anistreplase) unless a high risk of embolism is observed.[24] Presently, these guidelines recommend reduced dose IV UFH (60-U/kg bolus followed by a 12 U/kg/hour infusion) to augment the third generation fibrinolytics, followed by an activated partial thromboplastine time (aPTT) measurement to maintain an aPTT from 50 to 70 s.

Low Molecular Weight Heparin

ASSENT-3 (Table 13-2) compared IV enoxaparin along with full dose tenecteplase to TNK with UFH, or halfl dose TNK plus abciximab and UFH. The enoxaparin arm ($N = 2040$) had the lowest 30-day mortality rate (5.4%) than either of the other arms, although major bleeding was higher than in the UFH arm, the ICH rates were similar (0.9%).[17] In-hospital refractory ischemia or rein-

farction was lower in low molecular weight heparin (LMWH) group than in the UFH group, though not lower than the abciximab group. Results from ASSENT-3 suggest that substituting enoxaparin for UFH reduces 30-day mortality and the ischemic complications after STEMI, but increases the non-ICH bleeding rates. The authors noted that bleeding rates were significantly higher in those patients who were older than 75 years or had diabetes.[17]

The Heparin and Aspirin Reperfusion Therapy-II (HART-II) study compared IV UFH for 72 hours versus enoxaparin (30 mg IV, followed by 1 mg/kg SQ for 72 hours) as an adjunct to tPA in STEMI.[26] The primary and secondary outcomes measurements measured TIMI grade flow at 90 min and bleeding complications. In this small ($N = 393$) angiographic trial, the enoxaparin study arm resulted in 80.1% 90-min TIMI 3 flow versus 75.1% for UFH. Bleeding rates, including ICH were similar in both arms (1%). One-week reocclusion rates were lower for the enoxaparin arm (5.9%) than UFH (9.8%, $P = 0.12$). This pilot trial suggests that the IV enoxaparin may be an effective alternative to UFH in STEMI, although larger clinical data are required. No definitive recommendations are made for the routine use of LMWH in STEMI, although SQ enoxaparin is recommended as an alternative to UFH for non-ST-elevation MI. Trials are in progress to elucidate the appropriate role of LMWH (enoxaparin) as an alternative front-line strategy versus UFH in STEMI.

OPTIMIZING CARE

Consideration of Timing of Thrombolytic Administration

Early administration of thrombolytics provides the best outcomes. In a metaanalysis by Boersma et al., administration of a thrombolytic within 1 hour from symptom onset saved 65 lives per 1000. At 3 hours, the number of lives saved dropped to 26 per 1000, emphasizing the need for expedient decision making and drug delivery. Delays in thrombolytic administration reduce the effectiveness of the drug and negatively impacts patient outcomes. Timing therefore, is an important consideration to thrombolytic delivery. Delays in administration contribute more to worse outcomes than the choice of thrombolytic agent.

The National Heart Attack Alert Program (NHAAP) described four-time intervals responsible for most of the delays in thrombolytic administration[28]—time of arrival (door), time to ECG and identification of AMI (data), time to determine which AMI management strategy (thrombolytics vs. PCI, decision), and time of commitment to the chosen strategy (drug vs. PCI). A review of the NRMI data from 1990 to 1999 showed a significant reduction in each of these time intervals during the 1990s.[5] Delays at any of the time intervals prevent the AMI patient from expeditious treatment, resulting in an increased risk for mortality. A metaanalysis of 50,246 STEMI patients from 1983 to 1993 found that the benefit of thrombolytic therapy when started within 1 hour of symptom onset resulted in 60–80 additional lives saved at 1 month per 1000 patients treated.[27] From 1 to 3 hours, the additional lives saved dropped to 30–50 additional lives saved per 1000 treated. The relative reduction in mortality was significantly higher in those treated within 2 hours (44%) versus those treated later (20%), further supporting the data that early thrombolytic administration is a leading factor in determining outcomes after thrombolysis. Extrapolating these trials, Collins et al. reported that the absolute death risk reduction after thrombolysis was lowest (3%) when the drug was administered within 6 hours of symptoms. From 7 to 12 hours, the absolute reduction decreased to 2%.[29] Each hour of delay to thrombolysis results in a 16% absolute reduction in death benefits.

Although a 30-min door-to-drug time has been suggested by the ACC and the AHA,[24] this target interval has not been achieved in any large study to date. Hospital systems and national surveillance advocates closely monitor time to thrombolytics as the "sine quo non" benchmark for effective AMI management. The Society of Chest Pain Centers and Providers, a multidisciplinary group tasked to develop and promote chest pain centers, recommends a predetermined chest pain algorithm (e.g., AMI pathway) for chest pain as part of the center's core competency required for accreditation.[30]

Patient Eligibility

Clinically, patients presenting with chest discomfort (or its equivalent) and critical coronary stenosis with either elevated markers of necrosis (total creatinine phosphokinase [CK], or cardiac-specific CK-MB subform, and troponin T or I) or have electrocardiographic changes suggesting STEMI are eligible candidates for fibrinolytics. The goal of the acute care practitioner is to identify those AMI patients who do qualify for fibrinolytic therapy, and to start the therapy immediately. Eligibility requirements for AMI therapy exclude patients with massive bleeding, recent major surgery, and stroke. The practitioner should be familiar with all fibrinolytic eligibility criteria (Table 13-3) and should document the patient's eligibility or exclusion as well as the time of evaluation.

Table 13-3. Contraindications for Use of Fibrinolytics

Absolute
- Cerebrovascular events within 1 year
- Active internal bleeding, not including menses
- Known intracranial neoplasm, arteriovenous malformation, or aneurysm
- Suspected aortic dissection

Relative
- Blood pressure >180/110 mmHg
- Use of anticoagulants with an international normalized ratio >2.0
- Known bleeding diathesis
- Noncompressible vascular punctures
- Prolonged cardiopulmonary resuscitation (>10 min)
- Prior gastrointestinal hemorrhage
- Pregnancy
- Recent trauma including intracranial or intraspinal
- Major surgery within 3 weeks
- History of prior cerebrovascular accident or known intracranial pathology not covered in contraindications
- Active peptic ulcer
- History of chronic hypertension, uncontrolled hypertension
- Diabetic hemorrhagic retinopathy or other hemorrhagic ophthalmic conditions
- Age greater than 75 years
- Significant hepatic dysfunction
- Any condition where significant life-threatening bleeding is likely

Bleeding

Excessive bleeding resulting in adverse outcomes, such as stroke, remains the most devastating complication of thrombolytic therapy. All randomized trials include bleeding as a complication of thrombolytics. The results are reported as ICH or stroke, major bleeding (defined as severe or prolonged bleeding and/or requiring blood transfusion), and minor bleeding. Pooled data identified four independent predictors for increased risk of ICH: age >65, weight <70 kg, hypertension on admission, and use of tPA over SK.[31] History of prior cerebrovascular disease or hypertension, and the use of tPA over SK have further been identified as risk factors for ICH. The most common site for spontaneous bleeding, however, was in the GI tract.[9] ICH and major bleeding rates from the major trials are listed in Table 13-2. Other predictive models suggest that female gender and history of stroke also increase the risk for ICH after thrombolysis.

Choice of Thrombolytics Based on Convenience

The advantages to bolus thrombolytic therapy include ease of administration, ensured administration of the drug, reduced nursing time, and lower potential error in administration. Disadvantages include the all-or-nothing phenomenon since the bolus cannot be reversed or stopped after drug administration, and cost. Table 13-1 lists the common fibrinolytics, their mode of administration, and recommended starting doses.

Weight-Based Thrombolytics

Estimating weight-based fibrinolytics are another potential cause for medical error. Estimating thrombolytic dosing in the TIMI 10B and ASSENT-1 trials resulted in a 3.4% dosing error for tPA and 1.3% for TNK.[32] TNK's single weight-adjusted bolus resulted in lower dosing error than alteplase's bolus and infusion. ICH and death rates were similar between TNK groups with estimated and actual weights. Angeja et al., after analyzing the ASSENT data, concluded that estimating weight-based fibrinolytics for acute STEMI did not result in significantly higher bleeding complications.[33] Thirty-day mortality was significantly higher in patients whose weights were estimated on arrival, presumably because sicker patients could not be weighted on arrival. SK, tPA, and TNK require weight basing, while rPA does not.

Fibrin Specificity

Thrombolysis results in the degradation of not only fibrinogen but also numerous clotting factors. Trials have associated higher bleeding rates after thrombolysis with administration of a nonfibrin selective fibrinolytic SK and IV UFH. As a result, SK and IV UFH are not recommended in combination for STEMI.[24] TNK is the most fibrin-specific thrombolytic, followed by alteplase, and rPA. SK and anistreplase are not fibrin specific. Table 13-1 outlines the relative fibrin specificity of the agents. Fibrin specificity may be associated with lower bleeding complications and higher angiographic patency rates. However, trials are lacking to definitively show clinical superiority between fibrinolytics based on fibrin specificity alone.

SUMMARY: THROMBOLYTIC THERAPY

Thrombolytic therapy remains a first-line strategy for STEMI. Ongoing trials with adjunctive drugs (LMWHs,

platelet disablers and inhibitors, anticoagulants, and so on) and pharmacoinvasive strategies may further refine the role of thrombolytics in AMI. The acute care physician should be aware of the complications associated with thrombolytic therapy, most notably hemorrhage, and should risk stratify each candidate before starting therapy. Timing is the most important consideration in thrombolysis. Predetermined AMI pathways reduce decision time, decrease medical error, and increase efficiency in the emergency department. PCI may be more desirable than thrombolysis, especially in the elderly, but only if it can be delivered expeditiously. Finally, close coordination of care between the emergency department or prehospital provider and the cardiologist is necessary to define the best reperfusion strategy for the AMI patient.

REFERENCES

1. Weitz JI. Pharmacology. In: Kandarpa K (ed.), *Disease State Compendium: Clinical Applications of Fibrinolytics.* Online CME sponsored program through the University of Minnesota, 2002:26–30.
2. Kwaan H. Thrombolytic therapy—old and new. In: Green D (ed.), *Anticoagulants: Physiologic, Pathologic, Pharmacologic.* Orlando, FL: CRC Press, 1994:258–270.
3. Majerus PW, Tollefson DM. Anticoagulant, thrombolytic, and antiplatelet drugs. In: Goodman LS, Gillman A (eds.), *The Pharmacologic Basis of Therapeutics.* New York: McGraw-Hill, 2001:1579–1538.
4. Hermann HC. Triple therapy for acute myocardial infarction: Combining fibrinolysis, platelet IIb/IIIa inhibition, and percutaneous coronary intervention. *Am J Cardiol* 2000; 85:10c–16c.
5. Tiefenbrunn AJ, Chandra NC, French WJ, et al. Clinical experience with primary percutaneous transluminal coronary angioplasty compared with alteplase (recombinant tissue-type plasminogen activator) in patients with acute myocardial infarction (NRMI-2). *J Am Coll Cardiol* 1998;31(6):1240–1245.
6. Berger PB, Ellis SG, Holmes DR Jr., et al., for the GUSTO II Investigators. Relationship between delay in performing direct coronary angioplasty and early clinical outcome in patients with acute myocardial infarction: Results from the global use of strategies to open occluded arteries in Acute Coronary Syndromes (GUSTO-IIb) trial. *Circulation* 1999;100(1):14–20.
7. Gruppo Italiano per lo Studio della Sopravvivenza nell'Infarto Miocardico. GISSI-2: A factorial randomised trial of alteplase versus streptokinase and heparin versus no heparin among 12,490 patients with acute myocardial infarction. *Lancet* 1990;336(8707):65–71.
8. The TIMI Study Group. The thrombolysis in myocardial infarction (TIMI) trial. *N Engl J Med* 1985;312:932–936.

9. An International randomized trial comparing four thrombolytic strategies for acute myocardial infarction. The GUSTO investigators. *N Engl J Med* 1993;329(10):673–682.

10. Simes RJ, Topol EJ, Holmes DR, et al., for the GUSTO-1 Investigators. Link between the angiographic substudy and mortality outcomes in a large randomized trial of myocardial reperfusion: Importance of early and complete infarct artery reperfusion. *Circulation* 1995;91:1923–1928.

11. Randomized, double blind comparison of reteplase double-bolus administration with streptokinase in acute myocardial infarction (INJECT): Trial to investigate equivalence. International Joint Efficacy Comparison of Thrombolytics Committee. *Lancet* 1995;346:329–336.

12. Bode C, Smalling RW, Berg G, et al. Randomized comparison of coronary thrombolysis achieved with double-bolus reteplase (recombinant plasminogen activator) and front-loaded, accelerated alteplase (recombinant tissue plasminogen activator) in patients with acute myocardial infarction: The RAPID II investigators. *Circulation* 1996;94:891–898.

13. A comparison of reteplase with alteplase for acute myocardial infarction: The Global Use of Strategies to Open Occluded Coronary Arteries (GUSTO III) investigators. *N Engl J Med* 1997;337:1118–1123.

14. Single-bolus tenecteplase compared with front loaded alteplase in acute myocardial infarction: The ASSENT-2 double blinded randomized trial. The ASSENT-2 Investigators. *Lancet* 1999;354:716–722.

15. TNKase [package insert]. South San Francisco, CA: Genentech Inc., 2000.

16. Topol EJ, GUSTO V Investigators. Reperfusion therapy for acute myocardial infarction with fibrinolytic therapy or combination reduced fibrinolytic therapy and platelet glycoprotein IIb/IIIa inhibition: The GUSTO V randomised trial. *Lancet* 2001;357(9272):1905–1914.

17. Efficacy and safety of tenecteplase in combination with enoxaparin, abciximab, or unfractionated heparin: The ASSENT-3 randomized trial in acute myocardial infarction. *Lancet* 2001;358:605–612.

18. Stone GW, Cox D, Garcia E, et al. Normal flow (TIMI-3) before mechanical reperfusion therapy is an independent determinant of survival in acute myocardial infarction: Analysis from the primary angioplasty in myocardial infarction trials. *Circulation* 2001;104(6):636–641.

19. Hermann HC, Moliterno DJ, Ohman EM, et al. Facilitation of early percutaneous coronary intervention after reteplase with or without abciximab in acute myocardial infarction: Results from the SPEED (GUSTO-4 Pilot) Trial. *J Am Coll Cardiol* 2000;36(5):1489–1496.

20. Ailes FF for the GRACIA-2 Group. Randomized trial comparing primary PCI versus facilitated intervention (TNK + Stenting) in patients with STEMI. Vienna, Austria: Presented at the European Society of Cardiology Congress, Aug 30–Sept 3, 2003.

21. Dauerman HL, Sobel BE. Synergistic treatment of ST-segment elevation myocardial infarction with pharmacoinvasive recanalization. *J Am Coll Cardiol* 2003;42(4):646–651.

22. Second International Study of Infarct Survival (ISIS-2) Collaborative Group. Randomized trial of intravenous streptokinase, oral aspirin, both or neither among 17–187 cases of suspected acute myocardial infarction. *Lancet* 1998;ii:349–360.

23. Antiplatelet Trialists Collaboration. Collaborative overview of randomized trials of antiplatelet therapy I: Prevention of death, myocardial infarction, and stroke by prolonged antiplatelet therapy in various categories of people. *Br Med J* 1994;308:81–106.

24. A Report of the American College of Cardiology/American Heart Association Task Force on Practice Guidelines (Committee on Management of Acute Myocardial Infarction) *Circulation* 1999;100:1016–1030.

25. A randomized, blinded, trial of clopidogrel versus aspirin in patients at risk for ischaemic events (CAPRIE): CAPRIE Steering Committee. *Lancet* 1996;348:1329–1339.

26. Ross AM, Molhoek P, Lundergan C, et al., for the HART II Investigators. Randomized comparison of enoxaparin, a low-molecular-weight heparin, with unfractionated heparin adjunctive to recombinant tissue plasminogen activator thrombolysis and aspirin: Second trial of heparin and aspirin reperfusion therapy (HART II). *Circulation* 2001;104(6):648–652.

27. Boersma E, Maas AC, Deekars JW, et al. Early thrombolytic treatment in myocardial infarction: Reappraisal of the golden hour. *Lancet* 1996;348:771–775.

28. Rodrique BB. The NHAAP: Making the most of thrombolytic therapy. *Am Fam Physician* 1994;49(4):723–724.

29. Collins R, Peto R, Baigent BM, et al. Aspirin, heparin, and thrombolytic therapy in suspected acute myocardial infarction. *N Engl J Med* 1997;336:847–860.

30. SCPCP.org (website)/personal communication.

31. Simoons MI, Maggioni AP, Knatterud G, et al. Individual risk assessment for intracranial hemorrhage during thrombolytic therapy. *Lancet* 1993;342:523–528.

32. Murphy SA, Gibson CM, Van de Werf F, et al. Comparison of errors in estimating weight and in dosing of single bolus tenecteplase with tissue plasminogen activator (TIMI 10B and ASSENT 1). *Am J Cardiol* 2002;90:51–54.

33. Angeja BG, Alexander JH, Chin R, et al. Safety of the weight-adjusted dosing regime of tenecteplase in the ASSENT-Trial. *Am J Cardiol* 2001;88:1240–1245.

14

EMS
Prehospital Thrombolytics

Assaad J. Sayah

HIGH YIELD FACTS

- Early thrombolysis improves outcome in acute myocardial infarction (AMI).
- The delivery of thrombolytic agents in the prehospital setting has been shown to be safe and feasible.
- Prehospital thrombolysis significantly reduces delays in treatment even in urban settings with short transport times.
- Prehospital thrombolysis should even be considered in systems offering primary percutaneous coronary intervention (PCI).

INTRODUCTION

Acute myocardial infarction is the leading cause of death in the United States and most western civilized nations. There are more than 1.5 million AMI cases each year in the United States, resulting in almost 500,000 deaths, half of them occurring before patients received therapy.[1] Aggressive reperfusion therapy of patients with acute ST-segment elevation myocardial infarction (STEMI) leads to improved patient outcome.[2]

In AMI, reperfusion of the occluded artery is associated with an improvement in survival, smaller infarct size, and a reduction in the extent of left ventricular dysfunction. Furthermore, use of thrombolytic therapy is highly time dependent: the earlier it is administered, the more beneficial it is. Thus, the focus of both prehospital and emergency department (ED) management of patients with STEMI is on rapid identification and treatment.[2] Given the critical relationship between the time to successful reperfusion and outcomes in the treatment of patients with acute STEMI, administering fibrinolytic therapy prior to hospital arrival could significantly reduce the time between symptom onset and successful reperfusion.[3–6]

IMPORTANCE OF TIME TO TREATMENT

Time from the onset of symptoms to treatment is one of the key factors that influence the clinical outcome of patients presenting with AMI. Particularly in the first two hours from symptom onset, relatively small delays in treatment carry substantial implications for the outcome of the patient with AMI.[3–6] Approximately 65 lives are saved per 1000 treated when patients are thrombolysed within 1 hour of symptom onset.[6] The number drops to about 29 lives saved per 1000 treated at 2–3 hours after symptom onset (Fig. 14-1). In the first 90 min of symptoms starting therapy 30 min earlier results in additional 10–30 lives saved per 1000 treated.[6] Each minute matters; for every half hour delay in thrombolytic administration, the mortality rate rises by approximately 2%.

Delays from symptom onset to reperfusion can be attributed to many reasons including patient delays in contacting 911, transportation delays, in-hospital evaluation delays, and intervention/perfusion delays.[1,7,8] Overcoming each of these delays poses a unique challenge. Over the years, we have been able to impact the duration of each of these delays and improve the time to reperfusion in many ways. This includes public education and media campaigns, evolution of the 911 and emergency medical systems, constructing AMI protocols, providing better drugs, and instituting early in-hospital interventions. Despite many years of medical and operational advances, the median time from symptom onset until the initiation of thrombolysis remains about 2.5–3 hours.[9] Quality initiatives within EDs have reduced the door to drug times to a system "ideal" of around 30 min, with little opportunity for further incremental time reduction.[1] Even with prehospital ECG and emergency medical service (EMS) prearrival notification, it seems unlikely that the "door to needle" time can be reduced much below 20 min without compromising patient assessment.

Although we have succeeded in treating patients within 20–30 min from hospital arrival, the challenge remains to reperfuse these patients in the shortest time from symptom onset. The fact is that the patient's first medical contact is often with EMS and not in the ED. One way to further save valuable time and potentially improve outcome is to thrombolyse patients with STEMI from the time of first medical contact, even before arrival to the hospital when possible.

PREHOSPITAL STUDIES

Prehospital administration of a lytic agent has been the subject of numerous studies. Consistent findings across

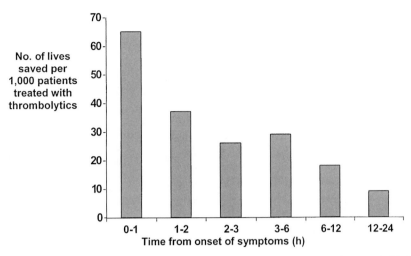

Fig. 14-1. Absolute 35-day mortality reduction vs. time to treatment from onset of symptoms. (Source: Modified with permission from reference 6.)

multiple trials demonstrate time savings with prehospital thrombolysis, ranging between 33 and 130 min, depending on the setting.[10,11] A meta analysis of six randomized trials involving 6434 patients, showed that prehospital lysis resulted in a shorter time to therapy (104 min vs. 162 min) and a 17% reduction in the odds of death, but was not affected by whether the on-scene evaluation is conducted by a physician or paramedical personnel.[11] Such benefit appears to come without any detectable difference in the risk of major bleeding or adverse cardiovascular events with prehospital therapy, as compared to in-hospital therapy.[10–12]

The specific trials included in this meta analysis included a double-blinded trial conducted by the European Myocardial Infarction Project Group (EMIP), and was the largest to evaluate the efficacy of prehospital thrombolysis.[10] In this study, patients who received thrombolysis in the prehospital arena were treated 60 min earlier and had a significant reduction in cardiac mortality (8.3% vs. 9.8%). In the Myocardial Infarction Triage and Intervention Trial (MITI), those treated within the first 70 min after symptom onset had better left ventricular function and improved survival.[12] Notably, the prehospital strategy in MITI increased the proportion of patients treated within that window by approximately four- to fivefold. The Grampian Region Early Anistreplase Trial (GREAT) showed a significant reduction in mortality at 1 year (10.4% vs. 21.6%) and at 5 years (25% vs. 36%) for patients treated in the prehospital field.[13,14] This benefit

remained significant at 10 years for patients who had ECG criteria consistent with AMI.[15]

The early Retavase (ER)-thrombolysis in myocardial infarction (TIMI) 19 study tested the feasibility of prehospital initiation of the bolus fibrinolytic reteplase, and determined the time saved by prehospital reteplase in the setting of contemporary emergency cardiac care.[16] In this trial of 20 emergency medical systems in urban, suburban, and rural areas in the United States and Canada, emergency medical technicians (EMTs) enrolled patients suspected of having AMI under the supervision of a remote medical control physician, based on symptoms, history, vital signs, examination, inclusion and exclusion criteria, and field 12-lead ECG findings. Patients with STEMI were lysed within a median of 31 min after EMS arrival, in comparison to 63 min for in-hospital lysis in a control group, resulting in a time saved of 32 min ($P < 0.0001$). By 30 min after first medical contact, 49% of patients had received the initial bolus of rPA, compared with only 5% of control patients ($P < 0.0001$) (Fig. 14-2). Further analysis identified that patients might benefit from prehospital thrombolytics when total field management time and/or door-to-drug time is greater than 20 min. ER-TIMI 19 demonstrated that fibrinolysis can be initiated safely and successfully while, in transit to a hospital by an EMT, using modern communications equipment and fibrinolytic agents.

More recently, in the ASSENT-3 PLUS study, more than 1600 prehospital thrombolysed patients had a

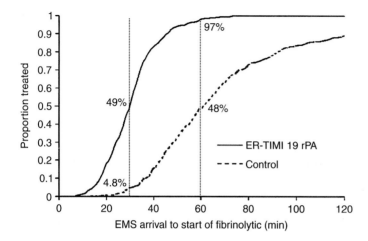

Fig. 14-2. Cumulative distribution of time to initiation of fibrinolytic from emergency medical service (EMS) arrival for patients treated with prehospital reteplase (rPA) vs. in-hospital fibrinolytic. ER-TIMI 19 = early Retavase thrombolysis in myocardial infarction 19 trial. (Source: Modified with permission from reference 16.)

median treatment time of 38 min from first EMS contact, and 115 min from symptom onset.[17] Additionally, the median treatment delay was shortened by 47 min as compared with the ASSENT-3 in-hospital trial, which used identical inclusion criteria.

BARRIERS TO PREHOSPITAL LYSIS

Despite consistent evidence that prehospital thrombolysis reduces time to treatment,[10–13] and potential improved survival,[11] a number of barriers have historically hindered the widespread development of prehospital thrombolytic programs. EMS personnel must accurately diagnose STEMI, identify appropriate patients for thrombolysis, and be able to administer a potentially complicated drug regimen outside the hospital. Over the past two decades, advances in prehospital care have been related to improved technology, pharmaceuticals, paramedic training, and implementation of evidence-based care.

Advances in technology have made rapid evaluation of the patient with suspected STEMI possible in the field.[1,18,19] Performance of prehospital 12-lead ECGs has been shown to reduce time to treatment and perhaps improve survival among patients with STEMI.[20] Furthermore, communication technology with widespread cell phone and radio coverage has been instrumental in improving field to hospital communication and 12-lead ECG transmission.[1,2] Paramedical personnel using prehospital ECG and standardized checklists, while in communication with a medical control physician, can rapidly identify fibrinolytic-eligible patients with accuracy equivalent to that achieved

in the ED.[21–25] ECGs can be transmitted to the receiving hospital, where the emergency physician can interpret the trace and provide direct advice and authorization for thrombolysis, via a two-way communication link.[16] Such progress has reinforced the notion that the continuum of emergency cardiac care begins at the first medical contact with the patient, and opened the opportunity for rapid identification and earlier treatment of patients with STEMI.

Another barrier to implementation of prehospital thrombolysis has been the logistical complexity of administering a weight-based, continuous infusion thrombolytic agent. However, the advent of bolus thrombolytics that are not weight dosed has simplified the complicated operational logistics of prehospital lysis.[16,17,26]

Prehospital fibrinolysis was investigated in numerous trials and has been the standard of care in many European countries for as long as 17 years.[27] The concept has not received widespread acceptance in North America for many reasons, including lack of interest and support of hospitals, cardiologists, and ED physicians, who generally do no perceive that the prehospital treatment of patients is their priority.[27] This is further exacerbated by the fragmented nature of the U.S. Emergency Medical System and the high cost of providing such therapy.

PREHOSPITAL LYSIS AND PRIMARY PCI

A systematic review of many trials comparing primary PCI and in-hospital fibrinolysis for patients with STEMI, showed a 30-day lower mortality for patients treated with primary PCI.[28] However, immediate primary PCI is not universally available, which imposes additional delays that could diminish its clinical benefits. The pathophysiologic evidence of increasing myocardial necrosis with time, coupled with registry and trial data, underscores the detrimental impact of treatment delay for both mechanical and pharmacologic reperfusion modalities.[27] Currently, fewer than 20% of patients with STEMI are treated with primary PCI.[29] Thus, thrombolytic therapy remains the mainstay of therapy for STEMI, partly due to the fact that the majority of hospitals lack primary PCI capabilities.

Initial trials suggested possible harm from early PCI, if thrombolytic therapy were given first.[30,31] With improved PCI techniques, newer stents and agents, future trials may demonstrate a wider role for thrombolysis followed by PCI. It has been suggested that "rescue" PCI may improve the outcome of patients who receive prehospital thrombolysis, but do not achieve good coronary arterial (TIMI 3) flow.[32] The CAPTIM trial compared prehospital thrombolysis (with rescue angioplasty when needed) to primary PCI in 840 patients with STEMI, and showed no significant difference in patient outcome between the two strategies.[33] In addition, patients who received prehospital thrombolysis in CAPTIM had a lower incidence of early-onset cardiogenic shock, presumably by promoting earlier reperfusion in patients prone to develop this complication.

Prehospital thrombolysis may also improve the likelihood of a patient receiving PCI by allowing initial reperfusion management of the patient and bypassing of non-PCI facilities to transport the patient to a facility with PCI capabilities. Getting the artery open quickly is critical for optimal outcomes. In addition, many interventional cardiologists would like to see some sort of chemical reperfusion in advance, simply because it is much easier to work with an open artery in the cardiac catheterization laboratory.

DISCUSSION

The data available to date support consideration of prehospital thrombolytic programs for a broad base of emergency medical systems. The findings of ER-TIMI 19 demonstrate that even with continued progress in the reduction of door-to-drug times, a prehospital thrombolytic program significantly saves time if either field management or door-to-drug times exceed 20 min.[16] In light of the compelling rationale for treatment as early as possible, and evidence that thrombolysis can be administered accurately and safely in the field, it appears that if the necessary infrastructure to support prehospital thrombolysis is in place, there is little reason to delay treatment, even if the temporal gains for any one patient may be modest.

Prehospital thrombolysis significantly saves time, even in an urban environment with a relatively short transport time.[16,17,34] This gain is mainly due to the elimination of in-hospital delays, which are significant in many cases.[16,34] A delay of at least 20 min is common as soon as a patient is unloaded from an ambulance. Prehospital administration allows thrombolysis to be given at the time where there is the greatest benefit. With training and support, paramedics will be able to provide effective thrombolysis to save lives and reduce mortality.

EMS is an integral part of the management of the patient with AMI. Regional protocols need to be established to triage patients to various destinations based on patient condition and resource availability. Point of entry plans need to be designed to guide EMS personnel to appropriate destinations based on geographical transportation constraints including extrication, traffic, and other potential transport delays, to centers with 24/7 emergent PCI availability. Future management of patients with STEMI may favor a strategy that includes early prehospital thrombolysis and triage, or eventual transfer, to hospitals that offer primary PCI.

The current therapeutic and EMS technological and logistical environments are ripe for the introduction of prehospital thrombolysis. Prehospital lytics should be seriously considered in any system that is currently choosing in-hospital lysis as the primary mode of reperfusion therapy. We need to redefine traditional boundaries and allow thrombolysis to be started by the first provider qualified to diagnose AMI, including adequately trained paramedics.

Prehospital lysis should even be considered in systems that offer PCI as the primary modality of in-hospital reperfusion. It is portable, safe, and proven to work for patients where PCI is delayed. Combination therapies that include full or partial prehospital lysis, followed by PCI, should also be considered to maximize patient outcome and system efficiencies. For systems where primary angioplasty is not immediately available, the ideal reperfusion strategy may consist of prehospital thrombolysis, followed by transfer for angioplasty, for patients in whom thrombolysis has failed.

Many trials have shown that prehospital thrombolysis is safe and operationally feasible with a protocol driven approach, and may lead to improved outcome when given early after symptom onset. Prehospital management for STEMI should include timely recognition, aggressive stabilization, initiation of therapy including thrombolysis if applicable, management of pain and complications, and selective triage to cardiac centers with rapid intervention capabilities.

UNRESOLVED ISSUES

- The ideal interface between pharmacologic and mechanical reperfusion.

- The value of selective triage of patients with STEMI by EMS to facilities offering primary PCI.

- The role of prehospital combination therapy and/or partial thrombolysis in mitigating the delays of extending transport time and bypassing non-PCI capable facilities.

REFERENCES

1. Cannon CP, Sayah AJ, Walls RM. ER TIMI-19: Testing the reality of prehospital thrombolysis. *J Emerg Med* 2000;19: 21S–25S.

2. Cannon CP, Sayah AJ, Walls RM. Prehospital thrombolysis: An idea whose time has come. *Clin Cardiol* 1999; 22(8 Supp):10–19.

3. GISSI Investigators. Effectiveness of intravenous thrombolytic treatment in acute myocardial infarction. Gruppo Italiano per lo Studio della Streptochinasi nell'Infarto Miocardico (GISSI). *Lancet* 1986;1:397–402.

4. Honan MB, Harrell FE Jr., Reimer KA, et al. Cardiac rupture, mortality and the timing of thrombolytic therapy: A meta-analysis. *J Am Coll Cardiol* 1990;16:359–367.

5. Fibrinolytic Therapy Trialists' (FTT) Collaborative Group. Indications for fibrinolytic therapy in suspected acute myocardial infarction: collaborative overview of early mortality and major morbidity results from all randomised trials of more than 1000 patients. *Lancet* 1994;343:311–322.

6. Boersma E, Maas AC, Deckers JW, et al. Early thrombolytic treatment in acute myocardial infarction: reappraisal of the golden hour. *Lancet* 1996;348:771–775.

7. Cannon CP, Antman EM, Walls R, et al. Time as an adjunctive agent to thrombolytic therapy. *J Thromb Thrombolysis* 1994;1:27–34.

8. Cannon CP Braunwald E. GUSTO, TIMI and the case of rapid reperfusion. *Acta Cardiol* 1994;49:1–8.

9. Wallentin L. Reducing time to treatment in acute myocardial infarction. *Eur J Emerg Med* 2003;24:28–66.

10. European Myocardial Infarction Project Group. Prehospital thrombolytic therapy in patients with suspected acute myocardial infarction. *N Engl J Med* 1993;329:383–389.

11. Morrison LJ, Verbeek PR, McDonald AC, et al. Mortality and prehospital thrombolysis for acute myocardial infarction: A meta-analysis. *JAMA* 2000;283:2686–2692.

12. Weaver WD, Cerqueira M, Hallstrom AP, et al. Prehospital-initiated vs hospital-initiated thrombolytic therapy. The Myocardial Infarction Triage and Intervention Trial. *JAMA* 1993;270:1211–1216.

13. GREAT Group. Feasibility, safety, and efficacy of domiciliary thrombolysis by general practitioners: Grampian region early anistreplase trial. *Br Med J* 1992;305:548–553.

14. Rawles JM. Quantification of the benefit of earlier thrombolytic therapy: Five-year results of the Grampian Region Early Anistreplase Trial (GREAT). *J Am Coll Cardiol* 1997;30:1181.

15. Rawles J. GREAT: 10 year survival of patients with suspected acute myocardial infarction in a randomized comparison of prehospital and hospital thrombolysis. *Heart* 2003;89:563.

16. Morrow DA, Antman EM, Sayah A, et al. Evaluation of the time saved by pre-hospital initiation of reteplase for ST elevation MI: Results of the Early Retevase (ER) TIMI 19 Trial. *J Am Coll Cardiol* 2002;40(1):71–77.

17. Wallentin L, Goldstein P, Armstrong PW, et al. Efficacy and safety of tenecteplase in combination with the low-molecular-weight heparin enoxaparin or unfractionated heparin in the prehospital setting: the Assessment of the Safety and Efficacy of a New Thrombolytic Regimen (ASSENT)-3 PLUS randomized trial in acute myocardial infarction. *Circulation* 2003;108(2):135–142.

18. Task Force of the The European Society of Cardiology and The European Resuscitation Council. The pre-hospital management of acute heart attacks. Recommendations of a Task Force of the The European Society of Cardiology and The European Resuscitation Council. *Eur Heart J* 1998;19: 1140–1164.

19. Hutter AM Jr., Weaver WD. 31st Bethesda Conference. Emergency cardiac care. Task force 2: Acute coronary syndromes: Section 2A—Prehospital issues. *J Am Coll Cardiol* 2000;35:846–853.

20. Canto JG, Rogers WJ, Bowlby LJ, et al. The prehospital electrocardiogram in acute myocardial infarction: Is its full potential being realized? National Registry of Myocardial Infarction 2 Investigators. *J Am Coll Cardiol* 1997;29: 498–505.

21. Karagounis L, Ipsen SK, Jessop MR, et al. Impact of field-transmitted electrocardiography on time to in-hospital thrombolytic therapy in acute myocardial infarction. *Am J Cardiol* 1990;66:786–791.

22. Aufderheide TP, Hendley GE, Thakur RK, et al. The diagnostic impact of prehospital 12-lead electrocardiography. *Ann Emerg Med* 1990;19:1280–1287.

23. Gibler WB, Kereiakes DJ, Dean EN, et al. Prehospital diagnosis and treatment of acute myocardial infarction: a north-south perspective. The Cincinnati Heart Project and the Nashville Prehospital TPA Trial. *Am Heart J* 1991;121:1–11.

24. Aufderheide TP, Keelan MH, Hendley GE, et al. Milwaukee Prehospital Chest Pain Project—Phase I: Feasibility and accuracy of prehospital thrombolytic candidate selection. *Am J Cardiol* 1992;69:991–996.

25. Pitt K. Prehospital selection of patients for thrombolysis by paramedics. *Emerg Med J* 2002;19(3):260–263.

26. Llevadot J, Giugliano RP, Antman EM. Bolus fibrinolytic therapy in acute myocardial infarction. *JAMA* 2001;286: 442–449.

27. Welsh RC, Ornato J, Armastrong PW. Prehospital management of acute ST-elevation myocardial infarction: A

time for preappraisal in North America. *Am Heart J.* 2003;145(1):1–8.

28. Weaver WD, Simes RJ, Betriu A, et al. Comparison of primary coronary amgioplasty and intravenous fibrinolytic therapy for acute myocardial infarction: A quantitative review. *J Am Coll Cardiol* 1997;278:2093–2098.

29. Eagle KA, Goodman SG, Avezum A, et al. for the GRACE Investigators. Practice variation and missed opportunities for reperfusion in ST-segment-elevation myocardial infarction: findings from the Global Registry of Acute Coronary Events (GRACE). *Lancet* 2002;359:373–377.

30. Comparison of invasive and conservative strategies after treatment with intravenous tissue plasminogen activator in acute myocardial infarction. Results of the thrombolysis in myocardial infarction (YIMI) phase II trial. The TIMI Study Group. *N Engl J Med* 1989;320:618.

31. Immediate vs delayed catheterization and angioplasty following thrombolytic therapy for acute myocardial infarction. TIMI II A results. The TIMI Research Group. *JAMA* 1988;260:2849.

32. Juliard, JM, Himbert D, Critofini P, et al. A matched comparison of the combination of prehospital thrombolysis and standby rescue angioplasty with primary angioplasty. *Am J Cardiol* 1999;83:305.

33. Bonnefoy E, Lapostolle F, Leizorovics A, et al. Primary angioplasty versus prohospital fibrinolysis in acute myocardial infarction: a randomized study. *Lancet* 2002;360:825–829.

34. Dussoix P, Olivier R, Vitali V, et al. Time savings with prehospital thrombolysis in an urban area. *Eur J Emerg Med* 2003;10(1):2–5.

15

Combination Therapy for ST-Segment Elevation Myocardial Infarction

Chadwick Miller
James W. Hoekstra

HIGH YIELD FACTS

- Combination therapy refers to the addition of glycoprotein IIb/IIIa inhibitor therapy to lower dose fibrinolytic therapy for patients withST-segment elevation myocardial infarction.
- Evidence suggests combination therapy improves coronary patency rates and small vessel perfusion, and prevents coronary reocclusion compared to fibrinolytic therapy alone.
- Recent clinical trials have investigated half dose fibrinolytic therapy with full dose glycoprotein IIb/IIIa inhibitor therapy in patients with ST-segment elevation myocardial infarctions.
- Global Utilization of Strategies to Open Occluded Coronary Arteries V (GUSTO V) and the Assessment of the Safety and Efficacy of a New Thrombolytic Regimen (ASSENT)-3 Investigators found decrease in refractory ischemia and reinfarctionfor patients treated with combination therapy compared to standard fibrinolytic therapy alone.
- GUSTO V and ASSENT-3 demonstrated no difference in mortality and revealed increased bleeding complications in patients treated with combination therapy compared to fibrinolytic therapy alone.

INTRODUCTION

The treatment of ST-segment elevation myocardial infarction has changed dramatically since the reperfusion era. With the excitement of new developments have come discussions about ideal reperfusion strategies. Fibrinolytic therapy sparked debate over protocols, time to treatment, and appropriate fibrinolytic candidates. Simultaneously, the debate over percutaneous coronary intervention versus fibrinolysis arose and continues to be discussed. Recently, the introduction of glycoprotein IIb/IIIa inhibitor therapy has again fueled research over protocols, appropriate patients, and the medications with which they should be treated.

Fibrinolytic therapy is very attractive for treatment of ST-segment elevation myocardial infarction patients. With introduction of the bioengineered products, their ease of administration has been greatly improved. Their administration provides a rapid, efficacious alternative for patients who present to many hospitals that do not have cardiac catheterization available. Furthermore, fibrinolytic therapy can be performed rather expeditiously when compared to mobilizing a cardiac catheterization laboratory.

However, in patients with ST-segment elevation myocardial infarctions, the infarct-related artery reperfusion rate with fibrinolytic therapy and standard dose heparin is only 50–60%. In addition, the reocclusion rate after fibrinolytic therapy approximates 10–15%, leading to high rates of recurrent myocardial infarction and "rescue" percutaneous coronary intervention. The unreliable success of fibrinolytic therapy has led to investigations of pharmacologic strategies to improve the efficacy of fibrinolytic therapy. Glycoprotein IIb/IIIa inhibitors block the glycoprotein IIb/IIIa receptor on the platelet surface, inhibit the binding of fibrinogen, and ultimately inhibit thrombus formation. In patients undergoing percutaneous coronary intervention, studies have shown a relative risk reduction of 31–83% in death or MI for patients treated with glycoprotein IIb/IIIa inhibitor therapy compared to patients treated with aspirin and heparin alone.[1–3] As a result, the use of glycoprotein IIb/IIIa inhibitor therapy in patients undergoing high-risk percutaneous coronary intervention in non ST-segment elevation myocardial infarction is a class Ia recommendation in the American College of Cardiology (ACC)/American Heart Association (AHA) guidelines.[4] The quest for higher reperfusion rates and lower reocclusion rates in fibrinolytic therapy, the improved outcomes seen with glycoprotein IIb/IIIa inhibitor therapy in patients undergoing percutaneous coronary intervention, and a strong physiologic basis led to the investigation of combination therapy.

PATHOPHYSIOLOGY

Overview

The most common mechanism for ST-segment elevation myocardial infarction is the thrombotic occlusion of an epicardial coronary vessel. Thrombosis is usually the result of a long process of atherosclerotic plaque development, inflammation, and subsequent rupture. Plaque rupture leads to exposure of the plaque contents and subendothelium to the circulating blood, activating the coagulation cascade, and leading to thrombus formation.[5] The extent of coronary occlusion is dependent on the nature of the resulting thrombus.

Pathophysiologic Rationale for Combination Therapy

As a result of plaque rupture, platelets bind in response to the exposed collagen and tissue factor. Platelet activation causes release of mediators that attract additional platelets. Furthermore, platelet activation leads to the expression of glycoprotein IIb/IIIa receptors on the platelet surface. Glycoprotein IIb/IIIa receptors, the final common pathway for platelet aggregation, bind circulating fibrinogen and lead to further platelet aggregation.[6] The fibrinogen and platelet aggregate, or "white thrombus," is responsible for primary hemostasis at the plaque rupture site.[7] Simultaneously, activation of the coagulation cascade leads to thrombin formation[7] which converts fibrinogen to active fibrin, and ultimately produces a cross-linked fibrin mesh. The dense fibrin mesh traps red blood cells producing the "red thrombus," and accounts for secondary hemostasis. Aspirin, thienopyridines (clopidogrel and ticlopidine), and glycoprotein IIb/IIIa inhibitors inhibit platelet function and thus work to prevent the white thrombus (Fig. 15-1). Heparin products such as unfractionated heparin and low molecular weight heparin work within the coagulation cascade and thus prevent the red thrombus. Fibrinolytic drugs, as their name implies, lyse fibrin and are useful after formation of the red thrombus.

Fibrinolytic therapy is useful for dissolving fibrin and restoring patency to a thrombosed epicardial, or coronary, vessel. However, despite its powerful "thrombolytic" effects, it is less effective in the platelets within the white thrombus due to plasminogen activator inhibitor (PAI)-1, a very potent natural inhibitor of fibrinolysis. Furthermore, fibrinolysis can produce a local hypercoagulable state. The dissolution of fibrin leads to increased exposure of thrombin. Exposed thrombin stimulates the production of more thrombin and also has a very potent platelet

aggregation effect.[6] The net result may be increased amounts and activities of both thrombin and platelets (Fig. 15-2). Without inhibition of platelets, the local environment is conducive to expansion of the platelet-rich, fibrinolytic-resistant, white thrombus which is predisposed to reocclusion.[8] Clinically this may account for the 10% rate of reocclusion after fibrinolytic therapy despite using heparin products.

Although restoration of epicardial flow is linked to outcome, recent evidence suggests mortality is also linked to small vessel perfusion. The open artery hypothesis, that treatment of acute coronary syndrome (ACS) need only to focus on opening the epicardial vessel,[9,10] has not proven completely true. In fact, this theory is likely a simplistic view of myocardial infarction that discounts the role of the myocardial microcirculation in treatment. This is supported by the lack of mortality benefit between fibrinolytic regimens despite one regimen proven to have superior epicardial patency rates.[11–14] Further, there is a strong inverse association between myocardial microcirculatory flow and mortality after fibrinolytic therapy.[15] These findings have added to the theory of microvascular "no reflow"[16] that refers to the dysfunction of the myocardial microvasculature in acute myocardial infarction. Although "no reflow" is likely caused by multiple mechanisms, the microembolization of plaque contents and platelet thrombi is likely responsible, in part, for the destruction.[17] Drawing the clinical correlation, microcirculatory flow can be assessed angiographically as a myocardial blush and lack of microcirculatory flow is demonstrated electrocardiographically as persistent ST-segment elevation. This theory of microcirculatory flow has gained even more strength from study results showing reduced mortality associated with early resolution of ST-segment elevation,[18] suggesting reperfusion of the microcirculation. A recent study also demonstrated the presence of "no reflow," and thus destruction of the microcirculation, is associated with an increased incidence of congestive heart failure, malignant arrhythmias, and cardiac death.[19]

The exaggerated platelet aggregation effect produced by fibrinolytic therapy, along with microembolization of platelet thrombi causing destruction to the microcirculatory flow, suggests antiplatelet therapy during myocardial infarction treatment could be improved. The addition of glycoprotein IIb/IIIa inhibitor therapy to fibrinolytic therapy could negate an increase in platelet aggregation and prevent expansion of the white thrombus. This mechanism may account for the reduction in angiographically evident thrombus seen in patients with ACS undergoing combination therapy when compared to patients treated with

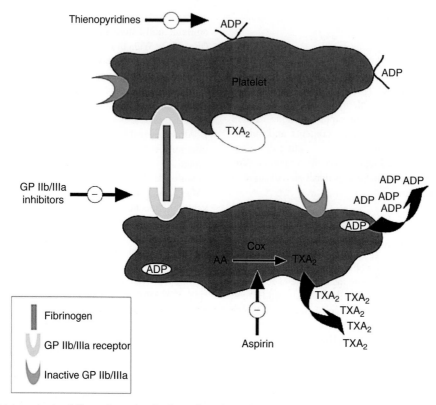

Fig. 15-1. Platelet activation follows atherosclerotic plaque disruption and consists of conformational changes, increased expression of glycoprotein (GP) IIb/IIIa receptors, and degranulation with release of prothrombotic substances such as thromboxane A$_2$ (TXA$_2$) and adenosine diphosphate (ADP). Aspirin, thienopyridines, and GP IIb/IIa receptor inhibitors block various pathways of thrombus formation. AA indicates acetylsalicylic acid; COX, cyclooxygenase. (Source: Jneid H, Bhatt DL, Corti R, et al. Aspirin and clopidogrel in acute coronary syndromes: Therapeutic insights from the CURE study. *Arch Intern Med* 2003;116:1145–1153.)

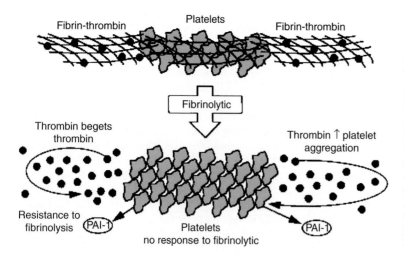

Fig. 15-2. Prothrombotic effects of fibrinolytic therapy. Coronary thrombus is composed of a platelet core with fibrin-thrombin admixture (Top). After fibrinolytic therapy, there is exposure of free thrombin, which autocatalytically begets more thrombin and strongly promotes platelet aggregation (Bottom). Platelets themselves are resistant to fibrinolytic therapy and furthermore secrete large amounts of PAI-1, which is a potent antagonist to fibrinolysis. (Source: Topol EJ. Toward a new frontier in myocardial reperfusion therapy: Emerging platelet preeminence. *Circulation* 1998;97: 211–218.)

fibrinolytic therapy alone.[18] The addition of glycoprotein IIb/IIIa inhibitor therapy to fibrinolytic therapy could also prevent microembolization of platelet thrombi during plaque rupture explaining the improvement in microcirculatory flow observed with combination therapy compared to fibrinolytic therapy alone.[18]

CLINICAL TRIALS OF COMBINATION THERAPY

Concepts Leading to Combination Therapy Clinical Trials

The benefits of combination therapy from a pathophysiologic view are well established. The clinical testing of combination therapy was fueled by the pathophysiologic basis and these conceptual advantages:

1. Given that the patency rate of fibrinolytic therapy is only 50–60%, the addition of glycoprotein IIb/IIIa inhibitor therapy could yield large improvements in epicardial infarct-related artery patency and thus improve mortality.

2. Combination therapy could increase myocardial microcirculation and thus reduce mortality.

3. The addition of glycoprotein IIb/IIIa inhibitor therapy could prevent reocclusion and thus reinfarction after fibrinolytic therapy.

4. Patients who do not achieve patency after fibrinolytic therapy are often transferred to interventional-equipped facilities for rescue percutaneous coronary intervention. Because glycoprotein IIb/IIIa inhibitor therapy improves outcomes in patients undergoing percutaneous coronary intervention therapy, early institution of glycoprotein IIb/IIIa inhibitor therapy could afford protection for patients needing rescue percutaneous coronary intervention.

5. The dose of heparin or fibrinolytic agents could be reduced and theoretically could reduce the incidence of bleeding complications.

Early Clinical Trials of Combination Therapy with Full Dose Fibrinolytic Therapy

The combination therapy concept was first tested in animal models such as the canine model by Yasuda et al.[8] The study compared combination therapy to fibrinolytic therapy alone in platelet-rich coronary occlusions and demonstrated dramatic success. Success in animal models led to the development of combination therapy trials in humans. The early combination therapy trials, Thrombolysis and Angioplasty in Myocardial Infarction (TAMI-8),[20] Integrilin to Minimize Platelet Aggregation and Combat Thrombosis in Acute Myocardial Infarction (IMPACT-AMI),[21] and Platelet Aggregation Receptor Antagonist Dose Investigation and reperfusion Gain in Myocardial infarction (PARADIGM),[22] all compared full dose fibrinolytic therapy in combination with glycoprotein IIb/IIIa inhibitor therapy to fibrinolytic therapy alone. One of the earliest human trials, the TAMI-8 protocol, demonstrated improved coronary patency in patients treated with combination therapy. The IMPACT-AMI trial demonstrated significant improvements in TIMI grade 3 flow (complete perfusion) at 90 min for the highest dose glycoprotein IIb/IIIa inhibitor group when compared to the fibrinolytic therapy group (66% vs. 39%, $P = 0.006$) as well as a significant decrease in the time to ST-segment recovery. No increase in bleeding was noted in these trials. The PARADIGM trial was designed similar to the previous studies. However, in contrast, there was no significant difference seen in clinical outcomes including a combined efficacy endpoint. The PARADIGM trial also demonstrated an increase in bleeding complications noted in the combination therapy group compared to controls.

Reduced Dose Fibrinolytic Combination Therapy Trials with Angiographic Outcome Measures

The early clinical trials, using full doses of fibrinolytic therapy, suggested combination therapy for patients with ST-segment elevation myocardial infarction improves coronary patency and improves microcirculatory flow. The TIMI 14,[23] Strategies for Patency Enhancement in the Emergency Department (SPEED),[24] INtegrilin and low dose ThROmbolysis in Acute Myocardial Infarction (INTRO AMI),[25] and INTEGRIlin and Tenecteplase for acute myocardial Infarction (INTEGRITI)[26] trials investigated the role of reduced dose fibrinolytic therapy in combination with the glycoprotein IIb/IIIa inhibitor therapy and used angiographically defined outcome measures.

The TIMI 14 trial enrolled 818 patients with ST-segment elevation myocardial infarction and was designed as an angiographic study to determine the impact of abciximab on the reperfusion of occluded coronary arteries. The first phase consisted of a dose-finding phase where full dose fibrinolytic therapy with alteplase was compared to abciximab alone, or in combination with reduced dose alteplase or streptokinase. The second phase was for dose confirmation, testing the best regimen from the first phase. The second phase also compared low dose and very low dose heparin with combination therapy. The primary outcome was TIMI grade 3 flow at 90 min. Secondary outcomes included TIMI grade 3 flow at 60 min and a microcirculatory assessment measured as TIMI frame counts at 60 and 90 min.

Results from the TIMI 14 trial demonstrated patients treated with the combination therapy of half dose alteplase and abciximab demonstrated significantly higher TIMI grade 3 flow rates at 90 min (77% vs. 62%, $P = 0.02$). Secondary outcomes for the combination of abciximab and reduced dose alteplase revealed a significant improvement in TIMI grade 3 flow rates at 60 min (72% vs. 43%, $P = 0.0009$) with rates of hemorrhage similar to the fibrinolytic therapy group (7% vs. 6%).

These encouraging results were followed by the SPEED trial that looked at the fibrinolytic drug reteplase in combination with the glycoprotein IIb/IIIa inhibitor abciximab. The phase A was designed for dose exploration as various doses of reteplase were administered. Phase B tested the fibrinolytic dose that appeared superior in the first phase. Heparin doses were also explored with two different heparin bolus and infusion regimens.

In phase B of the SPEED trial, the reteplase dose of 5 U + 5 U was used in combination with abciximab and heparin at either a 40 U/kg bolus and infusion or a 60 U/kg bolus and infusion. These patients were compared to a control group that received reteplase 10 U + 10 U and a 70 U/kg heparin bolus and infusion. TIMI grade 3 flow at 60–90 min was the primary outcome and was achieved in 61% of the combination therapy with 60 U/kg heparin group, 51% of the combination therapy with 40 U/kg heparin group, and 47% of the fibrinolytic therapy and heparin control group ($P = 0.05$ for combination therapy with 60 U/kg heparin group vs. control group). Major bleeding complications in phase B, although not reaching statistical significance, were seen more often in the combination therapy groups when compared to the control (9.8% vs. 3.7%).

The INTRO AMI trial compared the combination of eptifibatide and half dose alteplase to full dose alteplase alone. The trial was also designed with dose-finding and dose-confirmation phases, and all patients received standard therapy including aspirin and 60 U/kg heparin bolus followed by infusion. Phase A compared different doses of eptifibatide including single versus double boluses. Phase B randomized patients to either control (full dose alteplase) or one of two experimental groups (50 mg alteplase plus double bolus eptifibatide 10 min apart and higher dose infusion, or double bolus eptifibatide 30 min apart and lower dose infusion). The

primary endpoints measured were TIMI grade 3 flows at 60 min and major bleeding.

Phase B of INTRO AMI demonstrated improved TIMI grade 3 flow at 60 min for combination therapy. The group that received the accelerated eptifibatide dosing with half dose alteplase had 56% TIMI grade 3 flow compared to 40% for the full dose alteplase group ($P = 0.04$) and demonstrated improved corrected TIMI frame counts suggesting improved microvascular flow. Of note, there were no significant differences seen for the low dose eptifibatide group as compared to the control. Bleeding complications using the phase B protocols demonstrated major hemorrhage rates (excluding coronary artery by-pass grafting [CABG]-related bleeding) of 8% for the low dose eptifibatide combination therapy group, 11% for the high dose eptifibatide combination therapy group, and 6% for the alteplase group.

The INTEGRITI trial, similar to the INTRO AMI trial, compared eptifibatide used in combination therapy but differed by using the fibrinolytic drug tenecteplase in reduced dose. The trial of 438 patients was also a two-phase study with phase A used for dose finding and phase B dose confirmation. Primary outcome measure was TIMI grade 3 flow at 60 min. The superior regimen in phase A, half dose tenecteplase with double bolus eptifibatide 10 min apart and a 2 µg/kg/min infusion, was compared to full dose tenecteplase in phase B. All patients received aspirin and a 60 U/kg heparin bolus followed by infusion.

The outcome differences from the INTEGRITI trial failed to reach statistical significance. However, in agreement with the previous trials, there was a trend for increased TIMI grade 3 flow at 60 min in the combination therapy group when compared to the tenecteplase alone group (59% vs. 49%, $P = 0.14$). Bleeding complications were increased with more major hemorrhage (7.6%) in the combination therapy group compared to the tenecteplase group (2.5%) although this did not reach statistical significance. There were no large differences in rates of intracranial hemorrhage.

The results of the TIMI 14, SPEED, INTRO AMI, and INTEGRITI trials demonstrated improved *angiographic outcomes* for combination therapy when compared to fibrinolytic therapy without glycoprotein IIb/IIIa inhibitors (Fig. 15-3). However, these trials also demonstrate an increased rate of bleeding that, although not statistically significant, potentially could be clinically important (Fig. 15-4). It is worthy noting Brener et al.'s observation that these studies are angiographic studies and thus are prone to increased rates of bleeding.[25] Brener et al. cite an 8–10% incidence of major bleeding in primary

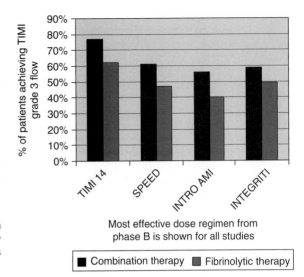

Fig. 15-3. Angiographic outcomes from the dose-confirmation phases of the combination therapy trials with angiographically defined endpoints. Primary outcome varies by study but is TIMI grade 3 flow at either 60 or 90 min.

Most effective dose regimen from phase B is shown for all studies

angioplasty studies and suggest the major hemorrhage rate for combination therapy may not be excessive. In the combination therapy treatment groups, the majority of bleeding seen was noted to be at the vascular access site. Since these four trials used angiographic outcome measures, many of these patients received mandatory angiography that in a real-world application may not be required. The trials also suggest the heparin bolus and infusion rates are related to the efficacy of combination therapy and possibly the bleeding complications. Looking at outcomes from the TIMI 14 trial, the very low dose

heparin group did not achieve the improved patency rates seen with the low dose heparin group but demonstrated a 1% major hemorrhage rate compared to 6 and 7% rates in the control and low dose heparin groups, respectively.

Combination Therapy Trials with Clinical Outcome Measures

In comparison to the angiographic studies, the Global Use of Strategies To Open occluded arteries (GUSTO V)[27] and ASsessment of the Safety and Efficacy of a New Thrombolytic Regimen (ASSENT-3)[28] trials were designed to look at the effect of combination therapy on clinical outcomes. The GUSTO V trial was a large, multicenter trial enrolling 16,588 patients with ST-segment elevation myocardial infarction into a randomized, open-label comparison of combination therapy with reteplase (half dose) plus abciximab versus reteplase (full dose) alone. All patients enrolled were given aspirin as well as heparin at a bolus of 60 U/kg and infusion of 7 U/kg for the combination therapy group and 5000 U bolus with an infusion of 1000 U/hour for the reteplase group. The primary endpoint was all-cause mortality (Table 15-1).

The results from GUSTO V revealed no significant difference in all-cause mortality at 30 days for the combination therapy group compared to the reteplase alone group (5.6% vs. 5.9%, $P = 0.43$). This finding also remained true at 1 year after randomization with no difference in mortality among both groups.[29] However, looking at secondary outcome findings, for the composite endpoint of death or recurrent infarction, a significant

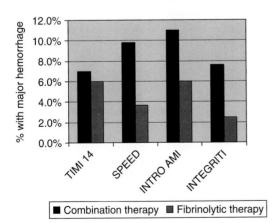

Fig. 15-4. Rates of major hemorrhage as defined by study investigators in the combination therapy trials with angiographic outcomes.

Table 15-1. Dosing Regimens for Combination Therapy in GUSTO V[27] and ASSENT-3[28]

Trial	Drug	Dose
GUSTO V	Aspirin	150–325 mg
	Heparin	60 U/kg bolus, infusion of 7 U/kg/h
	Abciximab	0.25 µg/kg bolus, infusion of 0.125 µg/kg/min for 12 h
	Reteplase	Two 5 U boluses, 30 min apart
ASSENT-3		
	Aspirin	150–325 mg
	Heparin	60 U/kg bolus, infusion of 12 U/kg/h
	Abciximab	0.25 µg/kg bolus, infusion of 0.125 µg/kg/min for 12 h
	Tenecteplase	15–25 U bolus (weight-based)

advantage was seen in the combination therapy group compared to the reteplase alone group (7.4% vs. 8.8%, $P = 0.0011$). Comparing rates of revascularization, the combination therapy group had a significantly lower rate of rescue percutaneous coronary intervention, or percutaneous coronary intervention within 6 hours (5.6% vs. 8.6%, $P < 0.0001$). The combination therapy group also had significant decreases at 7 days in rates of percutaneous coronary intervention (25.4% vs. 27.9%, $P < 0.0001$) and coronary artery bypass grafting (3.0% vs. 3.7%, $P = 0.013$) (Fig. 15-5).

However, the improved secondary outcomes seen in the combination therapy group came at the expense of increased bleeding complications. There was a 2.3% incidence of moderate or severe nonintracranial bleeding in the reteplase group compared to 4.6% in the combination therapy group ($P < 0.0001$). Although there was no difference between groups in intracranial hemorrhage in patients less than 75 years of age (0.4% vs. 0.5%, $P = 0.27$), there was an increase in intracranial hemorrhage in patients older than 75 years of age undergoing combination therapy (2.1% vs. 1.1%, $P = 0.069$). In addition, patients in the combination therapy group had a significant increase in the incidence of thrombocytopenia (2.9% vs 0.7%, $P < 0.0001$ for platelets <100,000) compared to the reteplase group[27] (Fig. 15-5).

The GUSTO V trial has several important findings. The mortality of all patients in the trial was very low at 5.9%. As explained by the GUSTO V investigators, the mortality is not only lower than that seen in the GUSTO III trial (7.5%) comparing two full dose fibrinolytic regimens, it is lower than that seen in any other trial of acute myocardial infarction.[27] Supporting combination therapy use, the rates of reinfarction and rescue percutaneous

coronary intervention were decreased in the combination therapy group. However, the rates of bleeding and thrombocytopenia were also increased with combination therapy, although the overall bleeding increase was small and the rate of 4.6% of moderate or severe bleeding seen in the combination therapy group is low compared to other trials. The increase in intracranial bleeding seen in the group over 75 years of age is another significant finding and, as such, the recommendation is to avoid combination therapy in this patient population.[14] Despite these points,

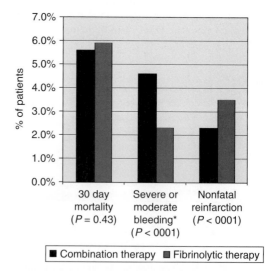

Fig. 15-5. Results from GUSTO V. Combination therapy = half dose reteplase + unfractionated heparin + abciximab. Fibrinolytic therapy = full dose reteplase + unfractionated heparin. The asterisk (*) denotes nonintracranial bleeding.

the fact remains that GUSTO V was a large, well-powered study that failed to detect a difference in mortality in patients treated with combination therapy compared to fibrinolytics alone. This suggests the improved angiographic outcomes seen in the earlier studies do not necessarily translate into improved mortality.

The ASSENT-3 trial[28] followed the results of GUSTO V and explored tenecteplase used in combination therapy with heparin and abciximab. The study enrolled 6095 patients with ST-segment elevation myocardial infarction and randomized the patients to one of three groups: full dose tenecteplase and unfractionated heparin, full dose tenecteplase and a low molecular weight heparin, and half dose tenecteplase with unfractionated heparin and abciximab. The last group, the combination therapy group, was administered heparin dosing at a 40 U/kg bolus and an infusion at 7 U/kg/hour. The primary outcomes were composite endpoints of efficacy (30-day death, recurrent in-hospital infarction, and refractory ischemia) and safety (efficacy endpoint plus major bleeding complications or intracranial hemorrhage) (Table 15-1).

The combination therapy group demonstrated a significant reduction in efficacy endpoints (11.1%) compared to the unfractionated heparin/fibrinolytic group (15.4%, $P < 0.0001$). However, similar to GUSTO V, the combination therapy group also had higher bleeding rates compared to the unfractionated heparin/fibrinolytic group (14.2% vs. 17.0%, $P = 0.014$). Also mirroring GUSTO V, at 30 days there was no difference in mortality. Furthermore, the improved endpoints came at the expense of increased bleeding with the combination therapy group experiencing significant increases in major bleeding complications and thrombocytopenia. Also, patients who were older than 75 years of age or were diabetic and received combination therapy had a major hemorrhage rate three times that of those patients treated with unfractionated heparin and fibrinolytic therapy (Fig. 15-6).

A post hoc analysis of the ASSENT-3 trial examined the relationship of the treatment groups to outcomes in those patients who underwent both elective and urgent, or rescue percutaneous coronary intervention.[30] Similar to GUSTO V, less patients required urgent percutaneous coronary intervention who were treated with combination therapy compared to the unfractionated heparin and fibrinolytic therapy group (9.1% vs. 14.3%, $P < 0.0001$). However, of those patients undergoing urgent percutaneous coronary intervention, mortality at 30 days and 1 year was increased in the combination therapy group. Furthermore, there was also a significant increase in major bleeding complications seen in the combination

therapy group undergoing percutaneous coronary intervention compared to the unfractionated heparin and fibrinolytic therapy group undergoing percutaneous coronary intervention. The authors point out that the effect of treatment in this analysis may have selected for a sicker population in the combination therapy group who underwent urgent percutaneous coronary intervention and may partially account for the findings. There were no differences in clinical outcomes seen among groups undergoing elective percutaneous coronary intervention.

SUMMARY OF THE COMBINATION THERAPY TRIALS

The need for aggressive platelet inhibition in patients with ST-segment elevation myocardial infarction is well grounded in theory. The addition of glycoprotein IIb/IIIa inhibitor therapy to fibrinolytic regimens should offset the hypercoagulable state induced by fibrinolytic therapy and prevent expansion of the white thrombus. Furthermore, the inhibition of platelet microembolization should improve myocardial microcirculation. Angiographic studies have demonstrated improved TIMI grade 3 flows but also have suggested an increase in bleeding complications. Taking the next step to demonstrating improved morbidity and mortality with combination therapy has proven difficult.

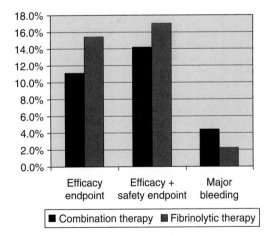

Fig. 15-6. Results from the ASSENT-3 trial. Efficacy endpoint is a composite of 30-day mortality, in-hospital reinfarction, and in-hospital refractory ischemia. Safety endpoint is composite of in-hospital intracranial hemorrhage or in-hospital major bleeding complications. Combination therapy = half dose tenecteplase + unfractionated heparin + abciximab. Fibrinolytic therapy = full dose tenecteplase + unfractionated heparin.

The ASSENT-3 and GUSTO V trials, designed to explore clinical outcomes in combination therapy, overall have disappointing results. The relatively large, clinical outcome-based studies failed to demonstrate a decrease in 30-day mortality. There was a decrease in recurrent myocardial infarction and refractory ischemia due to combination therapy, but at the expense of bleeding complications and thrombocytopenia. Importantly, both studies demonstrated a high rate of complications in those patients greater than 75 years of age and thus combination therapy is not recommended in this patient population.

Further studies are needed to address whether subgroups exist that may benefit from combination therapy. Other protocols also need to examine the effect of combination therapy on patients undergoing rescue percutaneous coronary intervention as well as the effect of low molecular weight heparin on combination therapy. With the evidence at hand, other options appear more promising in the reperfusion of patients with STEMI such as percutaneous coronary intervention facilitated by fibrinolytic therapy and/or glycoprotein IIb/IIIa inhibitors, or fibrinolytic therapy in concert with unfractionated heparin or low molecular weight heparin.

REFERENCES

1. Lincoff AM, Califf RM, Anderson KM, et al. Evidence for prevention of death and myocardial infarction with platelet membrane glycoprotein iib/iiia receptor blockade by abciximab (c7E3 Fab) among patients with unstable angina undergoing percutaneous coronary revascularization. *J Am Coll Cardiol* 1997;30:149–156.
2. PURSUIT Trial Investigators. Inhibition of platelet glycoprotein IIb/IIIa with eptifibatide in patients with acute coronary syndromes. Platelet glycoprotein IIb/IIIa in unstable angina: Receptor suppression using integrilin therapy. *N Engl J Med* 1998;339:436–443.
3. Platelet receptor inhibition in ischemic syndrome management in patients limited by unstable signs and symptoms (PRISM-PLUS) study investigators. Inhibition of the platelet glycoprotein IIb/IIIa receptor with tirofiban in unstable angina and non-Q-wave myocardial infarction. *N Engl J Med* 1998;338:1488–1497.
4. Braunwald E, Antman EM, Beasley JW, et al. ACC/AHA 2002 guideline update for the management of patients with unstable angina and non-ST-segment elevation myocardial infarction—summary article: A report of the American College of Cardiology/American Heart Association task force on practice guidelines (Committee on the Management of Patients With Unstable Angina). *J Am Coll Cardiol* 2002;40:1366–1374.
5. Rauch U, Osende JI, Fuster V, et al. Thrombus formation on atherosclerotic plaques: Pathogenesis and clinical consequences. *Ann Intern Med* 2001;134:224–238.
6. Topol EJ. Toward a new frontier in myocardial reperfusion therapy: Emerging platelet preeminence. *Circulation* 1998;97:211–218.
7. Jneid H, Bhatt DL, Corti R, et al. Aspirin and clopidogrel in acute coronary syndromes: Therapeutic insights from the CURE study. *Arch Intern Med* 2003;163:1145–1153.
8. Yasuda T, Gold HK, Leinbach RC, et al. Lysis of plasminogen activator-resistant platelet-rich coronary artery thrombus with combined bolus injection of recombinant tissue-type plasminogen activator and antiplatelet GPIIb/IIIa antibody. *J Am Coll Cardiol* 1990;16:1728–1735.
9. Braunwald E. Myocardial reperfusion, limitation of infarct size, reduction of left ventricular dysfunction, and improved survival. Should the paradigm be expanded? *Circulation* 1989;79:441–444.
10. Cannon CP. Importance of TIMI 3 flow. *Circulation* 2001;104:624–626.
11. The Global Use of Strategies to Open Occluded Coronary Arteries (GUSTO III) Investigators: A comparison of reteplase with alteplase for acute myocardial infarction. *N Engl J Med* 1997;337:1118–1123.
12. Bode C, Smalling RW, Berg G, et al. Randomized comparison of coronary thrombolysis achieved with double-bolus reteplase (recombinant plasminogen activator) and front-loaded, accelerated alteplase (recombinant tissue plasminogen activator) in patients with acute myocardial infarction. The RAPID II Investigators. *Circulation* 1996;94:891–898.
13. Smalling RW, Bode C, Kalbfleisch J, et al. More rapid, complete, and stable coronary thrombolysis with bolus administration of reteplase compared with alteplase infusion in acute myocardial infarction. RAPID Investigators. *Circulation* 1995;91:2725–2732.
14. Bhatt DL, Peacock WF, Hoekstra J, et al. Combination therapy for acute myocardial infarcation. The Cleveland Clinic, 2003 (Monograph).
15. Gibson CM, Murphy SA, Rizzo MJ, et al. Relationship between TIMI frame count and clinical outcomes after thrombolytic administration. Thrombolysis in Myocardial Infarction (TIMI) Study Group. *Circulation* 1999;99:1945–1950.
16. Ito H, Tomooka T, Sakai N, et al. Lack of myocardial perfusion immediately after successful thrombolysis. A predictor of poor recovery of left ventricular function in anterior myocardial infarction. *Circulation* 1992;85:1699–1705.
17. Reffelmann T, Kloner RA. The "no-reflow" phenomenon: Basic science and clinical correlates. *Heart* 2002;87:162–168.
18. Gibson CM, de Lemos JA, Murphy SA, et al. Combination therapy with abciximab reduces angiographically evident thrombus in acute myocardial infarction: A TIMI 14 substudy. *Circulation* 2001;103:2550–2554.
19. Morishima I, Sone T, Okumura K, et al. Angiographic no-reflow phenomenon as a predictor of adverse long-term outcome in patients treated with percutaneous transluminal coronary angioplasty for first acute myocardial infarction. *J Am Coll Cardiol* 2000;36:1202–1209.

20. Kleiman NS, Ohman EM, Califf RM, et al. Profound inhibition of platelet aggregation with monoclonal antibody 7E3 Fab after thrombolytic therapy. Results of the Thrombolysis and Angioplasty in Myocardial Infarction (TAMI) 8 Pilot Study. *J Am Coll Cardiol* 1993;22:381–389.

21. Ohman EM, Kleiman NS, Gacioch G, et al. Combined accelerated tissue-plasminogen activator and platelet glycoprotein IIb/IIIa integrin receptor blockade with integrilin in acute myocardial infarction: Results of a randomized, placebo-controlled, dose-ranging trial. *Circulation* 1997;95:846–854.

22. Combining thrombolysis with the platelet glycoprotein IIb/IIIa inhibitor lamifiban: Results of the platelet aggregation receptor antagonist dose investigation and reperfusion gain in myocardial infarction (PARADIGM) trial. *J Am Coll Cardiol* 1998;32:2003–2010.

23. Antman EM, Giugliano RP, Gibson CM, et al. Abciximab facilitates the rate and extent of thrombolysis: Results of the thrombolysis in myocardial infarction (TIMI) 14 trial. The TIMI 14 Investigators. *Circulation* 1999;99:2720–2732.

24. Strategies for Patency Enhancement in the Emergency Department (SPEED) Group. Trial of abciximab with and without low-dose reteplase for acute myocardial infarction. *Circulation* 2000;101:2788–2794.

25. Brener SJ, Zeymer U, Adgey AA, et al. Eptifibatide and low-dose tissue plasminogen activator in acute myocardial infarction: The integrilin and low-dose thrombolysis in acute myocardial infarction (INTRO AMI) trial. *J Am Coll Cardiol* 2002;39:377–386.

26. Giugliano RP, Roe MT, Harrington RA, et al. Combination reperfusion therapy with eptifibatide and reduced-dose tenecteplase for ST-elevation myocardial infarction. 1. Results of the integrilin and tenecteplase in acute myocardial infarction (INTEGRITI) Phase II Angiographic urial. *J Am Coll Cardiol* 2003;41:1251–1260.

27. Topol EJ. Reperfusion therapy for acute myocardial infarction with fibrinolytic therapy or combination reduced fibrinolytic therapy and platelet glycoprotein IIb/IIIa inhibition: The GUSTO V randomised trial. *Lancet* 2001; 357:1905–1914.

28. The Assessment of the Safety and Efficacy of a New Thrombolytic Regimen (ASSENT)-3 Investigators. Efficacy and safety of tenecteplase in combination with enoxaparin, abciximab, or unfractionated heparin: The ASSENT-3 randomised trial in acute myocardial infarction. *Lancet* 2001;358:605–613.

29. Lincoff AM, Califf RM, Van de Werf F, et al. Mortality at 1 year with combination platelet glycoprotein IIb/IIIa inhibition and reduced-dose fibrinolytic therapy vs conventional fibrinolytic therapy for acute myocardial infarction: GUSTO V randomized trial. *JAMA* 2002;288: 2130–2135.

30. Dubois CL, Belmans A, Granger CB, et al. Outcome of urgent and elective percutaneous coronary interventions after pharmacologic reperfusion with tenecteplase combined with unfractionated heparin, enoxaparin, or abciximab. *J Am Coll Cardiol* 2003;42:1178–1185.

16

Invasive Therapy for AMI/ACS

PCI and CABG

Gerard X. Brogan, Jr.

HIGH YIELD FACTS

- Optimal therapy for ST-elevation acute myocardial infarction (AMI) is primary percutaneous coronary intervention (PCI) when available in an appropriate time frame.
- High-risk acute coronary syndrome (ACS) patients benefit by aggressive antiplatelet and antithrombotic therapy in association with an early invasive approach.
- Non-high-risk patients should have early noninvasive diagnostic studies (stress, echo, and so on) to further evaluate the risk of coronary artery disease (CAD).

INVASIVE MANAGEMENT OF NSTEMI/UA

Two different treatment strategies, termed "early conservative" and "early invasive," have evolved for patients with unstable angina (UA)/non-ST elevation myocardial infarction (NSTEMI). In the *early conservative strategy*, coronary angiography is reserved for patients with evidence of recurrent ischemia (angina at rest or with minimal activity or dynamic ST-segment changes) or a strongly positive stress test, despite vigorous medical therapy. In the *early invasive strategy*, patients without clinically obvious contraindications to coronary revascularization are routinely recommended for coronary angiography and angiographically directed revascularization if possible.

Current American College of Cardiology (ACC)/American Heart Association (AHA) Practice Guidelines (See Table 16-1)

Class I

1. An early invasive strategy in patients with UA/NSTEMI and any of the following high-risk indicators.[1] (Level of Evidence: A)

   a. Recurrent angina/ischemia at rest or with low-level activities despite intensive anti-ischemic therapy

   b. Elevated troponin-t (TnT) or troponin-I (TnI)

   c. New or presumably new ST-segment depression

   d. Recurrent angina/ischemia with congestive heart failure (CHF) symptoms, an S3 gallop, pulmonary edema, worsening rales, or new or worsening MR

   e. High-risk findings on noninvasive stress testing

   f. Depressed left ventricular (LV) systolic function (e.g., ejection fraction [EF] less than 0.40 on noninvasive study)

   g. Hemodynamic instability

   h. Sustained ventricular tachycardia

   i. PCI within 6 months

   j. Prior coronary artery by-pass grafting (CABG)

2. In the absence of these findings, either an early conservative or an early invasive strategy in hospitalized patients without contraindications for revascularization. (Level of Evidence: B)

Class IIa

1. An early invasive strategy in patients with repeated presentations for ACS despite therapy and without evidence for ongoing ischemia or high risk. (Level of Evidence: C)

Class III

1. Coronary angiography in patients with extensive comorbidities (e.g., liver or pulmonary failure, cancer), in whom the risks of revascularization are not likely to outweigh the benefits. (Level of Evidence: C)

2. Coronary angiography in patients with acute chest pain and a low likelihood of ACS. (Level of Evidence: C.)

3. Coronary angiography in patients who will not consent to revascularization regardless of the findings. (Level of Evidence: C)

Randomized Studies Comparing Invasive Versus Conservative Strategies (See Table 16-2)

The TIMI-IIIB Trials

The Thrombolysis In Myocardial Ischemia (TIMI-IIIB) trials included 1473 patients with UA or non-Q-wave MI.[2]

This trial was a 2×2 factorial design comparing tissue plasminogen activator (tPA) with placebo and an early

Table 16-1. Recommendations for Patients Who May Benefit From Early Aggressive Management

Clinical factors predicting risk in the NSTE ACS

History
Frequent angina
Prior history of angina
Prolonged/ongoing (>20 min) angina
Ages >65 years
Prior beta-blocker use
Prior revascularization
Diabetes mellitus
Three risk factors for CAD (high cholesterol, plus
   family history of ongoing tobacco use)

Physical
Signs of heart failure (including S3 gallop, elevated neck
   veins, pulmonary rales) hypotension

Laboratory
ECG
ST-segment depression
Transient ST-segment elevation
Deep T-wave inversions (particularly during pain)
Cardiac markers
Elevated serum troponin I or T and/or creatine kinase-MB

Abbreviations: CAD = coronary artery disease; ECG = electrocardiogram; MB = myocardial band; NSTE ACS = non-ST-segment elevation acute coronary syndrome.
Source: Braunwald E, Antman EM, Beasley JW. ACC/AHA guidelines for the management of patients with unstable angina and non-ST-segment elevation myocardial infarction. A report of the American College of Cardiology/American Heart Association Task Force on Practice Guidelines (Committee on the Management of Patients With Unstable Angina). *J Am Coll Cardiol* 2000;36: 970–1062.

invasive strategy ($n = 740$) versus a conservative strategy ($n = 733$) within 48 hours of randomization. The invasive strategy involved cardiac catheterization, LV angiography, and coronary arteriography 18–48 hours after randomization. The PCI was performed in all lesions with >60% stenosis. CABG surgery was performed in the presence of significant left main coronary artery obstruction, three-vessel disease, and depressed LV function, or recurrent UA.

The conservative strategy involved initial medical therapy, with intervention only after ischemia was detected on stress testing at 6 weeks. All patients were treated with bed rest, oxygen, anti-ischemic medications (beta-blockade, calcium-channel blockade, and long-acting nitrates), aspirin, and heparin.

The primary outcome (combined death, nonfatal MI, or ischemia on stress testing) occurred in 18.1% of patients in the invasive strategy group and in 16.2% of patients in the conservative strategy group (a nonsignificant difference). In addition, there were no significant differences in any of the three individual endpoints. Of the patients randomized to the conservative strategy group, ST-segment depression on the qualifying electrocardiogram, prior aspirin use, and older age were independent predictors of primary outcome components.

VANQWISH

The Veterans Affairs Non-Q-Wave Infarction Strategies in Hospital (VANQWISH) trial[3] compared early and late clinical outcomes (death or recurrent MI) in patients randomly assigned to either early invasive strategy or conservative treatment. Patients treated with the early invasive strategy (heart catheterization followed by myocardial revascularization) had significantly worse clinical outcomes during the first year of follow-up than did those treated with a conservative strategy (intervention guided by rigorous ischemia management, noninvasive stress testing, and medical therapy). The number of patients who had one of the components of the primary endpoint was significantly higher in the invasive strategy group at hospital discharge (36 events vs. 15 events, $P = 0.004$), at 1 month (48 events vs. 26 events, $P = 0.012$), and at 1 year (111 events vs. 85 events, $P = 0.05$).[4] However, considering current use of stents and the rise of newer catheter-based techniques, these results must be interpreted in proper clinical context.

FRISC-II

The Fragmin and fast Revascularization during InStability in Coronary artery disease (FRISC-II) invasive trial[4] showed a significant event rate reduction favoring the invasive over the noninvasive strategy at 6 months in a subset of patients with UA and non-Q-wave infarction (Fig. 16-1). In the trial, 2457 patients in 58 Scandinavian hospitals were assigned to early invasive or noninvasive treatment with placebo-controlled low molecular weight heparin (LMWH) (dalteparin) for 3 months. In the invasive group, 96% of patients received angiography within 7 days; of those, 71% underwent revascularization within 10 days. For the noninvasive group, 10% received angiography within 7 days; of those, 9% went on to undergo revascularization procedures. At 6 months, the rate of death, MI, or both was 9.4% in the invasive group and 12.1% in the noninvasive group (risk ratio [RR], 0.78; 95% confidence interval, 0.62–0.98; $P = 0.031$).

However, the results favoring the invasive strategy were not uniformly shown among patient subsets in FRISC-II. In a substudy analysis of the influence of

Table 16-2. Early Invasive Vs. Early Conservative Approach to Non-ST-Elevation ACS[*]

Trial	N	Invasive Vs. Conservative	Comments
RITA-3 (2002)	1810	Death, MI, or refractory angina at 4 months (9.6% vs. 14.5%. $P = 0.001$). Mainly due to having refractory angina. No difference in death or MI between groups.	Angiography was performed within 48 h. Enoxaparin was the antithrombin in both groups. Discretionary use of GP IIb/IIIa inhibitors. Invasive approach resulted in less angina and fewer antianginal meds at follow-up.
FRISC-II (2002)	2457	1-year death (2.2% vs. 3.9%, $P = 0.016$), MI (8.6% vs. 11.6%, $P = 0.015$), death or MI (10.4% vs. 14.1%, $P = 0.005$); 2-year death (3.7% vs. 5.4%, $P = 0.038$), MI (9.2% vs. 12.7%, $P = 0.005$), death or MI (12.1% vs. 16.3%, $P = 0.003$)	In ACS patients treated with dalteparin (avg. 6 days prior to angiography), the invasive approach demonstrated clear benefit at 6 months, 1 year, and 2 years. Most PCI patients underwent coronary stenting.
TACTICS-TIMI 18 (2001)	2220	6-month death, MI, or readmission for ACS (15.9% vs. 19.4%, $P = 0.025$); 6-month death or MI (7.3% vs. 9.5%, $P < 0.05$). Similar benefit in men and women.	In ACS patients treated with tirofiban (avg. 22 h prior to angiography), the early invasive approach was superior to the early conservative approach. Most PCI patients underwent coronary stenting.
VANQWISH (1998)	920	Hospital death (4.5% vs. 1.3%, $P = 0.007$), death or MI (7.8% vs. 3.3%, $P = 0.004$); 1-year death (12.6% vs. 7.9%, $P = 0.025$), death or MI (24% vs. 18.6%, $P = 0.05$).	High mortality rate in the invasive group was due to unusually high (10.4%) 30-day mortality after CABG. Most PCI patients underwent PTCA.

[*]Early invasive approach = routine angiography and revascularization as appropriate; early conservative approach = angiography and revascularization for recurrent ischemia or high-risk finding on stress test.
Abbreviations: ACS = acute coronary syndrome; LOS = length of stay; MI = myocardial infarction; PCI = percutaneous coronary intervention; PTCA = percutaneous transluminal coronary (balloon) angioplasty; TVR = target-vessel revascularization.
Source: Califf RM, Fried M. In Califf RM (ed) *ACS Essentials*. Royal Oak, Michigan. Physicians Press 2003.

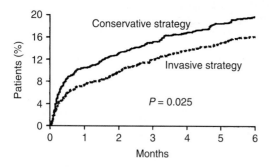

Fig. 16-1. Cumulative incidence of the primary endpoint of death, nonfatal myocardial infarction, or rehospitalization for an acute coronary syndrome during the 6-month follow-up period. The rate of the primary endpoint was lower in the invasive strategy group than in the conservative strategy group (15.9% vs. 19.4%; OR, 0.78; 955 CI, 0.62 to 0.97; $P = 0.025$).

troponin levels, 42% of patients were found to be troponin negative (<0.1 g/L).[5] The 6-month rate of death or MI was 8.3% in patients assigned to an invasive strategy versus 10.3% in those assigned to a conservative strategy ($P = $ ns).[6]

In the evaluation of patients who had ST-segment deviations on the admission electrocardiogram in FRISC-II, 418 patients had no demonstrable ST-T-wave changes. The relative risk of an unfavorable outcome (death or MI at 6 months) was actually slightly higher for patients in the invasive group. No significant benefit was shown with the invasive strategy in patients who had isolated T-wave inversion only. The early invasive strategy was not shown to be fully beneficial in 52% of patients who had either no electrocardiogram changes or T-wave inversion only. The true benefit of early invasive treatment, when evaluated by electrocardiography, was derived from the subset of patients with ST-segment depression MI.

Therefore, patients who were troponin negative and those who had no ST-T-wave changes or only isolated T-wave inversions (>50% of all patients) did not benefit from an invasive strategy.

TACTICS TIMI-18

The Treat angina with Aggrastat and determine Cost of Therapy with an Invasive or Conservative Strategy TIMI-18 (TACTICS TIMI-18) trial included 2220 patients with UA/NSTEMI.[5] Patients presenting with an accelerating pattern, prolonged or recurrent anginal pain at rest or minimal effort within the previous 24 hours, plus ischemia, electrocardiogram changes, elevated cardiac markers, or a history of prior CAD were included. Study subjects were immediately treated with aspirin, heparin, and a GP IIb/IIIa inhibitor (tirofiban) administered for 48–108 hours. Patients were then randomized to one of the following two groups: (a) catheterization and subsequent PCI/CABG within 4–48 hours; (b) conservative strategy with catheterization performed only if objective evidence showed recurrent ischemia or there was a positive exercise stress test.

At 6 months, the primary outcome (death, MI, and rehospitalization for ACS) occurred in 15.9% of the invasive strategy group and 19.4% of the conservative strategy group (odds ratio [OR], 0.78; $P = 0.025$). The rate of death or MI was also significantly lower in the invasive strategy group (7.3% vs. 9.5%; OR, 0.74; $P < 0.05$) (Fig. 16-2).

Subgroup analysis according to troponin-T status on admission revealed that the difference between the two strategies was largely due to a reduction in the primary outcome among troponin-T positive patients. In this subgroup, the invasive strategy was associated with a primary outcome rate of 14.3% compared with 24.2% for the conservative strategy (OR, 0.52; $P < 0.001$). The two strategies were comparable in their effects on the primary outcome in troponin-T negative patients. Patients with an intermediate or high TIMI UA risk score also benefited from an invasive over a conservative strategy. In patients with a low TIMI UA score, the two strategies were comparable.

RITA-3

The Randomized Intervention Trial of unstable Angina (RITA-3) study compared early intervention (angiography followed by revascularization) with a conservative strategy (antianginal and antithrombotic medications) in 1810 NSTE ACS patients in the United Kingdom.[7] All patients were treated with optimal antianginal and antiplatelet treatment, including enoxaparin. For the primary endpoint of death, MI, or refractory angina at 4 months, there was a 9.6% risk in the intervention group compared to 14.5% in the conservative group (RR, 0.66; $P = 0.001$).

This was mainly attributable to a halving of the incidence of refractory angina (defined as ischemic pain at rest or on minimum exertion, despite maximum medical treatment, associated with new cardiographic changes prompting revascularization within 24 hours or readmission to hospital after discharge) with the interventional strategy. For the coprimary endpoint of rates of death or MI at 1 year, the results were similar for both groups, but refractory angina and use of antianginal medications were significantly reduced in the early intervention group ($P = 0.0006$). This difference was also evident at 4 months ($P = 0.0001$).

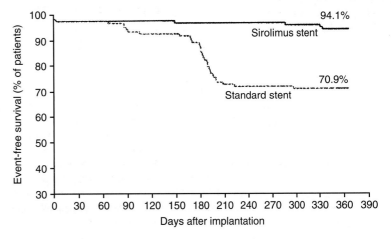

Fig. 16-2. Kaplan-Meier estimates of survival free of myocardial infarction and repeated revascularization among patients who received sirolimus-eluting stents and those who received standard stents. The rate of event-free survival was significantly higher in the sirolimus-stent group than in the standard-stent group ($P < 0.001$ by the Wilcoxon and log-rank tests).

A subanalysis of RITA-3 and FRISC-II found significant reductions in the composite of death and MI in men, but a trend to hazard was found for early intervention in women. This may be due to the fact that women tend to have more procedure-related complications than men and, with equivalent clinical presentations to men, usually have less CAD, and therefore less to gain from an invasive procedure.

Recommendations for Revascularization with PCI and CABG in Patients with UA/NSTEMI

Class I

1. CABG for patients with significant left main CAD. (Level of Evidence: A)

2. CABG for patients with three-vessel disease; the survival benefit is greater in patients with abnormal LV function (EF < 0.50). (Level of Evidence: A)

3. CABG for patients with two-vessel disease with significant proximal left anterior descending (LAD) CAD and either abnormal LV function (EF < 0.50) or demonstrable ischemia on noninvasive testing. (Level of Evidence: A)

4. PCI or CABG for patients with one- or two-vessel CAD without significant proximal LAD CAD but with a large area of viable myocardium and high-risk criteria on noninvasive testing. (Level of Evidence: B)

5. PCI for patients with multivessel coronary disease with suitable coronary anatomy, with normal LV function and without diabetes. (Level of Evidence: A)

6. Intravenous platelet GP IIb/IIIa inhibitor in UA/NSTEMI patients undergoing PCI. (Level of Evidence: A)

Class IIa

1. Repeat CABG for patients with multiple saphenous vein graft (SVG) stenoses, especially when there is significant stenosis of a graft that supplies the LAD. (Level of Evidence: C)

2. PCI for focal SVG lesions or multiple stenoses in poor candidates for reoperative surgery. (Level of Evidence: C)

3. PCI or CABG for patients with one- or two-vessel CAD without significant proximal LAD CAD but with a moderate area of viable myocardium and ischemia on noninvasive testing. (Level of Evidence: B)

4. PCI or CABG for patients with one-vessel disease with significant proximal LAD CAD. (Level of Evidence: B)

5. CABG with the internal mammary artery for patients with multivessel disease and treated diabetes mellitus. (Level of Evidence: B)

Class IIb

PCI for patients with two- or three-vessel disease with significant proximal LAD CAD, with treated diabetes or abnormal LV function, and with anatomy suitable for catheter-based therapy. (Level of Evidence: B)

Class III

1. PCI or CABG for patients with one- or two-vessel CAD without significant proximal LAD CAD or with mild symptoms or symptoms those are unlikely due to myocardial ischemia or who have not received an adequate trial of medical therapy and who have no demonstrable ischemia on noninvasive testing. (Level of Evidence: C)

2. PCI or CABG for patients with insignificant coronary stenosis (less than 50% diameter). (Level of Evidence: C)

3. PCI in patients with significant left main CAD who are candidates for CABG. (Level of Evidence: B)

Stents Versus PTCA

In more than 7000 patients with UA treated with stents or percutaneous transluminal coronary (balloon) angioplasty (PTCA), stents resulted in fewer in-hospital ischemic complications, including less death (1.5% vs. 2.6%, $P = 0.003$), recurrent angina (23.5% vs. 47.4%, $P < 0.00001$), Q-wave MI (0.4% vs. 1.9%, $P < 0.00001$), repeat PTCA (13.8% vs. 30.6%, $P < 0.00001$), and CABG (6.5% vs. 19.6%, $P < 0.00001$), but there was no difference in mortality at 1 year.[8] Further benefit on restenosis (but probably not death or MI) is likely to be achieved with drug-eluting stents that, in early trials, have led to 50–90% reductions in clinical and angiographic restenosis compared to standard stents.

CLINICAL RISK FACTORS AND RESPONSE TO ADJUNCTIVE THERAPY

By using both clinical information (history, physical, and electrocardiogram results) and biochemical methods (serum cardiac markers), risk stratification for ischemic complications in NSTE ACS patients can be reliably established, including the likelihood of recurrent instability, progression to MI, or even death[9–12] (Table 16-2). This approach can also ensure the optimal selection of therapeutic interventions for NSTE ACS patients, predicting the benefits of intravenous platelet GP IIb/IIIa receptor antagonism, or routine early invasive strategies.

The use of clinical risk scores to predict GP IIb/IIIa response was demonstrated in published data from two substudies of the Platelet Receptor Inhibition for ischemic Syndrome Management in Patients Limited by Unstable signs and Symptoms (PRISM-PLUS) trial. Using an exploratory analysis of clinical factors associated with patients from PRISM-PLUS, Sabatine and colleagues identified five clinical variables that could be used in an additive fashion to identify expected benefits to patients from the use of tirofiban.[10] These variables were advanced age, prior aspirin use, prior beta-blocker use, prior CABG, or ST-segment depression on the presenting electrocardiogram. Patients with 0 to 1 risk factors accrued no benefit; those with 2 or 3 risk factors accrued intermediate benefit; patients with 4 or 5 risk factors gained the most benefit. Similarly, Morrow and colleagues identified seven additive risk factors in developing the TIMI risk score: age >65 years, prior history of CAD, >3 coronary risk factors, ST-segment deviation, prior aspirin use within 7 days, frequent angina, or elevated serum markers of myocardial necrosis.[13] Using this risk score, they were able to predict the benefits of therapy with tirofiban in PRISM-PLUS, which were particularly strong in patients with scores >4.

PLATELET INHIBITORS AND PERCUTANEOUS REVASCULARIZATION

The three platelet GP IIb/IIIa inhibitors approved by the Food and Drug Administration based on the outcome of a variety of clinical trials are: abciximab (ReoPro), tirofiban (Aggrastat), and eptifibatide (Integrilin). The Evaluation of c7E3 for the Prevention of Ischemic Complications (EPIC), Evaluation of PTCA and Improve Long-term Outcome by c7E3 GP IIb/IIIa receptor blockade (EPILOG), C7e3 AntiPlatelet Therapy in Unstable REfractory angina (CAPTURE), and Evaluation of Platelet IIb/IIIa Inhibitor for STENTing (EPISTENT) trials investigated the use of abciximab; the PRISM, PRISM-PLUS, and Randomized Efficacy Study of Tirofiban for Outcomes and Restenosis (RESTORE) trials evaluated tirofiban; and the Integrilin to Minimize Platelet Aggregation and Coronary Thrombosis (IMPACT) and Platelet glycoprotein IIb/IIIa in Unstable angina: Receptor Suppression Using Integrilin Therapy (PURSUIT) trials studied the use of eptifibatide. All three of these agents interfere with the final common pathway for platelet aggregation. All have shown efficacy in reducing the incidence of ischemic complications in patients with UA.

In the EPIC trial, high-risk patients who were undergoing balloon angioplasty or directional atherectomy were randomly assigned to one of three treatment regimens: placebo bolus followed by placebo infusion for 12 hours;

weight-adjusted abciximab bolus (0.25 mg/kg) and 12-hour placebo infusion; or weight-adjusted abciximab bolus and 12-hour infusion (10 µg/min). In this trial, high risk was defined as severe UA, evolving MI, or high-risk coronary anatomy defined at cardiac catheterization. The administration of bolus and continuous infusion of abciximab reduced the rate of ischemic complications (death, MI, revascularization) 35% at 30 days (12.8% vs. 8.3%, $P = 0.0008$), by 23% at 6 months, and by 13% at 3 years. The favorable long-term effect was mainly due to a reduction in the need for bypass surgery or repeat PCI in patients with an initially successful procedure.

The administration of abciximab in the EPIC trial was associated with an increased bleeding risk and transfusion requirement. In the subsequent EPILOG trial, which used weight-adjusted dosing of concomitant heparin, the incidence of major bleeding and transfusion associated with abciximab and low-dose weight-adjusted heparin (70 U/kg) was similar to that seen with placebo.[14] The cohort of patients with UA undergoing PCI in the EPILOG trial demonstrated a 64% reduction (10.1–3.6%, $P = 0.001$) in the composite occurrence of death, MI, or urgent revascularization to 30 days with abciximab therapy compared with placebo (standard-dose weight-adjusted heparin).

The RESTORE trial was a randomized double-blind study that evaluated the use of tirofiban versus placebo in 2139 patients with UA or AMI, including patients with non-Q-wave MI who underwent PCI (balloon PTCA or directional atherectomy) within 72 hours of hospitalization.[15] Although the infusion of tirofiban (bolus of 10 µg/kg followed by a 36-hour infusion at 0.15 µg/kg/min) had no significant effect on the reduction in restenosis at 6 months, a trend was observed for a reduction in the combined clinical endpoint of death/MI, emergency CABG, unplanned stent placement for acute or threatened vessel closure, and recurrent ischemia compared with placebo at 6 months (27.1 % vs. 24.1%, $P = 0.11$).

The clinical efficacy of tirofiban was further evaluated in the PRISM-PLUS trial, which enrolled patients with UA/NSTEMI within 12 hours of presentation.[16] In patients who underwent PCI, the 30-day incidence of death, MI, refractory ischemia, or rehospitalization for UA was 15.3% in the group that received heparin alone compared with 8.8% in the tirofiban/heparin group. After PCI, death or nonfatal MI occurred in 10.2% of those receiving heparin versus 5.9% of tirofiban-treated patients.

Eptifibatide, a cyclic heptapeptide GP IIb/IIIa inhibitor, has also been administered to patients with ACS. In the PURSUIT trial, nearly 11,000 patients who presented with non-Q-wave MI or high-risk UA, were randomized to receive either unfractionated heparin (UFH) and aspirin (ASA) or eptifibatide, UFH, and ASA.[17] In patients undergoing PCI within 72 hours of randomization, eptifibatide administration resulted in a 31% reduction in the combined endpoint of nonfatal MI or death at 30 days (17.7% vs. 11.6%, $P = 0.01$).

The EPISTENT trial was designed to evaluate the efficacy of abciximab as an adjunct to elective coronary stenting[18]; approximately 2400 patients were randomized to either stent deployment with placebo, stent plus abciximab, or PTCA plus abciximab. Nineteen percent of the PTCA group had provisional coronary stent deployment for a suboptimal angioplasty result. All stented patients in this trial received oral ASA (325 mg) and oral ticlopidine (250 mg twice daily for 1 month). The adjunctive use of abciximab was associated with a significant reduction in the composite clinical endpoint of death, MI, or urgent revascularization. The 30-day primary endpoint occurred in 10.8% of the stent plus placebo group, 5.3% of the stent plus abciximab group, and 6.9% of the PTCA plus abciximab group. Most of the benefits from abciximab were related to a reduction in the incidence of moderate to large MI (CK greater than five times the upper limit of normal or Q-wave MI); these reductions occurred in 5.8% of the stent plus placebo group, 2.6% of the balloon plus abciximab group, and 2.0% of the stent plus abciximab group.

At 1 year of follow-up, stented patients who received bolus and infusion abciximab had reduced mortality rates compared with patients who received stents without abciximab (1.0% vs. 2.4%, representing a 57% risk reduction; $P = 0.037$). In diabetics, target-vessel revascularization at 6 months was markedly and significantly reduced (51%, $P = 0.02$) in stented patients who received abciximab compared with those who did not. Although a similar trend was also observed in nondiabetic patients, it did not reach statistical significance.

The Enhanced Suppression of Platelet Receptor GP IIb/IIIa using Integrilin Therapy (ESPRIT) trial was a placebo-controlled trial designed to assess whether eptifibatide improved the outcome of patients undergoing stenting.[19] Fourteen percent of the 2064 patients enrolled in ESPRIT had UA/NSTEMI. The primary endpoint (the composite of death, MI, target-vessel revascularization, and *bailout* GP IIb/IIIa inhibitor therapy) was reduced from 10.5 to 6.6% with treatment ($P = 0.0015$). There was consistency in the reduction of events in all components of the composite endpoints and in all major subgroups including patients with UA/NSTEMI major bleeding occurred more frequently in patients who received eptifibatide (1.3%) than in those who received placebo (0.4%, $P = 0.027$). However, no significant difference in transfusion rates occurred. At 1-year followup, death or MI occurred in 12.4% of placebo-track patients and 8.0% of eptifibatide-treated patients ($P = 0.001$).

The Tirofiban And Reopro Give similar Efficacy outcomes Trial (TARGET) randomized 5308 patients to tirofiban or abciximab before undergoing PCI with the intent to perform stenting.[20] The primary endpoint, a composite of death, nonfatal MI, or urgent target-vessel revascularization at 30 days occurred less frequently in those receiving abciximab than tirofiban (6.0% vs. 7.6%, $P = 0.038$). There was a similar direction and magnitude for each component of the endpoint. Eptifibatide has not been compared directly to either abciximab or tirofiban.

CORONARY ARTERY BYPASS GRAFTING

CABG is the preferred method of revascularization for patients with ACS and either significant left main obstruction or LV dysfunction (or possibly treated diabetes) plus three-vessel disease or two-vessel disease with proximal LAD involvement (Table 16-3). Since the risks of perioperative death (4%) and acute MI (10%) are high when CABG is performed on an urgent basis, efforts should be made to stabilize patients pharmacologically and, if needed, with intraaortic balloon pump (IABP) counterpulsation prior to surgical revascularization.

INTERVENTIONAL MANAGEMENT OF STEMI

Primary Stenting Versus Balloon Angioplasty (PTCA): Randomized Trials

The efficacy and safety of primary stenting have been evaluated in several prospective randomized trials[21,22] (Table 16-4). In Stent Primary Angioplasty in Myocardial Infarction (Stent-PAMI), 900 patients with acute MI were randomized to the Palmaz-Schatz heparin-coated stent or PTCA. Primary stenting resulted in less recurrent

Table 16-3. Indications for CABG in Acute MI

- Left main stenosis >50% with left anterior descending or left circumflex coronary infarct vessel
- Left main stenosis >75% with right coronary infarct vessel
- Severe proximal multivessel disease not suitable for PCI, especially if the infarct vessel is patent
- Severe multivessel disease with cardiogenic shock
- Failed mechanical reperfusion with infarct duration <6–12 h, a large area of jeopardized myocardium, and ongoing ischemic pain, especially in the presence of well-developed collaterals

Table 16-4. Randomized Trials of Stenting Vs. PTCA for Acute MI

Trial	*N*	Stent	Results (Stent Vs. PTCA)
CADILLAC (2002)	2082	MultiLink, MultiLink-Duet	Stents resulted in less clinical and angiographic restenosis but had no effect on death or MI. Abciximab prevented early thrombotic events but had no impact on restenosis.
STOPAMI (2002)	162	Stent + abciximab vs. tPA + abciximab	Compared to tPA, stents resulted in smaller infarct size ($P < 0.05$), better myocardial salvage ($P = 0.001$), and a trend toward less death or MI at 6 months (7.4% vs. 17.3%, $P = 0.053$).
STENTIM-2 (2000)	211	Wiktor	Stents resulted in less ARS (23.3% vs. 39.6%, $P < 0.05$) but no difference in procedural success, EFS, or TLR at 6 and 12 months.
FRESCO (2000)	150	GR	Stents resulted in less MACE (9% vs. 28%, $P < 0.01$) and ARS (17% vs. 43%, $P < 0.001$) at 6 months.
Stent-PAMI (1999)	900	HCPSS	Stents resulted in less TIMI-3 flow (89% vs. 93%, $P < 0.05$), less ischemic TVR at 6 months (7.7% vs. 17%, $P < 0.001$) and at 1 year (10.6% vs. 21%, $P < 0.0001$), less ARS at 6 months (23% vs. 35%, $P < 0.001$), and less MACE (17% vs. 24.8%, $P < 0.01$), but higher mortality at 1 year (5.8% vs. 3.0%, $P = 0.054$).
PASTA (1999)	136	PSS	Stents resulted in similar success (99% vs. 97%), less in-hospital MACE (6% vs. 19%, $P < 0.05$) and 1-year MACE (22% vs. 49%, $P < 0.001$), and less ARS at 6 months (17% vs. 37.5%, $P < 0.05$).

Abbreviations: ARS = angiographic restenosis; BPS = event-free survival; GR = Gianturco Roubin; HCPPS = heparin-coated Palmaz-Schatz stent; TLR = target lesion revascularization; MACE = major adverse cardiac events.

ischemia and restenosis, but TIMI-3 flow rates were lower and 6-month mortality was higher in the stent group. More recently, 2082 patients with acute MI were randomized to MultiLink stenting or PTCA (with or without abciximab) in Controlled Abciximab and Device Investigation to Lower Late Angioplasty Complications (CADILLAC). In contrast to Stent-PAMI, stenting resulted in better event-free survival at 6 months due to less clinical and angiographic restenosis. Abciximab reduced the rates of recurrent ischemia leading to early repeat target-vessel revascularization after PTCA or stenting and, in a recent systematic overview of Reopro in Acute myocardial infarction and Primary PTCA Organization and Randomized Trial (RAPPORT), Intracoronary Stenting and Antithrombotic Regimen trial (ISAR-2), Abciximab before Direct angioplasty and stenting in Myocardial Infarction Regarding Acute and Long-term follow-up (ADMIRAL), and CADILLAC, reduced the composite endpoint of death, MI, and revascularization at 6 months (Table 16-5). In a metaanalysis of 2844 patients in eight randomized trials of

PTCA versus stenting for acute MI, the composite endpoint of death, reinfarction, and target-vessel revascularization at 6 months was reduced by 46% with stents (14% vs. 26%, $P < 0.0001$). Sirolimus- and paclitaxel-eluting stents have led to dramatic reductions in restenosis compared to standard stents (<5% vs. 20–30%) (Table 16-6, Fig. 16-3), but they

Table 16-5. Abciximab as Adjunct to PCI for Acute MI[*]

Trial	No. of Patients	Abciximab (%)	Placebo (%)
ADMIRAL	300	22.8	33.8
CADILLAC	2082	13.9	16.2
ISAR-2	401	11.9	17.5
RAPPORT	483	28.2	28.1
Combined	3266	16.6*	19.8

[*]Death recurrent infarction or any target-vessel revascularization at 6 months. OR: 0.80, 95% CI: 0.67–0.97.

Table 16-6. Recent Drug-Eluting Stent Trials for Coronary Disease*

Study	Design	Late Loss	Restenosis	Clinical
RAVEL (2002) (*n* = 238)	Sirolimus-eluting Bx velocity stent vs. standard stent	− 0.01 mm vs. 0.80 mm (*P* < 0.001)	0% vs. 26% (*P* < 0.001); 0% vs. 47% in 44 diabetics (*P* = 0.002)	1-year MACE 5.8% vs. 28.8% (*P* < 0.001)
SIRIUS (2002) (*n* = 400 of 1101)	Sirolimus-eluting Bx velocity stent vs. standard stent	0.06 mm vs. 0.55 mm (*P* < 0.001)	2.0% vs. 31.1% at 8 months	9-month MACE 9.2% vs. 19.4% (*P* = 0.009)
ELUTES (2002) (*n* = 192)	Paclitaxel-eluting V—Flex plus stent without polymer (tested at 4 doses) vs. standard stent	0.10 mm vs. 0.73 mm (*P* = 0.002)	3.1% vs. 20.6% (*P* = 0.055)	30-day MACE 1.1% for drug stent; 1-year TLR 5% vs. 16%

*Results: drug-eluting stent vs. standard stent.
Abbreviations: Late loss = difference in minimum lumen diameter immediately after stenting and at follow-up (reflects degree of intimal thickening); MACE = major adverse cardiac events; MI = myocardial infarction, TLR = target lesion revascularization.

have yet to be evaluated in the setting of ST-elevation MI. The role of stents versus PTCA for culprit lesions in small (<2.5 mm) diameter vessels and SVGs is being evaluated.[23]

Primary stenting in conjunction with a GP IIb/IIIa inhibitor should be considered the routine reperfusion strategy for patients with acute ST-elevation MI, when available in an appropriate time frame. Based on available literature to date, appropriate is best defined as within 90 (ideally)–120 min. Direct transfer of patients from hospitals without cardiac catheterization facilities to those with such facilities (without fibrinolysis being initiated at the sending facility) is being suggested as the treatment of choice by some, if done within 3 hours.[24] The Comparision of Angioplasty and Pre-hospital Thrombolysis In acute Myocardial infarction (CAPTIM) study also suggests that patients who present within 2 hours of symptom onset may derive greater benefit from fibrinolysis versus transfer for primary PCI. The strategy requires rigorous prospective testing before being recommended as a standard.

Adjunctive Pharmacotherapy for PCI

Preprocedural Pharmacotherapy (Facilitated PCI)

The ability of fibrinolytic therapy to restore early patency prior to primary PTCA was evaluated in 606 patients with acute MI in Pravastatin in Acute Coronary Treatment (PACT).[25] The administration of tPA (50 mg IV bolus) immediately before angiography resulted in better TIMI-3 flow prior to PTCA (33% vs. 15%, *P* < 0.001) with less need for immediate intervention and no increase in bleeding complications, but preprocedural tPA had no impact on coronary blood flow, LV function, or clinical

outcome after PCI. Compared to patients not receiving tPA prior to hospital transport for urgent PCI in Primary Angioplasty in patients transferred from General community hospitals to specialized PTCA Units with or without Emergency thrombolysis (PRAGUE), administration of tPA prior to transport resulted in a higher rate of death, reinfarction, or stroke at 30 days (15% vs. 8%). The role for preprocedural (*upstream*) low-dose fibrinolytic therapy ± GP IIb/IIIa inhibitors continues to be investigated.

Intraprocedural pharmacotherapy

Aspirin and Clopidogrel

Prior to PCI, all patients should receive 325 mg of non-enteric-coated chewable aspirin followed by 75–325 mg

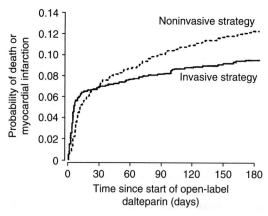

Fig. 16-3. Probability of death or myocardial infarction in invasive and noninvasive groups.

PO q24h long term. Patients undergoing stenting should also receive clopidogrel 300 mg PO followed by 75 mg PO q24h for up to 1 year.[26]

GP llb/IIIa Inhibitors

Trials of abciximab as an adjunct to primary PTCA (RAPPORT, CADILLAC) or stenting (ADMIRAL, CADILLAC) have demonstrated a reduction in events. In a metaanalysis of 1738 patients in three randomized trials of abciximab versus placebo as adjuncts to stenting for acute MI (CADILLAC, ADMIRAL, ISAR-2), the composite endpoint of death, reinfarction, and target-vessel revascularization at 6 months was reduced by 28% with abciximab (12% vs. 16.6%, $P < 0.001$). If abciximab is used, an IV bolus of 0.25 mg/kg is given at the start of the procedure followed by an IV infusion of 0.125 µg/kg/min (max. 10 µg/min) × 12 hours. If eptifibatide is used, an IV bolus of 180 µg/kg is given × 2 10 min apart followed by a 2.0 µg/kg/min infusion for 18–72 hours.

Heparin

Unfractionated heparin is usually given as a weight-adjusted IV bolus of 60–100 U/kg to achieve an intraprocedural ACT of 300–350 s. When abciximab is used, an IV heparin bolus of 60 U/kg is recommended to achieve a target activated clotting time (ACT) of 200–250 s. Prolonged heparin infusions following successful PCI are of no proven value. As an alternative to unfractionated heparin, LMWH may be easier to administer and associated with better clinical outcomes (ASSENT-3). Enoxaparin may be given as a 30 mg IV bolus followed by 1 mg/kg SQ q12h. (See sheath removal comments for enoxaparin.)

PROCEDURAL TECHNIQUE

Goals of Procedure

PTCA or stenting is performed on the infarct vessel to achieve a residual stenosis <30% and TIMI-3 flow. Emergency PCI is usually limited to the culprit vessel, but multivessel intervention may be indicated for patients in cardiogenic shock. IABP counterpulsation is often employed in patients with multivessel disease and ongoing ischemia, hypotension, pulmonary edema, or LV dysfunction. Following successful PCI, stable, low-risk patients can be managed in a step-down unit and can often be discharged on the third hospital day. Stress testing is not routinely performed after successful PCI.

Timing of sheath removal depends on several factors including whether or not a closure device is employed and the time and route of the last enoxaparin dose.

The sheath can be removed 6–8 hours after the last SQ dose of enoxaparin without a closure device or immediately if a closure device is used. The sheath can be removed 4 hours after the 0.3 mg/kg IV supplemental dose for the 8–12-hour group, as well as after the 1.0 mg/kg IV (0.75 mg/kg with a GP IIb/IIIa inhibitor) for the patients undergoing PCI >12 hours after their last SQ dose or who have not received any pretreatment.

Complications of PCI

Reperfusion Arrhythmias

Ventricular fibrillation and bradyarrhythmias are more common with right coronary artery (RCA) intervention. To minimize this risk, IV beta-blockers, low-osmolar ionic contrast, continuous monitoring of O_2 saturation, and adequate hydration are recommended prior to reperfusion of the RCA.

Bleeding Complications

Compared to fibrinolytic therapy, PCI is associated with less intracranial hemorrhage but more blood transfusions. Meticulous vascular access technique, monitoring of ACT levels, avoidance of postprocedural heparin, and early sheath removal are indicated to minimize bleeding complications. Newer closure devices and maintaining a target ACT of 200–250 s minimizes bleeding.

Ischemic Complications

Recurrent ischemia occurs in 10–15% of patients following PCI, and early reocclusion increases hospital mortality by threefold. Stents reduce ischemic complications (3% after stents vs. 15% after balloon angioplasty vs. 30% after lytics) and early reinfarction (<1% after stents vs. 1–2% after balloon angioplasty vs. 8% after lytics).

UTILITY OF PRIMARY PCI FOR CARDIOGENIC SHOCK

Patients in cardiogenic shock are usually taken to the catheterization laboratory for hemodynamic stabilization with an IABP, angiography, and emergency revascularization. Nonrandomized studies reported survival rates of 46–86% after PTCA compared to 30% after lytic therapy and 10% after medical therapy.[27–30] In Global Use of Strategies To open Occluded arteries (GUSTO-I), an aggressive revascularization strategy of PTCA or CABG was independently associated with improved survival at 30 days. More recently, in the SHould we emergently revasularize Occluded Coronaries for cardiogenic shocK (SHOCK) trial, 302 patients were randomized to an early invasive approach of emergency catheterization followed by immediate revascularization (PTCA or CABG) or an early conservative approach of initial medical stabilization followed by revascularization for recurrent ischemia. Revascularization was performed in 87% of patients in the invasive group and 34% of patients in the conservative group. One-year survival was 46.7% in the early revascularization group and 33.6% in the initial medical stabilization group ($P < 0.03$); benefit was apparent only for patients <75 years (survival 51.6% with early revascularization vs. 33.3% with initial medical therapy). At 1 year, 83% of survivors were in NYHA heart failure class I or II. These data support the use of immediate angiography, IABP counterpulsation, and emergency revascularization for cardiogenic shock, particularly in patients <75 years old.

COMMON CLINICAL QUESTIONS

Who Benefits from Early PCI?

Tailoring treatment to the level of risk remains a sound and proven approach to management. The FRISC-II and TACTICS TIMI-18 studies support the utility of troponin-T in risk stratification, although this is based on retrospective analysis. High-risk patients who are biomarker positive or have ST-segment depression are likely to benefit from a strategy of early revascularization. Low-risk patients are not likely to benefit from early revascularization, which accounts for 15–40% of all patients.

When is the Optimal Time to Intervene?

The optimal timing of PCI in the setting of intensive medical therapy remains ill defined. The FRISC-II study supports an interval of 4–6 days, but this is impractical according to current North American practice standards. The TACTICS TIMI-18 trial provides data to support this approach between 2–3 days postevent. There are no data from within 24 hours of symptom onset. Current ACC/AHA guidelines suggest that patients receive diagnostic catheterization within 48 hours.

Are Adjunctive Therapies Important?

Aggressive antiplatelet, antithrombin, and anti-ischemic therapy may be as important as revascularization. In FRISC-II, intervention was associated with early hazard,

with the survival curves crossing over between months 1 and 6. This phenomenon was not observed in the TACTICS TIMI-18 study, prompting the hypothesis that early hazard might be a consequence of inadequate platelet inhibition. Indeed, pharmacotherapy with GP IIb/IIIa platelet inhibition and LMWH may reduce clinical events whether an early invasive or early conservative strategy is followed.

Does the Catheterization Lab Volume of PCI Performed Relate to Long-Term Outcomes?

A cohort study of 25,222 patients undergoing PCI in 43 cardiac cathetorization labs in Pennsylvania from 1994 to 1995 was performed using the Pennsylvania health care cost containment council database. The association of laboratory volume within the hospital, 1- and 6-month events was estimated by use of multivariable analysis, adjusting for patient and procedural characteristics. Although a higher volume of procedure was associated with reduced in-hospital coronary bypass (or ratio 0.6 for 400 vs. less than 400 PCIs per year, 95% 0.4–0.8), it was not associated with CABG occurring within 1 month after discharge ($P = 0.71$). Laboratory volume was also not significantly associated with post-discharge composite 0.8–1.4) or 6 months ($P = 0.47$, OR 1.04, 95% composite 0.91–1.19). In addition, laboratory volume was not associated with rates of myocardial infarction ($P = 0.14$), death ($P = 0.28$), or the combined outcome of PCI, CABG, MI, or death ($P = 0.90$) at 1 month after hospital discharge. This study did confirm a volume/complication relationship for in-hospital CABG but it did not reveal an association between volume and postdischarge events.

CONCLUSION

The findings of the FRISC-II, TACTICS TIMI-18, and RITA-3 trials demonstrate improved clinical outcomes among intermediate and high-risk patients, especially those with positive biomarkers and/or ST-segment depression. For NSTE ACS patients who are clinically stable, and do not exhibit these high-risk features, stress myocardial perfusion imaging will help identify intermediate and high-risk groups. Aggressive pharmacologic treatment is indicated in all groups. This should include aspirin, heparin, and anti-ischemic therapy (IV NTG, beta-blockers, and/or calcium antagonists). The GP IIb/IIIa inhibitors should be used in intermediate or high-risk groups and non-Q-wave MI patients. The more widespread use of intracoronary stents with adjunctive antiplatelet, antithrombotic, and anti-ischemic therapy will yield optimal outcomes.

REFERENCES

1. Braunwald E, Antman EM, Beasley JW, et al. ACC/AHA guidelines for the management of patients with unstable angina and non-ST segment elevation myocardial infarction: A report of the American College of Cardiology/American Heart Association Task Force on Practice Guidelines (Committee on the Management of Patients with Unstable Angina). *J Am Coll Cardiol* 2000;36:970–1062.

2. The TIMI-IIIB investigators. Effects of tissue plasminogen activator and a comparison of early invasive and conservative strategies in unstable angina and non-Q-wave myocardial infarction. Results of the TIMI-IIIB trial. *Circulation* 1994;89:1545–1556.

3. Boden WE, O'Rourke RA, Crawford MH, et al., for the Veterans Affairs Non-Q-Wave Infarction Strategies in Hospital (VANQWISH) trial investigators. Outcomes in patients with acute non-Q-wave myocardial infarction randomly assigned to an invasive as compared with a conservative management strategy. *N Engl J Med* 1998;338:1785–1792.

4. Fragmin and Fast Revascularization during Instability in Coronary Artery Disease (FRISC-II) investigators. Invasive compared with non-invasive treatment in unstable coronary artery disease. FRISC-II prospective randomized multicenter study. *Lancet* 1999;354:708–715.

5. Cannon CP, Weintraub WS, Demopoulos LA, et al., for the TACTICS-Thrombolysis in Myocardial Infarction-18 investigators. Comparison of early invasive and conservative strategies in patients with unstable coronary syndromes treated with the glycoprotien IIb/IIIa inhibitor tirofiban. *N Engl J Med* 2001;344:1879–1887.

6. Lagerqvist B, Diderholm E, Lindahl B, et al. An early invasive treatment strategy reduces cardiac events regardless of troponin levels in unstable coronary artery (UCAD) with and without troponin-elevation: A FRISC-II sub-study. *J Am Coll Cardiol* 2001;37:492–498.

7. Fox KA, Poole-Wilson PA, Henderson RA, et al. Randomized intervention trial of unstable angina investigators. Interventional vs. conservative treatment for patients with unstable angina or non-ST elevation myocardial infarction: The British Heart Foundation RITA-3 randomized trial. Randomized Intervention Trial of unstable Angina. *Lancet* 2002;360:743–751.

8. Singh M, Holmes DR, Garratt KN, et al. Stents vs. conventional PTCA in unstable angina. *J Am Coll Cardiol* 1999;29A–33A.

9. Antman EM, Cohen M, Bernink PJ, et al. The TIMI risk score for unstable angina/non-ST elevation MI: A method for prognostication and therapeutic decision making. *JAMA* 2000;284:835–842.

10. Sabatine MS, Januzzi JL, Snapinn S, et al. A risk score system for predicting adverse outcomes and magnitude of benefit with glycoprotein IIb/IIIa inhibitor therapy in patients with unstable angina pectoris. *Am J Cardiol* 2001;88:488–492.

11. Boersma E, Pieper KS, Steyerberg EW. Predictors of outcome in patients with acute coronary syndromes without persistent ST-segment elevation. Results from an international trial of 9461 patients. The pursuit INVESTIGATORS. *Circulation* 2000;101:2557–2567.

12. Solomon DH, Stone PH, Glynn RJ, et al. Use of risk stratification to identify patients with unstable angina likeliest to benefit from an invasive vs. conservation management strategy. *J Am Coll Cardiol* 2001;38:969–976.

13. Morrow DA, Cannon CP, Rifai N, et al. Ability of minor elevations of troponins I and T to predict benefit from an early invasive strategy in patients with unstable angina and non-ST elevation myocardial infarction. Results from a randomized trial. *JAMA* 2001;286:2405–2412.

14. EPILOG Investigators. Platelet glycoprotein IIb/IIIa receptor blockade and low-dose heparin during percutaneous coronary revascularization. *N Engl J Med* 1997;336:1689–1696.

15. RESTORE Investigators. Effects of platelet glycoprotein IIb/IIIa blockade with tirofiban on adverse cardiac events in patients with unstable angina or acute myocardial infarction undergoing coronary angioplasty. Randomized Efficacy Study of Tirofiban for Outcomes and REstenosis. *Circulation* 1997;96:1445–1453.

16. Platelet Receptor Inhibition in Ischemic Syndrome Management in Patients Limited by Unstable Signs and Symnptoms (PRISM-PLUS) study Investigators. Inhibition of the platelet glycoprotein IIb/IIIa receptor with tirofiban in unstable angina and non-Q wave myocardial infarction (erratum appears in *N Engl J Med* 1998;339:45). *N Engl J Med* 1998;338:1488–1497.

17. PURSUIT Trial Investigators. Inhibition of platelet glycoprotein IIb/IIIa with eptifibatide in patients with acute coronary syndromes. The PURSUIT trial investigators platelet glycoprotein IIb/IIIa in unstable angina: Receptor suppression using integrilin therapy. *N Engl J Med* 1998;339:456–443.

18. EPISTENT Investigators. Randomized placebo-controlled and balloon-angioplasty-controlled trial to assess safety of coronary stenting with use of platelet glycoprotein IIb/IIIa blockade. Evaluation of platelet glycoprotein IIb/IIIa inhibitor for stenting. *Lancet* 1998;352:87–92.

19. Novel dosing regimen of eptifibatide in planned coronary stent implantation (ESPRIT): A randomized placebo-controlled trial. *Lancet* 2000;356:2037–2044.

20. Topol EJ, Moliterno DJ, JHerrmann HC, et al. Comparison of two platelet glycoprotein IIb/IIIa inhibitors, tirofiban and abciximab for the prevention of ischemic events with percutaneous coronary revascularization. *N Engl J Med* 2001;344:1888–1894.

21. Stone GW, Grines CL, Cox DA, et al. Comparison of angioplasty with stenting, with or without abciximab, in acute myocardial infarction. *N Engl J Med* 2002;346:957–966.

22. Januzzi JL, Chae CU, Sabatine MS, et al. Elevation in serum troponin I predicts the benefit of tirofiban. *J Thromb Thrombolysis* 2001;11:211–215.

23. Morice MC, Serruys PW, Sousa E, et al. A randomized comparison of a sirolimus-eluting stent with a standard

stent for coronary revascularization. *N Engl J Med* 2002;346:1773–1780.

24. Dalby M, Bouzamondo A, Lechat P, Montalescot G, et al. Transfer for primary angioplasty vs. immediate thrombolysts in acute myocardial infarction: A meta-analysis. *Circulation* 2003;108:1809–1814.

25. Ross AM, Coyne KS, Reiner JS, et al. A randomized trial comparing primary angioplasty with a strategy of short acting thrombolysis and immediate planned rescue angioplasty in acute myocardial infarction: The PACT trial. *J Am Coll Cardiol* 1999;34:1954–1962.

26. Steinhubl SR, Berger PB, Mann JT III, et al. Early and sustained dual oral antiplatelet therapy following percutaneous coronary intervention. The CREDO trial. *JAMA* 2002;288:2411–2420.

27. O'Neill WW, Erbel R, Laufer N, et al. Coronary angioplasty therapy of cardiogenic shock complicating acute myocardial infarction. *Circulation* 1995;72:III–309.

28. Holmes DR, Bates EF, Kleiman NS, et al. Contemporary reperfusion therapy for cardiogenic shock: The GUSTO-I trial experience. *J Am Coll Cardiol* 1995;26:668–674.

29. Hochmann JS, Boland J, Sleeper LA, et al. and the SHOCK Registry Investigators. Current spectrum of cardiogenic shock and effect of early revascularization on mortality. *Circulation* 1995;91:372–388.

30. Lee L, Erbel R, Brown TM, et al. Multicenter registry of angioplasty therapy of cardiogenic shock: Initial and long-term survival. *J Am Coll Cardiol* 1991;17:599–603.

17

The Chest Pain Center Concept

Andra L. Blomkalns
W. Brian Gibler

HIGH YIELD FACTS

- The initial patient examination, electrocardiogram, and initial cardiac marker levels alone are insufficient to determine if a patient is at risk for an acute coronary syndrome (ACS).
- Chest Pain Centers (CPC) are a safe and cost-effective method for the evaluation and risk assessment of the low-to-moderate emergency department (ED) patient with chest discomfort.
- CPCs require the collaboration of practitioners in emergency medicine, cardiology, and radiology.
- A variety of models for CPC exist and each model should be tailored to the specific institution and patient population.
- CPCs generally include initial assessment and risk stratification, monitoring over a period of time, serial assessment with cardiac markers, nuclear imaging, provocative testing, and appropriate follow-up for each patient.

INTRODUCTION AND RATIONALE

Each year in the United States, over six million patients present to the ED with complaints of chest discomfort or other symptoms consistent with potential acute manifestations of coronary artery disease (CAD).[1] A large percentage of these patients are admitted for further diagnostic workup, yet fewer than 20% are ultimately diagnosed with CAD. These potentially high-risk patients represent a significant opportunity for emergency medicine physicians to aid in the risk stratification and diagnosis of these undifferentiated patients. With hospital beds and inpatient resources rare and at a premium, these admissions can potentially be avoided by evaluating low-to-moderate risk patients with chest discomfort in CPCs.[2–5]

The tenants of a CPC are appropriate assessment and risk stratification, protocol zed evaluation and therapy, and in-patient admission and outpatient follow-up as appropriate. The protocols developed for CPCs must provide testing to evaluate every patient for three possibilities: myocardial necrosis, rest ischemia, and exercise-induced ischemia. Numerous studies in a several different hospital environments have proven the utility of the CPC and have strived to evaluate the patient for these possible conditions.[6–8]

OPERATIONAL ASPECTS OF A CHEST PAIN CENTER

One of the most challenging aspects of introducing a viable CPC is the organization and structure of its operation. For instance, to have an effective and efficient CPC, one must have:

1. Sufficient and dedicated space to evaluate and observe the patients
2. Nursing staff and other ED personnel that are knowledgeable and dedicated to this evaluation
3. Emergency physician staff that can still be responsible for these patients
4. Collaboration of cardiologist colleagues on the protocols, testing, follow-up, and admission procedures
5. Availability of nuclear cardiology and radiology colleagues for the emergent performance and reading of nuclear imaging studies
6. Laboratory personnel to run serial cardiac marker measurements
7. Primary care physicians who understand the scope and limitations of a CPC evaluation

A variety of physical models exist for CPCs. Several of these models are illustrated in Figs. 17-1 to 17-3. Each model takes into account the specific patient population, cardiologist collaboration, nuclear imaging availability, and ED resources to design the optimal CPC for that environment. It should be noted that each of these models are strikingly different. This reinforces that these centers should be individualized for each specific institution.

A special mention should be made that an essential component of a successful CPC is a nursing staff

Level	AMI risk	ACS risk	Strategy	Disposition
1	Very high	Very high	Fibrinolysis/ PCI	CCU
2	High	High	ASA, Heparin, NTG, IIb/IIIa	CCU
3	Moderate	Moderate	Markers + nuclear imaging	9-hour observation
4	Low	Mod or low	Nuclear imaging	Home and OP stress test
5	Very low	Very low	As needed	Home

Fig. 17-1. Medical College of Virginia CPC protocol.

dedicated to the care of these high-risk patients. These patients will require frequent assessment, close monitoring, noninvasive testing, serial cardiac marker testing, and ECG acquisition. Since the overall success of the unit depends on the strict adherence to the systematic evaluation protocol, nurse staffing is paramount. The nursing tasks involved with these protocols are generally in excess of those expected for a typical ED patient and may require additional training and staffing as appropriate for the individual institution and ED.

CARDIAC MARKER ASSESSMENT

Serial cardiac marker assessment is a key component of any CPC. These measurements and timely result reporting are integral to the success of these CPC protocols. Ideally,

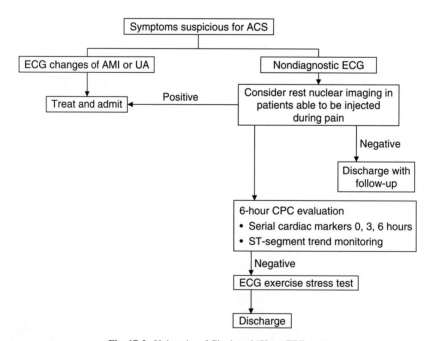

Fig. 17-2. University of Cincinnati "Heart ER" strategy.

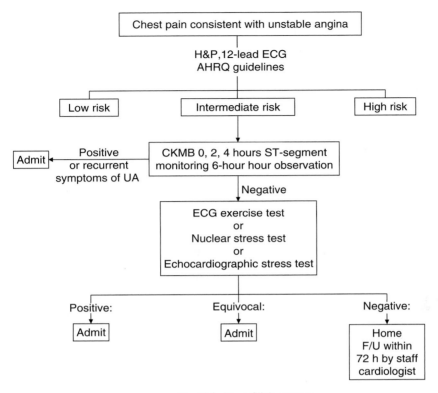

Fig. 17-3. Mayo Clinic strategy.

bedside point-of-care testing for cardiac biomarkers provides rapid data collection for these patients.[9]

In early CPC algorithms, Lee and colleagues' multicenter trial validated a 12-hour algorithm using creatinine phosphokinase (CK) and CK-MB in patients identified as "low-risk" through assessment of clinical characteristics in the ED.[10] Subsequently, Farkouh at al. demonstrated the use of a CPC protocol and CK-MB measurements for patients identified as intermediate risk for adverse cardiac events.[11]

Symptom onset to patient presentation is a crucial factor in the use of cardiac marker protocols. Marker release kinetics vary with time and as time to ED presentation may be as short as 90 min or as long as several days, no single biomarker determination is suitable for adequately "ruling out" myocardial necrosis.[12–14] The American Heart Association currently recommends serial cardiac biomarker determinations to increase sensitivity for detecting necrosis, rather than a single determination on ED presentation. Serial marker measurements and

comparison of marker elevation over 3–6 hours also improved sensitivity for myocardial infarction (MI).[15–17]

Serial CK/CK-MB protocols have largely become the diagnostic standard for acute myocardial infarction (AMI) in the CPC setting. Most of all studied protocols use a specific threshold, above which is diagnostic for AMI or ACS. Fesmire et al. studied a promising novel approach of change in CK-MB levels within the normal range over the course of ED evaluation. In his population of 710 CPC patients, a CK-MB increase or delta of 1.6 ng/mL over 2 hours was more sensitive for AMI than a second CK-MB drawn 2 hours after patient arrival (93.8% vs. 75.2%).[17]

Troponins I and T have revolutionized the risk stratification of chest pain patients in CPC protocols and now are a cornerstone of serial evaluation. They have been proved extremely valuable and sensitive in the diagnosis of myocardial necrosis.[18,19] In addition to diagnosis of myocardial necrosis in ACS, the troponins are valuable in risk stratification of both low- and high-risk patient populations. Troponin release kinetics mimic CK-MB, but elevated levels persist for days to weeks after AMI due to the breakdown of the contractile apparatus over this period.

The main issues surrounding the cardiac troponins include: (1) cutoff values for troponin I and (2) appropriately defining the time of chest pain onset in the context of the ED presentation. While exhaustive time and study have been performed to determine the more superior troponin, most large studies and analyses have determined that cTnI and cTnT can both identify patients at risk for adverse cardiac events.[18–21]

Cardiac TnT is detected at slightly lower serum levels than most cTnI assays and has proved valuable in the emergency setting for early identification of myocardial necrosis. The Global Use of Strategies To Open occluded arteries (GUSTO-II) investigators compared cTnI and cTnT in short-term risk stratification of ACS patients. This model compared troponins collected within 3.5 hours of ischemic symptoms.[22] Newby and colleagues found that cTnT showed a greater association with 30-day mortality ($\chi^2 = 18.0$, $P < 0.0001$) than cTnI ($\chi^2 = 12.5$, $P = 0.0002$). These authors concluded that cTnT is a strong, independent predictor of short-term outcome in ACS patients, and serial levels were useful in determining the risk of adverse cardiac events.[23]

Troponin applications in low-to-moderate risk patients presenting to EDs have shown similar encouraging results. Tucker et al. used a comprehensive marker strategy including myoglobin, CK-MB, troponin I, and troponin T in ED patients over 24 hours after arrival. As expected within the first 2 hours of presentation, CK-MB and myoglobin maintained better sensitivity. The troponins were useful only when measured 6 or more hours after arrival exhibiting sensitivities and specificities of 82 and 97% for troponin I and 89 and 84% for troponin T, respectively.[24] Troponin use seems to be more beneficial in later or delayed patient presentations. In a study of 425 patients using serial troponin I and CK-MB over 16 hours, Brogan et al. showed no increase in sensitivity or specificity between troponin and CK-MB in patients with symptoms <24 hours. However, in patients presenting with greater than 24 hours of symptoms, troponin I had a sensitivity of 100% compared to CK-MB (56.5%).[25]

Sayre et al. showed that patients with a troponin T level of 0.2 ng/L or greater were 3.5 times more likely to have a cardiac complication within 60 days of ED presentation.[26] In a CPC population, Newby et al. determined that cTnT positive patients had angiographically significant lesions (89% vs. 49%) and positive stress testing (46% vs. 14%)

more frequently than cTnT negative patients. Long-term mortality was also higher in cTnT positive patients (27% vs. 7%).[27] Johnson et al. studied a heterogeneous patient population admitted from an urban teaching hospital and found that cTnT was elevated in 31% of patients without MI who had major short-term complications as compared to CK-MB activity and mass.[19]

The recent publication of the "redefinition" of MI has brought troponin to the forefront of both diagnosis and risk stratification in this patient population.[28] In a reanalysis of the data from The Platelet IIb/IIIa Antagonism for the Reduction of Acute coronary syndrome events in a Global Organization Network (PARAGON-B), GUSTO IIa, and Chest Pain Evaluation by Creatine Kinase-MB, Myoglobin, and Troponin I (CHECKMATE) studies, patients with baseline troponin elevation without CK-MB elevation were found to be at increased risk for early and short-term adverse outcomes.[29–32]

It is likely that cardiac marker protocols will continue to evolve and various combinations of both new and traditional marker panels will appear. Additional markers such as brain natriuretic peptide (BNP), C-reactive protein (CRP), myeloperoxidase, and albumin cobalt binding assays have been investigated and have shown promising results as well.[33–38]

RADIONUCLIDE MYOCARDIAL PERFUSION IMAGING

It is clear that decision making for patients seen in the ED CPCs relies on appropriate risk stratification. Clinical factors and an ECG alone are not sufficient. For this reason, radionuclide myocardial perfusion imaging (RMPI) has taken a lead role in the evaluation of patients with potential ACS and is a cornerstone of many such protocols.[39]

There are important obstacles and considerations for RMPI. Traditionally, the major obstacles for radionuclide studies have included cost and accessibility. The perfusion agents have a 6–12-hour shelf life, and thus have to be prepared several times a day to be available for acute imaging. Also, the diagnostic sensitivity of myocardial perfusion imaging is in part dependent on the timing of injection in relation to chest pain. Timely evaluation of these patients requires immediate access to these studies and concomitant reading and reporting of the results. Collaboration with nuclear cardiology and radiology colleagues is paramount for this reason.

Initial protocols including RMPI used thallium-201 and were very successful.[40–42] While the sensitivity and specificity for the detection of patients with ACS were high, thallium has quickly been realized not to be the ideal radionuclide for ED CPC imaging. Thallium redistributes quickly and delayed imaging may not reflect significant perfusion abnormalities.

The subsequent availability of Tc-99m and its improved properties of not redistributing throughout the myocardium, further improved the stratification that could be achieved in the CPC. Initial studies using this radioisotope showed that this technology when applied to patients with typical anginal symptoms and a nondiagnostic ECG was very effective in differentiating between high- and low-risk patients.[43]

Since that time, several studies have confirmed the use of Tc-99m.[44–46] Tatum and colleagues found that patients with normal imaging findings had a 1-year event rate of 3% no MI or death compared to 42% with 11% experiencing MI and 8% cardiac death.[44] Duca and colleagues noted that rest sestamibi imaging had a better sensitivity with similar specificity to cardiac troponins[46]. Further studies determined that serial cardiac markers and RMPI could be complementary for the evaluation of these patients.[44–46] In most current CPC protocols, RMPI usually with Tc-99m sestamibi, is an integral part and disposition determining step in the patient's evaluation.

CHEST PAIN CENTER MODELS

Over the years, several manifestations of CPCs have evolved. Each of these models has been successfully adapted to specific institutions and patient populations. Any individual institution should carefully evaluate their patient population, physician expertise, physical structure, staffing model, and hospital environment to most adequately determine their optimal CPC protocol.

For instance, the University of Cincinnati Center for Emergency Care "Heart ER" was one of the first ED-based CPCs having been established in October 1991. Since then, over 2600 patients have been admitted to the Heart ER program and are considered to be a low-to-moderate risk cohort for ACS. Serial cardiac markers of CK-MB, myoglobin, and cTnT levels are drawn at 0, 3, and 6 hours. The original protocol used continuous ST-segment trend monitoring, which has since been discontinued. Graded exercise testing or Tc-99m sestamibi radionuclide scanning is now performed depending on the patient's functional status and test availability. Patients having negative evaluations in the Heart ER are released to home with careful follow-up as an outpatient.[12]

In the first 2131 consecutive patients evaluated over a 6-year period, 309 (14.5%) required admission and 1822 (85.5%) were released to home from the ED. Of admitted patients, 94 (30%) were found to have a cardiac cause for their chest pain. Follow up of 1696 patients discharged from the Heart ER to home yielded nine cardiac events (0.53%, CI 0.24–1.01%; 7 PTCA, 1 CABG, 1 death).[47] These data suggest that the Heart ER program provides a safe and effective means for evaluating low-to-moderate risk patients with possible ACS presenting to the ED.

Other institutions have also developed effective CPC strategies. The Medical College of Virginia has an elegant protocol which triages chest pain patients into five distinct levels (see Figs. 17-1 to 17-3).[44,48] Level 1 patients have ECG criteria for AMI while level 5 patients have clearly noncardiac chest discomfort. Triage level severity dictates treatment and further diagnostic measures. Intermediate level patients (levels 2 and 3) include individuals with variable probability of unstable angina (UA). These patients are admitted to the coronary care unit for the diagnosis of ACS while less acute patients (level 4) undergo serial biomarker determination and Tc-99m sestamibi radionuclide imaging from the ED.

The University of California at Davis protocol employs a novel use of immediate exercise treadmill testing without serial cardiac marker determination. In a recent study of 1000 patients, 13% were positive and 64% were negative for ischemia. The remaining 23% of the patients had nondiagnostic tests. There were no adverse effects of exercise testing and no mortality in each of the patient evaluation groups at 30-day follow-up. These authors concluded that immediate exercise testing of low-risk patients is safe and accurate for the determination of which patients can be safely discharged from the ED.[49]

Mayo Clinic separates patients into low-, intermediate-, and high-risk categories according to Agency for Health Care Policy Research (AHCPR) guidelines. Intermediate risk patients are evaluated with CK-MB levels at 0, 2, and 4 hours while undergoing continuous ST-segment monitoring and 6-hour observation. If this evaluation is negative, an ECG exercise test, a nuclear stress test, or an echocardiographic stress test is performed. Patients with positive or equivocal evaluations are admitted while patients with negative evaluations are discharged to home with a 72-hour follow-up.[11]

Lastly, Brigham and Women's Hospital divides patients into three groups: UA or AMI, possible ischemia, and nonischemic. Patients with UA or AMI are admitted while definitively nonischemic chest pain patients are discharged from the CPC. The intermediate, or "possible ischemia," group either undergoes exercise treadmill testing with a 6-hour period of observation or a 12-hour period of observation. At the end of the observation period, stable patients are discharged to home. Nichol et al.

evaluated the impact of this pathway approach in a retrospective cohort of 4585 patients and found that a 17% reduction in admissions and an 11% reduction in length of stay would occur if even fewer than 50% of eligible patients for observation and exercise testing had participated.[50]

From these protocols, it is apparent that each institution tailors CPC protocols to its patient population, expertise, and resource availability to meet the growing demands of chest pain evaluation. Each hospital and patient population represents a unique environment with specific needs and resources that must be reflected in the ultimate CPC design and implementation.

EDUCATION AND QUALITY MONITORING

One frequently overlooked advantage of the CPC is the potential to educate patients about CAD during their evaluation. For many patients, coming to the ED represents a key "interventional moment" where education about CAD and risk modification may be particularly effective.[51] Patients can view videos, read pamphlets, and ask questions related to their evaluation. Ultimately, these educational interventions may have a significant impact on the patient's lifestyle and medical care.

In general, protocol- and guideline-driven medicine is effective for the evaluation of multiple disease processes in the ED, chest discomfort included. Continuous quality improvement should be an integral part of the continued assessment of any CPC. Guidelines such as the 2002 ACC/AHA guidelines for non-ST-segment elevation myocardial infarction and UA must be reflected in any CPC protocol. Frequent quality assessment and intervention to improve the protocol must be part of the initial commitment to this type of unit.

GOING HOME—THE ROLE OF THE PRIMARY CARE PHYSICIAN

A collaborative relationship between emergency physicians, radiologist, and laboratorians can insure a consistent and effective evaluation of patients in the CPC. Finally, primary care physicians need to be supportive of the CPC and willing to have patients evaluated in this protocol-driven process. They must also be willing to complete the patient's evaluation in an outpatient setting.

Patients frequently require outpatient provocative testing, if not received in the CPC protocol, to further delineate their cardiac risk. These tests must be followed and acted upon by a primary care physician. Communication

between emergency physicians and the patient's primary care physician can assure careful follow-up and compliance after the CPC evaluation.

UNRESOLVED ISSUES

The most compelling "unresolved issue" surrounding the use of CPCs is the definition of the "ideal" protocol and "ideal" patient population for their enrollment. Unfortunately, there will likely be no resolution to this question. CPCs have to be individualized to patient populations and specific institutions. There is no "one-size-fits-all" protocol.

REFERENCES

1. Selker HP, Zalenski RJ, Antman EM, et al. An evaluation of technologies for identifying acute cardiac ischemia in the emergency department: A report from a National Heart Attack Alert Program Working Group. *Ann Emerg Med* 1997;29:13–87.
2. Pope JH, Aufderheide TP, Ruthazer R, et al. Missed diagnoses of acute cardiac ischemia in the emergency department. *N Engl J Med* 2000;342:1163–1170.
3. Nourjah P. *National Hospital Ambulatory Medical Care Survey: 1997 Emergency Department Summary. Advance Data from Vital and Health Statistics.* Hyattsville, MD: National Center for Health Statistics, 2001.
4. Kontos MC, Anderson FP, Schmidt KA, et al. Early diagnosis of acute myocardial infarction in patients without ST-segment elevation. *Am J Cardiol* 1999;83:155–158.
5. Graff LG, Dallara J, Ross MA, et al. Impact on the care of the emergency department chest pain patient from the chest pain evaluation registry (CHEPER) study. *Am J Cardiol* 1997;80:563–568.
6. Amsterdam EA, Lewis WR, Kirk JD, et al. Acute ischemic syndromes. Chest pain center concept. *Cardiol Clin* 2002;20:117–136.
7. Stein RA, Chaitman BR, Balady GJ, et al. Safety and utility of exercise testing in emergency room chest pain centers: An advisory from the Committee on Exercise, Rehabilitation, and Prevention, Council on Clinical Cardiology, American Heart Association. *Circulation* 2000;102:1463–1467.
8. Storrow AB, Gibler WB. Chest pain centers: Diagnosis of acute coronary syndromes. *Ann Emerg Med* 2000;35: 449–461.
9. Lee-Lewandrowski E, Corboy D, Lewandrowski K, et al. Implementation of a point-of-care satellite laboratory in the emergency department of an academic medical center. Impact on test turnaround time and patient emergency department length of stay. *Arch Pathol Lab Med* 2003;127:456–460.
10. Lee TH, Juarez G, Cook EF, et al. Ruling out acute myocardial infarction. A prospective multicenter validation of a 12-hour strategy for patients at low risk. *N Engl J Med* 1991;324:1239–1246.

11. Farkouh ME, Smars PA, Reeder GS, et al. A clinical trial of a chest-pain observation unit for patients with unstable angina. Chest Pain Evaluation in the Emergency Room (CHEER) Investigators. *N Engl J Med* 1998;339:1882–1888.

12. Gibler WB, Runyon JP, Levy RC, et al. A rapid diagnostic and treatment center for patients with chest pain in the emergency department. *Ann Emerg Med* 1995;25:1–8.

13. Lambrew CT, Bowlby LJ, Rogers WJ, et al. Factors influencing the time to thrombolysis in acute myocardial infarction. Time to thrombolysis substudy of the National Registry of Myocardial Infarction-1. *Arch Intern Med* 1997;157:2577–2582.

14. Newby LK, Rutsch WR, Califf RM, et al. Time from symptom onset to treatment and outcomes after thrombolytic therapy. GUSTO-1 Investigators. *J Am Coll Cardiol* 1996;27:1646–1655.

15. Gibler WB, Young GP, Hedges JR, et al. Acute myocardial infarction in chest pain patients with nondiagnostic ECGs: Serial CK-MB sampling in the emergency department. The Emergency Medicine Cardiac Research Group. *Ann Emerg Med* 1992;21:504–512.

16. Polanczyk CA, Lee TH, Cook EF, et al. Value of additional two-hour myoglobin for the diagnosis of myocardial infarction in the emergency department. *Am J Cardiol* 1999;83:525–529.

17. Fesmire FM, Percy RF, Bardoner JB, et al. Serial creatinine kinase (CK) MB testing during the emergency department evaluation of chest pain: Utility of a 2-hour delta CK-MB of +1.6 ng/ml. *Am Heart J* 1998;136:237–244.

18. Falahati A, Sharkey SW, Christensen D, et al. Implementation of serum cardiac troponin I as marker for detection of acute myocardial infarction. *Am Heart J* 1999;137:332–337.

19. Johnson PA, Goldman L, Sacks DB, et al. Cardiac troponin T as a marker for myocardial ischemia in patients seen at the emergency department for acute chest pain. *Am Heart J* 1999;137:1137–1144.

20. Ottani F, Galvani M, Ferrini D, et al. Direct comparison of early elevations of cardiac troponin T and I in patients with clinical unstable angina. *Am Heart J* 1999;137:284–291.

21. Ottani F, Galvani M, Nicolini FA, et al. Elevated cardiac troponin levels predict the risk of adverse outcome in patients with acute coronary syndromes. *Am Heart J* 2000;140:917–927.

22. Christenson RH, Duh SH, Newby LK, et al. Cardiac troponin T and cardiac troponin I: Relative values in short- term risk stratification of patients with acute coronary syndromes. GUSTO-IIa Investigators. *Clin Chem* 1998;44:494–501.

23. Newby LK, Christenson RH, Ohman EM, et al. Value of serial troponin T measures for early and late risk stratification in patients with acute coronary syndromes. The GUSTO-IIa Investigators. *Circulation* 1998;98:1853–1859.

24. Tucker JF, Collins RA, Anderson AJ, et al. Early diagnostic efficiency of cardiac troponin I and troponin T for acute myocardial infarction. *Acad Emerg Med* 1997;4:13–21.

25. Brogan GX Jr., Hollander JE, McCuskey CF, et al. Evaluation of a new assay for cardiac troponin I vs creatine kinase-MB for the diagnosis of acute myocardial infarction. Biochemical Markers for Acute Myocardial Ischemia (BAMI) Study Group. *Acad Emerg Med* 1997;4:6–12.

26. Sayre MR, Kaufmann KH, Chen IW, et al. Measurement of cardiac troponin T is an effective method for predicting complications among emergency department patients with chest pain. *Ann Emerg Med* 1998;31:539–549.

27. Newby LK, Kaplan AL, Granger BB, et al. Comparison of cardiac troponin T versus creatine kinase-MB for risk stratification in a chest pain evaluation unit. *Am J Cardiol* 2000;85:801–805.

28. Myocardial infarction redefined—a consensus document of The Joint European Society of Cardiology/American College of Cardiology Committee for the redefinition of myocardial infarction. *J Am Coll Cardiol* 2000;36:959–969.

29. Rao SV, Ohman EM, Granger CB, et al. Prognostic value of isolated troponin elevation across the spectrum of chest pain syndromes. *Am J Cardiol* 2003;91:936–940.

30. Newby LK, Storrow AB, Gibler WB, et al. Bedside multimarker testing for risk stratification in chest pain units: The chest pain evaluation by creatine kinase-MB, myoglobin, and troponin I (CHECKMATE) study. *Circulation* 2001;103:1832–1837.

31. Ohman EM, Armstrong PW, Christenson RH, et al. Cardiac troponin T levels for risk stratification in acute myocardial ischemia. GUSTO IIA Investigators. *N Engl J Med* 1996;335:1333–1341.

32. Newby LK, Ohman EM, Christenson RH, et al. Benefit of glycoprotein IIb/IIIa inhibition in patients with acute coronary syndromes and troponin t-positive status: The PARAGON-B troponin T substudy. *Circulation* 2001;103:2891–2896.

33. Sabatine MS, Morrow DA, de Lemos JA, et al. Multimarker approach to risk stratification in non-ST elevation acute coronary syndromes: Simultaneous assessment of troponin I, C-reactive protein, and B-type natriuretic peptide. *Circulation* 2002;105:1760–1763.

34. Gibler WB, Blomkalns AL, Collins SP. Evaluation of chest pain and heart failure in the emergency department: Impact of multimarker strategies and B-type natriuretic Peptide. *Rev Cardiovasc Med* 2003;4(Suppl 4):S47–S55.

35. Brennan ML, Penn MS, Van Lente F, et al. Prognostic value of myeloperoxidase in patients with chest pain. *N Engl J Med* 2003;349:1595–1604.

36. Russell CJ, Exley AR, Ritchie AJ. Widespread coronary inflammation in unstable angina. *N Engl J Med* 2003;348:1931.

37. Baldus S, Heeschen C, Meinertz T, et al. Myeloperoxidase serum levels predict risk in patients with acute coronary syndromes. *Circulation* 2003;108:1440–1445.

38. Bhagavan NV, Lai EM, Rios PA, et al. Evaluation of human serum albumin cobalt binding assay for the assessment of myocardial ischemia and myocardial infarction. *Clin Chem* 2003;49:581–585.

39. Klocke FJ, Baird MG, Lorell BH, et al. ACC/AHA/ASNC guidelines for the clinical use of cardiac radionuclide imaging—executive summary: A report of the American College of Cardiology/American Heart Association Task

Force on Practice Guidelines (ACC/AHA/ASNC Committee to Revise the 1995 Guidelines for the Clinical Use of Cardiac Radionuclide Imaging). *J Am Coll Cardiol* 2003;42: 1318–1333.

40. Wackers FJ, Lie KI, Liem KL, et al. Potential value of thallium-201 scintigraphy as a means of selecting patients for the coronary care unit. *Br Heart J* 1979;41:111–117.

41. Ben-Gal T, Zafrir N. The utility and potential cost-effectiveness of stress myocardial perfusion thallium SPECT imaging in hospitalized patients with chest pain and normal or non-diagnostic electrocardiogram. *Isr Med Assoc J* 2001; 3:725–730.

42. Hung J, Chaitman BR, Lam J, et al. Noninvasive diagnostic test choices for the evaluation of coronary artery disease in women: A multivariate comparison of cardiac fluoroscopy, exercise electrocardiography and exercise thallium myocardial perfusion scintigraphy. *J Am Coll Cardiol* 1984;4:8–16.

43. Hilton TC, Thompson RC, Williams HJ, et al. Technetium-99m sestamibi myocardial perfusion imaging in the emergency room evaluation of chest pain. *J Am Coll Cardiol* 1994;23:1016–1022.

44. Tatum JL, Jesse RL, Kontos MC, et al. Comprehensive strategy for the evaluation and triage of the chest pain patient. *Ann Emerg Med* 1997;29:116–125.

45. Kontos MC, Jesse RL, Anderson FP, et al. Comparison of myocardial perfusion imaging and cardiac troponin I in patients admitted to the emergency department with chest pain. *Circulation* 1999;99:2073–2078.

46. Duca MD, Giri S, Wu AH, et al. Comparison of acute rest myocardial perfusion imaging and serum markers of myocardial injury in patients with chest pain syndromes. *J Nucl Cardiol* 1999;6:570–576.

47. Storrow AB, Gibler WB, Walsh RA. An emergency department chest pain rapid diagnosis and treatment unit: Results from a six year experience. *Circulation* 1999;98:I-425.

48. Jesse RL, Kontos MC. Evaluation of chest pain in the emergency department. *Curr Probl Cardiol* 1997;22:149–236.

49. Amsterdam EA, Kirk JD, Diercks DB, et al. Immediate exercise testing to evaluate low-risk patients presenting to the emergency department with chest pain. *J Am Coll Cardiol* 2002;40:251–256.

50. Nichol G, Walls R, Goldman L, et al. A critical pathway for management of patients with acute chest pain who are at low risk for myocardial ischemia: Recommendations and potential impact. *Ann Intern Med* 1997;127:996–1005.

51. Bahr RD. The changing paradigm of acute heart attack prevention in the emergency department: A futuristic viewpoint? *Ann Emerg Med* 1995;25:95–96.

18

Stress Testing

J. Douglas Kirk
Deborah B. Diercks
Ezra A. Amsterdam

HIGH YIELD FACTS

> - The principle goal of stress testing, as part of an accelerated diagnostic protocol (ADP), is to identify patients with unrecognized acute coronary syndrome (ACS) while avoiding the unnecessary hospital admission of those without cardiovascular disease.
>
> - Stress testing provides important prognostic information. Patients deemed high risk typically benefit from coronary angiography and/or revascularization while those with normal test do not.
>
> - Although deviations in the ST segment ≥1 mm are used as diagnostic criteria for a positive test, other exercise-induced alterations indicative of an abnormal test include poor exercise capacity, angina, arrhythmias, or hypotension.
>
> - Treadmill stress testing or some form of provocative testing is a safe, effective, and necessary component of an ADP to thoroughly exclude ACS.
>
> - Fundamental to the safe application of early exercise testing is rigorous patient selection and recognition of low clinical pretest risk.
>
> - Although a common misconception, stress testing does have diagnostic and prognostic utility in patients recognized as low risk.
>
> - Immediate exercise testing distinguishes a very low-risk group and may allow ~80% of appropriately selected patients to be discharged from the emergency department.

INTRODUCTION

The evaluation of patients with chest pain presenting to the emergency department warrants a focused strategy because of the clinical volume and the potential consequences for the patient, physician liability, and the fiscal burden for the payer. Although extensively studied, safe, cost-effective management of these patients remains a challenge.[1,2] The principle goal in the evaluation of these patients is the recognition of those with ACS or other potentially life-threatening causes of chest pain.[3–5] Subsequent goals include prognostic assessment and reduction in costs associated with unnecessary hospitalization of patients without cardiovascular disease. Although ACS is the primary focus of the initial evaluation due to its potential morbidity and mortality, the majority of patients with acute chest pain in the emergency department have relatively benign causes including musculoskeletal, gastroesophageal, and anxiety disorders.[2] Physician concern for patient safety and the litigation potential for failure to recognize ACS has resulted in a low threshold of hospital admission to "rule out" life-threatening causes of chest pain.

This cautious approach has been supported by reports of failure to recognize ACS and its associated morbidity and mortality. The most recent of which suggests that 4% of patients with ACS are inadvertently discharged home.[6] This resulted in a nearly twofold increase in 30-day mortality compared to patients who were appropriately recognized. In addition, failure to recognize myocardial infarction (MI) has been the leading cause of malpractice awards against emergency physicians, thereby reinforcing this conservative approach.[7] Historically, management of patients with chest pain has been neither clinically optimal nor cost-effective. The need for a safe, accurate, and cost-effective method to evaluate these patients is paramount. The goal of such a strategy is apparent: reduce the unnecessary hospitalization of patients who do not have ACS without compromising the care of patients at risk. The development of chest pain units is a response to this need. The focus of these units has evolved to management of the lower-risk population that comprises chest pain patients without initial, objective evidence of myocardial injury or ischemia in whom an abbreviated evaluation can determine the need for admission or the safety of discharge.[8–12]

This approach is often referred to as an ADP. A cornerstone of the ADP is stress testing after a negative initial evaluation for MI or unstable angina. This chapter will focus on exercise electrocardiography (ECG) as the primary cardiac stress test in the context of the ADP.

METHODS OF STRESS TESTING

Clinical Application and Prognostic Assessment

Exercise testing is an important component of the diagnostic evaluation of patients with suspected coronary artery disease, regardless of the setting. The exercise test also provides critical prognostic information and is frequently used to predict future adverse cardiac events. Patients identified as high risk are typically referred for coronary angiography and revascularization if appropriate. Those with negative exercise tests benefit little from further aggressive evaluation. Exercise testing is most often performed with ECG monitoring alone, despite the proliferation of reportedly more accurate methods of stress imaging techniques used to define coronary artery disease, such as nuclear scintigraphy and echocardiography. These technological advances have resulted in a trend to use more costly procedures instead of the more affordable exercise ECG, which is still the procedure of choice in the majority of patients. Exceptions would include an inability to exercise, resting ECG abnormalities that would preclude accurate interpretation (left bundle branch block, paced rhythm, digoxin therapy, preexcitation, significant baseline ST-segment depression), or high pretest risk. The exercise ECG detects myocardial ischemia, a result of coronary artery obstruction and a mismatch of oxygen supply and demand. The accuracy of the test has been derived from studies that compare the ECG response to exercise with coronary angiography. Age, gender, chest pain characteristics, and cardiac risk factors are important determinants of pretest risk.[13,14] Bayes' theorem would suggest it is most useful in intermediate risk patients, as positive or negative tests in this group yield the greatest increment of information regarding the presence or absence of coronary artery disease, compared to test results in those with very high or low pretest probability of disease. Exercise testing may not be needed to diagnose coronary artery disease in patients with a high pretest probability of disease, although it may provide useful information for prognostic assessment. In such cases, proceeding directly to coronary angiography may be warranted. In patients with a low pretest probability of disease, a relatively high false positive rate may be expected and the results should be interpreted accordingly. However, in this low-risk group, the vast majority will have negative tests, without any suggestion of underlying coronary artery disease.

Diagnostic Criteria for a Positive Test

The American College of Cardiology (ACC)/American Heart Association (AHA) Task Force on Practice Guidelines published recommendations on exercise testing for risk stratification of patients with chest pain.[15] (Table 18-1). A number of studies have demonstrated that clinical and ECG responses to exercise can be useful in determining patients' risk. The usual ECG criteria for a positive test for myocardial ischemia are ≥1.0 mm horizontal or downsloping ST-segment deviation 80 ms after the J point. Other exercise-induced alterations that indicate an abnormal test and the need for further evaluation include angina, arrhythmias, and hypotension. Many exercise test variables are associated with an increased risk of future adverse outcomes[14,16] (Table 18-2). The occurrence of one or more of these variables identifies a high-risk group who may benefit from coronary angiography and revascularization. Comparison of exercise ECG results and coronary angiography suggest patients who develop ST depression at a low cardiac workload (Bruce stage I or II or heart rate <120 bpm) have a high probability of left main (25%) or three vessel (50%) disease and a poor prognosis.

Prognostic Tools

Treadmill scores are popular tools used to assess prognosis and compare patients or groups of patients. The most commonly used is the Duke Treadmill Score, which was derived from a cohort of 2758 patients who underwent exercise testing.[17] The Duke Score equals exercise time in minutes on a Bruce protocol, minus five times the ST-segment deviation in millimeters, minus four times the exercise-induced angina (0 = none, 1 = nonlimiting, and 2 = exercise limiting). Based on the score, patients are classified as low (score ≥ +5), moderate (score −10 to +4), and high (score ≤ −11) risk. In a study of 2842 patients undergoing exercise testing for risk assessment, prognosis was related to the risk category as determined by the Duke Score, even after adjustment for other clinical predictors of risk. Five-year survival was 65% in high-risk patients, 90% in moderate-risk patients, and over 97% in low-risk patients.[18]

The use of exercise scores as an additional management tool can add prognostic information to individual patients' clinical data, the importance of which is identification of patients who would likely benefit from coronary revascularization. This method of risk stratification is useful in the assessment of undifferentiated chest pain patients typically seen in the emergency department and can easily be incorporated into the management pathways of an ADP. Independent of the exercise ECG findings, patients with good exercise tolerance (>10 metabolic equivalents—METs) or a heart rate >160 bpm infrequently have three vessel (15%) or left main (1%) disease and have an

Table 18-1. Recommendations for Diagnosis of Obstructive Coronary Artery Disease with Exercise ECG Testing Without an Imaging Modality

Class I: Patients with an intermediate pretest probability of CAD based on age, gender, systems, including those with complete right bundle branch block or <1 mm of ST depression at rest (exceptions are listed below in classes II and III).

Class IIa: Patients with suspected vasospastic angina.

Class IIb:

1. Patients with a high pretest probability of CAS by age, gender, and symptoms.
2. Patients with a low pretest probability of CAS by age, gender, and symptoms.
3. Patients taking digoxin in whom ECG has <1 mm of baseline ST-segment depression.
4. Patients with ECG criteria for LV hypertrophy and <1 mm of baseline ST-segment depression.

Class III:

1. Patients with the following baseline ECG abnormalities:
   (a) Preexcitation (Wolff-Parkinson-White) syndrome
   (b) Electronically passed ventricular rhythm
   (c) Complete left bundle branch block
2. Patients with an established diagnosis of CAD due to prior MI or coronary angiography; however, testing can assess functional capacity and prognosis, as discussed in section III.

ACC/AHA classification

Class I: Conditions for which there is evidence and/or general agreement that a given procedure or treatment is useful and effective.

Class II: Conditions for which there is conflicting evidence and/or a divergence of opinion about the usefulness/efficacy of a procedure or treatment.

Class IIa: Weight of evidence/opinion is in favor of usefulness/efficacy.

Class IIb: Usefulness/efficacy less well established by evidence/opinion.

Class III: Conditions for which there is evidence and/or general agreement that the procedure/treatment is not useful and in some cases may be harmful.

Source: Adapted with permission from Gibbons RJ, Chatterjee K, Daley J, et al. ACC/AHA/ACP guidelines for the management of patients with chronic stable angina. *J Am Coll Cardiol* 1999;33:2092.

Table 18-2. Exercise Testing Variables that Predict a Poor Outcome

- ≥1 mm of downsloping or flat ST-segment depression
- ST-segment depression at a low cardiac workload or of prolonged duration
- Multiple leads with ST-segment depression
- Exercise-induced angina
- Fall in systolic blood pressure below baseline during exercise
- Poor exercise capacity
- ST-segment elevation
- Ventricular arrhythmias
- Chronotropic incompetence

excellent prognosis (1% mortality/year).[19] In a study of 6213 men who were referred for exercise testing and followed for 6 years, peak exercise capacity was the strongest predictor of mortality, regardless of the presence or absence of coronary artery disease.[16] Similar to poor peak exercise capacity, a generalized decrease in vagal tone is associated with an increase in all cause mortality. A delay in heart rate recovery after exercise, which is due to vagal reactivation, is defined as less than 12–18 bpm decrease at 1 min and is associated with a worse prognosis. A study of 2428 patients undergoing exercise testing with 6-year follow-up demonstrated a nearly twofold increase in adjusted mortality in patients with abnormal heart rate recovery.[20]

Distinguishing True Positive Stress Test

As previously discussed, a minority of patients undergoing stress testing in the emergency department or chest pain unit have positive tests. Although nearly half are later found to be false positives on further, more specific diagnostic testing, a significant number of these can be recognized during the initial exercise test. The degree of ST-segment deviation and at what point during exercise it occurs can be invaluable in determining its significance. The less the ST-segment deviation and the higher the cardiac workload (measured in exercise time, METs, or rate-pressure product [systolic blood pressure × heart rate]) at which it occurs, the more likely the test is a false positive.

A lack of corresponding clinical indicators, such as angina or poor exercise capacity that precludes further exercise suggests a false positive test. In addition, the relationship between the ST segment and heart rate during recovery is an important discriminating feature between true and false positive stress test.[21] If the ST-segment deviation starts to resolve as or before the heart rate begins to fall, this is highly suggestive of a false positive test. By contrast, ST-segment depression that is greater at the same heart rate during recovery as during exercise is predictive of a true positive test. The ST-heart rate loop depicts this relationship (Fig. 18-1). While the general rule is to follow-up a positive stress test with a more definitive study, one can appreciate that the likelihood of a true or false positive test can be reasonably predicted based on the characteristics of the initial stress test.

RECOGNITION OF LOW CLINICAL RISK

Fundamental to an approach that uses early stress testing in undifferentiated patients with chest pain is the identi-fication of those with low clinical risk on presentation to the emergency department. At the heart of this process is risk stratification, shifting the focus from diagnosis to prognosis. To be most efficient with resource utilization and diagnostic accuracy, it is critically important to match the risk of disease with the complexity or intensity of diagnostic testing. Identification of low-risk chest pain patients in the emergency department has the potential to obviate needless hospitalization and/or diagnostic testing, therefore improving resource utilization. There is significant evidence that among emergency department patients with chest pain, a low-risk group can be identified. These patients have a low occurrence of adverse cardiac events and neither require nor benefit from intensive care. Of patients admitted for "rule out MI," those with a probability of <5% of MI can generally be identified from the type of chest pain, cardiac history, and resting ECG.[22] Goldman et al. extended this approach in over 10,000 patients, demonstrating that the initial clinical assessment could distinguish those with <1% risk of adverse events[23] (Fig. 18-2). The initial ECG alone provides important prognostic data. Although not optimally sensitive for the diagnosis of MI, a normal ECG in patients with chest pain portends a favorable prognosis, with a high likelihood of a benign clinical course and fewer adverse events than in patients with abnormal ECGs.[24]

The reliable identification of low-risk groups is fundamentally important to the safety and feasibility of an ADP. These protocols usually incorporate a period of observation on telemetry monitoring while patients undergo serial ECGs and cardiac injury marker testing. In addition, most centers advocate noninvasive testing to detect coronary artery disease as part of this initial evaluation. This is typically some form of stress testing, used to elucidate

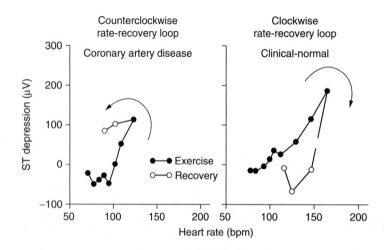

Fig. 18-1. Typical rate-recovery loops are shown for a clinically normal subject (right) and a patient with coronary artery disease (left). (Source: Adapted with permission from Okin PM, Kilgfield P. Heart rate adjustment of ST segment depression and performance of the exercise electrocardiogram: A critical evaluation. *J Am Coll Cardiol* 1995;25:1726–1736.)

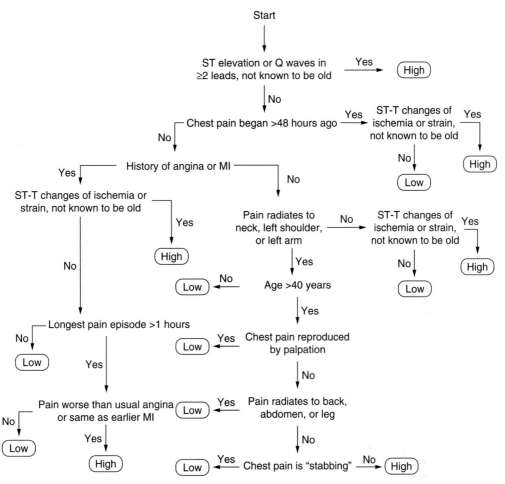

Fig. 18-2. Algorithm for evaluating patients with chest pain in the emergency room. The Goldman algorithm divides patients into groups at high risk (≥7%) and low risk (<7%) for an acute episode of myocardial ischemia. (Source: Adapted with permission from Zalenski RJ, McCarren M, Roberts R, et al. An evaluation of a chest pain diagnostic protocol to exclude acute cardiac ischemia in the emergency department. *Arch Intern Med* 1997;157:1085.)

evidence of inducible ischemia that may not be readily apparent on the resting ECG, especially in patients whose chest pain has resolved. The integration of stress testing into ADPs will be described in the next section.

EARLY STRESS TESTING

Current Guidelines

Although the standard treadmill exercise test is now an integral component of many ADPs, this is a recent development based on an accumulation of data during the past decade that has overcome initial concern regarding the

possible hazards of this technique in potentially unstable patients. Traditionally recommended after a prolonged symptom-free interval,[25] recent studies have demonstrated the safety and utility of early exercise testing in appropriately selected patients[8–12,26,27] and have provided the basis for firm support of this approach by expert panels. The 31st Bethesda Conference on Emergency Cardiac Care held in 1999 noted that "ADPs, including exercise testing as a key element, have been associated with reduced hospital stay and lower costs."[4] The absence of adverse effects and the accurate identification of low postdischarge prognostic risk were also recognized. This strategy is now reflected in the current ACC/AHA guidelines for the management of patients with suspected ACS, which advocate its use after completion of a negative ADP[3,28] (Table 18-3). During the last decade, recommendations for exercise testing in low-risk patients have progressed from a 48-hour period of clinical stability prior to testing, to expert consensus supporting its application after a much briefer interval. The evidence on which this consensus is based is described next.

Incorporating Stress Testing into an ADP

Although a variety of ADPs have been described, most are derived from the University of Cincinnati's Heart ER Program. This initial approach was based on a retrospective analysis of 1010 patients with chest pain who had an estimated 5% prevalence of ACS.[8] The protocol consisted of a 9-hour observation period in the emergency

Table 18-3. Guidelines for Exercise ECG Testing in the Emergency Department or Chest Pain Center

---

Requirements before exercise testing that should be considered:

- Two sets of cardiac enzymes at 4-h intervals should be normal
- ECG at the time of presentation and preexercise shows no significant change
- Absence of rest ECG abnormalities that would preclude accurate assessment of the exercise ECG
- From admission to the time, results are available from the second set of cardiac enzymes: patient asymptomatic, lessening symptoms, or persistent atypical symptoms
- Absence of ischemic chest pain at the time of exercise testing

Contraindications to exercise testing:

- New or evolving ECG abnormalities on the rest tracing
- Abnormal cardiac enzymes
- Inability to perform exercise
- Worsening or persistent ischemic symptoms from admission to the time of exercise testing
- Clinical risk profiling indicating imminent coronary angiography is likely

---

Source: Adapted with permission from Stein RA, Chaitman BR, Balady GJ. Safety and utility of exercise testing in emergency room chest pain centers: An advisory from the Committee on Exercise, Rehabilitation, and Prevention, Council on Clinical Cardiology, American Heart Association. *Circulation* 2000;102:1463.

department's chest pain center, during which time the patient underwent continuous ST-segment monitoring, serial measurement of CK-MB and ECGs, and a resting echocardiogram. Patients with evidence of cardiovascular disease on this stepwise approach were admitted to the hospital, while the remainder (791 patients) underwent exercise testing. The protocol had a negative predictive value of 98.7% and enabled 82% of the patients to be discharged from the emergency department. This approach led to compelling data from a number of subsequent studies, which suggested performing exercise testing as part of an ADP was safe and cost-effective.

Mikhail et al. evaluated 424 low-risk patients with mandatory exercise testing (some with cardiac imaging), assessing its safety, utility, and cost-effectiveness after 6–8 hours of serial cardiac injury marker testing.[10] At 5 months, there were no MIs or deaths in those with negative evaluations. Of the 44 (9%) of patients with subsequent final diagnoses of ischemic heart disease during follow up, all had a positive exercise test during initial evaluation, 24 (55%) of whom were identified only on stress testing. Evaluation in the chest pain unit with mandatory stress testing was associated with a cost-per-case savings of 62% for each patient who would otherwise have been admitted to the hospital.

Zalenski et al. prospectively evaluated 317 patients who presented to the emergency department with chest pain.[9] Patients with an obvious diagnosis of heart disease, clinical instability, or inability to perform exercise testing were excluded. Patients completed a 12-hour rule out MI protocol and those with negative evaluations (71%) underwent exercise testing. All patients, including those with negative exercise test were then admitted to establish a reference diagnosis by clinical outcome or further diagnostic testing for coronary artery disease (nuclear scintigraphy or coronary angiography). ACS was diagnosed in 30 (9.5%) of patients. The performance of the protocol, including the exercise test, compared to the reference diagnosis, revealed a sensitivity of 90% and negative predictive value of 98%; specificity was 51%. When the value of each component of the protocol was measured, the best performance was afforded by the combined use of CK-MB, ECG, and exercise testing, with particular incremental importance of the exercise test when analyzed by the receiver-operator curve. A cost analysis of a subset of 165 patients revealed a savings of 567 dollars per patient managed in the chest pain center, including the cost of exercise testing.

In a follow-up study to their initial report, 950 patients evaluated in the University of Cincinnati's Heart ER underwent exercise testing after the aforementioned

9-hour observation period.[29] This strategy demonstrated that patients with positive, nondiagnostic, and negative exercise test had cardiac event rates of 26%, 3%, and 0.9%, respectively, during 1-year follow-up. After adjustment, the relative risk of adverse events was 23 for a positive test and 4 for a nondiagnostic test compared to a negative test.

Polanczyk et al. reported their findings in 276 low-risk patients with chest pain who underwent exercise testing within 48 hours of presentation.[30] Twenty-six percent of these patients had a prior history of coronary artery disease. The test was performed within 12 hours in 7% of patients, at 12–24 hours in 45%, and after 24 hours in 48%. The Bruce treadmill protocol was employed in 84% of the patients and the modified version was used in 12%. A negative test was defined by achievement of at least three METs (1 stage of Bruce protocol) without evidence of ischemia. Positive tests were "those in which the results were interpreted as highly predictive of significant coronary disease and inconclusive tests were those consistent with but not diagnostic of ischemia" or without evidence of ischemia at a peak work of <3 METs. There were no adverse effects of exercise testing. The test was negative in 71% of patients, positive in 24%, and inconclusive in 5%. Outcome data were available at 6 months for 92% of the study group. Events during the follow-up period were defined as cardiac death, MI, or myocardial revascularization. During this interval, there was no mortality and the event rate in the negative exercise test cohort was 2% compared to 15% in those with abnormal (positive or nondiagnostic) tests. In the negative test group, compared to those with positive/nondiagnostic tests, there were also fewer repeat ED visits (17% vs. 21%, $P < 0.05$) and fewer readmissions (12% vs. 17%, $P < 0.01$). The negative predictive value of the exercise test was 98%; sensitivity and specificity were 73% and 74%, respectively. In addition to the documented prognostic utility of the exercise test, this study afforded other noteworthy features. The investigators demonstrated the safety of the early exercise test in patients with a history of coronary artery disease and their definition of test results yielded a low rate of inconclusive diagnoses, increasing the clinical utility of the test in clinical decision making.

Two studies randomized patients to an ADP, which included exercise testing versus usual care with hospital admission. In the rapid Rule Out of Myocardial Ischemia Observation (ROMIO) trial, investigators randomized 100 low-risk patients to either standardized inpatient care (control group) or an ADP (study group) that included 9 hours of serial cardiac injury marker measurement followed by exercise testing in those with negative

results.[10] In the study group, 49/50 patients had MI excluded and 44 underwent exercise testing. Negative test were found in 41/44 (93%) and 3/44 were positive (all false positives). At 1 month, there were no adverse cardiac events in either the study or control groups. Although this was a very low-risk population, the length of stay and associated costs in the study group were nearly half the control group, demonstrating the utility of this approach. In a prospective, controlled trial by the CHest pain Evaluation in the Emergency Room (CHEER) investigators, they similarly randomized patients with suspected ACS to a 6-hour chest pain observation unit protocol ($n = 212$) or standard inpatient care ($n = 212$).[12] Of the patients managed in the observation unit, those without evidence of ischemia or MI during serial ECG and cardiac injury marker testing underwent exercise testing, which was positive in 55 and negative in 97. Patients with negative tests were discharged home and those with positive tests were admitted to the hospital. At 1-month follow-up, adverse cardiac event rates trended lower in the observation unit group (3.8%) versus the inpatient group (8%). In addition, the length of stay was shorter and half the patients in the observation unit group avoided a hospital admission.

The impact of chest pain units compared to regular hospital care was analyzed by Graff and colleagues in the report of the CHEst Pain Evaluation Registry (CHEPER) study. Results were assessed in terms of the proportion of patients undergoing a complete rule out MI investigation, the number of missed MIs, and costs.[31] Outcomes in over 23,000 patients managed in eight chest pain observation units were compared with results in over 12,000 patients in five studies from hospitals without these units. Although data on exercise testing were not provided in the report, the authors note that all chest pain units complied with standards of the American College of Emergency Physicians[32] and the Clinical Practice Guidelines for management of unstable angina,[3] which include recommendations on exercise testing in their management algorithms. Chest pain units were associated with an increase in evaluations to rule out MI (67% vs. 57%, $P < 0.001$), a lower rate of missed MIs (0.4% vs. 4.5%, $P < 0.001$), and a lower admission rate (47% vs. 57%, $P < 0.001$). The latter effect equated to a potential for 2314 admissions avoided and over $4,000,000 saved.

Emerging from these studies[8–12,29–31] is recognition of the high frequency and excellent predictive value of negative exercise tests in patients identified as low risk. Further, although the positive predictive value is modest, positive tests are infrequent and result in the need for further evaluation in only small numbers of patients.

Therefore, the utility of this strategy is confirmed in its ability to safely and efficiently reduce unnecessary admissions in low-risk patients while avoiding inappropriate discharge in some patients with ACS otherwise not identified. Estimates of cost-effectiveness indicate the potential for substantial savings for similar reasons. The chest pain center is a relatively recent development and investigation is ongoing to determine optimal implementation of this concept. In this regard, as previously noted,[1,26,27] we have employed a unique approach to management of low-risk patients at our institution: the immediate exercise treadmill test (IETT).

Immediate Exercise Treadmill Testing

In the aforementioned studies, exercise testing was employed after a negative ADP evaluation, which by design incorporated a "cooling off" period in an observation setting. There were no adverse effects of exercise and the results were useful in determining accurate and safe disposition while preserving resources and limiting costs. Clinical outcomes were comparable to those of traditional inpatient evaluation.

Two early studies demonstrated the safety of exercise testing in low-risk patients in the emergency department setting, without the benefit of prolonged observation. Tsakonis et al. evaluated 28 patients "several hours" after hospital arrival with treadmill ECG using a symptom-limited modified Bruce protocol.[33] These patients had unexplained chest pain consistent with myocardial ischemia but normal baseline ECGs. The exercise test was negative in 23 patients and positive in 5. The latter group was admitted and the former were discharged after the exercise test. The authors report no cardiac morbidity or mortality at 6 months in the patients with negative exercise tests.

These findings were confirmed in the subsequent report of Kerns et al. who performed exercise testing in 32 emergency department patients with atypical chest pain, normal ECGs, and no cardiac risk factors.[34] Compared to a similar cohort of patients admitted for evaluation of atypical chest pain, those with negative results during emergency department exercise testing had a shorter length of stay (5.5 hours vs. 2 days) and lower costs ($467 vs. $2340). All patients had negative exercise tests and no evidence of coronary disease at 6 months follow-up. In addition to their small numbers, limitations of these two studies include the very low risk of the patients (none had been designated for admission), the lack of any positive tests in Kerns' study, and no further

evaluation for coronary artery disease in Tsakonis' patients with positive tests.

At the University of California, Davis, we have employed an IETT protocol (Table 18-4) in several thousand appropriately selected, low-risk patients with chest pain over the past decade. The IETT, in contrast to exercise testing after completion of an ADP, is performed without serial assessment of cardiac injury markers or

Table 18-4. Immediate Exercise Treadmill Test Protocol

Eligible patients
- All patients with chest pain suspicious of myocardial ischemia
- No other serious etiology for chest pain is considered or found (e.g., pulmonary embolism, aortic dissection, esophageal rupture)
- Clinically stable and without evidence of left ventricular dysfunction
- ECG normal or only minor nonspecific repolarization abnormalities

Exclusion criteria
- Inability to exercise adequately
- ECG abnormalities precluding accurate interpretation (e.g., bundle branch block, left ventricular hypertrophy with strain, or digitalis effect)

Emergency department evaluation
- Physical examination not suggestive of left ventricular dysfunction or significant valvular disease
- Equal arm blood pressures
- Chest radiograph not suggestive of aortic dissection or congestive heart failure
- Negative troponin I and myoglobin on arrival

ETT procedure (modified Bruce protocol)
- Test endpoints
  Symptoms limited
  Fall in systolic blood pressure $\geq$ 10 mmHg
  Coupling of ventricular ectopics
  Sustained supraventricular tachycardia
  1 mm ST-segment depression (horizontal or downsloping) or elevation 80 ms after the J point*

*Criteria for a positive test.
Abbreviations: ECG = electrocardiogram; ETT = exercise treadmill testing.
Source: Adapted with permission from Kirk JD, Diercks DB, Turnipseed SD, et al. Evaluation of chest pain suspicious for acute coronary syndrome: Use of an accelerated diagnostic protocol in a chest pain evaluation unit. *Am J Cardiol* 2000;85(5A):40B–48B.

prolonged observation in patients who are clinically stable and have normal or nondiagnostic ECGs. Our preliminary report in 93 patients suggested this approach was safe and had the potential for major cost savings.[26] The majority of patients had negative test and there were no complications from exercising patients with acute chest pain. A follow-up study of 212 patients extended this approach in several significant respects: (1) patients with a prior history of coronary artery disease were not excluded, (2) exercise testing was performed by attending physicians in our chest pain evaluation unit, not cardiologist, (3) serial cardiac injury markers were not measured, and (4) results were used for emergency department disposition.[27] There were no adverse affects of exercise testing. Of the 28 (13%) patients who had positive tests, 10 were diagnosed with unstable angina and 3 with MI on further testing. Negative exercise test were found in 125 (59%) and 59 (28%) were nondiagnostic (negative for ischemia but less than 85% age predicted maximum heart rate). All patients with negative exercise tests and 93% of those with nondiagnostic tests were discharged home from the emergency department. Follow up at 30 days revealed no adverse cardiac events in patients discharged from the emergency department. These data suggest that nearly 90% of these low-risk patients could be safely discharged home based on the results of IETT. This study demonstrated the safety of proceeding directly to exercise testing in rigorously selected patients on the basis of the initial presentation, without serial monitoring or cardiac injury markers. However, its limited numbers required a larger study for confirmation of the feasibility of this strategy.

A recent report from our group described this approach in the largest single center study of early exercise testing in low-risk patients with acute chest pain. The study group included a much larger (1000 patients) heterogeneous population of patients, including 7.5% with a prior history of coronary artery disease.[35] Similar to prior reports, the IETT was negative in 64%, positive in 13%, and nondiagnostic in 23%. Of these, 80% were safely discharged home from the emergency department after exercise testing. At 30 days, there were no mortality and cardiac events in the three groups included: negative test—1 MI; positive test—4 MI, 12 revascularizations; nondiagnostic test—7 revascularizations. Compared to a negative exercise test, the relative risk of a cardiac event or the diagnosis of coronary artery disease was 38 (95% CI = 9–161) for a nondiagnostic test and 114 (95% CI = 27–484) for a positive test. One limitation of employing IETT is the specialized equipment and personnel needed to perform the test. Historically, these tests have been performed by cardiologists who provide consultation to selected patients with negative findings during an ADP. Requiring this would limit the widespread applicability of exercise testing due to the lack of availability of cardiologists and the inherent delay associated with consultations in the emergency department. We examined the interreader reliability between cardiologist and chest pain evaluation unit staff physicians in IETT interpretation.[36] In 645 patients who underwent IETT, we compared the interpretations of each. Discrepancies were found in only 11 patients (1.7%), kappa = 0.9618. In the majority of cases, these discrepancies were clinically insignificant and resulted in no morbidity or mortality. These data suggest that noncardiologists, including internists or emergency physicians with specialized training in exercise testing, can reliably perform and interpret these studies. This is critically important to the timelines and generalizability of this procedure as a risk stratification tool.

Stress Testing in Special Groups

Evaluation of patients with an ADP or in an observation unit has traditionally only included those at low clinical risk of ACS. Patients with known coronary artery disease were typically not eligible by definition. Lewis et al. reported their experience in 100 patients with known coronary artery disease who underwent IETT.[37] There were no complications of testing despite a 23% rate of positive tests. ACS was found in seven patients who had positive exercise test and three with nondiagnostic test. Despite the increased prevalence of disease, more than half of the patients were discharged home from the emergency department with only one returning for coronary revascularization during 6-month follow-up.

Patients with diabetes have more extensive coronary artery disease and higher rates of adverse cardiac events. In some respects, type II diabetes is considered an equivalent to coronary artery disease. Not surprisingly, evaluating patients with diabetes in an observation unit has been met with some controversy due to a higher risk of ACS than in nondiabetics. Performing IETT in this group would presumably also raise concern, but preliminary data suggest these patients should not be excluded based solely on a history of diabetes.[38] Although diabetes was an independent predictor of abnormal tests and more diabetics were found to have ACS, there were no complications from exercise testing. Again, despite a higher prevalence of disease, these patients also appear to be safely and reliably evaluated with this approach.

Previous trials have indicated that beta-blockers and calcium-channel blockers decreased angina and may decrease blood pressure and maximum heart rate attained in patients with coronary artery disease undergoing exercise testing. There are conflicting data regarding an exercise test's utility in this group; therefore, patients are often excluded from exercise testing if taking one of these agents. This could potentially eliminate a number of patients from an ADP that incorporates exercise testing, in lieu of more expensive and time-consuming methods of evaluation. Diercks et al. reported data from 975 patients undergoing exercise testing for evaluation of acute chest pain, of which 176 were taking either a beta-blocker, calcium-channel blocker, or both.[39] Although patients on these agents were more likely to have a non-diagnostic exercise test (OR 2.1, 95% CI 1.5–3.1), the majority had a diagnostic study. Half the patients had abnormal exercise test (positive or nondiagnostic), 28% of whom were found to have adverse cardiac events or coronary artery disease during 30-day follow-up. There were no cardiac events or coronary artery disease found in those patients with negative test. This suggests that although the incidence of a nondiagnostic exercise test rises in patients on beta-blockers or calcium-channel blockers, the strategy maintains its usefulness in risk stratification.

Exercise testing should be considered as a reasonable option to evaluate a wide variety of patients in the emergency department or chest pain center despite the initial misconceptions that its diagnostic accuracy may be inadequate in certain groups or that some potentially higher-risk patients should be excluded from exercise testing solely on this basis, especially if their presentations are atypical.

SUMMARY

The value of chest pain centers in the assessment of low-risk patients presenting to the emergency department with symptoms suggestive of ACS is well established. A variety of ADPs have been developed within these units and studies over the last decade have demonstrated their utility in the safe, accurate, and cost-effective management of these patients. Stress testing has been a key component of these ADPs to complete the process of risk stratification, specifically to distinguish those patients who can be discharged from those who require admission. Most ADPs use a period of observation whereby serial ECGs and cardiac injury markers are obtained to exclude MI before proceeding to some form of stress testing. However, at the University of California, Davis, Medical Center, our approach includes IETT in appropriately selected patients without a traditional "cooling off" period of observation (Fig. 18-3). Although we do not advocate this strategy in all institutions or settings, extensive experience has validated this approach in a large, heterogeneous population. The optimal strategy for evaluating low-risk patients presenting to the emergency department with chest pain or other symptoms suggestive of ACS requires continuing study. Fortunately, stress testing is now established as an integral part of this process and should be considered a first-line strategy of risk stratification.

UNRESOLVED ISSUES

- *Should everyone with low-risk chest pain get a stress test?* No. There is a tendency to overuse diagnostic technology just because it is available. This leads to unnecessary expense, potentially causing an increase in cost as opposed to a cost savings measure. This may be further exacerbated by additional, more expensive testing as a result of an even higher false positive rate in patients at very low pretest risk. This decision requires clinical judgment with avoidance of stress testing in patients at very low risk. e.g., atypical chest pain in young women or in those with readily identifiable benign causes (musculoskeletal, gastroesophageal, or anxiety).

- *Does a negative stress test exclude CAD in patients with chest pain?* Although diagnosis and prognosis usually coincide, this is not always the case. Patients with single vessel disease or noncritical stenosis can have false negative exercise ECGs. However, in most instances, if applied in appropriate low-risk patients, a stress test that is negative or nonischemic with adequate exercise capacity and no symptoms is most consistent with a lack of critical CAD and more importantly, favorable prognosis.

- *How long are the results of a stress test applicable?* There is no simple answer, however, in appropriately selected low-risk patients,[23] a negative stress test, especially if good exercise capacity was demonstrated, has excellent 5-year prognosis.[17,18] A reasonable approach is that the stress test result is valid until a change in clinical status, e.g., description of pain now classic for angina, hemodynamic instability, or some objective measure of myocardial ischemia or injury (ECG or troponin) refutes the earlier findings of the stress test. In such cases, the stress test should be repeated, possibly with cardiac imaging or in patients with high-risk features on resting ECG or troponin testing, they should be referred for coronary angiography.

- *Should stress testing be done with cardiac imaging in all patients?* No. The majority of low-risk patients in our experience can be evaluated with exercise ECG alone. Myocardial scintigraphy or echocardiography adds expense and in most cases is unnecessary. The exceptions would be in patients with uninterpretable ECGs and those unable to exercise.

- *Should patients undergo a "formal rule out" with serial cardiac injury markers prior to stress testing?* Although the data are growing, there is no consensus about what constitutes an adequate observation time or the optimal selection or timing of cardiac injury markers needed to exclude MI (see Chap. 8). Our experience with IETT in rigorously selected low-risk patients suggest testing is safe and effective after a single set of markers (troponin/myoglobin) drawn at presentation. Using this approach, those patients

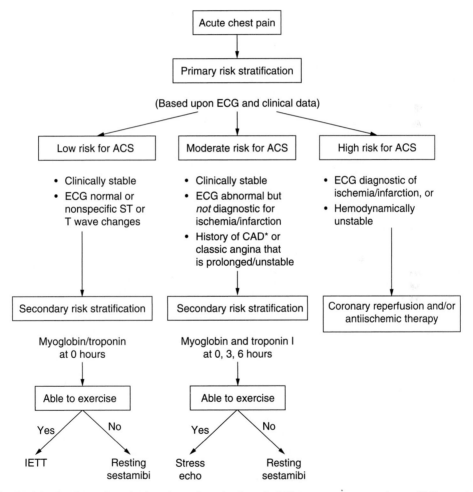

Fig. 18-3. Algorithm for diagnostic testing in a chest pain evaluation unit. ACS = acute coronary syndrome; CAD = coronary artery disease; ECG = electrocardiogram; Echo = echocardiography; IETT = immediate exercise treadmill test; resting sestamibi = resting technetium-99m sestamibi myocardial perfusion imaging. Asterisk (*) indicates patients with a history of CAD and atypical chest pain who have a normal ECG may be candidates for IETT. (Source: Adapted with permission from Kirk JD, Diercks DB, Turnipseed SD, Amsterdam EA. Evaluation of chest pain suspicious for acute coronary syndrome: Use of an accelerated diagnostic protocol in a chest pain evaluation unit. *Am J Cardiol* 2000;85:40B–48B.)

with ACS not identified at presentation are accurately identified by stress testing without any complications. A more conservative approach may include serial cardiac injury marker testing over a 4–6 hours period prior to stress testing.

REFERENCES

1. Kirk JD, Diercks DB, Turnipseed SD, et al. Evaluation of chest pain suspicious for ACS: Use of an ADP in a chest pain evaluation unit. *Am J Cardiol* 2000;85(5A):40B–48B.
2. Amsterdam EA, Lewis WR, Kirk JD, et al. Acute ischemic syndromes: Chest pain center concept. *Cardiol Clin* 2001;20(1):117–136.
3. Braunwald E, Antman E, Beasley JW, et al. ACC/AHA guidelines for the management of patients with unstable angina and on-ST segment elevation myocardial infarction. *J Am Coll Cardiol* 2000;36:970–1062.
4. Hutter AM, Amsterdam EA, Jaffe AS. Task force 2: ACSs: Section 2B-Chest discomfort evaluation in the hospital, 31st Bethesda Conference. *J Am Coll Cardiol* 2000;35: 853–862.
5. Lee TH, Goldman L. Evaluation of the patient with acute chest pain. *N Engl J Med* 2000;342:1187–1195.
6. Pope JH, Aufderheide TP, Ruthazer R, et al. Missed diagnoses of acute cardiac ischemia in the emergency department. *N Engl J Med* 2000;342:1163.
7. Karcz A, Holbrook J, Burke MC, et al. Massachusetts emergency medicine closed malpractice claims: 1988–1990. *Ann Emerg Med* 1993;22:553–559.
8. Gibler WB, Runyon JP, Levy RC, et al. A rapid diagnostic and treatment center for patients with chest pain the emergency department. *Ann Emerg Med* 1995;25:1–8.
9. Zalenski RJ, Rydman RJ, McCarren M, et al. Feasibility of a rapid diagnostic protocol for an emergency department chest pain unit. *Ann Emerg Med* 1997;29:99–108.
10. Mikhail MG, Smith FA, Gray M, et al. Cost-effectiveness of mandatory stress testing in chest pain center patients. *Ann Emerg Med* 1997;29:88–98.
11. Gomez MA, Anderson JL, Karagounis LA, et al. An emergency department-based protocol for rapidly ruling out myocardial ischemia reduces hospital time and expense: Results of a randomized study (ROMIO). *J Am Coll Cardiol* 1996;28:25–33.
12. Farkouh ME, Smars PA, Reeder GS, et al. A clinical trial of a chest-pain observation unit for patients with unstable angina: Chest pain evaluation in the emergency room (CHEER) investigators. *N Engl J Med* 1998;339:1882–1888.
13. Chaitman BR. The changing role of the exercise electrocardiogram as a diagnostic test for chronic ischemic heart disease. *J Am Coll Cardiol* 1986;8:1195.
14. Weiner DA, Ryan TJ, McCabe CH, et al. Prognostic importance of a clinical profile and exercise test in medically treated patients with coronary artery disease. *J Am Coll Cardiol* 1984;3:772.
15. Gibbons RJ, Balady GJ, Bricker JT, et al. ACC/AHA 2002 guideline update for exercise testing: Summary article: A report of the American College of Cardiology/American Heart Association Task Force on Practice Guidelines (Committee to Update the 1997 Exercise Testing Guidelines). *Circulation* 2002;106:1883.
16. Myers J, Prakash M, Froelicher V, et al. Exercise capacity and mortality among men referred for exercise testing. *N Engl J Med* 2002;346:793.
17. Mark DB, Hlatky MA, Harrell FE Jr., et al. Exercise treadmill score for predicting prognosis in coronary artery disease. *Ann Intern Med* 1987;106:793.
18. Shaw LJ, Peterson ED, Shaw LK, et al. Use of a prognostic treadmill score in identifying diagnostic coronary disease subgroups. *Circulation* 1998;98:1622.
19. McNeer JF, Margolis JR, Lee KL, et al. The role of the exercise test in the evaluation of patients for ischemic heart disease. *Circulation* 1978;57:64.
20. Cole CR, Blackstone EH, Pashkow FJ, et al. Heart-rate recovery immediately after exercise as a predictor of mortality. *N Engl J Med* 1999;341:1351.
21. Okin PM, Kligfield P. Heart rate adjustment of ST segment depression and performance of the exercise electrocardiogram: A critical evaluation. *J Am Coll Cardiol* 1995; 25:1726–1735.
22. Lee TH, Cook EF, Weisberg M, et al. Acute chest pain in the emergency room: Identification and examination of low-risk patients. *Arch Intern Med* 1985;145:65.
23. Goldman L, Cook EF, Johnson PA, et al. Prediction of the need for intensive care in patients who come to emergency departments with acute chest pain. *N Engl J Med* 1996; 334:1498.
24. Brush JE Jr., Brand DA, Acampora D, et al. Use of the initial electrocardiogram to predict in-hospital complications of acute myocardial infarction. *N Engl J Med* 1980;312:1137–1141.
25. Braunwald E, Jones RH, Mark DB, et al. Diagnosing and managing unstable angina. Agency for Health Care Policy and Research. *Circulation* 1994;90:613–622.
26. Lewis WR, Amsterdam EA. Utilities and safety of immediate exercise treadmill test of low-risk patients admitted to the hospital for suspected AMI. *Am J Cardiol* 1994;74:987–990.
27. Kirk JD, Turnipseed SD, Lewis WR, et al. Evaluation of chest pain in low risk patients presenting to the emergency department: The role of immediate exercise testing. *Ann Emerg Med* 1998;32:1–7.
28. Stein RA, Chaitman BR, Balady GJ. Safety and utility of exercise testing in emergency room chest pain centers: An advisory from the Committee on Exercise, Rehabilitation, and Prevention, Council on Clinical Cardiology, American Heart Association. *Circulation* 2000;102:1463.
29. Diercks DB, Gibler WB, Liu T, et al. Identification of patients at risk by graded exercise testing in an emergency department chest pain center. *Am J Cardiol* 2000;86(3):289–292.
30. Polanczyk CA, Johnson PA, Hartley LH, et al. Clinical correlates and prognostic significance of early negative exercise

tolerance test in patients with acute chest pain seen in the hospital emergency department. *Am J Cardiol* 1998;81:288.

31. Graff LG, Dallara, J, Ross MA, et al. Impact on the care of the emergency department chest pain patients from the chest pain evaluation registry (CHEPER) study. *Am J Cardiol* 1997;80:563.

32. Graff L, Joseph T, Andelman R, et al. American College of emergency Physicians Information Paper: Chest pain units in emergency departments: A report from the short-term observation services section. American College of Emergency Physicians. *Am J Cardiol* 1995;76(14):1036–1039.

33. Tsakonis JS, Shesser R, Rosenthal R, et al. Safety of immediate treadmill testing in selected emergency department patients with chest pain: A preliminary report. *Am J Emerg Med* 1991;9:557–559.

34. Kerns JR, Shaub TF, Fontanarosa PB. Emergency cardiac stress testing in the evaluation of Emergency department patients with atypical chest pain. *Ann Emerg Med* 1993; 22:794–798.

35. Amsterdam EA, Kirk JD, Diercks DB, et al. Immediate exercise testing for assessment of clinical risk in patients presenting to the emergency department with chest pain: Results in 1,000 patients. *J Am Coll Cardiol* 2002;40:251–256.

36. Kirk JD, Turnipseed SD, Diercks DB, et al. Interpretation of immediate exercise treadmill test: Inter-reader reliability between cardiologist and noncardiologist in a chest pain evaluation unit. *Ann Emerg Med* 2000;36:10–14.

37. Lewis WR, Amsterdam EA, Turnipseed SD, et al. Immediate exercise testing of low risk patients with known coronary artery disease presenting to the emergency department with chest pain. *J Am Coll Cardiol* 1999;33(7):1843–1847.

38. Diercks DB, Kirk JD, Onisko N, et al. Patients with diabetes can undergo immediate exercise treadmill testing in a chest pain evaluation unit. *Acad Emerg Med* 2003 (Abstract).

39. Diercks DB, Kirk JD, Turnipseed SD, et al. Utility of exercise treadmill testing in patients on beta-blockers and calcium channel blockers in a chest pain evaluation unit. *Am J Cardiol* 2002;90:882–885.

19

Cutting Edge Imaging Technologies for Identifying and Risk Stratifying Suspected Acute Coronary Syndrome Patients in the Emergency Department

Joseph P. Ornato
James L. Tatum
Michael C. Kontos

INTRODUCTION

Over 7.5 million Americans have had an acute myocardial infarction (AMI)[1] and there are an estimated 1.1 million new cases each year.[2] A variety of treatment options (e.g., fibrinolysis, antiplatelet therapy, percutaneous coronary angioplasty) are available that can reduce mortality and morbidity, particularly for patients with acute ST-segment elevation myocardial infarction (STEMI), but the effectiveness of these therapies diminishes rapidly within the first several hours following symptoms onset.[3] There is increasing evidence that aggressive, time-sensitive treatment of "high-risk" patients with a non-STEMI ACS, such as unstable angina or non-STEMI, can also affect outcome favorably.[4]

There are two major goals for evaluating ED patients who present with a possible ACS: (1) STEMI, non-STEMI, and unstable angina detection and (2) risk stratification. Because the "standard evaluation," consisting of a history, physical examination, and an ECG, can only identify 60–70% of these patients initially, emergency physicians can benefit from the use of various new cutting edge imaging technologies. The purpose of this chapter will be to describe four emerging technologies: (1) radionuclide MPI; (2) coronary calcium scoring using electron beam computerized tomography (EBCT); (3) cardiac magnetic resonance imaging (MRI); and (4) electrocardiographic ST-segment body map imaging.

RADIONUCLIDE MYOCARDIAL PERFUSION IMAGING

SPECT using ^{99m}technetium sestamibi or tetrofosmin is becoming increasingly popular for evaluating suspected ACS patients who have a normal or nondiagnostic ECG in the ED.[5–12] Both agents are taken up actively by the myocardium in proportion to blood flow, functioning like "chemical microspheres." MPI can identify MI and ACS patients accurately, and it can help to risk stratify chest pain patients.[5,9,12–20]

HIGH YIELD FACTS

- The diagnostic accuracy of acute myocardial perfusion imaging (MPI) in the evaluation of emergency department (ED) chest pain patients has sensitivities of 90–100%, and negative predictive values >99% for excluding acute coronary syndrome (ACS) and the occurrence of short-term cardiac events.

- Single photon emission computerized tomography (SPECT)-gated MPI is most accurate when patients are injected during active chest pain, but even if delayed by 6 hours, the sensitivity is significantly higher than that of the initial electrocardiogram (ECG) (35%).

- In males younger than 44 and females younger than 59, fewer than 25% of patients have detectable calcium. In contrast, even in an asymptomatic population, the majority of men older than 50 and women older than 65 have coronary calcium.

- Newer magnetic resonance imaging scanners have the potential to visualize coronary arteries, measure coronary flow reserve noninvasively, and detect significant atherosclerotic narrowing in the left main and left anterior descending (LAD) coronary arteries.

- Eighty-lead body surface ECG mapping may provide better detection of acute ischemia in those areas where the standard 12-lead ECG is insensitive (e.g., the posterior left ventricle, right ventricle).

Studies examining the diagnostic accuracy of acute MPI in the evaluation of ED chest pain patients have consistently found sensitivities of 90–100%, and negative predictive values >99% for excluding ACS and the occurrence of short-term cardiac events.[21–26] Although most studies were performed with sestamibi, comparable results have been obtained with tetrofosmin.[26] This high negative predictive value allows for the safe ED discharge of lower-risk patients in a time frame significantly shorter than a standard chest pain evaluation unit (CPEU) admission.

In contrast to prior studies, Tatum et al. examined the utility of a chest pain evaluation strategy in which acute MPI was used to further risk stratify lower-risk chest pain patients.[27] A total of 1187 consecutive patients who presented with a chief complaint of chest pain seen in the ED at Virginia Commonwealth University Medical Center in Richmond, VA were included in the analysis. Within 60 min of presentation, each patient was assigned to one of five levels on the basis of his or her risk of MI or ACS: level 1, ST-elevation MI; level 2, non-ST-elevation MI/ACS; level 3, probable ACS; level 4, possible ACS; and level 5, noncardiac chest pain. In the lower-risk levels (3 and 4), immediate resting MPI was used as a risk stratification tool alone (level 4) or in combination with serial markers (level 3). Sensitivity of immediate resting MPI for MI was 100% (95% confidence interval [CI], 64–100%) and specificity 78% (74–82%). In patients with abnormal imaging findings, risk for MI (7% vs. 0%, $P < 0.001$; relative risk [RR], 50; 95% CI, 2.8–2.89) and for MI or revascularization (32% vs. 2%, $P < 0.001$; RR, 15.5; 95% CI, 6.4–36) was significantly higher than in patients with normal imaging findings. During 1-year follow-up, patients with normal imaging findings ($n = 338$) had an event rate of 3% (revascularization) with no MI or death (combined events: negative predictive value, 97%; 95% CI, 95–98%). Patients with abnormal imaging findings ($n = 100$) had a 42% event rate (combined events: RR, 14.2; 95% CI, 6.5–30; $P < 0.001$), with 11% experiencing MI and 8% cardiac death. It was concluded that a comprehensive risk stratification strategy employing SPECT-gated MPI could help emergency physicians to triage low-risk chest pain patients.

Although observational studies indicated that rest MPI was a valuable technique, it remained to be proven in a randomized-controlled trial in a prospective fashion. To address this limitation, Udelson et al. conducted a prospective, randomized-controlled trial to determine the accuracy and cost-benefit of MPI in the ED at seven academic medical centers and community hospitals.[5] Between July 1997 and May 1999, 2475 adult ED patients with chest pain or other symptoms suggestive of acute cardiac ischemia and with a normal or nondi-

agnostic initial ECG were randomly assigned to receive either the usual ED evaluation strategy ($n = 1260$) or the usual strategy supplemented with results from acute resting Tc-99m sestamibi SPECT-gated MPI ($n = 1215$). Results were interpreted in real time by local staff physicians and were provided to the ED physician for incorporation into clinical decision making. MPI reduced unnecessary hospitalizations significantly among patients without acute ischemia without reducing appropriate admission for patients with acute ischemia. There were no differences in ED triage disposition decisions between acute MI or ACS patients receiving standard evaluation and those whose evaluation was supplemented by a sestamibi scan in patients without an acute MI or ACS ($n = 329$). Among patients with acute MI ($n = 56$), 97% versus 96% were hospitalized (RR, 1.00; 95% CI, 0.89–1.12), and among those with ACS ($n = 273$), 83% versus 81% were hospitalized (RR, 0.98; 95% CI, 0.87–1.10). In non-ACS patients ($n = 2146$), hospitalization was 52% with usual care versus 42% with sestamibi imaging (RR, 0.84; 95% CI, 0.77–0.92).

An important advantage of acute MPI compared to markers is the ability to define the risk area. This can be large, even in the absence of ischemic ECG changes. In a study of 141 patients, lower-risk patients diagnosed with MI after undergoing ED MPI, the ischemic risk area ranged from 0 to 62% of the left ventricle, with a mean risk area of $18 \pm 11\%$, a value similar to that of patients with inferior ST-elevation MI.[6] Patients with an entirely normal ECG had relatively large risk areas ($16 \pm 12\%$).[28]

These studies have established the effectiveness of technetium-based MPI for the evaluation of chest pain patients. Its major role is in the evaluation of lower-risk patients who do not have ischemic ECG changes or high-risk clinical features. Recent ACC/AHA/ANSC guidelines indicate that when used for the assessment of risk in possible ACS patients with nondiagnostic ECG, MPI is a class IA recommendation.[29] The guideline stipulates that it is most appropriate in patients who have "possible" ACS following an initial triage based on the symptoms, ECG, and history. In this situation, rest MPI is useful for identifying patients at high risk who should be admitted and those at low risk who can be discharged home.

Despite the obvious advantages of this technique, a number of limitations of acute MPI should be recognized. SPECT-gated MPI is most accurate when patients are injected during active chest pain.[30] However, the test can remain abnormal for several hours following transient myocardial ischemia even when normal flow is restored in an epicardial coronary artery.[31] In an early study, Bilodeau et al. reported a 96% sensitivity of MPI for detecting coronary artery disease (CAD) in 25 patients imaged during chest pain.[32] When the same patients were reinjected later (while pain free), the sensitivity was 65%. In both cases, the sensitivity was significantly higher than that of the initial ECG (35%). Kontos et al. found no difference in sensitivity for identifying patients with acute MI, significant CAD, or the need for revascularization when patients with and without symptoms were injected within 6 hours of their last symptomatic episode.[18]

An alternative strategy for evaluating patients who are chest pain free, which uses dual isotope imaging with thallium and sestamibi, was initially validated by Alazraki and colleagues[33] and modified by Fesmire et al.[34,35] Low-risk patients who are pain free at the time of initial evaluation are injected with thallium and undergo immediate imaging. If negative, stress MPI is performed right after. For moderate risk patients but still having a nonischemic ECG, Fesmire et al. added a rapid MI exclusion protocol using serial marker testing over 2 hours prior to stress testing.[34,35] The use of dual imaging allows testing to be completed in a rapid fashion. This protocol has the advantage of completing the patient work-up in a short time period without intervening discharge. However, to be feasible, it requires a stress laboratory with the flexibility to add additional tests on short notice, which may not be applicable to high volume laboratories.

A common misconception is that the perfusion defects resulting from ischemia should resolve quickly after resolution of ischemia. In contrast to stress testing in which decreased flow occurs transiently, flow abnormalities often persist in patients with ACS. Ischemia in patients with ACS is caused by thrombotic occlusion, which in conjunction with complex coronary morphology results in further coronary blood flow reductions.[36,37] Another potential mechanism was demonstrated by Fram et al. who found persistent perfusion abnormalities following successful percutaneous coronary intervention (PCI) in patients injected with ^{99m}Tc sestamibi at varying time intervals after PCI.[31] This study suggests that transient ischemia induces alterations that persist even after flow is returned to normal.

Although studies have consistently demonstrated a high sensitivity, acute MPI is imperfect. There is a minimal amount of myocardium that needs to be ischemic before it can be detected by current imaging technologies. This is approximately 3–4% of the left ventricle.[38] Because most prior studies included small numbers of patients who had MI, estimates of sensitivity were wide. This was addressed in a large cohort of 141 patients diagnosed with CK-MB MI. The overall sensitivity, 89% (95% CI, 83–94%), was slightly lower than reported in prior studies, but likely provides a more accurate estimate of the technology's true sensitivity.[11]

In recognition of its superior sensitivity and specificity compared to other cardiac markers, troponin has become the new gold standard for diagnosing MI. As might be expected, when compared to a more sensitive marker, such as troponin, sensitivity of MPI is lower. In a large study of 266 consecutive patients who underwent acute rest MPI who had TnI elevations detected on serial sampling after undergoing our standard chest pain evaluation protocol, we found a sensitivity of only 75%.[39] An important consideration is that despite being negative, MPI could still identify these patients as lower risk, as the absence of perfusion abnormalities predicted a smaller MI. For example, among the 66 patients with negative MPI, 37 (56%) had a peak CK-MB of <8 ng/mL, which was the former institutional threshold value for MI, and therefore would previously considered to have unstable angina, not MI. Similarly, almost three quarters of patients with negative MPI had peak CK values <300 U/L. In addition, patients with negative MPI but elevated TnI had higher ejection fractions ($55 \pm 15\%$ vs. $47 \pm 12\%$, $P < 0.01$) and were less likely to have significant disease (62% vs. 83%, $P < 0.01$) than those with positive MPI.

MPI should be considered complementary, rather than competitive, with cardiac markers since the latter cannot identify ischemia in the absence of myocardial necrosis. Because of this, the sensitivity of MPI for identifying nonnecrosis events, such as revascularization or significant CAD is higher than that of troponin.[20,40] In addition, rest MPI results are generally available within 1–2 hours after injection. In contrast, markers of myocardial necrosis such as troponin are not detectable in the blood until several hours after the damage has occurred. To achieve a high sensitivity, sampling of cardiac markers must be performed over an 8–9-hour period.[30,41]

The ability to provide imaging 24 hours a day may be difficult. The hours in which this technology is available can be extended by having the ED physician or radiology technician inject the patient. Imaging can be performed hours later by an on-call technologist because of the lack of redistribution.

The inability to determine whether a perfusion defect is a result of acute MI, acute ischemia, or prior ischemia could be considered a limitation. However, in all these cases they identify a high-risk cohort in whom further evaluation is required. Despite the addition of costly technology, routine use of MPI in the ED setting for evaluating suspected ACS patients appears to be cost-effective. Several observational studies estimated significant cost savings due to changes in disposition made based on the results from acute MPI, as well as a reduction in the performance of coronary angiography in low-risk patients.[42,43] In addition, the large, randomized, multicenter clinical trial conducted by Udelson et al. showed that aggressive use of MPI in the ED can be highly cost-effective, reducing overall cost per patient by approximately $70 due to the higher number of individuals who could be discharged home safely directly from the ED.[5,44]

CORONARY CALCIUM SCORING

Coronary artery calcification is almost invariably associated with atherosclerotic plaque formation.[45] This can be detected and accurately quantified using EBCT. The prevalence of angiographic disease in patients without detectable coronary calcium is less than 1%, regardless of age or sex in individuals who have a low risk of cardiovascular events.[46,47] This has obvious implications for the evaluation of the low-risk chest pain patient.

Until recently, EBCT's primary use has been to screen asymptomatic individuals who have coronary risk factors for the presence of developing coronary atherosclerosis. EBCT has a diagnostic accuracy similar or superior to exercise treadmill testing for identifying angiographically significant CAD.[48,49] Shavelle et al. studied 97 patients who underwent technetium stress testing, treadmill-ECG, and EBCT coronary scanning within 3 months of coronary angiography for the evaluation of chest pain.[49] The RR of obstructive angiographic CAD for an abnormal test was higher for EBCT (4.53) than either treadmill-ECG (1.72) or technetium stress (1.96). The low specificity of EBCT (47%) was improved by the addition of treadmill-ECG (83%, $P < 0.05$). Schmermund et al. examined to 323 patients with a normal rest ECG and no history of CAD who were referred for coronary angiography.[48] The sensitivity of exercise treadmill testing was 50% with a specificity of 84%, compared with EBCT sensitivities ranging from 78 to 90% and specificities of 69 to 82%, depending on the calcium score cut point chosen. The calcium score also correlates with the degree of ischemia shown on SPECT-gated MPI regardless of age or gender.[50]

The limited availability and cost of an EBCT scanner is a potential limitation to its applicability. However, software has been developed which can be added to multidetector computed tomography (MDCT) for coronary calcification. Thus, coronary calcium quantitation can be extended to the large number of hospitals that currently have MDCT. MDCT has been found to have a high diagnostic accuracy for detecting coronary calcium[51] and was similar to EBCT in comparative studies.[52]

Given the high association of coronary calcium with atherosclerosis, it is not surprising that a potential application would be for evaluating low-risk chest pain patients. Current experience with EBCT for risk stratification of suspected ACS patients in the ED is limited to a few small case series. Laudon et al. conducted a prospective observational study of 105 women aged 40–65 years and men aged 30–55 years who presented to the ED with angina-like chest pain requiring admission to the hospital or chest pain observation unit.[8] All patients underwent EBCT along with other cardiac testing (treadmill exercise testing in 58, coronary angiography in 25, radionuclide stress testing in 19, and echocardiography in 11). Results of EBCT and cardiac testing were negative for both in 53 patients (53%), positive for both in 14 (14%), positive for tomography and negative for cardiac testing in 32 (32%), and negative for tomography and positive for cardiac testing in only 1 patient. This positive test result, on a treadmill exercise test, was ruled a false positive by an independent staff cardiologist. Two other female patients with normal exercise sestamibi or coronary angiography and EBCT findings also had false positive treadmill exercise results. The sensitivity of EBCT was 100% (95% CI, 77–100%), with a negative predictive value of 100% (95% CI, 94–100%). Specificity was 63% (95% CI, 54–75%). McLaughlin et al. found that EBCT had a 98% negative predictive value in 137 patients without a history of CAD who presented to the ED with chest pain. EBCT was negative in 36% of these patients, one of whom had an acute MI.[53]

One limitation pertinent to evaluating chest pain patients is the high frequency of coronary calcium in asymptomatic patients. In males younger than 44 and females younger than 59, fewer than 25% of patients have detectable calcium. In contrast, even in an asymptomatic population, the majority of men older than 50 and women older than 65 have coronary calcium. This likely contributed to the low specificity found in prior studies.[8,53]

Another limitation of coronary calcium is that it may not detect fissure or erosion of noncalcified plaque.[54,55] Studies have confirmed that coronary calcium is not invariably present in patients with MI. Pohle et al. measured coronary calcium in 1032 patients under 60 years of age diagnosed with MI.[56] Patients with MI had a coronary calcium score greater than the 50th percentile in 87%, and was above the 90th percentile in 61%. However, 5% of patients with MI had no detectable calcium. Similar results were reported by Mascala et al.[57] in 120 patients diagnosed with MI.[57] Coronary calcium was absent in 6 of 120 patients (5%). Importantly, however, only one had obstructive disease on angiography, suggesting that the MI in these patients occurred from a mechanism different from traditional plaque rupture.

The use of rest MPI in conjunction with ECG overcomes this limitation. Therefore, optimal usage of this imaging technique may be in younger patients in whom rest MPI is negative. A low-risk calcium score would negate the need for subsequent stress testing. When used in low to intermediate risk patients, this approach could be cost-effective.[57] The advantage of this diagnostic strategy is that entire risk stratification process can be completed in just a few hours—24 hours a day. In addition, coronary calcium scoring may provide better long-term prediction of coronary events than stress testing.

CARDIAC MAGNETIC RESONANCE IMAGING

Cardiac MRI is an exciting new technology, which has the potential to complete the entire stress evaluation in one setting. Ischemia and infarction can be detected with a high sensitivity, by the presence of wall motion abnormalities. Newer contrast agents allow assessment of perfusion. If this initial evaluation is negative, dobutamine stress MRI could then be performed. Newer scanners have the potential to visualize coronary arteries, measure coronary flow reserve noninvasively, and detect significant atherosclerotic narrowing in the left main and LAD coronary arteries.[58] Early studies indicate that this is possible. In one study, Hundley et al. performed dobutamine stress echocardiography in 153 patients in whom standard echocardiographic windows were considered suboptimal.[58] Sensitivity and specificity were both 83% in the challenging to image patient group. In another study, Hundley et al. studied 30 subjects (23 men, 7 women, age 36–77 years) who underwent MRI of the left main and LAD coronary arteries as well as measurement of flow in the proximal, middle, or distal LAD both at rest and after intravenous adenosine. Immediately thereafter, contrast coronary angiography and intracoronary Doppler assessments of coronary flow reserve were performed. There was a statistically significant correlation between MRI assessments of coronary flow reserve and (a) assessments of coronary arterial stenosis severity by quantitative coronary angiography and (b) invasive measurements of coronary flow reserve ($P <$ 0.0001 for both). In comparison to computer-assisted quantitative coronary angiography, the sensitivity and specificity of MRI for identifying a stenosis >70% in the distal left main or proximal/middle LAD arteries was 100% and 83%, respectively.

There has been limited experience with the use of cardiac MRI for evaluating patients with suspected ACS in the ED setting. The largest published series to date is from Kwong et al. who evaluated the diagnostic performance of MRI prospectively in 161 consecutive patients.[21] Enrollment required 30 min of chest pain compatible with myocardial ischemia and an ECG that was not diagnostic of an acute MI. MRI was performed at rest within 12 hours of presentation and included perfusion, left ventricular function, and gadolinium-enhanced MI detection. MRI was interpreted qualitatively and analyzed quantitatively. The sensitivity and specificity, respectively, for detecting ACS were 84% and 85% by MRI, 80% and 61% by an abnormal ECG, 16% and 95% for strict ECG criteria for ischemia (ST depression or T-wave inversion), 40% and 97% for peak troponin I, and 48% and 85% for a thrombolysis in myocardial infarction (TIMI) risk score ≥3. The MRI was more sensitive than strict ECG criteria for ischemia ($P < 0.001$), peak troponin I ($P < 0.001$), and the TIMI risk score ($P = 0.004$), and MRI was more specific than an abnormal ECG ($P < 0.001$). Multivariate logistic regression analysis showed MRI was the strongest predictor of ACS and added diagnostic value over clinical parameters ($P < 0.001$).

Although these results are quite promising, widespread clinical use of MRI in an ED setting is limited by its relatively high cost and the fact that there is low availability of equipment and trained personnel.[22] Since there are no portable systems, cardiac MRI cannot be performed in the ED or at the patient's bedside. Monitoring of patients who potentially have MI is problematic. Cardiac MRI will need to be compared with proven and cost-effective techniques like echocardiography and MPI in large, randomized clinical trials before it can be considered seriously as a tool for emergency physicians in evaluating suspected ACS patients.

ST-SEGMENT BODY MAPPING

The traditional evaluation of ED patients with chest pain or other symptoms suggesting acute cardiac ischemia relies heavily on the patient's history, physical examination, and the standard 12-lead ECG. This approach fails to identify approximately 2% of MI patients and another 2% of those with unstable angina.[2] Such "missed ACS" patients are at relatively high risk of death and/or complications for the next 4–6 weeks following ED discharge.[2,19,23–26]

The standard 12-lead ECG has been the principal tool used to diagnose ACS patients in real time at the bedside since the 1940s. Unfortunately, the 12-lead ECG has significant limitations. The sensitivity of a single 12-lead ECG for diagnosing AMI or unstable angina is relatively poor due to the fact that leads do not cover the lateral, true posterior, and right ventricular locations comprehensively.[59]

A number of strategies have been explored in an effort to increase the diagnostic value of the standard ECG. For example, varying the ST-segment elevation diagnostic criteria can alter the sensitivity and specificity of the ECG substantially. Menown et al. found that the "optimum" model (>1 mm ST-segment elevation in >1 inferior or lateral lead, or >2 mm ST-segment elevation in >1 anteroseptal lead) could correctly classify 83% of subjects with chest pain (56% sensitivity, 94% specificity for acute MI). The degree of ST-segment elevation required to diagnose acute MI in the theoretical model influenced the ECG's sensitivity (45–69%) and specificity (81–98%) markedly.

Performing serial 12-lead ECGs offer modest improvement compared to interpretation of just the initial tracing.[7] The use of additional leads can increase ECG sensitivity for detecting acute MI slightly in both right ventricular and posterior locations.[59-62] Brady et al. examined the diagnostic and therapeutic impact of performing a 15-lead ECG on the management of 595 ED chest pain patients.[59] Although the 15-lead ECG provided a more complete description of myocardial injury, it did not significantly alter the ED diagnosis, initial therapy, or hospital disposition in these adult chest pain patients. Zalenski et al. assessed the accuracy of posterior (V_7 to V_9) and right ventricular (V_4R to V_6R) leads compared with the standard 12-lead ECG in a prospective clinical trial of patients with suspected acute MI.[62] Of 533 study patients, 345 (64.7%) had an acute MI and 24.8% received fibrinolytic therapy. Posterior and right ventricular leads increased sensitivity for acute MI by 8.4% ($P = 0.03$) but decreased specificity by 7.0% ($P = 0.06$). The authors concluded that the standard ECG is not optimal for detecting STEMI, but its accuracy is improved only moderately by the addition of posterior and right ventricular leads.

Until recently, body surface mapping was limited by the inability of computer technology to process multiple leads simultaneously and display the results in a simple-to-interpret, intuitive format. Computer processing limitations necessitated the use of two-dimensional, static, black and white displays. Modern body surface mapping can be used to look for ischemia and/or infarction in suspected ACS patients. At present, the most mature diagnostic platform available for clinical use in the United States is the PRIME ECG 80-lead body surface mapping system.

The body surface mapping ECG system uses 80 leads (64 on the chest and 16 on the back) to collect data (Fig. 19-1). The 80-lead body surface mapping ECG system leads are screen-printed in conductive silver ink onto a disposable vest made up of clear plastic strips that combine at

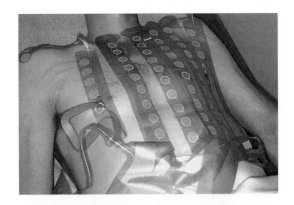

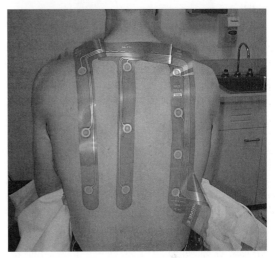

Fig. 19-1. Application of the 80-lead body surface mapping ECG electrodes.

the base to form a single connection. The vest is applied by removing a paper backing to reveal self-adhesive hydrogel pads at each electrode site. The strips can be positioned and secured in 5–7 min, just a few minutes longer than the time needed to acquire a standard 12-lead ECG.

After the strips are in place, the vest is connected to the 80-lead body surface mapping ECG's computer diagnostic unit, and data collection begins. All 80 leads are recorded simultaneously. The device measures the degree of ST-segment elevation or depression in each of the leads and uses algorithms to develop a three-dimensional representation of the human torso on a computer screen. The torso will remain green in color if there is no significant ST-segment elevation or depression (as would be the case in a normal, healthy individual) (Fig. 19-2). Deviations from the 95% CI for normal values at each point on the human

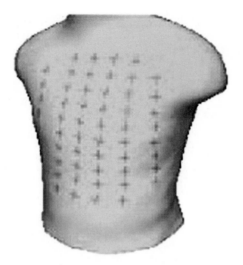

Fig. 19-2. Eighty-lead body surface mapping ECG in a normal healthy person.

chest and abdomen are represented on the screen in red (ST-segment elevation) or blue (ST-segment depression). The degree of ST-segment elevation or depression is represented by the color intensity.

Menown et al. compared the ability of an early version of the 80-lead body surface mapping ECG system with a standard 12-lead ECG to correctly classify 314 patients with chest pain.[63] This early version of the 80-lead body surface mapping ECG system correctly classified 123/160 MI patients (sensitivity 77%) as having an infarction and 131/154 non-MI patients (specificity 85%) as not having an MI.

Since then, much progress has been made in refining the diagnostic criteria for differentiating a normal tracing from normal variants, cardiac ischemia, MI, and a host of other electrocardiographic abnormalities. Ornato et al.[64] conducted a prospective, multicenter, international evaluation of whether the 80-lead body surface mapping ECG system could detect more acute STEMI cases than standard 12-lead ECGs in chest pain patients presenting to hospital EDs in the United States, Northern Ireland, and England. A trained technician at each site performed an ECG and an 80-lead body surface mapping ECG on all consenting adult ED chest pain patients in whom MI or ischemia was suspected clinically. During the study period, 647 patients had an 80-lead body surface mapping ECG recorded along with a standard 12-lead ECG. The most common locations of MI, defined clinically or by biomarker, missed by ECG but detected

by an 80-lead body surface mapping ECG were: (1) CK-MB-MI: 1 septal, 4 posterior (1 infero-posterior), 1 inferior; (2) clinical-MI: 1 septal, 8 posterior (3 infero-posterior), 1 inferior; and (3) TROP-MI: 2 septal, 9 posterior (3 infero-posterior), 1 inferior. The incidence of extensive right ventricular involvement in inferior STEMI detected by an 80-lead body surface mapping ECG but missed by standard ECG was: CK-MB-MI 2/9 (22%), TROP-MI 2/9 (22%), clinical definition of MI 6/18 (33%). The 80-lead body map correctly identified 93% of STEMI cases compared to only 57% with the standard 12-lead ECG ($P < 0.008$). Specificity was not significantly different between the two techniques (95% vs. 97%, body map vs. 12-lead ECG, respectively).

In another study, Menown et al. performed an 80-lead body surface mapping ECG and a standard 12-lead ECG on 62 patients with inferior wall MI.[65] ST-segment elevation >0.1 mV occurred in 26 patients (42 in V_2R or V_4R compared with 36 patients (58%) in >1 electrode on the regional right ventricular map ($P = 0.0019$). ST elevation >0.1 mV occurred in 1 patient (2%) in V_7 or V_9 compared with 17 patients (27%) in >1 electrode on the regional posterior map ($P = 0.00003$). ST-segment elevation >0.05 mV occurred in 6 patients (10%) in V_7 or V_9 compared with 22 patients (36%) in >1 electrode on the regional posterior map ($P = 0.00003$). Patients with ST-segment elevation on the regional RV and/or posterior maps had a trend toward a larger infarct size (mean peak creatinine kinase 1789 ± 226 vs. 1546 ± 392 mmol/L; $P =$ ns). Body surface mapping better classified patients with inferior wall MI accompanied by right ventricular and/or posterior wall involvement when compared with right ventricular or posterior chest leads.

A number of other potential uses for the 80-lead body surface mapping ECG system are emerging. The device can detect reperfusion after treatment with fibrinolytic drugs, and subsequent reocclusion (if it occurs). In a study comparing the ability of the 80-lead body surface mapping ECG system, and the standard 12-lead ECG to detect reperfusion after fibrinolytic therapy in acute MI patients, the 80-lead body surface mapping ECG system identified 97% of patients who achieved reperfusion and 100% of those who did not based on coronary angiographic results as the "gold standard."[66] The 12-lead ECG identified only 59% of patients who achieved reperfusion and only 50% of those who did not.

The ECG body surface mapping can also detect acute MI accurately despite the presence of left bundle branch block.[67] Studies are under way to better define its use in diagnosing ACS patients and during stress testing.

CONCLUSIONS

New cutting edge imaging technologies offer great promise in assisting emergency physicians to diagnose and risk stratify suspected ACS patients. Radionuclide MPI is the most mature technology discussed in this chapter and is being using increasingly throughout the United States in larger EDs. The use of coronary calcium scoring using EBCT, cardiac MRI, and electrocardiographic ST-segment body map imaging are best described as promising but needing further study.

REFERENCES

1. American Heart Association. *2002 Heart and Stroke Statistical Update*. Dallas, TX: American Heart Association National Center, 2002.
2. Pope JH, Aufderheide TP, Ruthazer R, et al. Missed diagnoses of acute cardiac ischemia in the emergency department. *N Engl J Med* 2000;342(16):1163–1170.
3. Cannon CP. Time to treatment: A crucial factor in thrombolysis and primary angioplasty. *J Thromb Thrombolysis* 1996;3(3):249–255.
4. Braunwald E, Antman EM, Beasley JW, et al. ACC/AHA guideline update for the management of patients with unstable angina and non-ST-segment elevation myocardial infarction—2002: Summary article: A report of the American College of Cardiology/American Heart Association Task Force on Practice Guidelines (Committee on the Management of Patients With Unstable Angina). *Circulation* 2002; 106(14):1893–1900.
5. Udelson JE, Beshansky JR, Ballin DS, et al. Myocardial perfusion imaging for evaluation and triage of patients with suspected acute cardiac ischemia: A randomized controlled trial. *JAMA* 2002;288(21):2693–2700.
6. Kontos MC, Kurdziel K, McQueen R, et al. Comparison of 2-dimensional echocardiography and myocardial perfusion imaging for diagnosing myocardial infarction in emergency department patients. *Am Heart J* 2002;143(4):659–667.
7. Lau J, Ioannidis JP, Balk EM, et al. Diagnosing acute cardiac ischemia in the emergency department: A systematic review of the accuracy and clinical effect of current technologies. *Ann Emerg Med* 2001;37(5):453–460.
8. Laudon DA, Vukov LF, Breen JF, et al. Use of electron-beam computed tomography in the evaluation of chest pain patients in the emergency department. *Ann Emerg Med* 1999;33(1):15–21.
9. Kosnik JW, Zalenski RJ, Shamsa F, et al. Resting sestamibi imaging for the prognosis of low-risk chest pain. *Acad Emerg Med* 1999;6(10):998–1004.
10. Kontos MC, Schmidt K, Nicholson CS, et al. Myocardial perfusion imaging with technetium-99m sestamibi in patients with cocaine-associated chest pain. *Ann Emerg Med* 1999;33(6):639–645.
11. Kontos MC, Arrowood JA, Jesse RL, et al. Comparison between 2-dimensional echocardiography and myocardial perfusion imaging in the emergency department in patients with possible myocardial ischemia. *Am Heart J* 1998; 136(4 Pt 1):724–733.
12. Tatum JL, Jesse RL, Kontos MC, et al. Comprehensive strategy for the evaluation and triage of the chest pain patient. *Ann Emerg Med* 1997;29(1):116–125.
13. Varetto T, Cantalupi D, Altieri A, et al. Emergency room technetium 99m sestamibi imaging to rule out acute myocardial ischemic events in patients with nondiagnostic electrocardiograms. *J Am Coll Cardiol* 1993;22(7):1804–1808.
14. Hilton TC, Thompson RC, Williams HJ, et al. Technetium-99m sestamibi myocardial perfusion imaging in the emergency room evaluation of chest pain. *J Am Coll Cardiol* 1994; 23(5):1016–1022.
15. Christian TF, Gibbons RJ. Myocardial perfusion imaging in myocardial infarction and unstable angina. *Cardiol Clin* 1994;12(2):247–260.
16. Tatum JL, Ornato JP, Jesse RL, et al. A diagnostic strategy using Tc-99m sestamibi for evaluation of patients with chest pain in the emergency department. *Circulation* 1994;90:1367.
17. Heller GV, Herman SD, Travin MI, et al. Independent prognostic value of intravenous dipyridamole with technetium-99m sestamibi tomographic imaging in predicting cardiac events and cardiac-related hospital admissions. *J Am Coll Cardiol* 1995; 26(5):1202–1208.
18. Kontos MC, Jesse RL, Schmidt KL, et al. Value of acute rest sestamibi perfusion imaging for evaluation of patients admitted to the emergency department with chest pain. *J Am Coll Cardiol* 1997;30(4):976–982.
19. Jesse RL, Kontos MC. Evaluation of chest pain in the emergency department. *Curr Probl Cardiol* 1997; 22(4):149–236.
20. Kontos MC, Jesse RL, Anderson FP, et al. Comparison of myocardial perfusion imaging and cardiac troponin I in patients admitted to the emergency department with chest pain. *Circulation* 1999;99(16):2073–2078.
21. Kwong RY, Schussheim AE, Rekhraj S, et al. Detecting acute coronary syndrome in the emergency department with cardiac magnetic resonance imaging. *Circulation* 2003; 107(4):531–537.
22. Soman P, Bokor D, Lahiri A. Why cardiac magnetic resonance imaging will not make it. *J Comput Assist Tomogr* 1999; 23(Suppl 1):S143–S149.
23. Storrow AB, Gibler WB. Chest pain centers: Diagnosis of acute coronary syndromes. *Ann Emerg Med* 2000; 35(5):449–461.
24. Karcz A, Korn R, Burke MC, et al. Malpractice claims against emergency physicians in Massachusetts: 1975–1993. *Am J Emerg Med* 1996;14(4):341–345.
25. Graff L. Missed MI diagnosis. *Ann Emerg Med* 1994; 23(1):141–142.
26. McCarthy BD, Beshansky JR, D'Agostino RB, et al. Missed diagnoses of acute myocardial infarction in the emergency

department: Results from a multicenter study. *Ann Emerg Med* 1993;22(3):579–582.

27. Tatum JL, Jesse RL, Kontos MC, et al. Comprehensive strategy for the evaluation and triage of the chest pain patient [see comments]. *Ann Emerg Med* 1997;29(1):116–125.

28. Kontos MC, Kurdziel KA, Ornato JP, et al. A nonischemic electrocardiogram does not always predict a small myocardial infarction: Results with acute myocardial perfusion imaging. *Am Heart J* 2001;141(3):360–366.

29. Wackers FJ, Brown KA, Heller GV, et al. American Society of Nuclear Cardiology position statement on radionuclide imaging in patients with suspected acute ischemic syndromes in the emergency department or chest pain center. *J Nucl Cardiol* 2002;9(2):246–250.

30. Kontos MC, Tatum JL. Imaging in the evaluation of the patient with suspected acute coronary syndrome. *Semin Nucl Med* 2003;33(4):246–258.

31. Fram DB, Azar RR, Ahlberg AW, et al. Duration of abnormal SPECT myocardial perfusion imaging following resolution of acute ischemia: An angioplasty model. *J Am Coll Cardiol* 2003;41(3):452–459.

32. Bilodeau L, Theroux P, Gregoire J, et al. Technetium-99m sestamibi tomography in patients with spontaneous chest pain: Correlations with clinical, electrocardiographic and angiographic findings. *J Am Coll Cardiol* 1991;1:1684–1691.

33. Alazraki NP, Krawczynska EG, Kosinski AS, et al. Prognostic value of thallium-201 single-photon emission computed tomography for patients with multivessel coronary artery disease after, revascularization (the Emory Angioplasty versus Surgery Trial [EAST]. *Am J Cardiol.* 1999 Dec 15;84(12):1369–1374.

34. Fesmire FM, Hughes AD, Fody EP, et al. The Erlanger chest pain evaluation protocol: A one-year experience with serial 12-lead ECG monitoring, two-hour delta serum marker measurements, and selective nuclear stress testing to identify and exclude acute coronary syndromes. *Ann Emerg Med* 2002;40(6):584–594.

35. Fesmire FM, Hughes AD, Stout PK, et al. Selective dual nuclear scanning in low-risk patients with chest pain to reliably identify and exclude acute coronary syndromes. *Ann Emerg Med* 2001;38(3):207–215.

36. Emre A, Ersek B, Gursurer M, et al. Angiographic and scintigraphic (perfusion and electrocardiogram-gated SPECT) correlates of clinical presentation in unstable angina. *Clin Cardiol* 2000;23(7):495–500.

37. Koch KC, vom Dahl J, Kleinhans E, et al. Influence of a platelet GPIIb/IIIa receptor antagonist on myocardial hypoperfusion during rotational atherectomy as assessed by myocardial Tc-99m sestamibi scintigraphy. *J Am Coll Cardiol* 1999;33(4):998–1004.

38. O'Connor MK, Hammell T, Gibbons RJ. In vitro validation of a simple tomographic technique for estimation of percentage myocardium at risk using methoxyisobutyl isonitrile technetium 99m (sestamibi). *Eur J Nucl Med* 1990;17(1/2):69–76.

39. Kontos MC, Fratkin MJ, Jesse RL, et al. Rest myocardial perfusion imaging results in patients with troponin I elevations. *J Am Coll Cardiol* 2002;39:332A.

40. Duca MD, Giri S, Wu AH, et al. Comparison of acute rest myocardial perfusion imaging and serum markers of myocardial injury in patients with chest pain syndromes. *J Nucl Cardiol* 1999;6(6):570–576.

41. de Winter RJ, Koster RW, Sturk A, et al. Value of myoglobin, troponin T, and CK-MB mass in ruling out an acute myocardial infarction in the emergency room. *Circulation* 1995;92(12):3401–3407.

42. Kontos MC, Schmidt KL, McCue M, et al. A comprehensive strategy for the evaluation and triage of the chest pain patient: A cost comparison study. *J Nucl Cardiol* 2003;10(3):284–290.

43. Radensky PW, Hilton TC, Fulmer H, et al. Potential cost effectiveness of initial myocardial perfusion imaging for assessment of emergency department patients with chest pain. *Am J Cardiol* 1997;79(5):595–599.

44. McGuire DK, Hudson MP, East MA, et al. Highlights from the American Heart Association 72nd Scientific Sessions: November 6 to 10, 1999. *Am Heart J* 2000;139(2 Pt 1): 359–370.

45. McCarthy JH, Palmer FJ. Incidence and significance of coronary artery calcification. *Br Heart J* 1974;36(5):499–506.

46. Haberl R, Becker A, Leber A, et al. Correlation of coronary calcification and angiographically documented stenoses in patients with suspected coronary artery disease: Results of 1,764 patients. *J Am Coll Cardiol* 2001;37(2):451–457.

47. Raggi P, Callister TQ, Cooil B, et al. Identification of patients at increased risk of first unheralded acute myocardial infarction by electron-beam computed tomography. *Circulation* 2000;101(8):850–855.

48. Schmermund A, Mohlenkamp S, Stang A, et al. Assessment of clinically silent atherosclerotic disease and established and novel risk factors for predicting myocardial infarction and cardiac death in healthy middle-aged subjects: Rationale and design of the Heinz Nixdorf RECALL Study. Risk Factors, Evaluation of Coronary Calcium and Lifestyle. *Am Heart J* 2002;144(2):212–218.

49. Shavelle DM, Budoff MJ, LaMont DH, et al. Exercise testing and electron beam computed tomography in the evaluation of coronary artery disease. *J Am Coll Cardiol* 2000;36(1):32–38.

50. He ZX, Hedrick TD, Pratt CM, et al. Severity of coronary artery calcification by electron beam computed tomography predicts silent myocardial ischemia. *Circulation* 2000; 101(3):244–251.

51. Broderick LS, Shemesh J, Wilensky RL, et al. Measurement of coronary artery calcium with dual-slice helical CT compared with coronary angiography: Evaluation of CT scoring methods, interobserver variations, and reproducibility. AJR *Am J Roentgenol* 1996;167(2):439–444.

52. Carr JJ, Crouse JR 3rd, Goff DC Jr., et al. Evaluation of subsecond gated helical CT for quantification of coronary

artery calcium and comparison with electron beam CT. *AJR Am J Roentgenol* 2000;174(4):915–921.

53. McLaughlin VV, Balogh T, Rich S. Utility of electron beam computed tomography to stratify patients presenting to the emergency room with chest pain. *Am J Cardiol* 1999; 84(3):327–328.

54. O'Rourke RA, Brundage BH, Froelicher VF, et al. American College of Cardiology/American Heart Association Expert Consensus document on electron-beam computed tomography for the diagnosis and prognosis of coronary artery disease. *Circulation* 2000;102(1):126–140.

55. O'Rourke RA, Brundage BH, Froelicher VF, et al. American College of Cardiology/American Heart Association Expert Consensus Document on electron-beam computed tomography for the diagnosis and prognosis of coronary artery disease. *J Am Coll Cardiol* 2000;36(1):326–340.

56. Pohle K, Ropers D, Maffert R, et al. Coronary calcifications in young patients with first, unheralded myocardial infarction: A risk factor matched analysis by electron beam tomography. *Heart* 2003;89(6):625–628.

57. Mascola A, Ko J, Bakhsheshi H, et al. Electron beam tomography comparison of culprit and non-culprit coronary arteries in patients with acute myocardial infarction. *Am J Cardiol*. 2000 Jun 1;85(11):1357–1359.

58. Hundley WG, Hamilton CA, Clarke GD, et al. Visualization and functional assessment of proximal and middle left anterior descending coronary stenoses in humans with magnetic resonance imaging. *Circulation* 1999;99(25):3248–3254.

59. Brady WJ, Hwang V, Sullivan R, et al. A comparison of 12- and 15-lead ECGS in ED chest pain patients: Impact on diagnosis, therapy, and disposition. *Am J Emerg Med* 2000;18(3):239–243.

60. Wung SF, Drew B. Comparison of 18-lead ECG and selected body surface potential mapping leads in determining maximally deviated ST lead and efficacy in detecting acute myocardial ischemia during coronary occlusion. *J Electrocardiol* 1999;32(Suppl):30–37.

61. Zalenski RJ, Cooke D, Rydman R, et al. Assessing the diagnostic value of an ECG containing leads V4R, V8, and V9: The 15-lead ECG. *Ann Emerg Med* 1993;22(5):786–793.

62. Zalenski RJ, Rydman RJ, Sloan EP, et al. Value of posterior and right ventricular leads in comparison to the standard 12-lead electrocardiogram in evaluation of ST-segment elevation in suspected acute myocardial infarction. *Am J Cardiol* 1997;79(12):1579–1585.

63. Menown IB, Patterson RS, MacKenzie G, et al. Body-surface map models for early diagnosis of acute myocardial infarction. *J Electrocardiol* 1998;31(Suppl):180–188.

64. Ornato JP, Menown IB, Riddell JW, et al. 80-lead body map detects acute ST-elevation myocardial infarction missed by standard 12-lead electrocardiography. *J Am Coll Cardiol* 2002;39(5):332A.

65. Menown IB, Allen J, Anderson JM, et al. Early diagnosis of right ventricular or posterior infarction associated with inferior wall left ventricular acute myocardial infarction. *Am J Cardiol* 2000;85(8):934–938.

66. Menown IB, Allen J, Anderson JM, et al. Noninvasive assessment of reperfusion after fibrinolytic therapy for acute myocardial infarction. *Am J Cardiol* 2000;86(7):736–741.

67. Menown IB, Mackenzie G, Adgey AA. Optimizing the initial 12-lead electrocardiographic diagnosis of acute myocardial infarction. *Eur Heart J* 2000;21(4):275–283.

20

Ventricular Dysrhythmias

Jason Knight
John Sarko

HIGH YIELD FACTS

- Because of the difficulty in distinguishing between ventricular tachycardia (VT) and supraventricular tachycardia (SVT) with aberrant conduction, wide complex tachycardia should be treated as VT.

- Patients who present with syncope or near syncope who have a right bundle branch block pattern with ST elevations in leads V_1 to V_3 on the ECG may have had an episode of torsades des pointes and must be admitted for electrophysiology testing to rule out the Brugada syndrome.

- Treat torsades des pointes with magnesium and overdrive pacing, and remember to correct any underlying abnormalities that may have precipitated it.

- Unstable patients with VT and all patients with ventricular fibrillation (VF) must be treated immediately with cardioversion/defibrillation. The longer the VF is allowed to exist, the more difficult it is to convert.

INTRODUCTION

The evaluation and management of ventricular arrhythmias have undergone dramatic changes in recent years. New data have changed the way emergency physicians and cardiologists diagnose and treat ventricular arrhythmias in the emergency department. The morbidity and mortality of specific ventricular dysrhythmias has been further elucidated and the risk-benefit ratio of antiarrhythmic drug treatment has been changed based on studies such as the Cardiac Arrhythmia Suppression Trial (CAST) trial.[1] A thorough understanding of the diagnosis and treatment of ventricular dysrhythmias is a necessary skill for practicing emergency physicians.

NORMAL CARDIAC CONDUCTION

Normal depolarization and impulse conduction is central to maintaining cardiac output. There are two types of cells found in the heart: (1) cells responsible for impulse generation and conduction and (2) cells responsible for contraction. Depolarization of the myocardium begins in the sinoatrial (SA) node. The SA node is located in the anterosuperior portion of the right atrium. Blood supply to the SA node is through the SA nodal artery, which arises from the right coronary artery (RCA) in 55% of the population, the circumflex in 35% of people, and both in 10%. The SA node is innervated by the sympathetic and parasympathetic nervous systems.

The impulse is generated by a specialized group of cells that have the ability to depolarize spontaneously. The initial depolarization of the SA node is not seen on the ECG; the P wave is generated when the impulse spreads throughout the atria. There is not a specific conduction system in the atria to convey the SA node impulse to the atrioventricular (AV) node. The impulse is transmitted by adjacent depolarization of atrial myofibrils. Approximately halfway through the P wave, the impulse reaches the AV node. The second half of the P wave is due to left atrial depolarization.

In a normal heart, the atria and the ventricles are electrically isolated from each other except at the AV node. The AV node is located in the atrial septum near the apex of the triangle of Koch. Blood supply to the AV node is from the AV nodal artery, which arises from the posterior descending artery (PDA) in 80% of the population, from the circumflex in 10% of people, and from both in 10%. The AV node is innervated by the sympathetic and parasympathetic nervous systems. Conduction through the AV node accounts for the majority of the PR interval.

Intraatrial and infranodal conduction times are minor contributors to the overall PR duration. After emerging from the AV node, the impulse is conducted through the Bundle of His. From there, the impulse travels down the right and left bundle branches, their fascicles, and to the Purkinje network, which causes ventricular contraction.

MECHANISMS OF DYSRHYTMIAS

Abnormal rhythms can fairly simplistically be described as being due to disorders of impulse formation, disorders of impulse conduction, or a combination of both. Current diagnostic tools do not always allow precise determination of the type of mechanism responsible for the observed rhythm. Some rhythms can be initiated by one mechanism and propagated by another.

Disorders of Impulse Formation

Automaticity

Normal automaticity: Automaticity is the ability of a cell to depolarize and generate an impulse spontaneously, without prior stimulation.[2] Specialized cells of the heart (e.g., the SA node) are capable of spontaneously depolarizing. These are responsible for the spontaneous cardiac rhythm, and the rhythm is called an automatic rhythm. Abnormal rhythms may arise when these cells depolarize at an abnormal rate or when cells usually suppressed by the faster pacemaking cells become no longer suppressed and are allowed to depolarize spontaneously. These are known as dysrhythmias resulting from normal automaticity, because the ionic mechanism leading to depolarization is normal, but occurring at a faster or slower rate. An example is the ventricular escape beat seen when the sinus and AV nodes fail to depolarize the ventricles. Previously suppressed, Purkinje cells become able to depolarize at their own intrinsic rate of 20–40/min.

Abnormal automaticity: Purkinje cells do not normally depolarize the heart because their rate of depolarization is slow and suppressed by impulses from the SA node. Normal ventricular myocardial cells do not develop automaticity. Under certain conditions these cells can develop an abnormal type of automatic firing. This occurs when their resting membrane potential is altered (during phase 4 of the cardiac cycle). The resting potential is raised from −80 mV to between −70 and −50 mV, allowing spontaneous depolarization, even of cells not ordinarily capable of spontaneous depolarization. Accelerated idioventricular rhythm (AIVR) due to ischemia from a myocardial infarction can be caused by this mechanism.

They only are evident when the rate of the abnormal focus is faster than the usual pacemaker.

Triggered Activity

After-potentials are responsible for triggered rhythms.[3] These are fluctuations in the membrane voltage that can depolarize the cells. They are dependent on a preceding action potential or series of action potentials, and they are not automatic rhythms. These depolarizations can occur before or after complete repolarization of the membrane and are called early or late after-depolarizations, respectively. Early after-depolarizations occur while repolarization is still occurring, and may be related to reactivation of calcium channels. Early after-depolarizations may prolong repolarization time (if they do not depolarize the cell) and may be involved in the prolonged QT syndrome and the initiation of torsades de pointes. Late after-depolarizations appear to be related to intracellular calcium overload and a secondary release of calcium from the sarcoplasmic reticulum. Digitalis toxicity is a common cause of delayed after-depolarizations. Ventricular tachycardia arising from the right ventricular outflow tract (RVOT) may be due to delayed after-depolarizations.

Disorders of Impulse Conduction

Prolonged Conduction Time

An impulse may take a longer time than normal to depolarize the heart for several reasons. Conduction may be slowed, as can be seen with cardioactive drugs or through an area of ischemic tissue. It may also be seen as a normal response of cardiac tissue, as when a premature complex is conducted slowly through the AV node. Slow conduction may be generalized throughout the heart, or limited to an anatomic region. Conduction may also be prolonged because the pathway of depolarization is lengthened and abnormal, even though conduction is occurring at a normal speed. A premature ventricular contraction (PVC) is an example of this, as the pathway for ventricular activation is lengthened. Prolonged conduction is most important in creating reentry pathways.

Blocked Conduction

An impulse may be blocked for many reasons. It may reach an area of the heart that is inexcitable because it is in a refractory state or because of disease. For example, scar tissue cannot conduct an impulse. The impulse itself may not be strong enough to propagate itself.

Unidirectional Block with Reentry

In some instances an impulse is able to propagate itself indefinitely. This most often occurs with the development of a reentry pathway. Most important tachydysrhythmias such as SVT or monomorphic VT use such a path. Reentry can theoretically occur with normal conduction velocity if the reentrant path is long enough, but essentially all reentrant rhythms require the presence of an area with prolonged conduction.

When the same stable reentrant circuit is used, the rhythm is said to be due to ordered reentry. This may be a distinct anatomic pathway (as seen with accessory pathways), or a functional pathway, with properties of the myocardial cells slowing conduction, or a combination of both. When the order of reentry is random, impulses propagate in ever-changing pathways. Circuits here are functional. Ventricular fibrillation is an example of this.

Disorders of Both Impulse Formation and Conduction

Parasystole

An area of the heart may be able to generate impulses independent of the normal sinus impulse. Either automaticity or triggered activity can initiate the impulse. If there is a unidirectional block that allows this depolarization to be conducted to the rest of the heart, then it will depolarize the heart, preventing the normal sinus impulse from depolarizing it. Both this ectopic impulse and the normal sinus impulse can then depolarize myocardium and two foci will be seen on the ECG.

VENTRICULAR FIBRILLATION

Etiology and Risk Factors

Ventricular fibrillation is a life-threatening arrhythmia that must be rapidly recognized and treated. This arrhythmia is characterized by disorganized and irregular multifocal contractions occurring in the ventricular myocardium (Fig. 20-1). There is no effective or coordinated ventricular pumping activity and cardiac output is compromised. If resuscitation is not begun within 4–6 min, death will be inevitable. Patients with true VF do not have a measurable blood pressure or pulse. If a patient is awake and alert, has a blood pressure, and/or has a pulse, lead placement should be checked and artifact should be eliminated.

The ECG in VF is characterized by a fine to coarse irregular oscillating pattern with no discernible organized cardiac activity. P waves, QRS complexes, and T waves are absent. Brown et al. have demonstrated that the coarseness of the waveform of VF is correlated with the likelihood of successful defibrillation and subsequent survival, and appears to correlate with coronary blood flow.[4] When the ECG shows "fine" fibrillation waves, defibrillation efforts are rarely successful. Animal data suggest that the coarseness of the fibrillation waveform may be increased by epinephrine. Definitive studies in humans are ongoing.

The onset and propagation of VF is intimately related to myocardial calcium load. The accumulation of calcium in cardiac myocytes can cause delayed after-depolarization to occur, initiating VF.[5] Also contributing to this is calcium-induced cell-to-cell uncoupling. The resulting slowed conduction can permit a reentry phenomenon to develop. VF itself can increase intramyocyte calcium and this can maintain the dysrhythmia. Successful termination (chemical or electrical) lowers intracellular calcium levels and unsuccessful defibrillation does not.[6] As calcium overload continues, defibrillation thresholds increase.[6] Thus, it is important to defibrillate a patient as early as possible after the onset of VF.

Primary VF occurs spontaneously without prolonged hemodynamic compromise. Secondary VF is seen in evolving ischemia, left ventricular failure, and cardiogenic shock. Most cases are associated with coronary artery disease (CAD). Digoxin toxicity, quinidine toxicity, hypoxia, hypothermia, chest trauma, electrolyte abnormalities, SWAN-GANZ catheters, and pacemaker malfunctions may also lead to VF. Rapid ventricular rates seen with preexcitation syndromes can degenerate into VF, and overdrive pacing can also induce the dysrhythmia. In ischemic heart disease, VF is usually preceded by VT although, in some cases, no inciting cardiac dysrhythmia or event occurs.

Predictors of VF include ischemia, decreased left ventricular systolic function, 10 or more PVCs per hour on telemetry, inducible or spontaneous VT, hypertension with left ventricular hypertrophy, smoking, male gender,

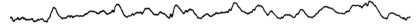

Fig. 20-1. Ventricular fibrillation. There is an absence of organized atrial or ventricular activity. Instead, irregular complexes are of varying shape and amplitude.

obesity, elevated cholesterol, age greater than 55 for males and 65 for females, and alcohol abuse.

Seventy-five percent of patients with out-of-hospital cardiac arrest have VF as their initial rhythm. Of patients who are successfully resuscitated, 75% have significant CAD. Twenty to thirty percent of patients have transmural infarctions. Patients without an ischemic etiology for VF are at greater risk than patients with an ischemic etiology for sudden death. Patients who have an MI associated with VF have a 2% 1-year recurrence rate of VF.

Treatment

Ventricular fibrillation rarely converts to a stable cardiac rhythm spontaneously. Cardiopulmonary resuscitation (CPR) should be initiated as soon as possible because there is little to no cardiac output during fibrillation of the myocardium. Defibrillation should occur immediately after the rhythm is recognized. The longer the dysrhythmia is present, the more difficult it is to terminate, and the greater the energy required.[6]

Successful defibrillation is accomplished by passing adequate electrical current (amperes) through the heart. Current flow is dependent on energy (Joules) and impedance (resistance) to flow. Transthoracic impedance is influenced by the energy selected, electrode size, skin coupling, the distance between the two electrodes, the number of previous shocks, paddle pressure or skin contact, and the phase of ventilation. Average chest wall impedance is 70–80 Ω with a range from 15 to 150 Ω. If impedance is high, low energy shocks are ineffective and a higher voltage may be necessary. Transthoracic impedance can be reduced by firm pressure on manual paddles and the use of a coupling gel. If skin pads are used, the chest should be thoroughly dried prior to electrode placement to ensure adequate contact by the adhesive pads.

One electrode should be placed over the anterior aspect of the sternum. The other electrode can be placed adjacent to the left nipple or on the back in the left infrascapular location. If a patient has large breasts, the electrodes are best placed to the right of the upper sternum and under or lateral to the left breast.

The American Heart Association (AHA) recommends that initial defibrillation attempts begin with 200 J of energy and be delivered as a nonsynchronous shock.[7] If 200 J are unsuccessful, then the energy should be increased to 300 J and then 360 J. All additional shocks should be administered at 360 J or the equivalent biphasic energy levels. Adgey et al. prospectively had an 80–95% success rate using an initial voltage of 200 J if the patient weighed less than 90 kg.[8]

If three successive shocks are unsuccessful in converting the rhythm, then 1 mg of epinephrine should be administered followed by another shock at 360 J. Epinephrine has been shown to cause a more vigorous and coarse fibrillation wave that is more susceptible to defibrillation. Epinephrine's effect is most likely due to increased coronary blood flow and positive inotropy. Epinephrine may be repeated every 3–5 min. Vasopressin (40 U) may be used instead of epinephrine. If defibrillation and epinephrine fail, then there is an increased likelihood of severe acidosis and hypoxemia. Attempts should be made to correct these two entities through intubation and effective CPR. High-dose epinephrine seemed promising in early studies, but larger trials failed to show a benefit.

The administration of sodium bicarbonate is no longer a universal recommendation in Advanced Cardiac Life Support (ACLS) protocols, and now has an AHA evidence rating of IIB. Clinical trials have failed to show a benefit of sodium bicarbonate therapy in cardiac arrest situations, and the deleterious effects of worsening metabolic acidosis, hypernatremia, and hyperosmolality have all been reported. Sodium bicarbonate is usually administered as a 1 mg/kg bolus.

If there is no response to cardioversion and epinephrine or VF is recurrent, then IV lidocaine or amiodarone should be considered (Table 20-1). Lidocaine is administered at a dose of 1.0–1.5 mg/kg IV bolus. Amiodarone is given as a 150–300 mg bolus over 10 min. A 1–2 mg/min infusion for 6 hours follows, and then it is decreased to 0.5–1 mg/min for 6–24 hours. Studies have shown that amiodarone yields a slightly higher rate of spontaneous return of circulation, but no difference in mortality or survival to hospital discharge has been detected.[9] The AHA states that amiodarone is an alternative to lidocaine for VF, but does not endorse either drug as "first line." The combination of amiodarone and lidocaine together can be proarrhythmogenic.

Procainamide and bretylium have also been used in patients with VF. Procainamide is given as a 20 mg/kg dose infused at a rate less than 50 mg/min. A significant side effect of procainamide is hypotension. Bretylium has been advocated for use in hypothermic patients with VF. Beta-blockers have also been used by some authors for VF secondary to acute myocardial infarction (AMI) and ongoing ischemia with some success.

Ventricular fibrillation due to hyperkalemia should be rapidly recognized and quickly treated. Intravenous calcium should be given to stabilize the cardiac membrane potential and counter-act the adverse effects of potassium. Insulin, glucose, albuterol, sodium bicarbonate, and

Table 20-1. Doses of Antiarrhythmic Drugs in Ventricular Fibrillation

Initial drug	
Epinephrine	1 mg Q 3–5 min
Vasopressin	40 U once
Secondary drug	
Amiodarone	300 mg bolus then a 1–2 mg/min infusion. May repeat dose of 150 mg bolus
Lidocaine	1.5 mg/kg bolus then a 2–4 mg/min drip. Repeat bolus once if needed
Procainamide	17 mg/kg bolus at 30 mg/min
Bretylium	5 mg/kg bolus IV
Sodium bicarbonate	1 mg/kg bolus

Kayexalate may all be useful in lowering the potassium level. Hyperkalemic cardiac arrest is an indication for pacing.

Although a precordial thump and cough CPR has been shown to be effective for VT, these maneuvers have been shown to have little, if any, efficacy in VF.[10,11]

VENTRICULAR TACHYCARDIA

Description and Etiology

Ventricular tachycardia is defined by a run of three or more successive ectopic ventricular complexes that occur at a rate greater than 100 bpm. It is arbitrarily defined as sustained or nonsustained, with sustained VT lasting for longer than 30 s or requiring termination because of patient instability (Figs. 20-2 and 20-3). Table 20-2 describes the characteristics of VT seen on ECG. Mechanisms include triggered activity with reentry, but other mechanisms can provoke it as well. Ventricular tachycardia can have one or multiple sites of origin; depending on the type of VT the rate can vary from 70 to 250 complexes per minute, and the QRS contours can vary or be uniform.[12]

Ventricular flutter is characterized by a sawtooth or zigzag pattern without discernible P waves, QRS complexes, or T waves. The differences between VT and ventricular flutter are of intellectual interest; ventricular flutter is treated as VT. Bidirectional VT is described by QRS complexes with alternating polarity in a single lead. Alternating VT is identified by QRS complexes alternating in height with constant polarity. Digoxin toxicity and severe ischemic disease can cause alternating and bidirectional VT. Polymorphic VT is characterized by QRS complexes with different morphologies in the same lead (see below). Torsades de points or twisting of the points is a variant of polymorphic VT.

Repetitive monomorphic VT is uncommon. Repetitive salvos of nonsustained VT is separated by a few sinus impulses. The ventricular rate is usually between 100 and 150 although rates as high as 200 have been reported. Repetitive monomorphic VT is more common in women and is usually benign.[13] Treatment is undertaken when structural heart disease is present, palpitations are poorly tolerated by the patient, or patients experience severe light-headedness, near syncope, or syncope. Calcium-channel blockers and beta-blockers are the mainstays of

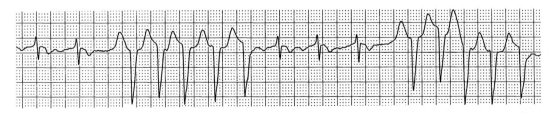

Fig. 20-2. Nonsustained ventricular tachycardia. Brief runs of VT are seen that have the same shape and terminate spontaneously.

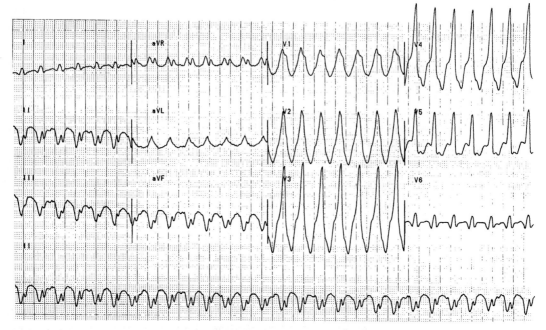

Fig. 20-3. Ventricular tachycardia. Wide complex QRS tachycardia at a rate of 174/min is seen. The QRS duration is 272 ms, and the QRS complexes show concordance in the precordial leads.

treatment. Catheter ablation also has a high rate of success.[14]

Nonsustained monomorphic VT is characterized by salvos of three to five consecutive impulses or nonsustained VT of six impulses or up to 30 s. Patients with nonsustained VT are at high risk for fatal arrhythmias. Patients with poor ejection fractions and organic heart disease who have runs of nonsustained VT have the highest risk for sudden death. Implantable cardioverter-defibrillator therapy has been shown to decrease mortality in one randomized-controlled trial.[15]

Table 20-2. ECG Characteristics of Ventricular Tachycardia

- Wide QRS complexes (5% of patients will have narrow complexes)
- Rate greater than 100
- Regular rhythm although some beat to beat variation may occur
- QRS axis is typically constant

The most common causes of monomorphic VT are AMI and ischemic heart disease. Other causes include hypertrophic cardiomyopathy, mitral valve prolapse, and drug toxicity (digoxin, procainamide, quinidine, and sympathomimetics). Hypoxia, alkalosis, hypomagnesemia, hypocalcemia, and hyperkalemia increase the likelihood of VT.

Distinguishing VT from SVT with Aberrancy

It can be difficult to distinguish monomorphic VT from SVT with aberrancy. Wide QRS complexes only indicate that conduction through the ventricle is abnormal. It does not indicate the origin of the complexes. Conduction may be originating above the ventricle, and traveling to the ventricle via an accessory pathway. A bundle branch block may also preexist, and other mechanisms may be involved as well. A few criteria are useful in making this discrimination (Table 20-3). It is important to remember that VT is the most common cause of a wide complex tachycardia, and if in doubt, the rhythm should be treated as VT.

Several authors have attempted to identify criteria to help differentiate VT from SVT with aberrant conduction.

Table 20-3. Useful Criteria to Distinguish SVT with Aberrant Conduction from VT

- Favoring ventricular tachycardia
  - Fusion beats[*]
  - Capture beats[*]
  - AV dissociation[*]
  - A postectopic pause
  - Constant coupling intervals
  - No response to vagal maneuvers
  - QRS duration > 0.14 ms
  - QRS concordance in precordial leads
  - Advanced age, history of MI or CHF, and CABG
- Favoring SVT with aberrant conduction
  - Preceding ectopic P wave
  - A varying BBB
  - Varying coupling intervals
  - May respond to vagal maneuvers

[*]These criteria provide strong presumptive evidence for VT.

Wellens identified a set of criteria that were suggestive of SVT with aberrant conduction or VT (Table 20-4).[16] The criteria consist of data obtained from the clinical history, physical examination, and ECG. The data set may be useful to formulate a preliminary assumption of VT or SVT with aberrant conduction, but should not be relied on to definitively differentiate these two clinical entities. Subsequent studies in emergency department settings have shown that these criteria have poor interobserver reliability and are generally not helpful.

Brugada et al. derived four questions to analyze ECG morphology in patients with a wide complex, regular tachycardia (Fig. 20-4).[17] The criteria focus on identifying specific ECG criteria consistent with VT, and if those criteria are not met, the diagnosis defaults to SVT with aberrancy. Although the initial study reported a sensitivity of 99% and a specificity of 97% in differentiating VT from SVT with aberrant conduction, subsequent studies by both cardiologists and emergency physicians have found that the sensitivity is closer to 75–80%.

Griffith's algorithm is somewhat the reverse of the Brugada criteria (Table 20-5).[18] The algorithm applies morphologic criteria to identify SVT with aberrant conduction and any of the answers to the questions are "no," then the diagnosis defaults to VT.

Because of the high degree of uncertainty involved in differentiating SVT with aberrant conduction from VT, all patients should be treated presumptively as VT.

Treatment

The treatment of a patient with monomorphic VT depends on stability. Unstable patients are those with

Table 20-4. Features Helpful in Distinguishing Ventricular Tachycardia from Supraventricular Tachycardia with Abnormal Conduction (Wellens Criteria)

	Ventricular Tachycardia	SVT with Aberrant Conduction
Clinical features	Age > 50 Prior MI, CHF, CABG, MVP, or ischemia History of VT	Age < 35 MVP History of SVT
Physical examination	Cannon A waves Variation in atrial pulse Variable first heart sound	None
ECG	Fusion beats	P waves before QRS Complexes
	QRS > 0.14 s Extreme LAD (<30 degrees) No response to vagal maneuvers AV dissociation	QRS < 0.14 s Axis normal or slightly abnormal Slows or terminates with vagal maneuvers
Specific QRS pattern	V_1: R, qR, or RS V_6: S, rS, or Qr Concordance[*]	V_1: rSR′ V_6: qRs

[*]Primary deflection of precordial QRS complexes are all positive or all negative.

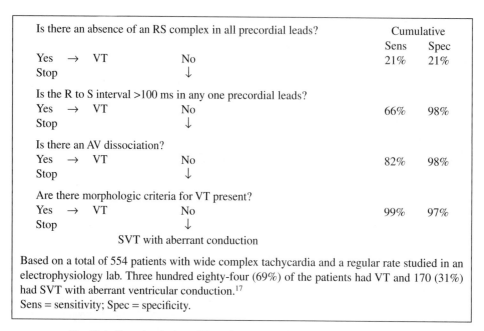

Is there an absence of an RS complex in all precordial leads?		Cumulative	
		Sens	Spec
Yes → VT	No	21%	21%
Stop	↓		
Is the R to S interval >100 ms in any one precordial leads?			
Yes → VT	No	66%	98%
Stop	↓		
Is there an AV dissociation?			
Yes → VT	No	82%	98%
Stop	↓		
Are there morphologic criteria for VT present?			
Yes → VT	No	99%	97%
Stop	↓		
	SVT with aberrant conduction		

Based on a total of 554 patients with wide complex tachycardia and a regular rate studied in an electrophysiology lab. Three hundred eighty-four (69%) of the patients had VT and 170 (31%) had SVT with aberrant ventricular conduction.[17]

Sens = sensitivity; Spec = specificity.

Fig. 20-4. Brugada criteria to differentiate SVT with aberrant conduction from VT.

hypotension, chest pain, altered mental status, or unconsciousness.

Patients with VT who are unstable but have a palpable pulse should be cardioverted with synchronous shocks delivered at an initial voltage of 100 J. Ninety percent of patients will convert with this energy level. VT can be converted with energy as low as 10 J and almost all patients convert with an energy of 100 J. ACLS guidelines recommend that pulseless patients with VT be cardioverted with a nonsynchronous 200-J shock.

Patients with VT who present for medical attention with stable vital signs can be treated with antiarrhythmic drugs or cardioversion. Due to the pain involved in electrical cardioversion, most physicians will attempt conversion with pharmacologic agents first. Multiple agents have been shown to convert VT, and may be useful in patients with SVT with aberrant conduction (Table 20-6). Calcium-channel blockers and beta-blockers should be avoided in all patients with a wide complex tachycardia. These drugs can accelerate the heart rate and decrease the blood pressure without converting the patient's rhythm.

Adenosine has been advocated by some authors to differentiate SVT with aberrant conduction from VT. A small percentage of patients with VT will convert to a normal

Table 20-5. Griffith's Criteria for the Diagnosis of Wide QRS Complex Tachycardia with Regular Rhythm

Step 1: Determine the morphologic classification of the wide QRS complexes: RBBB vs. LBBB.

Step 2: Apply criteria for normal forms of either RBBB or LBBB. A negative answer to ANY of the three questions is inconsistent with a RBBB or a LBBB and the diagnosis defaults to VT.

QRS complexes consistent with RBBB:

1. Is there an rSR′ morphology in lead V_1?
2. Is there an RS complex in V_6 (may have a small septal Q wave)?
3. Is the R/S ratio in lead $V_6 > 1$?

QRS complexes consistent with a LBBB:

1. Is there an rS or QS complex in leads V_1 and V_2?
2. Is the onset of the QRS to the nadir of the S wave in lead $V_1 < 70$ ms?
3. Is there an R wave in lead V_6, without a Q wave?

Table 20-6. Medical Management of Ventricular Tachycardia

Lidocaine: 1–1.5 mg/kg bolus followed by an infusion at 1–4 mg/min. Bolus may be repeated to a total of 3 mg/kg.
Amiodarone: 150 mg IV over 10 min. Repeat once in 10 min if needed. Then 1 mg/min for 6 h, followed by
    0.5 mg/min for 18 h.
Procainamide: 17 mg/kg infusion at a rate less than 50 mg/min IV followed by an infusion at 1–4 mg/min[*]
    a. Loading dose is 12 mg/kg in patients with congestive heart failure.
    b. Infusion rate is 1.4 mg/kg/h in patients with renal insufficiency.
    c. When the dysrhythmia is suppressed, start an infusion.

---

[*]The infusion should be stopped if patients develop hypotension or QRS widening of greater than 50% of the baseline interval.

rhythm with adenosine. Adenosine has an extremely short half-life and does not appear to harm patients with SVT with aberrant conduction or VT. Because not treating VT with appropriate pharmacotherapy can lead to malignant arrhythmias and sudden death, most authors do not recommend the routine use of adenosine in these patients.

Cough may reverse the arrhythmia of VT without defibrillation. Repeated coughing has been shown in case reports to maintain the conscious state by raising intrathoracic pressure.[19,20]

Conversion of VT using a precordial thump has been reported in patients with VT. There are scattered case reports of decompensation with precordial thumps in patients with a pulse. They should be reserved for patients without a pulse when defibrillation is not available.

POLYMORPHIC VENTRICULAR TACHYCARDIA

This type of VT is diagnosed when a wide complex tachycardia with varying QRS shapes or heights is seen. These tachydysrhythmias tend to be more unstable than monomorphic VT. They tend to degenerate into VF more frequently, occur at faster rates, and more often are associated with symptoms such as syncope. Polymorphic VT also does not usually last as long as monomorphic VT, self-terminating or degenerating into VF. Polymorphic VT is classified based on whether the QT interval is prolonged or normal.

Polymorphic Ventricular Tachycardia with a Normal QT Interval

Most cases of polymorphic VT with a normal QT interval occur in the setting of CAD and myocardial ischemia. The ECG usually shows signs of ischemia or infarction. Treatment is the same as for monomorphic VT, and revas-

cularization should be undertaken, even though it may not be sufficient to prevent recurrences.[21]

Idiopathic Polymorphic Ventricular Tachycardia

Idiopathic polymorphic VT has been reported in patients with normal hearts and normal QT intervals. Authors have classified idiopathic polymorphic VT into several different groups.[22] One group of patients had persistent ST elevation despite the absence of cardiac ischemia or CAD (Brugada syndrome). Another group had exercise-induced ventricular arrhythmias that were responsive to beta-blocker therapy. The third group had PVC-induced polymorphic VT and a high incidence of sudden death that was not altered by beta-blocker therapy. Verapamil demonstrated some benefit in patients in the third group.

Brugada Syndrome

This is a syndrome characterized by a right bundle block, incomplete right bundle block or right bundle block pattern, ST elevation in the right precordial leads, and symptoms of sudden death or syncope.[23] Originally thought to be limited to males of Southeast Asian descent, it has been found in both genders and many ethnic groups. No associated structural heart disease has been described, and patients do not have CAD. The defect is believed to be due to abnormal cardiac sodium channels, coded for a gene on chromosome 3. Adolescent and young males are at highest risk for sudden death and the disease has a familial pattern. Affected patients develop polymorphic VT, associated with a normal QT interval. The best treatment available to date in patients with the inherited form is an implantable cardioverter-defibrillator.[24]

The ECG findings of Brugada syndrome can also develop in response to medications and electrolyte abnormalities. Procainamide, flecainide, diphenhydramine, propoxyphene, cyclic antidepressants, and cocaine have provoked it. Severe hyperkalemia and hypercalcemia have also been noted to cause the ECG findings.

At this time, recommendations for evaluation of the patient with the Brugada ECG are based on expert opinion and studies of follow-up of patients with and without symptoms. No controlled trials of differing regimens exist. Patients who present with symptoms or a family history of sudden death and the ECG findings of Brugada syndrome should be admitted for electrophysiologic (EP) testing. Those who develop the ECG abnormality because of medications or electrolyte disturbances should be admitted and observed until the causative factors have been treated. Those who have the ECG pattern discovered incidentally and have no risk factors probably have the same risk of sudden death as those without the ECG findings and do not need admission or EP testing.[25]

Polymorphic Ventricular Tachycardia with a Prolonged QT Interval (Torsades de Pointes)

Torsades de pointes is a type of polymorphic VT in which the QRS complexes change morphology from beat to beat. The QRS peaks seem to twist around an isoelectric baseline [Fig. 20-5(a) and (b)]. The rate is typically 200–250 bpm. Torsades de pointes is distinguished from polymorphic VT by the presence of a prolonged QT interval on a baseline ECG. The prolonged QT interval may be seen on all beats, or only on the beat preceding the onset of the VT.[12] Torsades

de pointes can occur as a result of a congenitally prolonged QT interval, or can be due to an acquired QT interval prolongation, usually due to medications, though other etiologies are possible (Table 20-7). The dysrhythmia can self-terminate, and then recur after a period of normal complexes. It can also degenerate into VF.

Early after-depolarizations appear to initiate the dysrhythmia, and it is perpetuated most likely by reentry, abnormal automaticity, or triggered activity.[12]

Congenital Prolonged QT Syndrome

The congenital cause of prolonged QT syndrome has an incidence 1:10,000 to 1:15,000. There is an equal male:female gender distribution and the average age of symptom onset is 14 years old. Sixty percent of patients with congenital prolonged QT syndrome have a family history of sudden death. Untreated mortality has been reported to be as high as 50%. With appropriate therapy the mortality rate can be decreased to as low as 10%.

Congenital prolonged QT syndrome is an inherited disease and at least five chromosomal abnormalities have been identified. The molecular defects involve membrane sodium and potassium ion channel proteins and lead to abnormal function.

Two clinical patterns exist. Jervell and Lange-Nielsen (JLN) syndrome has an autosomal recessive inheritance pattern. The disorder is characterized by bilateral sensorineural deafness at birth and a long QT. Romano-Ward

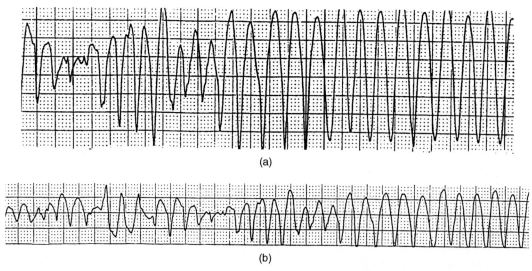

(a)

(b)

Fig. 20-5. (a) Torsades de pointes. Wide complex tachycardia with QRS complexes of varying heights, give the appearance of a "twisting around the points." (b) Torsades de pointes. The runs of torsades de pointes are shorter than seen in part A. (Source: Courtesy of Lawrence Klein, MD.)

Table 20-7. Congenital and Acquired Causes of QT Prolongation

Congenital causes
  Jervell and Lange-Nielsen Syndrome (JLN)
  Romano-Ward Syndrome (RW)

Acquired causes
  Medications
    Class I antiarrhythmics
    Class III antiarrhythmics: sotalol, ibutilide
    Phenothiazines
    Haloperidol
    Tricyclic antidepressants
    Macrolide antibiotics: erythromycin
    Trimethoprim-sulfamethoxazole
    Antihistamines
    Ionic contrast media
    Cisapride
    Certain azole antifungals: ketoconazole
    Hypothyroidism

Electrolyte abnormalities
  Hypokalemia
  Hypomagnesemia
  Hypocalcemia
  Cerebrovascular events: Subarachroid Hemorrhage (SAH)
  Myocardial infarctions
  Ischemia
  Starvation diets
  Organophosphate poisoning
  Myocarditis
  Severe CHF

Mitral valve prolapse

syndrome is an autosomal-dominant disease that is associated with normal hearing.

Patients with LQTS have heterogeneous repolarization in the ventricular myocardium. Electrocardiographic findings in the prolonged QT syndrome include a corrected QT interval greater than 460 ms, QT dispersion, T-wave alternans, T-wave morphology changes, and bradycardia. T-wave alternans is a marker of significant electrical instability and these patients have a high incidence of torsades de points. The T-wave morphology may also be biphasic, bifid, or notched similar to a T-U wave fusion. Patients with LQTS may also present with sinus pause and inappropriate bradycardia for age. The positive predictive value of a QT_c greater than 460 ms is 92% and the negative predictive value is 94%.[26] The degree of QT prolongation

varies with time in the same patient. There is no clear correlation between the degree of QT prolongation and syncope and the incidence of sudden death.

The diagnosis of the long QT syndrome is made by combining ECG findings, clinical characteristics, and family history. A scoring system was developed to assist in determining a patient's probability of having the disease.[27] It incorporates ECG abnormalities, QT_c duration, presence or absence of syncope or deafness, and family history into a single score. Exercise testing can be useful in unclear cases; it can lengthen the QT interval, supporting the diagnosis.

Symptoms vary from light-headedness to syncope and sudden death, and symptoms usually begin in adolescence or childhood. Symptoms develop in response to sympathetic stimulation: exercise, emotional stress, anger, fright. Recurrent episodes of syncope, relative bradycardia, female sex, family history of sudden death, and a QT_c interval of greater than 600 ms are risk factors for sudden death.[28]

Immediate treatment involves IV magnesium, maintenance of potassium levels, and temporary overdrive pacing. Long-term treatment options begin with beta-blockers in the maximum tolerated dose. Second-line modalities include pacemaker or cardioverter-defibrillator implantation. Pacing at higher than usual rates, such as 80 bpm is used when bradycardia is a prominent feature of the syndrome. Cardioverter-defibrillators are placed when the initial presentation is cardiac arrest, or when beta-blockade and pacing fail to control symptoms. Left cardiac sympathetic sympathectomy, previously used to prevent tachycardia, has mostly given way to the use of pacemakers or cardioverter-defibrillators. Treatment has reduced 5-year mortality to about 6%,[29] but the adjusted annual mortality rate is 4.5%, even with treatment.[30]

Treatment of Polymorphic Ventricular Tachycardia

Treatment of polymorphic VT depends on whether the baseline QT interval is prolonged or not. Because of this it is better to reserve the term "torsades de pointes" to that polymorphic VT which occurs in the setting of a prolonged QT interval. If torsades de pointes is present, then IV magnesium is the preferred agent for first-line treatment. Two grams over 5–10 min, followed by another 2 g, if needed, is the dosing. Successful termination of torsades occurs within 5 min in 75% of patients. Greater than 95% of patients terminate their malignant rhythms by 15 min. Rapid infusion of magnesium can cause significant hypotension so the patient's blood pressure should be monitored closely.

Ventricular overdrive pacing follows the magnesium, at a rate of 80–120 bpm. Bradycardia should be corrected

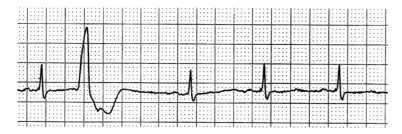

Fig. 20-6. A premature ventricular complex. Note the wide QRS complex, absence of a preceding P wave, T-wave orientation opposite to the QRS direction, and compensatory pause.

with temporary pacing. Pacing is probably the preferred modality in bradycardic patients if the inciting cause of torsades is unknown. Class Ia, Ic, and III antidysarrhythmics should not be used, as they can increase the QT interval. Lidocaine and phenytoin (class Ib) can be used. A search for the underlying cause should be made and corrected. Patients with torsades de pointes due to medications should be observed until at least 2–3 half-lives of the offending drug have elapsed, and the QT interval has returned to normal.

If the baseline QT interval is not prolonged, then torsades de pointes is not present, and standard measures for VT can be used. Unstable patients in either scenario should be treated with cardioversion. When the decision is difficult to make, clinical features may help decide if torsades de pointes is present or not.

PREMATURE VENTRICULAR CONTRACTIONS

A PVC is defined as a ventricular contraction originating in the ventricular myocardium with no preceding premature P wave. PVCs may originate from single or multiple foci, and may have similar (uniform) or different (multiform) shapes to the QRS complex (Figs. 20-6 and 20-7). They may

exhibit varying or fixed coupling intervals to the preceding beat. Bigeminy is noted when a PVC follows a normal complex in a paired pattern (Fig. 20-8). Trigeminy is defined as the pattern seen when a PVC follows two normal complexes. A PVC pair or couplet is seen when two PVCs occur together, and a triplet is the presence of three PVCs in succession. Almost any mechanism can produce a PVC. Variable coupling can be due to triggered activity, changing conduction in a reentrant circuit, or parasystole. Reentry and triggered activity can produce fixed coupling.[12] It is usually difficult to determine which mechanism is occurring. Table 20-8 shows characteristics of a typical PVC.

Premature ventricular complexes are very common and occur in patients with and without heart disease. Common causes of PVCs include AMI, ischemic heart disease, digoxin toxicity, congestive heart failure (CHF), hypokalemia, alkalosis, hypoxia, and sympathomimetic drugs. Stress, excessive use of caffeine, alcohol, or tobacco can provoke them, as can exercise in some patients. A grading system has been devised to classify PVCs based on their frequency and pattern (Table 20-9). Symptoms depend on the rate of PVCs, current patient activity, duration, and underlying comorbidities. Palpitations, light-headedness, dizziness, syncope, angina, and CHF can all be seen.[12]

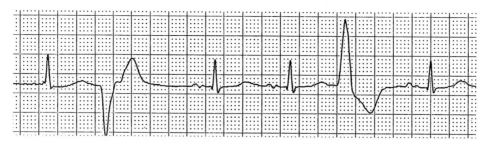

Fig. 20-7. Multiform premature ventricular complexes. The QRS contours of the PVCs are wide, opposite in direction to each other, and have a different shape compared to the normally conducted beats.

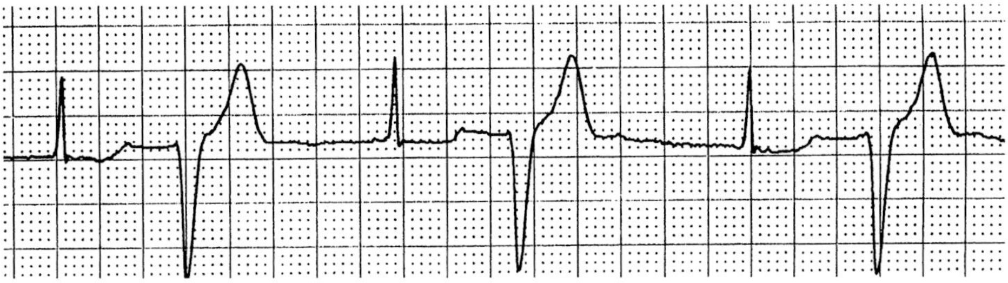

Fig. 20-8. Bigeminy. The PVCs are paired to each sinus beat, with a fixed coupling interval.

Studies have indicated that the frequency of PVCs correlates with the degree of ischemic heart disease, although controversy exists as to whether PVCs are independent risk factors for adverse events. Two or more PVCs in a row appears to increase the risk of malignant arrhythmias in patients with CAD. PVCs are also markers of electrical instability in patients with acute MI, but the presence or absence of PVCs does not correlate with the development of VF. Late-coupled PVCs have a higher incidence of the R on T phenomenon and VT compared to early-coupled PVCs. Recent randomized-controlled clinical trials in postmyocardial infarction patients using amiodarone showed no benefit on total mortality.[31,32] The CHF-STAT trial which randomized ischemic versus nonischemic myopathies to amiodarone or placebo showed no mortality benefit.[33] Beta-blockers have evolved as the treatment of choice for symptomatic PVCs after MI although no randomized-controlled trials have demonstrated benefit.

PVCs are also frequently seen in patients with transient ischemic attacks. PVCs in these patients have a high risk of degenerating into sustained VT and VF. Primary treatment should be aimed at reversing the ischemia. Intravenous lidocaine or procainamide has been given with some success to suppress the PVCs.

Severe heart failure and acute pulmonary edema may also cause frequent PVCs especially during low output states or during periods of decompensation. Treatment should be aimed at improving the patient's hemodynamic status. Intravenous lidocaine and procainamide have been used while the patient's hemodynamic state is being stabilized, but drugs may not have a significant effect until the patient's hemodynamic status is improved.

Premature ventricular complexes frequently accompany acute and subacute pericarditis and myocarditis. Premature ventricular complexes rarely decompensate to VT and VF in these clinical conditions even in the presence of heart failure. In patients without VT and VF, antidysrhythmic drugs can be given orally. Oral therapy is continued for a minimum of 2 months.

Most PVCs do not require pharmacotherapy or treatment. A few studies have indicated that treatment of frequent or multifocal PVCs in the setting of acute MI reduces the risk of VT and fibrillation, but meta analyses and analysis of the literature as a whole do not suggest a benefit in mortality. Of note, randomized trials of post-MI patients have shown that antiarrhythmic drugs paradoxically increase the risk of cardiac arrest and sudden death. The CAST study clearly demonstrated that post-MI

Table 20-8. ECG Characteristics of PVCs

- Premature and wide QRS complex
- No preceding P wave
- The ST segment and T wave of the PVC is directed opposite the QRS complex
- Most PVCs do not affect the sinus node so there is usually a full postectopic pause after the PVC
- The PVC may occur between two sinus beats
- PVCs may occur at a fixed time after a sinus beat
- PVCs can induce atrial contraction through retrograde conduction, so a retrograde P wave may be observed

Table 20-9. Grading System for PVCs

Grade	ECG Characteristics
I	Uniform PVCs < 30/h
II	Uniform PVCs > 30/h
III	Multiform PVCs
4a	Couplets (2 consecutive PVCs)
4b	Triplets (3 or more consecutive PVCs)
5	R on T PVCs

patients with PVCs treated with flecainide or encainide had a higher mortality than patients not treated with an antiarrhythmic.[1] Therefore, we recommend that treatment of asymptomatic patients with PVCs should be done in consultation with a cardiologist.

Most patients with PVCs will respond to IV lidocaine administered at a loading dose of 1–1.5 mg/kg followed by a 2–4 mg/min drip. Procainamide or amiodarone may also be used if the PVCs are refractory to lidocaine. The dose of amiodarone is 150 mg IV bolus followed by a 1–2 mg/min infusion. The loading dose of procainamide is 17 mg/kg followed by an infusion of 1–4 mg/min. Both lidocaine and procainamide can have significant adverse side effects, especially with improper dosing.

Chronic PVCs are very common in patients with advanced idiopathic dilated cardiomyopathy and hypertrophic cardiomyopathy. Both groups have a significant risk of sudden death. Some reports indicate that more than 90% of patients with dilated cardiomyopathy have frequent PVCs and over 50% have salvos or nonsustained VT.[34,35] Efficacy of antiarrhythmic therapy in these two groups of patients is unclear. If patients are placed on antiarrhythmics, it is recommended that patients be hospitalized due to the proarrythmogenic properties of these medications. One study showed that an angiotensin converting enzyme (ACE) inhibitor has a favorable effect on the hemodynamic state in heart failure and decreases ventricular ectopy.[36]

Management of chronic PVCs in the presence of heart disease differs from the management of PVCs in acute cardiac conditions. There is an increased risk of sudden death and total death rate in patients with chronic ischemia, hypertensive heart disease, and cardiomyopathies.[34,35,37–43] Frequent PVCs, salvos, and nonsustained runs of VT in conjunction with a low ejection fraction further increase the risk of sudden death. Bigger et al. observed a 42% mortality in post-MI patients with nonsustained VT and salvos with an EF less than 30% compared to a 2-year mortality of 12% for patients with a normal EF and salvos or nonsustained runs of VT.[41] The use of amiodarone may reduce the risk of sudden death in post-MI patients who have frequent PVCs.[44] In patients with chronic PVCs and no evidence of heart disease there is no evidence that antiarrhythmic drugs improve morbidity and mortality.

If one chooses to use antidysrhythmic drugs, selecting the best agent is difficult. Class IA drugs are moderately effective but have a higher incidence of allergic reactions, uncomfortable side effects, and torsades des pointes. Class IB agents do have some efficacy and their proarrhythmogenic side effects are lower, but they also have a relatively high incidence of uncomfortable side effects. Class IC agents are very effective in reducing ventricular ectopy, but they are now contraindicated based on the CAST data.[1] Class III agents also can be proarrhythmogenic and precipitate torsades although amiodarone seems to have lower incidence of torsades compared to the IA agents. The incidence of torsades with sotalol is dose-dependent unlike the class I agents, which are idiosyncratic. Class IV agents have no role in the treatment of chronic PVCs. Data on combining antidysrhythmic drugs are limited.

IDIOVENTRICULAR RHYTHM AND ACCELERATED IDIOVENTRICULAR RHYTHM

Idioventricular rhythm (IVR) is a ventricular escape rhythm (Fig. 20-9), and AIVR usually occurs with an underlying supraventricular rhythm. The rate is 20–40 bpm (IVR) and 40–110 bpm (AIVR). Both can occur when the atria or AV node fail to depolarize the ventricles (e.g., complete AV node block). AIVR occurs as a rule in patients with cardiac disease. AMI and digitalis toxicity are the common precipitating events. AIVR can also develop in patients with an underlying supraventricular beat; as a result, competition between the supraventricular and ectopic ventricular impulses can occur, and fusion beats are commonly seen. The P wave may come closer and closer to the QRS complex at the same time the shape of the QRS complex changes to its wide ventricular

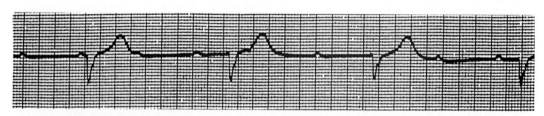

Fig. 20-9. Idioventricular rhythm. Wide QRS complexes, with the T-wave direction opposite to that of the QRS direction, is seen. Complete heart block is present. (Source: Courtesy of Lawrence Klein, MD.)

contour, and then disappears into it. This rhythm is also commonly seen when thrombolytics are given for an AMI, and if it occurs, thrombolytics should be continued. Episodes typically last 3–30 s. Most episodes are benign and do not require treatment. Frequently, accelerating the sinus rate, with atropine, or pacing, is all that is needed. Patients who depend on the atrial component of ventricular filling (atrial kick) may suffer symptoms due to this rhythm. Treatment can also be considered when AIVR occurs with VT. Suppression of the dysrhythmia can also be undertaken with the same drugs used to treat VT. Enhanced automaticity is the mechanism suspected of producing AIVR.

An IVR, on the other hand, is usually too slow to maintain adequate cardiac output and treatment is more frequently needed. These represent escape beats—the heart is attempting to maintain a degree of cardiac output, and the patient depends on these complexes for survival. Suppressive treatment (e.g., lidocaine) may therefore lead to asystole. Atropine and pacing are usually required, as well as correction of the underlying cause (AMI, complete heart block, cardiac tamponade, hemorrhage). CPR may be needed as well.

Agonal Ventricular Rhythm

An agonal rhythm describes an irregular ventricular rhythm with a slow rate (under 20 bpm), usually without associated ventricular contractions (Fig. 20-10). The QRS complexes become slower and broader with time. It represents a dying heart. CPR is required.

VENTRICULAR PARASYSTOLE

Ventricular parasystole is characterized by an ectopic pacemaker in the ventricle that competes with the sinus node. The ectopic pacemaker usually has fixed rate, but every depolarization does not necessarily initiate a ventricular contraction. Exit block occurs when the ventricle has previously depolarized and the next impulse arrives during the ventricle's refractory phase.

ECG characteristics of parasystole include variation in the coupling interval between the sinus beat and the ectopic beat, the presence of fusion beats, and regular occurrence of the ectopic contraction. The contractions will march out except for contractions suppressed by exit block. Long rhythm strips may be necessary to differentiate parasystole from isolated PVCs.

Parasystole can be caused by ischemic heart disease, AMI, electrolyte disturbances, and hypertensive heart disease. The activity and rhythm disturbances of the ectopic ventricular pacemaker are usually benign and do not require treatment. Some patients will develop VT and fibrillation. Symptomatic patients should be treated with antiarrhythmic medications.

UNRESOLVED ISSUES

Should amiodarone be the first-line drug used to treat VT or VF, stable or unstable? Lidocaine has been used for decades to treat VT and VF, and the evidence for its efficacy is sparse.[45] Two studies appeared recently examining the treatment of out-of-hospital VF not responsive to three attempts at defibrillation. One compared amiodarone to placebo and found that 44% of the amiodarone-treated patients survived to hospital admission versus 34% of the placebo-treated patients.[46] Because of criticism of this study another trial was undertaken to compare amiodarone to lidocaine.[9] It found that amiodarone did result in a higher proportion of patients surviving to admission: 22.8% versus 12%. However, in neither study did more amiodarone patients survive to discharge from the hospital. This lack of survival, together with the cost of amiodarone, has led many to continue using lidocaine as the first-line drug, despite the AHA giving amiodarone a class IIb rating for this indication.

Other studies have shown that procainamide,[47] sotalol,[48] and amiodarone [49] are better than lidocaine at terminating stable VT. It seems reasonable, based on these studies, to use one of these other agents in patients with sustained VT. In VF, either lidocaine or amiodarone can be used. Amiodarone may become the drug of choice in the future when neurologic treatments are developed that are better able to preserve brain function.

Does VT respond to adenosine, calcium-channel blockers, or vagal maneuvers? There is a widespread

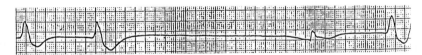

Fig. 20-10. Agonal rhythm. Slow, wide QRS complexes along with a long episode of asystole illustrate this terminal rhythm. (Source: Courtesy of Lawrence Klein, MD.)

belief that drugs and procedures used to terminate supraventricular dysrhythmias do not successfully treat dysrhythmias of ventricular origin, and that as a result, response of a wide QRS complex tachycardia to these treatments indicates that the rhythm is of supraventricular origin. This is only a myth; there is ample literature that indicates that some types of VT respond to these maneuvers.

VT originating in the RVOT or left ventricular outflow tract (LVOT) can respond to adenosine.[50–53] It is believed that triggered activity due to a cyclic AMP-mediated mechanism accounts for this dysrhythmia. VT arising from the RVOT also responds to verapamil. RVOT-associated VT is typically seen on the ECG as a left bundle branch pattern and an inferior axis in the frontal plane. LVOT-associated VT usually is seen on the ECG as showing a pattern of right bundle branch block with a superior axis.

Fascicular tachycardia (left septal VT), which may occur when a fascicle of the left bundle branch acts as a reentrant pathway, often responds to verapamil (but not to adenosine).[54] It is believed to be due to triggered activity.

Vagal maneuvers have also been reported to terminate VT originating in the RVOT.[51]

Therefore, wide complex tachycardias that respond to drugs used to treat supraventricular dysrhythmias may still be VT. Comparison of the QRS complexes to those of an old ECG may be helpful, but if any doubt exists, patients should be treated as having VT.

Should vasopressin or epinephrine be the first drug given in cardiac arrest? In an attempt to improve the survival of patients in cardiac arrest, other drugs have been studied. Vasopressin was found in animal studies to increase coronary blood flow and myocardial oxygen availability, and to increase the chances of successful resuscitation. In addition, survivors of cardiac arrest were found to have high endogenous vasopressin levels than those who died. Studies on humans, though have not been as encouraging.

The most recent study and largest to date, examined 1186 patients who suffered out-of-hospital arrest. Patients with VF, pulseless electrical activity (PEA), or asystole were given up to two doses of vasopressin (40 U) 3 min apart. No differences were found in return of spontaneous circulation, survival to hospital admission, or survival to hospital discharge.[55] A subgroup of patients with asystole did have a higher survival to hospital admission rate, but again, no difference in ultimate survival was noted.

Two other studies, one of patients suffering out-of-hospital VF, and the other of patients with in-hospital

arrest (VF, PEA, asystole) found conflicting results. The out-of-hospital arrest study, by Lindner and colleagues, found more patients given a single dose of vasopressin survived to hospital admission and were alive at 24 hours, than those given epinephrine.[56] There were no differences between groups in those discharged alive from the hospital. This was a very small study (20 patients per group).

When patients experiencing an in-hospital arrest were given one dose of vasopressin or epinephrine, no differences in any outcomes were found.[57]

The AHA, in the 2000 guidelines on resuscitation, allows the use of one dose of vasopressin instead of epinephrine for the initial treatment of VF or pulseless VT when initial attempts at defibrillation have failed. Further research is needed to determine if vasopressin will provide better outcomes, but the initial research is not promising.

REFERENCES

1. Echt D, Leibson P, Mitchell L, et al. Mortality and morbidity in patients receiving encainide, flecainide, or placebo: The Cardiac Arrhythmia Suppression Trial. *N Engl J Med* 1991;324:781.
2. Waldo AL, Witt AL. Mechanisms of cardiac arrhythmias and conduction disturbances. In: Fuster V, Alexander RW, O'Rourke RA, et al. (eds.), *Hurst's the Heart*, 10th ed. New York: McGraw-Hill, 2001, pp. 753–767.
3. Rubart M, Zipes DP. Genesis of cardiac arrhythmias: Electrophysiological considerations. In: Braunwald E, Zipes DP, Libby P (eds.), *Braunwald: Heart Disease: A Textbook of Cardiovascular Medicine*, 6th ed. Philadelphia, PA: W.B. Saunders, 2001, pp. 680–684.
4. Brown CG, Dzwoncyk R, Martin DR. Physiologic measurement of the ventricular fibrillation ECG signal: Estimating the duration of ventricular fibrillation. *Circulation* 1993; 22:70–74.
5. Lakatta EG, Guarnieri T. Spontaneous myocardial calcium oscillations: Are they linked to ventricular fibrillation? *J Cardiovasc Electrophysiol* 1993;4(4):473–489.
6. Zaugg CE, Wu ST, Barbosa V, et al. Ventricular fibrillation-induced intracellular Ca2+ overload causes failed electrical defibrillation and post-shock reinitiation of fibrillation. *J Mol Cell Cardiol* 1998;30(11):2183–2192.
7. Anonymous. Guidelines 2000 for Cardiopulmonary Resuscitation and Emergency Cardiovascular Care. Part 6: Advanced cardiovascular life support: Section 2: Defibrillation. The American Heart Association in collaboration with the International Liaison Committee on Resuscitation. *Circulation* 2000;102(8 Suppl):I90–I94.
8. Adgey AAJ, Patton JN, Campbell NP, et al. Ventricular defibrillation: Appropriate energy levels. *Circulation* 1979; 60:2–23.

9. Dorian P, Cas D, Schwartz B, et al. Amiodarone as compared with lidocaine for shock-resistant ventricular fibrillation. *N Engl J Med* 2002;346(12):884–890.

10. Miller J, Tresch D, Horwitz L, et al. The precordial thump. *Ann Emerg Med* 1984;13:791.

11. Caldwell G, Millar G, Quinn E, et al. Simple mechanical methods for cardioversion: Defense of the precordial thump and cough version. *Br Med J* 1985;291:627.

12. Olgin JE, Zipes DP. Specific arrhythmias: Diagnosis and treatment. In: Braunwald E, Zipes DP, Libby P (eds.), *Braunwald: Heart Disease: A Textbook of Cardiovascular Medicine*, 6th ed. Philadelphia, PA: W.B. Saunders, 2001, pp. 855–871.

13. Buxton AE, Marchlinski FE, Doherty JU, et al. Repetitive monomorphic ventricular tachycardia; Clinical and electrophysiologic characteristics in patients with and without organic heart disease. *Am J Cardiol* 1984;54:997–1002.

14. Klein LS, Shih HT, Hackett FK, et al. Radiofrequency catheter ablation of ventricular tachycardia in patients without structural heart disease. *Circulation* 1992;85:1666–1674.

15. Moss AM, Hall WJ, Cannom DS, et al., for the Multicenter Automatic Defibrillator Implantation Trial Investigators. Improved survival with an implanted defibrillator in patients with coronary disease at high risk for ventricular arrhythmia. *N Engl J Med* 1996;335:1933–1940.

16. Wellens HJ, Bar FW, Lie KI. The value of the electrocardiogram in the differential diagnosis of a tachycardia with a widened QRS complex. *Am J Med* 1978;64(1):27–33.

17. Brugada P, Brugada J, Mont L, et al. A new approach to the differential diagnosis of a regular tachycardia with a wide QRS complex. *Circulation* 1991;83(5):1649–1659.

18. Griffith MJ, Garratt CJ, Mounsey P, et al. Ventricular tachycardia as default diagnosis in broad complex tachycardia. *Lancet* 1994;343(8894):386–388.

19. Criley JM, Blaufuss AN, Kissel GL. Cough induced cardiac compression. *JAMA* 1976;236:1246–1250.

20. Wei JY, Greene HL, Weisfeldt ML. Cough-facilitated conversion of ventricular tachycardia. *Am J Cardiol* 1980;45:174–176.

21. Passman R, Kadish A. Polymorphic ventricular tachycardia, long Q-T syndrome, and torsades de Pointes. *Med Clin North Am* 2001;85(2):321–241.

22. Eisenberg S, Scheinman M, Dullet N, et al. Sudden cardiac death and polymorphous ventricular tachycardia in patients with normal QT intervals and normal systolic cardiac function. *Am J Cardiol* 1995;75:687–692.

23. Brugada P, Brugada J. Right bundle branch block, persistent ST segment elevation and sudden cardiac death: A distinct clinical and electrocardiographic syndrome. A multicenter report. *J Am Coll Cardiol* 199;20(6):1391–1396.

24. Myerburg RF, Kloosterman EM, Castellanos A. Recognition, clinical assessment, and management of arrhythmias and conduction disturbances. In: Fuster V, Alexander RW, O'Rourke RA, et al. (eds.), *Hurst's the Heart,* 10th ed. New York: McGraw-Hill, 2001, pp. 848–852.

25. Littmann L, Monroe MH, Kerns WP, et al. Brugada syndrome and "Brugada sign": Clinical spectrum with a guide for the clinician. *Am Heart J* 2003;145(5):768–778.

26. Farhy RD. Long QT syndrome. In: Marso SP, Griffin BP, Topol EJ (eds.), *Manual of Cardiovascular Medicine.* Philadelphia, PA: Lippincott Williams & Wilkins, 2000, p. 320.

27. Schwartz PJ, Moss AJ, Vincent GM, et al. Diagnostic criteria for the long QT syndrome. An update. *Circulation* 1993;88(2):782–784.

28. Moss AJ, Schwartz PJ, Crampton RS, et al. The long QT syndrome: Prospective longitudinal study of 328 families. *Circulation* 1991;84:1136–1144.

29. Schwartz PJ, Locati EH, Moss AJ, et al. Left cardiac sympathetic denervation in the therapy of congenital long QT syndrome. A worldwide report. *Circulation* 1991;84(2):503–511.

30. Park MK. Syncope. In: Park MK (ed.), *Pediatric Cardiology for Practitioners*, 4th ed. St. Louis, MO: Mosby, 2002, p. 459.

31. Julian DG, Camm AJ, Frangin G, et al., for the European Myocardial Infarct Amiodarone Trial Investigators. Randomized trial of effect of amiodarone on mortality in patients with left-ventricular dysfunction after recent myocardial infarction: EMIAT. *Lancet* 1997;349:667–674.

32. Cairns JA, Connolly SJ, Roberts R, et al., for the Canadian Amiodarone Myocardial Infarction Arrhythmia Trial Investigators. Randomized trial of outcome after myocardial infarction in patients with frequent or repetitive ventricular premature depolarizations. CAMIAT. *Lancet* 1997;349:675–682.

33. Singh SN, Fletcher RD, Fisher SB, et al. Amiodarone in patients with congestive heart failure and asymptomatic ventricular arrhythmia. Survival trial of antiarrhythmic therapy in congestive heart failure. *N Engl J Med* 1995;333:77–82.

34. Maskin CS, Siskin SJ, LeJemtal TH. High prevalence of nonsustained ventricular tachycardia in severe congestive heart failure. *Am Heart J* 1983;207:896–901.

35. Chakko CS, Gheorghiade M. Ventricular arrhythmias in severe heart failure: Incidence, significance, and effectiveness of antiarrhythmic therapy. *Am Heart J* 1985;109:497–504.

36. Webster MWI, Fitzpatrick MA, Nicholis MG, et al. Effect of enalapril on ventricular arrhythmias in congestive heart failure. *Am J Cardiol* 1985;56:566–569.

37. Moss AJ, Schnitzler R, Green R, et al. Ventricular arrhythmias 3 weeks after acute myocardial infarction. *Ann Intern Med* 1971;75:837–841.

38. Vismara LA, Amsterdam BA, Mason DT. Relation of ventricular arrhythmias in the late-hospital phase of acute myocardial infarction to sudden death after hospital discharge. *Am J Med* 1975;59:6–12.

39. Ruberman W, Weinblatt E, Goldberg JD, et al. Ventricular premature complexes and sudden death after myocardial infarction. *Circulation* 1981;64:297–305.

40. Schulze RA, Strauss HW, Pitt B. Sudden death in the year following myocardial infarction: Relationship of ventricular premature contractions in the late hospital phase and left ventricular ejection fraction. *Am J Med* 1977;62:192–199.

41. Bigger JT, Fleiss JL, Lleiger R, et al., and the multicenter postinfarction research group. The relationships among ventricular arrhythmias, left ventricular dysfunction, and mortality in the 2 years after myocardial infarction. *Circulation* 1984;69:250–258.

42. Meinertz T, Hofmann T, Kasper W, et al. Significance of ventricular arrhythmias in idiopathic dilated cardiomyopathy. *Am J Cardiol* 1984;53:902–907.

43. Holmes J, Kubo SH, Cody RJ, et al. Arrhythmias in ischemic and nonischemic dilated cardiomyopathy: Prediction of mortality by ambulatory electrocardiography. *Am J Cardiol* 1985;55:146–151.

44. Cairns JA, Connolly SJ, Roberts R, et al. Randomised trial of outcome after myocardial infarction in patients with frequent or repetitive ventricular premature depolarisations: CAMIAT. Canadian Amiodarone Myocardial Infarction Arrhythmia Trial Investigators. *Lancet* 1997;349(9053):675–682.

45. Nasir N Jr., Taylor A, Doyle TK, et al. Evaluation of intravenous lidocaine for the termination of sustained monomorphic ventricular tachycardia in patients with coronary artery disease with or without healed myocardial infarction. *Am J Cardiol* 1994;74(12):1183–1186.

46. Kudenchuk PJ, Cobb LA, Copass MK, et al. Amiodarone for resuscitation after out-of-hospital cardiac arrest due to ventricular fibrillation. *N Engl J Med* 1999;341(12):871–878.

47. Gorgels AP, van den Dool A, Hofs A, et al. Comparison of procainamide and lidocaine in terminating sustained monomorphic ventricular tachycardia. *Am J Cardiol* 1996; 78(1):43–46.

48. Ho DS, Zecchin RP, Richards DA, et al. Double-blind trial of lignocaine versus sotalol for acute termination of spontaneous sustained ventricular tachycardia. *Lancet* 1994;34:18–23.

49. Somberg JC, Bailin SJ, Haffajee CI, et al. Intravenous lidocaine versus intravenous amiodarone (in a new aqueous formulation) for incessant ventricular tachycardia. *Am J Cardiol* 2002;90(8):853–859.

50. Yeh SJ, Wen MS, Wang CC, et al. Adenosine-sensitive ventricular tachycardia from the anterobasal left ventricle. *J Am Coll Cardiol* 1997;30(5):1339–1345.

51. Markowitz SM, Litvak BL, Ramirez de Arrellano EA, et al. Adenosine-sensitive ventricular tachycardia: Right ventricular abnormalities delineated by magnetic resonance imaging. *Circulation* 1997;96(4):1192–1200.

52. Lee KL, Lauer MR, Young C, et al. Spectrum of electrophysiologic and electropharmacologic characteristics of verapamil-sensitive ventricular tachycardia in patients without structural heart disease. *Am J Cardiol* 1996; 77(11):967–973.

53. Wilber DJ, Baerman J, Olshansky B, et al. Adenosine-sensitive ventricular tachycardia. Clinical characteristics and response to catheter ablation. *Circulation* 1993;87(1):126–134.

54. Griffith MJ, Garratt CJ, Rowland E, et al. Effects of intravenous adenosine on verapamil-sensitive "idiopathic" ventricular tachycardia. *Am J Cardiol* 1994;73(11): 759–764.

55. Wenzel V, Krismer AC, Arntz HR, et al. A comparison of vasopressin and epinephrine for out-of-hospital cardiopulmonary resuscitation. *N Engl J Med* 2004;350:105–113.

56. Lindner KH, Dirks B, Strohmenger HU. Randomised comparison of epinephrine and vasopressin in patients with out-of-hospital ventricular fibrillation. *Lancet* 1997;349:535–537.

57. Stiell Ig, Herbert PC, Wells GA, et al. Vasopressin versus epinephrine for inhospital cardiac arrest: A randomized controlled trial. *Lancet* 2001;358:105–109.

21

Atrial Arrhythmias

Daniel J. Walters
Lala M. Dunbar

HIGH YIELD FACTS

- Narrow complex tachyarrhythmias at a rate >200 beats/min may involve an accessory pathway of conduction and should *not* be treated with digoxin, verapamil, adenosine, or beta-blockers as hemodynamic instability may occur.

- Atrial fibrillation (AF) or atrial flutter (Aflutter) in the setting of Wolff-Parkinson White syndrome (WPW) should be treated with IV antiarrhythmics, such as IV ibutilide, procainamide, flecainide, propafenone, or amiodarone.

- Unless specifically contraindicated, chronic anticoagulation therapy with warfarin is indicated in *all* patients with atrial fibrillation at high risk of stroke, regardless of whether sinus rhythm is restored.[18,20,24,25,31]

- Risk factors for stroke include history of prior ischemic stroke, transient ischemic attack, or systemic thromboembolism, age >75 years, heart failure, left ventricular dysfunction (ejection fraction less than 0.35), valvular heart disease, a history of hypertension, or diabetes mellitus.[19,26–31]

- Rate control is an acceptable alternative to rhythm control in the long-term management of AF with respect to relief of symptoms, thromboembolic complications, quality of life, and overall survival.[18,20–23,25]

- Warfarin is the only intervention or drug therapy that has been shown to improve survival in patients with AF by reducing the risk of death up to 33%.[31]

INTRODUCTION

Arrhythmia is the commonly accepted term for any rhythm other than regular sinus rhythm. This chapter will focus on atrial tachyarrhythmias with an observed ventricular rate >100 beats/min and a QRS complex duration less than 0.12 s. Some of the arrhythmias described are not of atrial origin, but rather originate from a focus outside the atria including the AV node or His bundle. For this reason, the term supraventricular tachycardia (SVT) will be used in favor of atrial arrhythmia to describe this large group of arrhythmias. AF and Aflutter will be discussed separately to highlight their unique electrophysiologic properties and clinical management.

MECHANISMS OF ARRHYTHMIAS

The most common mechanism accounting for these abnormal rhythms is a problem with impulse *conduction* known as reentry. Reentry mechanisms are the result of uneven conduction through a circuit in a self-perpetuating circular movement of impulse activity. For reentry to occur, two conduction pathways must exist with different rates of conduction. Problems with impulse *formation*, termed automaticity, can also occur but much less often. An arrhythmia due to a problem of automaticity implies that an ectopic pacemaker originating somewhere in the conduction system below the SA node is now functioning as the cardiac rate and rhythm pacemaker. The specific type of arrhythmia seen with either of these mechanisms depends on the anatomic origin, pathway, and electrical characteristics of the aberrant impulses.

CLASSIFICATION OF SUPRAVENTRICULAR TACHYCARDIAS

Sinus Tachycardia

Sinus tachycardia (ST) is a narrow complex regular rhythm with a ventricular rate that is not usually in excess of 170 beats/min in adults and 225 beats/min in infants and children, if the AV node is functioning normally. The P waves all have the same morphology. ST is a manifestation of a physiologic stressor such as infection, hypovolemia, hypoxemia, anemia, metabolic or endocrine derangements, or possibly a toxicologic cause. Patients are neither symptomatic nor unstable as a direct result of the arrhythmia itself. As such, antiarrhythmic drugs, AV-nodal blocking agents, and electrical cardioversion (EC) typically play no role in the treatment of these patients. Recognizing and alleviating the underlying physiologic cause will also treat the arrhythmia. Adenosine or carotid sinus massage (CSM) if used will slowly decrease the rate, which will then increase again in a continuous, graded manner. If the patient is symptomatic or is beginning to show signs of end-organ dysfunction, beta-blockers are recommended (e.g., symptomatic hyperthyroidism).

Paroxysmal Supraventricular Tachycardia

The term paroxysmal supraventricular tachycardia (PSVT) describes intermittent or paroxysmal variants of SVT characterized by abrupt onset and termination patterns. Patients typically present with complaints of palpitations, dizziness, chest discomfort, dyspnea, and fatigue. These arrhythmias are rarely associated with underlying structural heart disease. The most common causes of PSVT are AV-nodal reentrant tachycardia (AVNRT) and AV-reentrant tachycardia (AVRT). Junctional tachycardias (JT), SA-nodal reentrant tachycardia (SNRT), and atrial tachycardias (AT) are other less common causes of PSVT accounting for fewer than 10% of observed cases.[1] AVNRT accounts for nearly two-thirds of cases of PSVT and is the result of dual conduction pathways within the AV node and surrounding perinodal atrial tissue. The reentrant circuit consists of a tract capable of antegrade conduction and one in which only retrograde ventriculoatrial conduction is possible. AVRT results from an aberrant conduction circuit that involves the normal AV-nodal conduction pathway as well as an accessory pathway or AV-bypass tract, which independently bridges the atrium and ventricle. This is known as a preexcitation syndrome. The most common preexcitation syndrome is the WPW. The diagnosis of WPW is usually made when a tachyarrhythmia coexists with preexcitation. AVRT is the presenting rhythm in nearly 80% of symptomatic patients presenting with WPW[2] (see Section *Tachycardias Associated with Preexcitation Syndromes*). Conduction over these pathways occurs primarily in an antegrade or retrograde direction, though bidirectional conduction may also occur. Conduction in AVRT is further described as either orthodromic or antidromic. Orthodromic AVRT, which accounts for most cases of AVRT, is characterized by antegrade conduction across the AV node with retrograde conduction via the accessory pathway. In antidromic AVRT, the antegrade conduction pathway uses the accessory pathway while the retrograde pathway is usually across the AV node itself. The bypass tract allows 1:1 conduction to occur from the atria to the ventricles. During sinus rhythm, both types of AVRT are associated with wide, aberrant QRS complexes. During an episode of tachycardia, however, with orthodromic conduction only

retrograde conduction occurs and the QRS complexes become narrow on ECG. This is not seen with antidromic conduction in which the QRS complex stays wide. SNRT is a rare cause of PSVT that is the result of a reentrant circuit in the area of the SA node that produces P waves identical to those seen during sinus rhythm. This tachyarrhythmia is usually initiated and terminated by a premature atrial contraction (PAC). It is clinically indistinguishable from ST except for its abrupt onset and termination.

Inappropriate Sinus Tachycardia

Inappropriate sinus tachycardia (IST) is a ST in which no identifiable anatomic or physiologic abnormality or stimulus can be found to explain the tachycardia. These patients have a resting heart rate of >100 beats/min and inappropriate heart rate increases in response to minimal activity. IST is a diagnosis of exclusion for which all other causes of tachycardia must first be ruled out. No specific treatment is required though beta-blockers can be used in patients who are symptomatic.

Atrial Tachycardia

Atrial tachycardias are regular SVTs in which atrial activity originates from an ectopic focus that is outside of the SA node but above the AV node. P-wave morphology is different from that seen in sinus rhythm. The underlying mechanism accounting for the observed arrhythmia is variable. Reentrant mechanisms are more likely in patients with underlying atrial diseases, while enhanced automaticity is often observed in patients with otherwise healthy cardiac tissue. AT due to enhanced automaticity tends to be gradual in onset and termination. This is a classic presentation of digitalis toxicity in which an AV block is seen concomitantly. This arrhythmia is often exacerbated by hypokalemia. Reentrant forms of AT tend to be paroxysmal, usually initiated by a PAC. Previously known as paroxysmal atrial tachycardia (PAT), this term is no longer used and this arrhythmia is now referred to simply as a PSVT. Reentrant AT is a rare cause of PSVT. Clinically, AT can be indistinguishable from ST. Discrete atrial activity exists with a P-wave morphology that is different from that seen in sinus rhythm. Unless a comparison tracing of sinus rhythm is available, this difference may go undetected. On ECG tracing, the rhythm is regular with a ventricular rate of 140–220 beats/min. The AV node does not play a role in the initiation or maintenance of these arrhythmias; thus, the atrial to ventricular conduction ratio is usually 1:1

unless an AV block coexists. Medical treatment of both incessant and paroxysmal AT is the same as for other SVTs but is generally found to be less successful in controlling symptoms or terminating the arrhythmia. In patients unsuccessfully treated by drug therapy, catheter ablation of the ectopic focus is the best therapy.[3]

Multifocal Atrial Tachycardia

Multifocal atrial tachycardia (MAT) is a subset of AT. Unlike the other arrhythmias in this classification, MAT does not have a regular ventricular rhythm. On ECG, an irregular ventricular rhythm with no recognizable pattern (irregularly irregular) is observed. By definition, a diagnosis of MAT requires that at least three different ectopic P-wave morphologies be identified in addition to the sinus P wave. MAT is often misdiagnosed as AF but the observed ventricular rates are rarely as rapid as seen with AF and P waves are discernible. MAT is most often associated with severe underlying pulmonary disease and other metabolic and electrolyte abnormalities. Correction of these physiologic abnormalities often terminates the arrhythmia and is therefore the initial approach to treatment.

Junctional Tachycardia

Paroxysmal JT is an uncommon cause of PSVT and the most commonly observed type of JT. It is the result of an ectopic focus of conducting tissue from within either the AV node or His bundle. Although this arrhythmia is usually the result of enhanced automaticity, reentrant mechanisms can occur, but less frequently. Clinically, paroxysmal JT is characterized by the abrupt onset and termination of a narrow complex regular tachyarrhythmia with an observed ventricular rate of 110–250 beats/min. Surface ECG manifestations can be variable as neither the atrium nor ventricle is required for the initiation or propagation of this arrhythmia. Atrioventricular dissociation is often present and the rhythm can frequently appear irregular, being mistaken for AF. Ectopic P waves are present but typically indiscernible, as they are often concealed within the QRS complexes. If visualized, the P waves have an inverted appearance, due to retrograde atrial depolarizations. Paroxysmal JT presents most commonly in young adults and usually carries a benign prognosis. It is usually exercise or stress related and is observed in patients with both structurally normal hearts and in those with congenital abnormalities. Patients are frequently symptomatic and if left untreated can develop tachycardia-induced cardiomyopathy. Medical therapy is only infrequently successful and catheter ablation is usually required for long-term management.

Nonparoxysmal JT is a benign arrhythmia that is usually a response to severe underlying physiologic abnormality such as hypokalemia, digoxin toxicity, cardiac ischemia, or hypoxemia. It is typically the result of a high junctional focus of enhanced automaticity that causes an incessant arrhythmia characterized by a gradual onset and termination pattern. Clinically, a regular narrow complex tachycardia with a ventricular rate that is rarely greater than 120 beats/min is observed. Correcting the underlying physiologic abnormality typically results in termination of the observed arrhythmia.

Tachycardias Associated with Preexcitation Syndromes

Ventricular preexcitation refers to early depolarization of the ventricles as a result of electrical activation via an alternative pathway before the arrival of an impulse via the normal AV-conduction pathway.[4] The cause is an anatomic cardiac abnormality that allows aberrant or accessory pathway conduction to occur through an AV-bypass tract. The most common preexcitation syndrome is the WPW in which an accessory conduction pathway known as the Bundle of Kent exists. Classically, on ECG tracing WPW is characterized by a shortened PR interval (<0.12 s). This is due to a *delta wave*, which appears as a slurred upstroke at the initial part of the QRS complex and is the result of early ventricular depolarization via the AV-bypass tract. The QRS complex also appears widened (>0.10 s) because it represents a fusion tracing of the abnormal preexcitation wave and the normal AV-conduction wave. Even in the absence of these classic ECG findings, any symptomatic patient presenting with a paroxysmal tachycardia at a rate greater than 200 beats/min should raise suspicion to the existence of a preexcitation syndrome with an accessory pathway of conduction. A diagnosis of WPW syndrome is typically reserved for situations in which both preexcitation and a tachyarrhythmia coexist. The most commonly observed rhythm of symptomatic patients presenting with a WPW syndrome is AVRT accounting for nearly 80% of cases. In these patients, the accessory pathway is required to both initiate and sustain the arrhythmia. Other rhythms observed in patients presenting with WPW include AT, AF, Aflutter, and rarely AVNRT. In these patients, the bypass tract functions as another pathway of conduction but is not required to initiate nor sustain the arrhythmia. AF or Aflutter occurring in patients with preexcitation syndromes can be potentially fatal. Rapid ventricular rates can cause the rhythm to degenerate to ventricular fibrillation and sudden death. In these patients, treatment with antiarrhythmic agents is preferred over the use of AV-nodal blocking agents (see Step 6). Catheter ablation strategies are being used increasingly in the long-term management of pre-excitation-mediated tachyarrhythmias.

CLINICAL APPROACH TO SUPRAVENTRICULAR TACHYCARDIAS

The following stepwise approach to arrhythmia evaluation gives a basic framework by which all SVTs, including AF and Aflutter, can be evaluated and treated.

Step 1—Stable Versus Unstable

The initial evaluation of a symptomatic patient is to determine whether the patient is hemodynamically stable or unstable as a direct result of the tachyarrhythmia itself. The signs and symptoms of an unstable patient include evidence of end-organ dysfunction including cardiac ischemia, hypotension, congestive heart failure, or mental status changes. Emergent treatment with electrical DC cardioversion is indicated if the arrhythmia is identified as the main factor responsible for the patient's hemodynamic instability and prompt pharmacologic measures are ineffective. It should be noted that an unstable patient in ST or any arrhythmia whose underlying mechanism is one of enhanced automaticity, such as MAT, will not respond to treatment with EC and is therefore not indicated in these situations. Instead, identification and treatment of the underlying cause will stabilize the patient and typically resolve the observed arrhythmia. While preparing for cardioversion an initial attempt should be made to identify and treat any rapidly reversible factors that may be contributing to a patient's instability (e.g., pneumothoraces, hyperthermia, drug intoxication, hypovolemia, hypoxia). If this cannot be readily accomplished, with immediate stabilization of the patient, treatment with EC is indicated. In symptomatic yet stable patients, a more systematic approach can be taken in evaluating and treating the arrhythmia.

Step 2—ECG Analysis

During any observed tachyarrhythmia, a 12-lead ECG should always be obtained prior to initiating treatment. If this is not possible due to a patient's hemodynamic instability and need for emergent EC, at the very least a long rhythm strip from the cardiac defibrillator unit should be obtained. In hemodynamically stable patients, all aspects of the clinical presentation should be reviewed including a thorough history and focused physical examination. SVTs are typically narrow complex with a QRS

duration <0.12 s. If a wide complex SVT is observed that is not of ventricular origin, consider the presence of either a concomitant bundle branch block or a preexcitation syndrome with an accessory conduction pathway (see Section *Tachycardias Associated with Preexcitation Syndromes*). Both can account for a widened QRS complex. If a firm diagnosis of SVT cannot be made and the arrhythmia cannot be easily differentiated from VT, then the patient should be treated as if the arrhythmia were of ventricular origin. Once the diagnosis of an SVT has been made, the tachycardia can be further characterized to identify the specific arrhythmia present.

Step 3—Regular or Irregular Ventricular Rhythm

The tachyarrhythmia should be assessed first for ventricular rhythm regularity. Most narrow complex tachyarrhythmias are associated with a regular rhythm such as ST, PSVT, AT, and Aflutter. Only MAT, AF, or one of the preceding regular rhythms with a variable conduction block, has an irregular rhythm. A long rhythm strip or increased paper speed may help in making the determination of regularity. For paroxysmal arrhythmias, recording the pattern of onset or termination of the rhythm can be helpful. If the rhythm is irregular, the ECG should be scrutinized for a pattern. If no pattern exists then the diagnosis is either MAT or AF. If the rhythm is irregular yet a distinct pattern is discernible then the arrhythmia is likely a normally regular arrhythmia such as Aflutter with variable AV-nodal conduction and block.

Step 4—Determining Atrial Activity

If the rhythm is irregular and discrete P waves are not discernible, the rhythm is likely AF. An irregular rhythm in which discrete P waves are visible is likely MAT. Arrhythmias with a regular ventricular rhythm and discrete P waves include ST, PSVT, AT, or Aflutter. Although P waves may exist during an observed rapid tachyarrhythmia, they may not always be seen on an ECG tracing due to the rapid ventricular rate. This is often seen with the common causes of PSVT including AVRT, and AVNRT. During these arrhythmias, P waves are often superimposed on the QRS complex and thus not identified. The rapid ventricular rates obscure the electrical baseline making it nearly impossible to evaluate the arrhythmia for discrete atrial activity. ST, PSVT, AT, Aflutter, and even AF can all look very similar on ECG tracings when observed ventricular rates are greater than 180 beats/min. To further characterize these narrow complex tachyarrhythmias in which P waves cannot be clearly identified, vagal maneuvers such as CSM or IV adenosine can be used diagnostically to slow the ventricular rate allowing visualization of atrial activity (see Step 6). Once discrete atrial activity has been identified, P-wave morphology can be evaluated.

Step 5—Analyzing P-Wave Morphology

If the P-wave morphology is identical to that seen in normal sinus rhythm, the arrhythmia is ST, IST, SNRT. If the P-wave morphology is different from that in sinus rhythm the possible arrhythmias include PSVT, AT, MAT, or Aflutter. Ectopic P waves of at least three different morphologies are required to make a diagnosis of MAT.

Step 6—General Approach to Medical Treatment

After attempting to identify the type of arrhythmia present, an initial effort should be made to identify and treat any reversible underlying causes for the tachyarrhythmia. Hypovolemia should always be considered as a possible cause of any SVT, especially in the young. Fever, anemia, hypoxemia or impaired oxygen delivery (including abnormal hemoglobin states), relative sympathetic excess, drug intoxication, endocrinologic disease (especially thyroid), metabolic derangements, ischemia, infections, and inflammatory causes (including myocarditis and pericarditis) should also be considered. Other precipitating factors such as excessive caffeine, alcohol, or nicotine use if present should also be eliminated. Some arrhythmias are classically associated with specific disease processes, which once identified and treated will result in resolution of the arrhythmia (e.g., ST, AT, and MAT). MAT is most often associated with pulmonary disease and hypoxemia and is readily amenable to treatment.

If an underlying cause for the arrhythmia is not easily identified or amenable to treatment, vagal maneuvers such as CSM, or IV adenosine are the first-line choices of therapy for symptomatic patients. They both act to slow SA-nodal activity and increase AV-nodal conduction delay, which can be therapeutic as well as diagnostic. The observed outcome depends on the underlying electrophysiologic mechanism responsible for the arrhythmia being treated. Any SVT that *must* involve the SA or AV node in their conduction circuit will often terminate completely as seen with SNRT and most cases of PSVT including AVRT and AVNRT. Patients with ST and IST will demonstrate a temporary decrease in the observed ventricular rate, which then reaccelerates back to baseline. During certain arrhythmias in which the AV node is not required to initiate or sustain the arrhythmia, the induced AV-conduction delay may help unmask discrete atrial

activity that was previously indiscernible. This can play a diagnostic role, helping to differentiate the tachyarrhythmias of AT, AF, and Aflutter. In some instances no effect is seen. Regardless of the outcome, the observed effect can provide valuable information. Short-term side effects of adenosine which patients should be warned about include dyspnea, flushing, chest pain, and a feeling of extreme anxiety that is likely due to the induced period of brief asystole that can sometimes last for 5 or more seconds. Caution should be used when treating patients with reactive airway disease as bronchospasm can be induced. Theophylline directly antagonizes the effect of adenosine and treatment with another agent should be considered. Adenosine use can rarely precipitate AF in some patients, which although usually transient, may be problematic if a concurrent preexcitation syndrome is present.

In patients with preserved LV function requiring further treatment, ventricular response rates can be controlled with beta-blockers and nondihydropyridine calcium-channel blockers (Table 21-1). Any SVT that has a conduction circuit involving the AV node will be amenable to treatment with agents that block AV-node conduction. Digoxin can also be used for rate control but it has a slower onset of action and therefore should not be used as a first-line agent. It may play more of a role in patients with refractory arrhythmias, impaired LV function, or for maintenance therapy. Intravenous magnesium sulfate may be used as adjunctive therapy to decrease ventricular rates. Antiarrhythmic agents such as procainamide, sotalol, propafenone, flecainide, and amiodarone though indicated should be used with caution because of their proarrhythmic effects and potential to cause hypotension (Table 21-2). Amiodarone is the preferred antiarrhythmic agent if LV dysfunction or signs of heart failure are present concurrently. Overdrive atrial pacing is also an option.[5] Electrical DC cardioversion is rarely needed except in unstable patients, but may be used when other treatment modalities are unable to terminate the arrhythmia. Emergent and elective EC should be attempted starting at 50–100 J with concurrent conscious sedation. EC plays no role in treating AT caused by digitalis toxicity. With digitalis toxicity as the cause of the arrhythmia, correcting hypokalemia, using digoxin-specific Fab and IV magnesium may help.

Caution

Drugs that slow AV-nodal conduction such as adenosine, digoxin, calcium-channel blockers, and beta-blockers, should be used cautiously in patients with conduction via a suspected accessory pathway. Rapid ventricular rates

Table 21-1. Intravenous and Oral Pharmacologic Agents for Ventricular Rate Control in Patients with Atrial Arrhythmias

Drug	Oral Dosage	IV Dosage	Side Effects
Adenosine	NA	6 mg bolus; may repeat with 12 mg twice	Flushing, chest pain, dyspnea, anxiety, hypotension
Digoxin	0.25 mg load every 2 h up to 1.5 mg, then 0.125–0.5 mg/day	0.25–0.5 mg load, then 0.25 mg every 2 h to a maximum of 1.5 mg	Heart block, bradycardia, digoxin toxicity with GI and visual disturbances
Diltiazem	120–360 mg/day in divided doses or as an extended release preparation	0.25 mg/kg over 2 min, repeat with 0.35 mg/kg, then infuse at 5–20 mg/h	Hypotension, heart block, heart failure
Esmolol	NA	0.5 mg/kg over 1 min, then 0.05–0.2 mg/kg/min infusion	Hypotension, heart block, heart failure, asthma, bradycardia, sexual dysfunction
Metoprolol	25–100 mg twice daily or daily as an extended release preparation	2.5–15 mg every 5–15 min up to 3 doses	Hypotension, heart block, heart failure, asthma, bradycardia, sexual dysfunction
Propranolol	80–240 mg in divided doses or as an extended release preparation	0.15 mg/kg	Hypotension, heart block, heart failure, asthma, bradycardia, sexual dysfunction
Verapamil	240–480 mg/day in divided doses or as an extended release preparation	0.075–0.15 mg/kg over 2 min	Hypotension, heart block, heart failure, constipation, peripheral edema

greater than 200 beats/min should alert the clinician to this possibility (see Section *Tachycardias Associated with Preexcitation Syndromes*). These agents may enhance conduction via the accessory path; thus, increasing the ventricular rate paradoxically from that observed prior to the intervention. If a patient has a preexcitation syndrome and a narrow complex tachycardia with a rate that is <200 beats/min, treatment is the same as for other SVTs. Patients in AF or Aflutter with a widened QRS complex and a preexcitation syndrome like WPW (see Section *Tachycardias Associated with Preexcitation Syndromes*) will usually have an observed ventricular rate >200 beats/min.[6] These patients should *never* be treated with digoxin, verapamil, adenosine, or beta-blockers. Use of these agents could increase conduction through the accessory pathway resulting in exceedingly high ventricular rates that could cause the rhythm to deteriorate to ventricular tachycardia, fibrillation, or even sudden death.[7-9] These patients should be treated as if VT were present. EC or drug therapy with antiarrhythmics such as IV ibutilide, procainamide, or flecainide is recommended.[10,11] These drugs slow conduction and prolong the refractoriness of the accessory conduction pathway. If concurrent LV dysfunction exists, EF <35%, amiodarone is the preferred alternative.

Disposition of any patient presenting with a symptomatic SVT depends mainly on the type of arrhythmia present, severity of symptoms, presence of any serious underlying medical illnesses, and treatment course. Many adult patients can be safely discharged from the emergency department (ED) with appropriate follow up if their arrhythmia was associated with benign symptoms and easily terminated. Patients with serious underlying medical illnesses, advanced age, recurrent symptoms, or any evidence of hemodynamic instability should be admitted to the hospital for further monitoring and evaluation. Outpatient ambulatory Holter or event monitoring, and echocardiography should be considered in anyone discharged to home that has not been previously evaluated, or in patients whose symptoms are paroxysmal. Referral to an arrhythmia specialist for electrophysiology studies is indicated in patients with severe symptoms such as syncope, patients with paroxysmal arrhythmias, and in all patients with evidence of preexcitation syndromes such as WPW.

ATRIAL FLUTTER

Atrial flutter is characterized by regular atrial depolarizations at a rate of 250–350 beats/min. The usual

Table 21-2. Intravenous and Oral Antiarrhythmic Agents for the Acute and Long-Term Management of Patients with Atrial Arrhythmias

Drug	Oral Dosage	IV Dosage	Side Effects
Amiodarone	800–1600 mg daily for 7–14 days or 10 g total, then 200–400 mg daily maintenance dose	5–7 mg/kg over 20–60 min, then 1.2–1.8 g/day IV infusion until 10 g total given, then 200–400 mg/day maintenance dose	Proarrhythmic, thyroid, skin, CNS, and liver abnormalities, pulmonary toxicity, GI upset, hypotension
Disopyramide	100–200 mg tid-qid	NA	Proarrhythmic, anticholinergic effects
Dofetilide	0.1–0.5 µg bid (should follow use of Ibutilide)	NA	Proarrhythmic, negative inotrope, adjust dose for renal function
Flecainide	50 mg bid to maximum 300 mg/day	1.5–3 mg/kg over 10–20 min	Proarrhythmic, CNS disturbances, rapidly conducting atrial flutter
Ibutilide	NA	0.015–0.02 mg/kg over 10 min, may repeat to maximum dose of 2 mg	Pro-arrhythmic, headache, chest pain, dizziness
Procainamide	2–4 g daily in divided doses	50 mg/min; to total 18 mg/kg (12 mg/kg if CHF)	Proarrhythmic, hypotension, lupus, agranulocytosis, GI upset, rapidly conducting atrial flutter
Propafenone	150–300 mg tid	1.5–2 mg/kg over 10–20 min	Proarrhythmic, GI upset, metallic taste, CNS disturbances, rapidly conducting atrial flutter
Quinidine	200–300 mg initially may repeat every 1 h until 1.5 g given	NA	Proarrhythmic, GI upset, rashes
Sotalol	80–240 mg bid	100 mg over 10 min	Proarrhythmic, bradycardia, fatigue

mechanism is a reentrant atrial conduction circuit, although an abnormal automatic mechanism is possible. AV-nodal conduction protects against the 1:1 conduction of these rapid atrial impulses directly to the ventricles by 2:1, 3:1, or even higher ratio AV blocks. On surface ECG, the rapid atrial depolarizations give a sawtooth pattern to the baseline known as flutter waves. These are best seen in the inferior leads (II, III, aVF) or in lead VI. The classic A flutter pattern is a 2:1 AV-conduction ratio with a 150 beat/min regular ventricular rate. A flutter with a variable AV-conduction block ratio is also possible which clinically results in an irregular ventricular rhythm that is nearly indistinguishable from AF. On ECG, the flutter waves can be difficult to discern often making the rhythm indistinguishable from ST or PSVT. Vagal maneuvers or IV adenosine can be used diagnostically to temporarily slow SA-nodal activity or increase the block ratio at the AV node, which temporarily decreases the observed ventricular rate and may unmask the flutter waves. A flutter is most commonly seen in older individuals and is almost always an indication of underlying disease. Patients are usually symptomatic as a result of the rapid heart rate as well as the underlying disorder or physiologic abnormality that precipitated the arrhythmia. A flutter is often associated with chronic cardiac and pulmonary disease or as a response to acute cardiac or pulmonary strain as seen with myocardial ischemia, pulmonary embolism, chronic obstructive pulmonary disease exacerbations, or hyperthyroidism. Common presenting symptoms include chest pain, palpitations, dizziness, fatigue, dyspnea, and rarely syncope. The initial workup for a patient with suspected A flutter includes serum chemistries and blood counts, thyroid function studies, an ECG, and CXR. Patients should also have an echocardiogram to assess underlying cardiac disease, atrial size, and risk for thromboembolic complications. Transesophageal echocardiography (TEE) is most sensitive for detecting atrial thrombus formation. Holter or event monitoring may be useful if symptoms are paroxysmal.

Treatment Options for Atrial Flutter

Treatment of Aflutter focuses on the following issues: ventricular rate control, restoration of sinus rhythm, treatment of underlying disease processes, and the prevention of thromboembolic complications. The optimal outcome of treatment is the restoration and maintenance of sinus rhythm. Although Aflutter is an electrically unstable rhythm that usually converts spontaneously to either AF or normal sinus rhythm, hemodynamic instability can occur necessitating emergent evaluation and treatment with EC. Low energy can be used (25–50 J) but higher energy has been recommended (100–200 J) to avoid converting the rhythm to AF.[12] Less energy may be required if biphasic shock modalities are used in place of monophasic shocks. In stable patients not requiring immediate EC, treatment of Aflutter can proceed in the following stepwise approach. As an underlying disease process or physiologic abnormality often precipitates Aflutter, an initial attempt should be made to treat any reversible physiologic abnormalities that can be identified. This intervention alone may result in resolution of the arrhythmia, obviating the need for further treatment. Although vagal maneuvers and IV adenosine may play a diagnostic role in the initial evaluation of a patient with suspected Aflutter, neither plays a therapeutic role once the diagnosis has been made. In symptomatic yet stable patients, rate control strategies represent the first-line of treatment in the ED aimed at reducing patient symptoms caused by the rapid ventricular rates observed. Rate control can be accomplished with AV-nodal blocking agents such as IV calcium-channel blockers (verapamil, diltiazem), or IV beta-blockers (metoprolol, esmolol) (Table 21-1). These agents should not be used in patients with severe heart failure, and should be used cautiously in patients with SA-node dysfunction, preexcitation syndromes, hypotension, or high degree preexisting AV block. Digoxin can be used if heart failure or hypotension is present and may be used in combination with beta-blockers and calcium-channel blockers. In general, rate control strategies are less effective in patients with Aflutter compared to other types of atrial arrhythmias and should not be considered definitive treatment in the management of this arrhythmia. Rate control is only a means to reduce patient symptoms until sinus rhythm can be safely restored. Rhythm control is the preferred treatment outcome in the management of Aflutter. Elective cardioversion can be accomplished either electrically or chemically using any of a variety of antiarrhythmic agents (Table 21-2). The strategy of chemical cardioversion is to depress the initiating premature atrial beats or to prolong the atrial refractory period. Ibutilide is the antiarrhythmic drug of choice. Its use carries the risk of

QT prolongation and torsades de pointes, thus close patient monitoring is a necessity. Caution should be exercised when using flecainide, propafenone, or procainamide for rhythm control. By slowing atrial rates, these agents can cause 1:1 AV conduction to occur which may paradoxically increase the observed ventricular rate and precipitate life-threatening symptoms. When these agents are used, AV-nodal blocking agents *must* be used concurrently. The antiarrhythmic agents also play a role in the long-term management of patients requiring suppressive therapy to maintain sinus rhythm and prevent recurrences. Overdrive atrial pacing is also an established means of converting Aflutter to sinus rhythm. Radiofrequency ablation of the reentrant circuit is another treatment option that has gained popularity because of the substantial recurrence rate of Aflutter in patients after cardioversion alone and the potential toxicity of long-term therapy with prophylactic antiarrhythmic drugs.

Thromboembolic events are possible with Aflutter. Although atrial blood flow rates are greater than those seen in AF, they are less than the rates seen in normal sinus rhythm. This may predispose to clot formation. Despite reduced flow rates, active atrial contractions still occur during Aflutter, which is not the case in AF. This makes atrial thrombus formation less likely. In one study, patients with isolated Aflutter had a risk that was found to be no different from that of the control population.[13] In another study, the risk of thromboembolic events in patients with Aflutter and AF concurrently was found to be the same as for patients with AF alone.[14] Unfortunately, AF and Aflutter often occur in the same patient, making thromboembolic risk stratification and anticoagulation recommendations even more difficult to ascertain. Well-designed, clinical trials to assess the role of antithrombotic therapy in patients with Aflutter are lacking, so antithrombotic guidelines for patients with AF are often extended to include those patients with Aflutter as well[2] (see Section *Treatment Options for Atrial Fibrillation*).

ATRIAL FIBRILLATION

Atrial fibrillation is the most common sustained arrhythmia with a prevalence that increases with age from 0.5% in adults aged less than 60 to more than 6% in those 80 and older.[15] Underlying heart disease including hypertension, heart failure, myocardial ischemia, and valvular heart disease (particularly mitral disease) predispose to AF, though it may occur in patients with no detectable cardiac disease, designated as "lone" AF. An underlying predisposing condition exists in more than 90% cases of AF. Thyrotoxicosis, binge alcohol use called the "holiday heart syndrome," surgery, pulmonary embolism, and electrocution are other acute causes of AF that usually resolve with treatment of the underlying condition. Autonomic instability with either increased vagal or sympathetic tone can also trigger AF in a susceptible patient. Physiologically, AF is the loss or replacement of organized, regular atrial tissue depolarizations with chaotic, unorganized depolarizations. The result is the replacement of sinus P waves with rapid fibrillatory F waves that vary in size, shape, and timing. The F waves can be coarse, medium, or fine with no correlation existing between the type of F waves observed and the etiology of the arrhythmia, or size of the atria.[16] On surface ECG, AF is recognized by F waves, giving an undulating appearance to the ECG baseline and an irregularly irregular ventricular pattern. When AV conduction is normal, a narrow complex tachyarrhythmia is observed while a wide complex tachyarrhythmia may occur when accessory conduction pathways exist, or in the presence of a bundle branch block. Regardless of the underlying physiologic mechanism, this chaotic, disorganized activity can lead to hemodynamic compromise and thromboembolic complications, which result in significant morbidity, mortality, and economic burden. The prognosis for patients younger than 60 years of age with no evidence of underlying cardiopulmonary disease can be benign, but worsens with increasing age and the prevalence or development of cardiac abnormalities. Nearly 17% of all cases of stroke occur in patients with a history of AF, while patients with recurrent AF carry a total mortality rate approximately double that of people with normal sinus rhythm.[17]

Although AF represents a heterogeneous group of clinical entities, general classifications based on patterns of disease presentation can be made. Four main categories or types of AF have been described.[18] AF can be designated as a "first-detected episode" or "recurrent" if two or more episodes have occurred. Recurrent AF can be further divided into "paroxysmal" if it terminates spontaneously or "persistent" when sustained, requiring cardioversion to restore sinus rhythm. Persistent AF is designated as "permanent" when cardioversion fails or is not attempted. Recurrent AF is a chronic disease process regardless of whether sinus rhythm is restored. Once classified as persistent, the resumption of sinus rhythm does not change the designation and patients maintain the same risks of thromboembolism and death.[18] This classification scheme does not include AF due to a reversible cause.

Clinically, patients often present with complaints of chest pain, dyspnea, palpitations, fatigue, dizziness, and syncope. On physical examination, irregularly irregular pulses, irregular venous jugular pulsations, and variations in the loudness of the first heart sound characterize AF. Capturing the arrhythmia on ECG tracing is diagnostic. Unfortunately, paroxysmal forms of the disease may require longer monitoring periods through the use of an event or Holter monitor. Patients are usually symptomatic as a direct result of the rapid ventricular rates that can be achieved with this arrhythmia. Although atrial rates in AF can range from 350 to 500 beats/min, the observed ventricular rates are usually significantly less. The AV node is normally the only conducting pathway between the atria and ventricles and exerts a protective mechanism against 1:1 conduction of the rapid atrial impulses directly to the ventricles. While ventricular rates as high as 200 beats/min can be seen with a normally functioning AV node, rates greater than 200 beats/min strongly suggest a bypass of the AV nodal pathway with aberrant conduction through either an accessory or preexcitation pathway (see Section *Tachycardias Associated with Preexcitation Syndromes*). Conduction via one of these alternate mechanisms can allow for ventricular rates as high as 300 beats/min to occur which poses a serious risk of myocardial ischemia, hemodynamic compromise, ventricular fibrillation, and sudden death. AV-nodal blocking agents such as digitalis, beta-blockers, or calcium-channel antagonists which are used to control ventricular rates in AF, do not block conduction over these accessory pathways and may even paradoxically increase it, and thus should not be used if these mechanisms are suspected (see Step 6).

In patients with new-onset AF, a comprehensive evaluation to determine the cause of their arrhythmia is appropriate. This includes a thorough history and physical examination, metabolic profile, blood tests of thyroid function, blood counts, an ECG, and CXR. Attempts should be made to determine the duration of symptoms, associated symptoms, prior episodes of AF, underlying risk factors, and any associated comorbidities. An echocardiogram is helpful to assess cardiac function, atrial sizes, and to detect thrombus formation. Although this evaluation does not always necessitate an inpatient evaluation, within the time constraints of a busy ED these patients are usually admitted for further treatment and to determine the underlying etiology of their arrhythmia.

Treatment Options for Atrial Fibrillation

Patients presenting to the emergency department with AF encompass a wide spectrum of clinical scenarios. Asymptomatic patients with a previous diagnosis of AF that is already adequately rate or rhythm controlled do not require any treatment on an emergent basis. These patients can be managed as outpatients, assuring that their anticoagulation needs are addressed to reduce their risk of thromboembolic complications. At the other end of the clinical spectrum are hemodynamically unstable patients presenting with rapid ventricular response rates requiring emergent cardioversion. Emergent dc cardioversion is indicated if AF is the main factor accounting for a patients' hemodynamic instability and prompt pharmacologic measures prove ineffective. Symptoms and signs of instability include decompensated heart failure, hypotension, altered mental status, angina, or ECG evidence of myocardial ischemia. Once indicated, emergent EC should not be delayed while waiting for prior anticoagulation. Unfractionated or low-molecular weight heparin can be given concurrently, followed by oral anticoagulation for at least 3–4 weeks after cardioversion to achieve an international normalized ratio (INR) of between 2 and 3.[19] Between these two clinical extremes are the majority of patients presenting for acute evaluation and treatment of symptomatic AF. The two major aspects of managing these patients are to minimize symptoms, and to reduce the risk of thromboembolic complications. Treatment to reduce symptoms can be accomplished by two fundamentally different approaches. The first approach is to restore sinus rhythm through either electrical or chemical cardioversion. The second approach is to permissively allow the abnormal rhythm to continue, focusing solely on minimizing patient symptoms by reducing the ventricular response rate. The restoration of sinus rhythm makes intuitive sense while a ventricular rate control approach has the advantage of avoiding highly potent and frequently toxic antiarrhythmic drugs. Although both treatment approaches have their advantages and disadvantages, supporters and critics, recent studies have failed to show any significant differences between the two approaches with respect to relief of symptoms, thromboembolic complications, quality of life, and overall survival.[20–23] The decision to initiate antithrombotic therapy in patients with AF represents a balance between efforts to prevent thromboembolic complications while attempting to avoid catastrophic hemorrhagic complications. Unless contraindicated, all patients with paroxysmal or persistent AF at increased risk for stroke should be anticoagulated with warfarin to achieve an INR of between 2 and 3, regardless of whether sinus rhythm is restored.[18–20,24,25] Patients considered to be at increased risk for stroke include those with prior ischemic stroke, transient ischemic attack, or systemic thromboembolism, age >75 years, heart failure, left ventricular dysfunction (ejection fraction less than 0.35), valvular heart disease, a history of hypertension, or diabetes mellitus.[19,26–31] In

patients with paroxysmal or persistent AF, age 65–75, in the absence of other risk factors, antithrombotic therapy with warfarin or aspirin 325 mg/day is recommended.[19] In patients <65 years with paroxysmal or persistent AF but no other risk factors, aspirin 325 mg/day is recommended.[19] Patients younger than 60 years of age with "lone AF" may require no therapy at all. Aspirin in a dose of 325 mg/day is acceptable alternative therapy in patients with contraindications to oral anticoagulation with warfarin. At present both rhythm control and rate control approaches can be considered first-line treatments in the management of AF. Failed attempts to restore sinus rhythm should not be looked upon as treatment failures.

Rate Control Strategies in the Treatment of Atrial Fibrillation

Ventricular rate control is the mainstay of the ED management of patients with symptomatic AF. Patient symptoms are optimally minimized with a reduction in heart rate to below 100 beats/min at rest and below 120 beats/min during exercise. Preferred first-line agents for rate control include IV calcium-channel blockers (verapamil or diltiazem), and beta-blockers (esmolol, metoprolol) (Table 21-1). These drugs decrease AV-nodal conduction, thus decreasing observed ventricular rates. In the presence of hypotension or underlying heart failure, IV digoxin is the preferred agent. IV amiodarone is also effective therapy for rate control in patients with "permanent" AF in whom attempts at cardioversion have been unsuccessful. Vagal maneuvers and IV adenosine do not have a therapeutic role in the management of AF. Caution should be exercised when treating any patient with an AV-nodal blocking agent if an accessory pathway of conduction is suspected. These agents do not block conduction over the accessory pathway and may even enhance conduction, potentially precipitating ventricular tachycardia, fibrillation, or even sudden death (see Step 6). In these patients, IV procainamide or ibutilide are the drugs of choice, as both will block conduction over the accessory pathway. Other agents that can be used in this setting include IV quinidine, disopyramide, and amiodarone.

Rhythm Control Strategies in the Treatment of Atrial Fibrillation

Cardioversion can be performed either emergently or on an elective basis. AF that has been present for >48 hours carries a significant risk of thromboembolism. Elective cardioversion should not be attempted without prior anticoagulation unless the arrhythmia duration is <48 hours, and the patient is at very low risk for thromboembolic complications, or a TEE study can be obtained immediately prior to cardioversion. A negative TEE study that fails to detect thrombus in the left atrium or left atrial appendage represents a safe alternative to anticoagulation for 3 weeks prior to cardioversion.[32] In all other cases, anticoagulation should be instituted for 3–4 weeks prior to cardioversion being attempted. Restoration of sinus rhythm can result in transient myocardial dysfunction known as "stunning" during which thrombus may form. For this reason, all patients undergoing cardioversion should be anticoagulated at the time of cardioversion and for at least 3–4 weeks after cardioversion, including those with a negative TEE screening study.[19,33] Unless a TEE can be obtained promptly, elective cardioversion is rarely part of the emergency department management of patients with AF due to the inherent difficulty in determining whether the arrhythmia duration is less than 48 hours. Elective cardioversion can be accomplished either pharmacologically (PC) or electrically (EC). Both carry the same risk of thromboembolism. EC is slightly more effective, but carries the risks of conscious sedation. The agents used for PC carry the risk of causing proarrhythmias such as torsades de pointes, ventricular tachycardia, or fibrillation. For this reason PC is usually recommended as an inpatient procedure where cardiac monitoring is possible and arrhythmias can be treated. PC is most effective if attempted within 1 week of arrhythmia onset. Preferred agents include ibutilide, dofetilide, amiodarone, propafenone, flecainide, quinidine, procainamide, and sotalol (Table 21-2). In patients with impaired LV function amiodarone is the preferred agent. These agents are also used to maintain sinus rhythm in select patients in whom the benefits of therapy outweigh the risks of long-term treatment with these potentially toxic agents. AV-nodal blocking agents *must* be used if cardioversion is attempted using flecainide, propafenone, or procainamide as these agents can rarely cause 1:1 AV conduction to occur which paradoxically increases the observed ventricular rate and may precipitate life-threatening symptoms. The success of EC depends on a number of variables including the voltage of the defibrillator capacitor, the position of the paddles, and transthoracic impedence. The energy level required is less and overall success is greater with anterior-posterior paddle configuration when compared to anterior-lateral configuration.[34] Cardioversion with 50 J has typically been recommended in the past but is rarely effective unless biphasic waveform modalities are used. As such, EC starting at 100–200 J is recommended for both emergent and elective cardioversion. Electrical cardioversion of patients with implanted pacemaker or defibrillator devices is safe in so far as the devices are checked for functioning before and after cardioversion. Paddles position should be as far from the device as possible. Elevations in CK-MB blood levels may occur after cardioversion and surface ECG tracings may demonstrate transient ST-segment elevations even without clinically significant myocardial damage having occurred.

UNRESOLVED ISSUES

Are rate control strategies equivalent to rhythm control in the management of all patients with AF? Recent studies have failed to demonstrate a difference between rate and rhythm control strategies with respect to relief of symptoms, thromboembolic complications, quality of life, and overall survival in the management of AF. Younger patients have been under-represented in these studies and it is unclear at this time whether rhythm control strategies may not be more appropriate in these patients. In younger patients with lone AF, new-onset AF, or paroxysmal AF without risk factors for stroke, there may be a preference to be maintained in sinus rhythm because of poor exercise tolerance and continued symptoms with rate control therapy. As well, the longer-term effects of remaining in AF with rate control therapy, particularly with regard to the structural remodeling of the myocardium, are unclear at this time. Further study is required to definitively answer this question.

Will ablative therapies replace both presently used rhythm control and rate control strategies as the preferred treatment of AF? Before rate control was known to be comparable to rhythm control in the long-term management of patients with AF, the endpoint of therapy was always to restore sinus rhythm. This led to the use of antiarrhythmic drugs often with a very narrow risk-benefit profile primarily due to their potential to be proarrhythmic. As a result, efforts were made to develop new ways of restoring sinus rhythm, which led to the development of ablative therapies to restore sinus rhythm. Today, with rate control being considered first-line treatment for AF, it is still unclear what role ablative therapies will play in the future. It is particularly unclear which patient populations would benefit most from attempts to cure their AF and restore sinus rhythm, thus continuing the debate over how to best treat AF.

Do all patients with new-onset AF require admission to the hospital for further evaluation? Stable patients who present with new-onset AF of less than 48 hours duration, that either spontaneously reverts to sinus rhythm or is cardioverted in the ED, and who are at low risk for stroke without underlying heart disease, may not require admission to the hospital and can be discharged from the ED to home safely.[35–37] In practice though, many of these same patients are admitted solely to rule out ACS. AF is rarely indicative of ACS in the absence of either chest pain or ECG changes consistent with ischemia or infarction. These patients can be safely discharged home and further evaluated as an outpatient unless there are other reasons beside the AF requiring an inpatient setting. These can include advanced age, significant comorbidities requiring treatment, and any patient with hemodynamic compromise that may be at risk for complications. Unfortunately, clinical practice does not always follow these recommendations making further study into this matter necessary.

Is there a role for angiotensin converting enzyme inhibitors (ACEIs) and angiotensin receptor blockers (ARBs) in the treatment of patients with left ventricular dysfunction (LVD) and concurrent AF? The incidence of AF in patients with LVD ranges from 2% to 50%, with the highest incidence occurring in those with the most severe symptoms. Clinical data suggest that patients with LVD and concurrent AF carry a worse prognosis with regard to increased rates of heart failure exacerbations, hospitalizations, and death.[38–41] Current treatment recommendations for patients with AF have failed to outline strategies specifically designed for patients with LVD and AF. An improved understanding of the pathophysiologic changes that predispose patients with LVD to the develop AF may lead to improved preventive and treatment strategies in the future. Recent insights into the basic mechanisms of AF suggest that activation of the renin-angiotensin system contributes to the development and maintenance of AF primarily through atrial remodeling. Treatment with an ACEI or ARB may attenuate this remodeling.[42–44] Results from recent studies support this hypothesis. In one study using animal models, atrial remodeling was reduced following treatment with an ACEI.[45] In another study, the incidence of AF in patients with LVD after acute myocardial infarction was reduced by 55% in patients treated with an ACEI versus a placebo.[46] In a third study, following cardioversion, patients treated with an ARB plus amiodarone had a lower rate of recurrence of AF than did patients treated with amiodarone alone.[47] Although their exact role is unknown at this time, the results are encouraging enough to suggest that ACEIs and ARBs will be used in the future to optimize the treatment of patients with LVD and concurrent AF.

REFERENCES

1. Trohman RG. Supraventricular tachycardia: Implications for the intensivist. *Crit Care Med* 2000;28:N129.
2. Blomstrom-Lundqvist C, Scheinman MM, Aliot EM, et al. ACC/AHA/ESC guidelines for the management of patients with supraventricular arrhythmias—executive summary: A report of the American College of Cardiology/American Heart Association Task Force on Practice Guidelines and the European Society of Cardiology Committee for Practice Guidelines (Writing Committee to Develop Guidelines for the Management of Patients With Supraventricular Arrhythmias): Developed in Collaboration With the NASPE—Heart Rhythm Society. *Eur Heart J* 2003;24(20):1857–1897.
3. Anguera I, Brugada J, Roba M, et al. Outcomes after radiofrequency catheter ablation of atrial tachyacardia. *Am J Cardiol* 2001;87:886–890.
4. Durrer D, Schuilenburg RM, Wellens HJJ. Pre-excitation revisited. *Am J Cardiol* 1970;25:690–697.
5. Peters RW. Overdrive atrial pacing for conversion of atrial flutter: Comparison of postoperative with nonpostoperative patients. *Am Heart J* 1999;137(1):100–103.
6. Al-Khatib SM. Clinical features of Wolff-Parkinson White syndrome. *Am Heart J* 1999;138(3 Pt 1):403–413.
7. Gulamhusein S, Ko P, Carruthers G, et al. Acceleration of the ventricular response during atrial fibrillation in the Wolff-Parkinson White syndrome after verapamil. *Circulation* 1982;65:348–354.
8. Sellers TD, Bashore TM, Gallagher JJ. Digitalis in the pre-excitation syndrome: Analysis during atrial fibrillation. *Circulation* 1977;56:260–267.
9. Stewart RB, Bardy GH, Green HL. Wide complex tachycardia: Misdiagnosis and outcome after emergent therapy. *Ann Intern Med* 1986;104:766–771.
10. Hohnloser SH, Zabel M. Short- and long-term efficacy and safety of flecainide acetate for supraventicular arrhythmias. *Am J Cardiol* 1992;70:3A–9A.
11. Glatter KA, Dorostkar PC, Yang Y, et al. Electophysiologic effects of ibultilide in patients with accessory pathways. *Circulation* 2001;104:1933–1939.
12. Pinski SL, Sgarbossa EB, Ching E, et al. A comparison of 50-J versus 100-J shocks for direct-current cardioversion of atrial flutter. *Am Heart J* 1999;137(3):439–442.
13. Biblo LA, Yuan Z, Quan KJ, et al. Risk of stroke in patients with atrial flutter. *Am J Cardiol* 2001;87:346.
14. Seidl K, Hauer B, Schwick NG, et al. Risk of thromboembolic events in patients with atrial flutter. *Am J Cardiol* 1998;82:580–583.
15. Go AS, Hylek EM, Phillips KA, et al. Prevalence of diagnosed atrial fibrillation in adults: National implications for rhythm management and stroke prevention: The anticoagulation and risk factors in atrial fibrillation (ATRIA) study. *JAMA* 2001;285:2370–2375.
16. Wagner, GS. *Marriot's Practical Electocardiography*, 10th ed, Lipincott Williams and Wilkins; Philadelphia, PA: 2001. p. 317.

17. Benjamin EJ, Wolf PA, D'Agostino RB, et al. Impact of atrial fibrillation on the risk of death: The Framingham Heart Study. *Circulation* 1998;98:946–952.

18. Fuster V, Ryden LE, Asinger RW, et al. ACC/AHA/ESC guidelines for the management of patients with atrial fibrillation: Executive summary. A report of the American College of Cardiology/American Heart Association Task Force on Practice Guidelines and the European Society of Cardiology Committee for Practice Guidelines and Policy Conferences (Committee to Develop Guidelines for the Management of Patients With Atrial Fibrillation): Developed in Collaboration With the North American Society of Pacing and Electrophysiology. *J Am Coll Cardiol* 2001;38:1231–1266.

19. Singer DE, Albers GW, Dalen JE, et al. Antithrombotic therapy in atrial fibrillation: The Seventh ACCP Conference on Antithrombotic and Thrombolytic Therapy. *Chest* 2004;126(3 Suppl):429S–456S.

20. Hohnloser SH, Kuck KH, Lilienthal J. Rhythm or rate control in atrial fibrillation:Pharmacological intervention in atrial fibrillation (PIAF): A randomized trial. *Lancet* 2000;356:1789–1794.

21. Van Gelder IC, Hagens VE, Bosker HA, et al. A comparison of rate control and rhythm control in patients with recurrent persistent atrial fibrillation. *N Engl J Med* 2002;347: 1834–1840.

22. Albers GW. Antithrombotic therapy for prevention and treatment of of ischemic stroke. *J Thromb Thrombolysis* 2001;12:19–22.

23. Snow V, Weiss KB, LeFevre M, et al. Management of newly detected atrial fibrillation: A clinical practice guideline from the American Academy of Family Physicians and the American College of Physicians. *Ann Intern Med* 2003;139:1009–1017.

24. Hart RG, Pearce LA, McBride R, et al. Factors associated with ischemic stroke during aspirin therapy in atrial fibrillation: Analysis of 2012 participants in the SPAF I-III clinical trials. *Stroke* 1999;30:1223–1229.

25. Atrial Fibrillation Investigators. Risk factors for stroke and efficacy of antithrombotic therapy in atrial fibrillation. Analysis of pooled data from five randomized controlled trials. *Arch Intern Med* 1994;154(13):1449–1457.

26. Klein EA. Assessment of cardioversion using transesophageal echocardiography (TEE) multicenter study (ACUTE I): Clinical outcomes at eight weeks. *J Am Coll Cardiol* 2000;36:324.

27. Black IW, Fatkin D, Sagar KB, et al. Exclusion of atrial thromus by transesophageal echocardiography does not preclude embolism after cardioversion of atrial fibrillation. A multicenter study. *Circulation* 1994;89:2509–2513.

28. Botto GL, Politi A, Bonini W, et al. External cardioversion of atrial fibrillation: Role of paddle position on technical efficacy and energy requirements. *Heart* 1999;82(6):726–730.

29. Dell'Ofrano JT, Kramer RK, Naccarelli GV. Cost-effective strategies in the management of atrial fibrillation. *Curr Opin Cardiol* 2000;15:23.

30. Domanovits H, Schillinger M, Thoennissen J, et al. Termination of resent-onset atrial fibrillation/flutter in the emergency department: A sequential approach with intravenous ibutilide and external electrical cardioversion. *Resuscitation* 2000;45:181.

31. Middlekauf HR, Stevenson WG, Stevenson LW. Prognostic significance of atrial fibrillation in advanced heart failure. A study of 390 patients. *Circulation* 1991;84:40–48.

32. Mathew J, Hunsberger S, Fleg J, et al. Incidence, predictive factors and prognostic significance of supraventricular tachy-arrhythmias in congestive heart failure [abstract]. *J Am Coll Cardiol* 1998;34(A Suppl):218A.

33. Nakashima H, Kumagai K, Urata H, et al. Angiotensin II antagonist prevents electrical remodeling in atrial fibrillation. *Circulation* 2000;101:2612–2617.

34. Allessie MA, Boyden PA, Camm AJ, et al. Pathophysiology and prevention of atrial fibrillation. *Circulation* 2001; 103:769–777.

35. Li D, Shinagawa K, Pang L, et al. Effects of angiotensin-converting enzyme inhibition on the development of the atrial fibrillation substrate in dogs with ventricular tachypacing-induced congestive heart failure. *Circulation* 2001;104:2608–2614.

36. Pedersen OD, Bagger H, Kober L, et al. Trandolopril reduces the incidence of atrial fibrillation after acute myocardial infarction in patients with left ventricular dysfunction. *Circulation* 1999;100:376–380.

37. Madrid AH, Bueno MG, Rebollo JMG, et al. Use of irbesartan to maintain sinus rhythm in patients with long-lasting persistent atrial fibrillation a prospective and randomized study. *Circulation* 2002;106:331–336.

22

Cardiac Conduction Blocks

Donald A. Moffa

HIGH YIELD FACTS

- There are no symptoms specific to sick sinus syndrome. Patients may be asymptomatic, but the most significant and threatening symptom is syncope or near syncope, and is experienced by 40–60%.
- Symptoms from sick sinus syndrome may be worsened by digitalis, verapamil, calcium-channel blockers, beta-blockers, clonidine, methyldopa, and antiarrhythmic agents.
- ECG changes predicting acute myocardial infarction in the presence of left bundle branch block with 90% specificity are:
  · ST-segment elevation greater than or equal to 1 mm in leads with a positive QRS.
  · ST-segment depression greater than or equal to 1 mm in lead V_1 through V_3.
  · ST-segment elevation greater than or equal to 5 mm in leads with a negative QRS.
- The Brugada syndrome is characterized by ST-segment elevation in leads V_1 through V_3, and right bundle branch block. Patients with Brugada syndrome are at risk for sudden death by ventricular tachycardia. The only proven therapy is automatic internal cardiac defibrillator (AICD) placement.

INTRODUCTION

Though not widely studied with epidemiologic rigor, emergency patients present with all conceivable cardiac conduction blocks and their attendant, diagnostic, and treatment challenges to the emergency physician. Cardiac conduction blocks can occur anywhere along the orthodromic electrical conduction pathway, and the extensive range of potential causes includes:

1. Presentation at birth with congenital conduction deficits linked to maternal circulating autoimmune antibodies
2. In association with systemic diseases such as collagen vascular disorders, amyloidosis, and systemic lupus erythematosus
3. As the sequelae of infections such as myocarditis or infective endocarditis
4. From injury to ganglionic plexi, the sinoatrial node, the atrioventricular node, or perinodal nerves
   a. Direct tumor infiltration
   b. Toxin damage as in the case of toxin from *Trypanosoma cruzi*
   c. Direct damage to nodal and conducting fibers
   d. Calcific changes, fibrosis, or periarteritis
   e. Hemorrhage (e.g., from diphtheria) and infarction
5. Autonomic imbalance, during stress testing
6. De novo as with the case of a minority (16%) of left bundle branch blocks that can accompany normal cardiac function without evidence or atherosclerotic coronary vascular disease.

Therefore, the physician must interpret a cardiac conduction abnormality with respect to the patient's presenting illness and by recognizing the underlying medical conditions that may influence or cause the abnormality. Recognizing and treating the patient in extremis supercedes immediate deliberation about underlying causes though they must be considered.

EPIDEMIOLOGY

The epidemiology of cardiac conduction blocks has not been studied in isolation, but some information about the prevalence and natural history of cardiac blocks has been studied in association with the illnesses with which they occur and in population-based studies. A review of a 5% sample of the Medicare Provider Analysis and Review Files characterizing 144,512 discharges from 1991 through 1998 for which the principal diagnosis was a conduction disorder or arrhythmia, annual hospitalizations for sinoatrial disorder, atrial flutter, atrial fibrillation, or ventricular fibrillation increased more rapidly than did the elderly Medicare beneficiary population. Sinoatrial node dysfunction, Mobitz type I second-degree block, and complete atrioventricular block all increased with patient age in this study.[1]

For hospitalized patients between the ages of 20 and 99, the prevalence of intraventricular conduction abnormalities detected by ECG show that White patients are significantly more likely than Black patients to have intraventricular block (15.2% vs. 8.6%), and hospitalized White men have the highest prevalence (16.8%) while hospitalized Black women have the lowest (6.5%).[2]

The incidence of left bundle branch block increases with age.[3] Approximately two-thirds (62%) of patients with bifascicular block, 78% of patients with left bundle branch block, and 56% of patients with right bundle branch block and left axis deviation will have coronary vascular disease.[4] The likelihood of developing complete heart block is highest for patients who have right bundle branch block and concomitant left axis deviation (4%/year) while mortality is highest for patients with left bundle branch block, first-degree atrioventricular block, and left axis deviation (43%/year).[4]

CARDIAC CONDUCTION SYSTEM ANATOMY

The cardiac conduction cycle begins when the sinoatrial node, first demonstrated histologically by Tawara in 1906, generates an electrical impulse that is conducted through the right atrium along two or perhaps three specialized conduction pathways to the atrioventricular node. One of these electrical approaches to the atrioventricular node is along the crista terminalis, the terminal crest of the right atrium that is a ridge of tissue along the internal surface of the right atrium to the right of the inlets of the superior and inferior venae cavae. The crista terminalis may become a site of secondary pacemaker activity or participate in the pathology of sick sinus syndrome[5] as it may have electrically active cells found outside the anatomic boundary of the sinoatrial node.

The impulse is conducted to the atrioventricular node, where the *classical conduction hypothesis* assumes that the atrial electrical impulse is conducted across the atrioventricular node by producing action potentials in a cell-to-cell fashion, and on through the His-Purkinje system, until the entire ventricular muscle is depolarized.[6] The second and less widely accepted theory of atrioventricular nodal conduction, the *modulated pacemaker hypothesis*, postulates that the atrioventricular node has an automaticity that is modulated by the advancing atrial depolarization front. In this case, the atrial impulse is not conducted through the atrioventricular node but only modifies the atrioventricular node's electrical impulse discharge rate to the His-Purkinje system.[7] This theory of atrioventricular nodal

conduction has largely been discounted in favor of the *classical conduction theory*.[6]

The junction formed by the atrioventricular nodal-His bundle shows anatomic variation.[5] Embryologically, specialized cells intermingle with ordinary muscle cells in the fetal heart up to a relatively late stage of fetal development, even during the time that the fetal electrocardiogram develops an adult atrioventricular conduction pattern.[5] These specialized cells, presumed to be of conduction tissue, may persist in fetal development despite the development of the fibrous cardiac skeletal rings separating atria and ventricles and despite the normal resorptive degradation of these accessory pathways.[5] Should they persist, they may remain as accessory conduction pathways in the developing heart.

There is no precise histologic differentiation between the atrioventricular node and the His bundle. Likewise, the boundary between the junction and the subjunctional or intraventricular specialized pathway is not histologically defined.[5] The atrioventricular node may penetrate the pars membranacea septi, the very small and completely membranous area of the intraventricular septum near the root of the aorta, while the His bundle and its bifurcations may be laterally displaced to either side or may lie intramurally, deep within the ventricular septum. Fibers from the His bundle appear to separate from a single stem and show the tendency to regroup into fairly discrete fascicles that are destined to become either the right or left bundle branch.[5]

Anatomic differences between the left and right bundle branches belie their susceptibility to pathology and make plain the extent each may be injured. The left bundle branch is a fan-like dispersion of Purkinje-like fibers. These fibers penetrate and run deep through the upper ventricular septum until they, more or less, coalesce and split into the anterior and posterior fascicles. The right bundle branch is a rather discrete condensation of ordinary-looking myocytes that runs a narrow course just beneath the right ventricular endocardium.[5] In this position, a small, focused insult to the region of the right bundle branch can produce a right bundle branch block evident on electrocardiogram whereas a larger and more diffuse lesion is required to produce a left bundle branch block. Even so, the right bundle branch is vulnerable to septal infarcts whereas the left bundle branch may be protected against anoxia by transendocardial oxygenation from arterial blood in the left ventricle.[5] Consequently, a left bundle branch block rarely signifies benign pathology. Although no correlation exists between traditional risk factors for ischemic heart disease and the subsequent development of left bundle branch block, once left bundle branch block is present, it signifies an increased likelihood of developing overt cardiovascular disease.[3]

CARDIAC CONDUCTION SYSTEM PATHOLOGY

The causes of cardiac conduction defects are many and can occur anywhere along the cardiac conduction system to cause the different forms of conduction block.[8] Clinical and histologic studies of the human conduction systems do not always correlate.[9] In general, the causes of conduction system dysfunction include mechanical and dystrophic factors, aging of the cardiac skeleton, infectious etiologies, acute and chronic ischemia, autoimmune disorders, locally impaired lymphatic and/or venous drainage, tumor invasion or influence on the conducting system, autonomic nervous system tone, toxins and medications, and myriad other genetic and familial conditions. Conduction system disorders may be the result of acute and chronic diseases of the myocardium, primary degradation of the conduction system, or changes in tissues surrounding the conduction system (e.g., the annulus, central fibers body, membranous septum, aortic valve, crest of ventricular system, bundle branches).[5]

MECHANICAL AND DYSTROPHIC FACTORS AFFECTING CONDUCTION

Calcification of valvular structures may interrupt electrical impulse conduction particularly at the atrioventricular node, where the main penetrating bundle of His is located near the noncoronary cusp of the aortic valve and near the base of the anterior leaflet of the mitral valve, both of which are subject to calcification, causing atrioventricular block.[10] Such calcific atrioventricular block can be caused by calcification from various disorders that cause hypercalcemia, where calcium may extend from a heavily calcified aortic or mitral valve.[11] Echocardiographic evidence shows the correlation between mitral annular calcification and conduction abnormalities.[12]

Myocardial fibrosis may also cause cardiac conduction block. Right ventricular biopsies, from patients less than 60 years of age who have atrioventricular block without apparent heart disease, showed evidence of myocardial fibrosis with either myocyte hypertrophy or disarray. In these cases, electrophysiologic testing did not correlate with the histopathologic findings or severity.[13] Lev's disease and Leanegre disease represents two distinct forms of "idiopathic bilateral bundle branch fibrosis" that

are characterized by slowing and progressive loss of conduction fibers without myocardial abnormalities.[10]

Apoptic cell death may account, to some extent, for the development of conduction system defects. Apoptosis (programmed cell death), partially under mitochondrial control, is seen in the sinus node in patients with complete heart block.[14] Histologic abnormalities consistent with apoptosis have been shown in individuals who develop progressive, complete heart block.[15]

INFILTRATIVE PROCESSES AFFECTING CONDUCTION

Patients with *amyloidosis* are prone to cardiac involvement of not only the contractile tissues but also the conduction system. In 25 patients with biopsy-proven amyloidosis and cardiac involvement, electrophysiologic testing showed that the functions of the sinoatrial and atrioventricular nodes were preserved in most patients, but that infra-Hisian (HV) conduction times were usually prolonged and that HV prolongation is the sole independent predictor of sudden death. It is not possible to record the HV interval on surface electrocardiogram in the presence of the narrow QRS complex in this group of patients who are prone to sudden death by complete atrioventricular block.[16]

Atrioventricular block is associated with the *collagen vascular disorders* systemic lupus erythematosus, dermatomyositis, scleroderma, rheumatoid arthritis, and ankylosing spondylitis.[17] Rheumatoid nodules may occur in the central fibrous body or cusps of the aortic valve, the aortic root, or in all of the structures.[18–21] The atrioventricular node, penetrating bundle, and bundle branches may be replaced with granulation tissue or fibrosis owing to the conduction disturbance.[17]

INFECTIOUS PROCESSES AFFECTING CARDIAC CONDUCTION

Extension of a valvular *infection* to surrounding portions of the myocardium and conduction system may be responsible for conduction block.[11] Conduction blocks may result from myocarditis caused by viral, bacterial, or fungal organisms.[11] The area of myocarditis may be focal.[22] Rarely, acute myocarditis will cause chronic atrioventricular block[17] although chronic block is more likely in patients with sarcoidosis or tuberculosis.[23] Other causes of acute atrioventricular block from myocarditis include acute rheumatic fever, diphtheria, Chagas disease,[10,24,25] and Coxsackie-B3.[26] The bundle branches are the most commonly involved structures followed by the atrioventricular node for infectious causes of cardiac conduction delay.[22]

NEOPLASTIC PROCESSES AFFECTING CARDIAC CONDUCTION

Tumors may affect cardiac conduction by causing direct impulse disruption at the atrioventricular node or the penetrating bundle from tumor mass or from diffuse tumor infiltration (e.g., leukemias).[11] Primary tumors of the heart that involve the conduction system may include rhabdomyosarcoma, fibroma, and nodular rhabdomyomata of tuberous sclerosis.[11] A mesothelioma may arise within the atrioventricular node causing cystic spaces with squamoid epithelial lining that disrupt conduction and present with atrioventricular block as the only clinical symptom.[11]

AUTOIMMUNE ANTIBODIES CAUSING CONGENITAL HEART BLOCK

Mothers with systemic lupus erythematosus or Sjögren syndrome are at particular risk for having children with *congenital heart block*.[27] Congenital atrioventricular block is a rare condition occurring in 1 out of every 20,000 births. Children of mothers with circulating *autoimmune antibodies* are more likely than children without to be born with a congenital cardiac conduction deficit. More than 85% of mothers giving birth to infants with congenital heart block are anti-Rho antibody positive, but only approximately 1% of babies with anti-Rho positive mothers develop congenital heart block.[28] Other antibodies purported to cause congenital heart block include antibodies against neonatal M1 muscarinic acetylcholine receptors in mothers with primary Sjögren syndrome,[29] antibodies against the calcium ion channel as studied in the murine model,[30,31] anti-5 HT4 receptor peptide antibodies against the serotonin-induced L-type calcium-channel activation in human atrial cells,[32] antisinus node and antiatrioventricular node antibodies,[33] and antibodies from autoimmunization to retrovirus-3 acquired during pregnancy.[34] Patients with antisinus node antibodies have a 10-fold higher risk of developing sick sinus syndrome, and patients with antiatrioventricular node antibodies have a threefold increased risk of developing atrioventricular block, both, compared to age-matched controls.[33]

The transplacental passage of antibodies that attack the fetal conduction system appears to have a direct influence on fetal and congenital conduction disturbances. The conduction deficit may be as innocuous as first-degree heart block or as profound as complete heart block.[35] The block is not always permanent. Second-degree heart block, on rare occasions, can revert to normal sinus rhythm, but complete atrioventricular block is irreversible in patients with congenital heart block and carries substantial morbidity and mortality with greater than 60% of affected children requiring lifelong cardiac pacing.[31]

MEMBRANE ION CHANNELS AND GENETICS AFFECTING CARDIAC CONDUCTION

Recent literature focuses much attention on alterations in membrane ionic channels responsible for the movement of sodium, potassium, and calcium into and out of the conducting cells. Alterations in these channel proteins can lead to either premature closing or prolonged opening of the ionic channels. These protein channels' structures are under genetic regulation. Cardiac conduction deficits have been linked to mutations of several genes including the *SCN5A* gene,[36–39] the *LMNA* gene,[40,41] the *DMPK* gene,[42,43] and other genes including those coding for the sodium channel,[44] the potassium channel,[45] and gap junctions[46,47] to name a few.

Mutations in the *SCN5A* gene (which encodes the cardiac sodium channel alpha subunit) are associated with the long QT3 subtype of long QT syndrome, Brugada syndrome (right bundle branch block and ST-segment elevation in V_1–V_3),[39] congenital 2:1 atrioventricular block,[48] and isolated progressive cardiac conduction defects (e.g., Leanegre disease).[49,50] Sudden unexpected death syndrome, originally described in Thai men, has the same ECG pattern as Brugada syndrome. Brugada syndrome is inherited in an autosomal-dominant fashion.[38] The sodium channel current causes rapid cellular membrane depolarization and is responsible for the action potential upstroke.[51] Normally, the sodium channel closes rapidly, but mutations in the SCN5a codon[39] makes a mutated subunit that causes the sodium channel to inactivate incompletely, thus, allowing a persistent inward sodium current during the plateau of the action potential which retards repolarization.[51] Myocardial conduction velocity will, therefore, slow in association with atrioventricular block.[37]

The *LMNA* gene is one of six autosomal disease genes implicated in familial dilated cardiomyopathy.[41] The *LMNA* gene encodes lamins A and C, alternatively spliced nuclear envelope proteins, and mutations in this gene cause four diseases: Emory-Dreifuss muscular dystrophy, limb girdle muscular dystrophy type 1B, Dunnigan-type familial partial lipodystrophy, and dilated cardiomyopathy. In patients of families with autosomal-dominant familial dilated cardiomyopathy and conduction system disease caused by mutation in this gene, the conduction deficit is most likely to manifest in the third, forth, or fifth decades of life as progressive conduction disease, ventricular dysrhythmias, left ventricular enlargement, and systolic dysfunction followed by death.[41] In fact, *LMNA* gene mutations may account for one-third of patients with dilated cardiomyopathy who have atrioventricular block for lack of other causes[52] and autosomal-dominant limb girdle muscular dystrophy with atrioventricular block.[40]

Myotonic dystrophy is the most common form of muscular dystrophy and is associated with progressive skeletal myopathy and atrioventricular conduction disturbances.[53] Myotonic dystrophy protein kinase (DMPK) is implicated in the regulation of membrane excitability.[53] The murine model demonstrates that mice deficient in the gene coding for DMPK show compromise in the atrioventricular node and His-Purkinje areas of the conduction system. Specifically, DMPK haplodeficient mice develop first-degree heart block similar to that observed in patients with myotonic dystrophy.[53] DMPK appears to regulate membrane excitability, and DMPK-deficient mice show late reopenings of cardiac muscle sodium channels causing resting membrane potential depolarization and prolonged action potential duration.[43]

MISCELLANEOUS CONDITIONS AFFECTING CARDIAC CONDUCTION

Other diseases and conditions associated with cardiac conduction defects include Alport syndrome (atrioventricular block),[54] Epstein anomaly (sick sinus syndrome, atrioventricular block),[55] Kearns-Sayre syndrome (complete atrioventricular block),[56] Emory-Dreifuss syndrome (atrioventricular block ranging from sinus bradycardia to complete atrioventricular block),[57] Fabry disease (complete atrioventricular block),[58] sarcoidosis (complete atrioventricular block),[59] HLA-B27-associated diseases (complete atrioventricular block),[60] obstructive sleep apnea (atrioventricular block),[61] and orthotopic heart transplantation (various conduction defects including complete atrioventricular block).[62]

Vagal surge from the autonomic nervous system may cause various forms of second-degree atrioventricular block for reasons that remain poorly understood. Vagal surge can cause simultaneous sinus slowing and first- and second-degree atrioventricular nodal block.[63] The

autonomic influence on the cardiac conduction system is sometimes evident during cardiac stress testing. Atrioventricular block developing during exercise stress testing is rare, but if it occurs, it suggests an abnormal His-Purkinje system (refractory to autonomic modulation) or ischemic heart disease.[64]

Cardiac conduction deficits may become apparent during procedures to isolate ischemic cardiac disease such as *exercise testing* or *heart catheterization.* Exercise-induced ventricular tachycardia with left bundle branch block may be assigned to two groups based on the initiating sequence of ventricular tachycardia on exercise. The first group exhibits a variable, long-short, RR interval prior to the onset of ventricular tachycardia, and the other shows patients without changes in cycling prior to ventricular tachycardia.[65] The ventricular tachycardia associated with a long-short RR sequence suggests the mechanism to be the late after depolarizations or reentry, is more often nonsustained, and may have a superior axis suggesting the origin of the ventricular tachycardia from the septum or body of the ventricle.[65] Ventricular tachycardia initiated without changes in cycling is more common and is more likely to have an inferior axis suggesting origination of the ventricular tachycardia in the ventricular outflow tract.[65] Left-sided heart catheterization can cause left bundle branch block though it is uncommon in patients with intact atrioventricular conduction.[66]

ELECTROLYTES, TOXINS, AND MEDICATIONS AFFECTING CARDIAC CONDUCTION

Ohmae, in 1981, recognized that hyperkalemia may depress conduction in the His-Purkinje system and induce complete heart block distal to the atrioventricular injunction.[66] The ECG in hyperkalemia may show right bundle branch block with type II second-degree atrioventricular block that may progress to bilateral bundle branch block and, ultimately, high-degree atrioventricular block.[67] Hyperkalemia can cause complete atrioventricular block, especially in renal patients, and is usually associated with QRS prolongation. Ventricular myocytes and the Purkinje system are thought to be more sensitive to the effects of hyperkalemia than are the sinoatrial and atrioventricular nodes.[68] The heart block from hyperkalemia may be temporary, amenable to treatment with temporary cardiac pacing.[69] Refractory hyperkalemia, associated with digoxin overdose, may present with complete atrioventricular block. In this case, the patient should not be treated with intravenous calcium, since elevated intracellular calcium levels may be present in digoxin toxicity. Instead, the patient should receive hemofiltration[70] or repeated intravenous dosing of recombinant Fab fragments, which will lower the effect of digoxin and reverse hyperkalemia.[71]

Patients with chronic renal insufficiency or endstage renal disease treated with sustained released verapamil hydrochloride show varying degrees of atrioventricular heart block, hypotension, hyperkalemia, metabolic acidosis, and hepatic dysfunction. Calcium-channel blockers must be used with caution in this patient population who should be monitored for adverse cardiovascular, metabolic, and hepatic side effects.[72] The combination of a *calcium-channel blocker* and a *beta-blocker* will very rarely cause cardiac conduction abnormalities and should be used with caution, or may not be suitable in patients with first-degree atrioventricular block.[73]

In an animal model of iron overload, hepatocellular decompensation can cause hyperlactatemia and hypercalcemia leading to progressive cardiac conduction defects and cardiac arrest.[74] Iron overload cardiomyopathy causes a reduction in the fast inward sodium current showing significantly slower conduction velocities, PR interval prolongation, QRS complex widening, and dysrhythmias.[75]

Other agents that may cause cardiac conduction deficits include cocaine (which may cause the transient Brugada pattern)[76] or epidural mepivacaine (which has been described to cause complete left bundle branch block),[77] and tricyclic antidepressants.[78]

THE CARDIAC CONDUCTION DEFECTS

Sick Sinus Syndrome

Lown, in 1967, first used the term *sick sinus syndrome*[79] that has come to describe several electrocardiographic features relating to sinoatrial node dysfunction. *Sick sinus syndrome* refers to a spectrum of cardiac dysrhythmias that includes sinus bradycardia, sinus arrest, sinoatrial block, and paroxysmal supraventricular tachyarrhythmias alternating with periods of bradycardia or asystole.[80]

The ECG in Sick Sinus Syndrome

The electrocardiogram may show:[81]

- Inappropriate sinus bradycardia
- Sinoatrial block, sinoatrial arrest, or both
- Cessation of sinus rhythm, or long pauses with failure of secondary pacemakers
- Replacement of sinus rhythm by ectopic atrial or junctional pacemaker

- Inappropriately prolonged suppression of sinus rhythm after cardioversion (spontaneous or electrical) from tachydysrhythmia or bradycardia alternating with tachycardia
- Paroxysmal or chronic atrial fibrillation from lack of sinoatrial node function

By convention, a sinus rate of less than 60 bpm defines bradycardia, although rates between 50 and 60 bpm or slower are commonly found in healthy individuals during rest or sleep and do not necessarily indicate sinus node dysfunction.[82] Marked, persistent sinus bradycardia, with sinus rate less than 40 bpm with little diurnal variability and pauses of greater than 2 s, indicate sinus node dysfunction.[83–85] Chronic atrial fibrillation is the endstage of sinus node dysfunction. Prior to this, the ECG may show sinus arrest, sinus pauses, atrial standstill, Wenckebach or Mobitz type II sinoatrial block, complete sinoatrial block (pauses indistinguishable from those secondary to sinus arrest), abnormal prolonged sinus pauses (abnormally slow rescue rhythms that are markers of sinus dysfunction),[86] paroxysmal supraventricular tachycardia that terminates in long pauses, or severe sinus bradycardia (bradycardia-tachycardia syndrome).[86,87] A sinoatrial pause greater than 3 s following carotid massage may indicate sick sinus syndrome.[81]

Pathophysiology of Sick Sinus Syndrome

Sick sinus syndrome can occur in all ages, including neonates,[88] but it occurs most commonly in the elderly (mean age 68 years), and affects both sexes equally.[89] Sick sinus syndrome can occur in virtually every cardiac disease that involves the sinus node.[81] Sclerodegenerative disease is most common cause involving the atrial, atrioventricular node, and the His-Purkinje system.[81] Coronary artery disease is not considered a major cause, though sinus node ischemia and local autonomic neural factors, in patients with myocardial infarction, may precipitate sick sinus syndrome. The nutrient blood vessel supplying the sinoatrial node is from a branch of the right coronary artery that is infrequently affected by atherosclerosis. However, it is possible that this branch is subject to dystrophic sclerosis or acute thrombosis causing infarction of the sinoatrial node and resulting in sinoatrial block or sudden cardiac death.[5] Temporary sinoatrial dysfunction may be caused by sinus node ischemia, surgical trauma, myocarditis, pericarditis, and a variety of drugs that affect sinoatrial conduction.[81] Other causes include mediastinal metastases from bronchial tumor (probably affecting external nerve plexuses), Chagasic heart disease (causing sinus node block with nodal ganglionic plexus damage), acute myocardial infarction, diphtheria (inflammation and hemorrhage of the sinus node), systemic lupus erythematosus (sinus node block, focal degeneration, fibrosis, periarteritis), damage to internodal and perinodal nerves or occlusion of the sinus node artery or both, and autonomic imbalance.[9,25]

Clinical Features of Sick Sinus Syndrome

There are no symptoms specific to sick sinus syndrome.[81] Patients with sick sinus syndrome are usually asymptomatic, though symptoms may be mild or nonspecific. The most significant and threatening symptom is syncope or near syncope, and is experienced by 40–60%.[90–95] The characteristic but uncommon feature of sick sinus syndrome is syncope at the end of paroxysmal supraventricular tachyarrhythmias caused by overdrive suppression of the sinus node ending in long sinus pauses.[81] Despite adequate pacing 20% of patients will have recurrent syncope,[94] which may indicate disease of the autonomic nervous system.[81]

The natural history of sick sinus syndrome is an erratic course with periods of normal sinus node function that alternates with abnormal behavior. It may progress slowly over more than 10 years, exemplifying from sinus bradycardia to various forms of exit block, until sinoatrial arrest or chronic atrial fibrillation occur.[81] However, some may show complete recovery. Symptoms that may be present for years or months include syncope, palpitations, and dizziness. Sick sinus syndrome may worsen congestive heart failure, angina pectoris, and cerebrovascular accidents.[96] Peripheral thromboembolism and stroke are possible.[97] Other symptoms include irritability, nocturnal wakefulness, memory loss, errors in judgment, lethargy, lightheadedness, generalized fatigue,[98,99] mild digestive disturbances, myalgia, periodic oliguria or edema, and mild intermittent dyspnea.[98]

Diagnostic Testing for Sick Sinus Syndrome

Methods of diagnoses are difficult since the disease shows a slow, erratic course with the rather vague symptoms. A greater than 3 s pause after carotid massage may imply the diagnosis of sick sinus syndrome.[81] Symptoms may be difficult to associate with ECG changes.[98] Atrial fibrillation with slow ventricular response may indicate sick sinus syndrome if it is found in the absence of medications that slow ventricular response (e.g., digoxin, quinidine, procainamide), and hyperkalemia may cause periodic sinus arrest or sinoatrial exit block in these patients. Holter

monitors are commonly used for diagnosis.[88] Sinus node dysfunction should be suspected if on physical examination isometric handgrip exercises, Valsalva maneuvers, or carotid massage produce abrupt sinus arrest of 3 s or longer.[96] Stress testing has a limited role in the diagnosis. In patients older than 60, maximum heart rate less than 65% of established norms for sex and age can differentiate patients with sinus node dysfunction from normals and those with chronotropic incompetence due to other myocardial diseases.[100] Sinus node recovery time, after overdrive right atrial pacing to 200 bpm, normally does not exceed 1.5 s after cessation of pacing.[81] If it is greater than 3 s, this increases the likelihood of sinus node dysfunction and the probability of neurologic symptoms.[81]

Treatment for Sick Sinus Syndrome

When selecting therapeutic options, the emergency physician should consider that symptoms from sick sinus syndrome may be worsened by digitalis, verapamil, calcium-channel blockers, beta-blockers, clonidine, methyldopa, and antiarrhythmic agents.[101]

Treatment for sick sinus syndrome is aimed at controlling morbidity and alleviating symptoms. Approximately one-third of patients with sinus bradycardia have symptoms severe enough to warrant therapy.[102] Drugs that suppress sinus node function should be avoided. Slow-release theophylline (550 mg/day) can increase resting heart rate by one-third and can prevent attacks of overt heart failure, but not syncope.[103] Most patients probably need anticoagulation because of the high-risk of systemic embolism.[104]

Pacemakers are widely accepted to reduce syncope and relieve symptoms,[81] especially since patients with sick sinus syndrome and right bundle branch block have increased risk of developing symptomatic high-degree atrioventricular block[88] Patients receiving a pacemaker should be treated by dual chamber pacing, because the addition of atrial pacing lowers the incidence of thromboembolic complications,[104–106] atrial fibrillation,[105–108] heart failure,[105,106,109,110] cardiovascular mortality,[103,104,109] and total morbidity.[106,107] Compared with 35 control subjects, dual chamber pacing showed significantly fewer episodes of syncope (6% vs. 23%) and overt heart failure (3% vs. 15%) but no difference in atrial tachyarrhythmias and thromboembolic events.[103]

As per the American College of Cardiology, American Heart Association, and the North American Society for Pacing and Electrophysiology (ACC/AHA/NASPE) 2002 guidelines for cardiac pacemakers; permanent pacing may not necessarily improve survival although it may relieve symptoms related to bradycardia.[80] Their recommendations are (see class table [p. i]):

Class I recommendations for permanent pacing in sinus node dysfunction include:[80]
- Symptomatic bradycardia including frequent sinus pauses that produce symptoms
- Symptomatic, chronotropic incompetence

Class IIa recommendations for permanent pacing include:[80]
- Spontaneous sinus node dysfunction or sinus node dysfunction resulting from drug therapy with heart rate less than 40 bpm that is clearly associated with significant symptoms from bradycardia though the actual presence of bradycardia has not been documented
- Unexplained syncope when major abnormalities of sinus node function are discovered or provoked in electrophysiologic testing

Prognosis for Sick Sinus Syndrome

Factors affecting survival are associated with myocardial ischemia, congestive heart failure, and systemic embolization.[93,111] Advanced age and the development of atrioventricular block, chronic atrial fibrillation, or systemic embolism contribute to morbidity.[81] Systemic embolism is much more frequent in unpaced patients with sick sinus syndrome than in age-matched controls (15.2% vs. 1.3%).[104]

ATRIOVENTRICULAR BLOCKS

Pathophysiology of Atrioventricular Blocks

The most common cause of chronic, acquired, atrioventricular block is progressive idiopathic fibrosis of the conduction system associated with age-related changes of the cardiac skeleton.[112] Atrioventricular block may result from various acute and chronic diseases of the myocardium, changes in structure surrounding the conduction system (affecting the annulus, central fibrous body, membranous septum, aortic valve, crest of ventricular system, or bundle branches), and primary degeneration of the conduction system.[9] Lyme disease is the most common cause of reversible atrioventricular block (usually nodal) in young individuals.[112]

Topographically, atrioventricular block may be classified as supra-Hisian (involving atria, atrioventricular node, and its approaches), infra-Hisian (represented by a prolonged HV interval on electrophysiologic testing), and split-His (not truly intra-Hisian but affecting the bifurcation or the bundle branches or both).[10] At autopsy of patients with atrioventricular block, the atrioventricular node, penetrating bundle, or both are affected 32% of the time, bifurcating bundle, right bundle, or left bundle 63% of the time, and areas above the atrioventricular node 2% of the time.[10] The causes are idiopathic (38%), associated with chronic atherosclerotic coronary heart disease (18%), calcific involvement (11%), dilated cardiomyopathy (13%), and other causes (20%).[10]

Atrioventricular Block Associated with Myocardial Infarction

Myocardial infarction usually affects the bundle branches (74%) rather than the atrioventricular node (6%) or penetrating bundle (20%),[10] but when it does, the prognosis is unfavorable and depends on the extent and location of the infarction.[10,113] Atrioventricular block in patients with posterior inferior infarctions are usually transient while atrioventricular block in patients with anterior anteroseptal infarctions are less common but carry a worse prognosis.[113] Complete atrioventricular block may be associated with a healed, remote myocardial infarction where both the conduction system and adjacent myocardium are replaced by fibrosis.[9]

First-Degree Atrioventricular Block

First-degree atrioventricular block describes a delay in the electrical impulse traversing the atrioventricular node, with a PR interval prolongation greater than 200 ms on the ECG or the rhythm strip. A normal PR interval is 120–200 ms. A PR interval consistently greater than 200 ms defines first-degree atrioventricular block, and is the most benign form of heart block. The prevalence of first-degree atrioventricular block in the young adult population ranges from 0.65 to 1.1%, and increases to 1.36% in people older than 50.[114]

The emergency physician must interpret first-degree atrioventricular block with respect to the patient's presenting complaints, medical history, electrolyte milieu, and medications. Because most causes of PR prolongation can also produce second- and third-degree atrioventricular block, those with ischemic heart disease may have this or other forms of heart block of any degree. Medications such as digitalis, amiodarone, beta-blockers, and calcium-channel blockers, can suppress atrioventricular nodal conduction. Ischemic heart disease, either chronic myocardial ischemia or acute myocardial infarction, can produce atrioventricular block of any degree and is particularly common with myocardial ischemia affecting the inferior wall, which shares a common arterial supply from the right coronary artery, with the atrioventricular node.[115]

The importance of this block may not be readily apparent. However, hemodynamic affects of first-degree atrioventricular block become important the closer atrial systole is to the preceding ventricular systole. In this case, the hemodynamic consequences approximate that of retrograde ventriculoatrial conduction, like that encountered in pacemaker syndrome[112] (see Chap. 23). Patients may be asymptomatic at rest only to become symptomatic with activity.[112] First-degree atrioventricular block with symptoms suggestive of pacemaker syndrome is a class IIb indication for pacing.[80] Dual chamber pacing improves symptoms when the PR interval is greater than 280 ms.[116]

Second-Degree Atrioventricular Block

Second-degree atrioventricular block is divided into type I and type II blocks determined by the behavior of the P wave with respect to the preceding PR intervals and can only be described provided there are at least two conducted P waves prior to the blocked QRS on ECG.

Type I Second-Degree Atrioventricular Block (Wenckebach or Mobitz Type I)

Type I second-degree atrioventricular block is defined electrocardiographically when a single, nonconducted sinus P wave is associated with *inconsistent* PR intervals preceding and following the blocked impulse provided there are at least two consecutive conducted P waves to determine the PR intervals' behavior.[63,117,118] The PR interval after the blocked P wave is *always shorter* than the PR interval before the block.[112] Progressive PR interval prolongation before the block may not occur because the PR intervals may shorten, stabilize, or show no preceding change anywhere in the PR interval sequence, but the PR interval after the block is always shorter.[112] If the practitioner follows these criteria, a slowing or increase in sinus rate should not cloud the ECG interpretation and diagnosis of type I second-degree atrioventricular block.[112]

Narrow QRS type I second-degree atrioventricular block usually occurs at the atrioventricular node, and can be physiologic, especially during sleep in individuals with high vagal tone.[112] After causes provoking this block have been excluded, these patients generally require no treatment.

Intra-Hisian narrow QRS type I second-degree atrioventricular block is rare but may be provoked by exercise in contrast to type I atrioventricular nodal block, which generally improves with exercise.[63] It is impossible to distinguish this form of block from atrioventricular nodal

block on ECG, but intra-Hisian block may be detected on electrophysiologic testing performed for other reasons. If electrophysiologic mapping shows diffuse conduction system disease, intra-Hisian type I atrioventricular block is then considered a class I indication for cardiac pacing.[63] Otherwise, the patient may be asymptomatic, the location of the block may go undetermined, and no treatment is warranted.

Type I second-degree atrioventricular block associated with bundle branch block occurs in the His-Purkinje system most of the time (60–70%), in the absence of acute myocardial infarction.[112] These patients should undergo electrophysiologic testing,[63] and permanent pacing is generally recommended.[112] The emergency physician who encounters a new Wenckebach pattern, in association with a bundle branch block, should diligently search for causes of diffuse conduction system disease (including myocardial infarction), and obtain cardiology consultation.

Type II Second-Degree Atrioventricular Block

Type II second-degree atrioventricular block is defined electrocardiographically as a single nonconducted sinus P wave, associated with a constant PR intervals before and after the blocked impulse, provided there are at least two consecutive conducted P waves prior to the blocked impulse to indicate the behavior of the PR interval.[63,117,118] The pause, including the blocked P wave, should equal two P-P cycles. Unlike type I second-degree atrioventricular block, the PR interval following the blocked P wave is either *normal or prolonged* but remains constant.[112] The diagnosis of type II block may not be possible in the presence of sinus arrhythmia, especially if it occurs during sinus slowing since high vagal tone may cause simultaneous sinus rate slowing and AV nodal conduction delay that may superficially resemble type II second-degree atrioventricular block.[112,119]

The location of type II second-degree atrioventricular block always occurs in His-Purkinje system[63,112] as its has not yet been demonstrated conclusively in the atrioventricular node.[112] The location of this block leads to a wide QRS complex (greater than or equal to 120 ms) in 70–80% of cases.[112] Type II second-degree atrioventricular block should be regarded as a class I indication for cardiac pacing regardless of QRS duration, symptoms, or chronicity.[120]

Fixed-Ratio Atrioventricular Block (2:1, 3:1, 4:1, ...)

Fixed-ratio block cannot be classified as either type I or type II second-degree atrioventricular block because only one PR interval precedes the blocked P wave or string of P waves. Therefore, a fixed-ratio atrioventricular block is considered an "advanced block."[117,118] The location of this advanced block can be either AV nodal or in the His-Purkinje system.[112] In the absence of acute myocardial infarction, advanced blocks with a wide QRS complex occur in the His-Purkinje system 80% of the time and in the atrioventricular node 20% of the time.[112] Infranodal blocks should be treated with cardiac pacing, but it is difficult to determine the location of the block by surface electrocardiogram. When a stable sinus rhythm with 1:1 atrioventricular conduction is suddenly followed by atrioventricular block of several impulses, and all the preceding and following PR intervals remain constant, infranodal block is strongly suggested, and hence, cardiac pacing should be urgently implemented.[112]

Complete Atrioventricular Block

Complete atrioventricular block occurs when there is a disconnection between the electrical activity of the atrium and that of the ventricle causing an escape ventricular rate that is slower than the normal sinus rate. The escape ventricular rhythm can either be junctional or ventricular in origin. Patients may be either symptomatic or asymptomatic. Asymptomatic complete atrioventricular block with ventricular escape rates >40 bpm is a class IIa indication for cardiac pacing.[80] Asymptomatic patients with neuromuscular diseases may require cardiac pacing earlier in the course of their disease even if a second-degree atrioventricular block has not yet developed.[120]

The emergency patient presenting with complete atrioventricular block must be quickly evaluated for cardiopulmonary and neurologic stability. The cause of the block is investigated, and arrangements for temporary pacing should be considered before the patient becomes hemodynamically or neurologically compromised. Complete heart block is a rare cause of syncope (2.4%) among elderly patients hospitalized and monitored for syncope.[121]

BUNDLE BRANCH BLOCKS

Normal, orthodromic atrioventricular conduction leads, first, to depolarization of the left side of the ventricular septum with depolarization spreading to the main mass of the left and right ventricles by way of the left and right bundle branches. The entire process produces a QRS complex of normal width on ECG of less than or equal to 100 ms.[122] Interruption in the electrical conduction down either of the bundle branches will produce the characteristic wide complex bundle branch block pattern on the ECG.

LEFT BUNDLE BRANCH BLOCK

Left Bundle Branch Anatomy

The His bundle passes through the membranous ventricular septum to divide into the right and left bundle branches.[123] The left bundle emerges from the His bundle as a structure ranging from approximately 1–14 mm in diameter as a branching meshwork though it sometimes remains a narrow structure for up to 1 cm before splitting into three relatively distinct fascicles.[124] There are multiple connections among the divisions.[125–127] The posterior fascicle is broader and branches earlier than the more narrow anterior fascicle. A third or septal segment may form from branches from each of these fascicles.[124] The anterior fascicle supplies the medial basilar area of the anterior papillary muscle of the mitral valve, and the posterior fascicle supplies the medial basal portion of the posterior papillary muscle.[124] Each fascicle terminates into a peripheral Purkinje network that interdigitates with individual myocardial cells.[124] The left bundle branch, anterior fascicle, and proximal right bundle branch share the same blood supply from the *left anterior descending artery* and from the *AV nodal artery* (from the right coronary artery).[124] The posterior fascicle receives its blood supply from the *AV nodal artery*, branches from the *posterior descending artery*, and from the *left circumflex artery*.[128] Therefore, The location of the bundle branch block or fascicular block should correlate, for example, with the blood vessel involved in the patient with coronary artery occlusion.

Left Bundle Branch Block Pathophysiology

Left bundle branch block is associated with atherosclerotic coronary artery disease, hypertension, aortic valvular disease, cardiomyopathies, syphilitic aortitis, aortic coarctation, patent ductus arteriosus, constrictive pericarditis, and may be seen in patients with an otherwise normal heart.[3,129] A structurally normal heart is found in 16% of patients with left bundle branch block.[129] Approximately 80% of patients with left bundle branch block have left ventricular hypertrophy.[124]

ECG Findings in Left Bundle Branch Block

Left bundle branch block affects the early phase of ventricular conduction, whereas right bundle branch block affects the terminal phase. With left bundle branch block, the ventricular septum depolarizes from right to left instead of from left to right. Left bundle branch block produces a delay in the total time available for left ventricular depolarization and contraction. Characteristic ECG findings in left bundle branch block are:[122]

- Loss of the normal septal R wave in lead V_1 (variation: V_1 may show an rS complex with a small R wave and a large S wave)
- Loss of the normal septal Q wave in lead V_6 (variation: V_6 may show an abnormally wide and notched R wave without an initial Q wave)
- QRS complex is abnormally prolonged, greater than 120 ms
- Lead V_6 shows a wide, positive R wave without a Q wave
- Right chest leads show a negative QS pattern (since left ventricular depolarization is electrically predominant producing greater voltages than the right ventricle)
- Discordant T waves are expected (T-wave inversion in right precordial leads may reflect primary abnormality, such as ischemia)
- Occasional notching to the point of the QS wave in lead V_1 giving a characteristic W shape
- Occasional notching to the point of the R wave in lead V_6 giving a characteristic M shape
- Lead V_1 usually shows a wide, negative QS complex or, rarely, a wide rS complex

Clinical Significance of Left Bundle Branch Block

QRS duration, QRS axis, and the ventricular gradient help distinguish *uncomplicated* from *complicated* left bundle branch block. Left bundle branch block is considered uncomplicated when the QRS duration is between 120 and 140 ms, the frontal plane QRS axis is normal, the displacement of ST segment and T wave are discordant (deflection is to the opposite direction) to the principal QRS deflection, and the ventricular gradient (or T-wave altering force) is normal.[129] Left bundle branch block is considered complicated when the QRS duration is >140 ms, left or right axis deviation may be present, the ST segment and the T wave are concordant (same direction) with the principal QRS deflection, and the ventricular gradient is abnormal. Complicated left bundle branch block implies more diffuse myocardial disease,

more widespread conduction system disease, and a greater degree of ventricular dysfunction.

QRS duration can predict the left ventricular function with 98% specificity. A QRS duration less than 140 ms predicts a normal end-diastolic volume index and normal ejection fraction. A QRS duration >170 ms predicts a depressed left ventricular ejection fraction.[130] In patients who have left bundle branch block associated with a dilated cardiomyopathy, the strongest predictor for a *nonischemic cause* of the dilated cardiomyopathy is left bundle branch block.[131] However, left bundle branch block is the strongest predictor of mortality in patients with dilated cardiomyopathy.[3]

Chest Pain and Left Bundle Branch Block

Patients with intermittent left bundle branch block will frequently develop chest discomfort at the onset of the dysrhythmia. This is thought to be related to paradoxical cardiac movement at the onset of the bundle branch block.[132–135] The left bundle branch block may be acceleration-dependent, and the chest pain may occur during exercise.[135] The chest discomfort is unlikely due to myocardial ischemia since it begins at the onset of left bundle branch block, and there are no antecedent ischemic ST-segment changes on ECG.[3]

When there is left bundle branch block in the setting of chest pain, the ECG diagnosis of acute myocardial infarction is difficult. Comparison with a prior ECG may help. Uncomplicated left bundle branch block is often characterized by ST-segment changes due to late repolarization in the left ventricle with respect to the right ventricle. ECG changes predicting acute myocardial infarction in the presence of left bundle branch block with 90% specificity are:[136]

- ST-segment elevation greater than or equal to 1 mm in leads with a positive QRS
- ST-segment depression greater than or equal to 1 mm in lead V_1 through V_3
- ST-segment elevation greater than or equal to 5 mm in leads with a negative QRS

Detecting myocardial ischemia and acute coronary syndrome in patients with left bundle branch block may not be apparent on ECG; myocardial perfusion during exercise testing may be of help. Nuclear testing in patients with left bundle branch block has a low specificity for detecting hemodynamically significant coronary artery disease in the left anterior descending coronary artery distribution.[137–139] Up to 80% of patients with left bundle branch block and a normal left anterior descending artery on angiogram have septal perfusion defects after exercise, and the septal abnormalities found are more prominent in patients who have achieved high peak heart rates during exercise. However, defects limited to the septum are the ones most likely to be false positive.[137]

Hemodynamic Effects of Left Bundle Branch Block

The hemodynamic implications of acute left bundle branch block are a consequence of endocardial activation and repolarization, which is reversed from normal orthodromic cardiac conduction. This causes a parallel rather than radial spread of the depolarization front toward the left ventricular wall. Hemodynamic consequences include unfavorable affects on systolic end-diastolic left ventricular performance. However, left ventricular dysfunction depends on underlying myocardial contractility. In patients with a normal heart, left bundle branch block causes deterioration of ventricular filling with minimal change in systolic performance. In patients with severely dilated cardiomyopathy, the clinical effects of left bundle branch block include an instantaneous and profound drop in myocardial performance, decline in arterial blood pressure, delay in the onset and termination of systolic ejection, shortening of the diastolic period, reduction in stroke volume, a compensatory rise in heart rate, and pulmonary edema.[140–143]

Patients with chronic left bundle branch block and dilated cardiomyopathy exhibit a reduced peak in left ventricular contractility, prolonged duration of the pulse pressure, delayed time to peak left ventricular contractility, and prolonged relaxation time,[144] which shortens the time for left ventricular filling, and thereby limits stroke volume.[145] Therefore, patients with left bundle branch and a dilated cardiomyopathy develop progressive left ventricular dilatation and mitral regurgitation.[131,146] It is not known whether left bundle branch block is the cause or the consequence of left ventricular dilatation.[3]

Prognosis for Patients with Left Bundle Branch Block

Prognostically, left bundle branch block in young, healthy men is generally benign, but in older patients it may indicate progressive degenerative disease of the ventricular myocardium. In patients with dilated cardiomyopathy, left bundle branch block is the strongest predictor of mortality, more so than the presence of the ventricular arrhythmias,

elevated right atrial pressure, left ventricular ejection fraction, atrial fibrillation, atrial flutter, or the presence of an S_3 gallop.[3]

FASCICULAR BLOCKS

A delay in electrical conduction down either the anterior or posterior fascicle of the left bundle branch is referred to as *fascicular block* or *hemiblock*. Fascicular blocks do not widen the QRS complex. Instead, they produce an axis deviation. *Left anterior fascicular block* causes a marked *left axis deviation* (QRS vector of −45 degrees or more). *Left posterior fascicular block* produces a marked *right axis deviation* (QRS vector +120 degrees or more). The QRS vector with respect to fascicular block is read in the frontal plane (i.e., extremity leads) in contrast to bundle branch blocks which are read on ECG in the precordial leads (i.e., leads V_1 through V_6).[122]

Left Anterior Fascicular Block

Left anterior fascicular block increases the normal QRS by 10–20 ms.[124] ECG findings in left anterior fascicular block include:

- Frontal plane QRS vector of −45 degrees (some consider −30 degrees) to −80 degrees
- QRS duration greater than or equal to 110 ms
- T wave in leads I and a VL less than or equal to 20 ms

Left anterior fascicular block may go unrecognized or cause problems interpreting the ECG for myocardial infarction. For example, left anterior fascicular block, which normally causes a left axis deviation, may be obscured by a large left lateral myocardial infarction that produces a right axis deviation. In this case, the left anterior fascicular block may be unrecognized unless prior ECGs showing the left anterior fascicular block are available for comparison. Conversely, left anterior fascicular block can mimic a high lateral infarction by creating a large T wave in leads I and aVL. Distinguishing this pattern from myocardial infarction, the Q wave is usually less than 40 ms and the R wave in lead II is not wide.[124] An anterior myocardial infarction may be masked by left anterior fascicular block by changing the infarction pattern QS complex into an RS pattern and correcting the T-wave abnormalities in the anterior precordial leads.[147–150]

The combination *left axis deviation* and *right bundle branch block* is the result of left anterior fascicular block and a block of the entire right bundle branch. This is described in many terms including "left the bundle branch block masquerading as right bundle branch block," bilateral bundle branch block, right bundle branch block with left parietal block, or right bundle branch block with left axis deviation,[124] and bifascicular block.

Left Posterior Fascicular Block

Left posterior fascicular block shifts QRS vector to the right by delaying activation of the inferior and rightward portion of the left ventricle supplied by the posterior fascicle. ECG findings in left posterior fascicular block include:[122]

- Rightward QRS vector of plus 120 degrees or more
- QRS width < 120 ms
- Usually an rS complex in lead I
- Usually a qR complex in leads II, III, and aVF
- More common causes of right axis deviation are excluded (e.g., right ventricular hypertrophy, chronic obstructive lung disease, lateral wall myocardial infarction, pulmonary embolism). In these cases, comparison with the previous ECG may be helpful

Compared with left anterior fascicular block, left posterior fascicular block is rare and most often occurs with right bundle branch block.[122] When the left posterior fascicular block is found, it probably represents more widespread disease than that associated with left anterior fascicular block.[124]

Right Bundle Branch Block

Right bundle branch block occurs when there is a delay in normal orthodromic conduction of electrical impulse down the right bundle. The bundle branch block may be incomplete or complete depending on the degree of that delay. Electrocardiographic criteria for right bundle branch block include:[151]

- QRS duration greater than or equal to 120 ms (incomplete right bundle branch block has QRS duration less than 120 ms)
- rsr′, rsR′, rSR′, or M shape with R′ usually greater than the initial R wave in leads V_1 and V_2
- Wide S wave in leads I, V_5, and V_6 with S-wave duration greater than R-wave duration or S-wave duration greater than 40 ms in adults (incomplete right bundle branch block has S-wave duration less than or equal to 40 ms)

Right Bundle Branch Anatomy

Right bundle branch block can be associated with both cardiac and noncardiac diseases or can occur in the normal individual. In contrast to the left bundle branch, the right bundle branch passes down the right ventricular septum as a long slender structure without proximal branching. The anatomic location and then structure of the right bundle branch makes it particularly susceptible to any damage to the ventricular septum, no matter how limited. An clinical example is the temporary right bundle branch pattern that develops on cardiac rhythm strip during Swan-Ganz catheter placement if the tip inadvertently impacts the ventricular septum.

Right Bundle Branch Block Pathophysiology

Right bundle branch block, associated with acute myocardial infarction, carries a high potential for progression to complete heart block and reflects extensive myocardial disease. The right bundle branch may necrose in proximal disease, causing persistent right bundle branch block, but if necrosis doesn't occur, then the bundle branch block is usually transient.[152] Right bundle branch block is commonly associated with dilated cardiomyopathy, and when associated with a superior axis deviation suggests more extensive myocardial damage.[151] Right bundle branch block can occur in the postsurgical patient, especially in those who have history of a repair of a tetralogy of Fallot, ventricular septal defect, ventriculotomy, resection of infundibulum muscles, or resection of the moderator band.[153] In patients who have had repair of a tetralogy of Fallot, right bundle branch block is commonly associated with left anterior hemiblock. Lenegre disease and Lev disease are degenerative diseases of the conduction system that occur with advancing age, and manifest initially as atrioventricular and intraventricular conduction blocks that gradually progress to complete heart block. A common feature of these two diseases is right bundle branch block with left anterior hemiblock.[17,154–156] Right bundle branch block can occur with pulmonary embolism which produces acute right-sided heart strain that may cause a right ventricular conduction delay.[122] If right bundle branch block occurs after cardiac bypass surgery, it does not have any specific implications.[122]

Clinical Significance of Right Bundle Branch Block

The patient who presents with syncope and right bundle branch block is more likely to have a distal lesion in the right bundle branch as opposed to a more proximal one.[157] Experimentally, measuring the delay between mitral valve closing, tricuspid valve closing, and pulmonary valve opening helps distinguish proximal from distal lesions in the right bundle. The delay between mitral valve closing and tricuspid valve closing indicates a proximal right bundle branch lesion. The delay between tricuspid valve closing and pulmonary valve opening is attributed to more distal block. Right bundle branch block is peripheral, rather than proximal, in 80%.[158] Therefore, the finding of right bundle branch block in patients without known cardiac disease cannot be regarded as benign until an appropriate cardiac evaluation is complete.

Right bundle branch block associated with myocardial infarction and left-sided hemiblock poses an increased risk of complete heart block and must be approached with caution. When this occurs, the emergency physician should be prepared to provide emergency cardiac pacing.[122] Otherwise, right bundle branch block by itself requires no specific treatment.

Bifascicular Block and Trifascicular Block

Considering the trifacicular ventricular conduction system (right bundle branch, left bundle branch becoming the left anterior and left posterior fascicles), bifascicular block occurs from electrical disruption of any two of the three fascicles, and trifasicular block occurs when all three fascicles are involved. Bifascicular block from a right bundle branch block and *left anterior hemiblock* on ECG will show a right bundle branch pattern with marked *left axis deviation*. Bifascicular block from right bundle branch block with *left posterior hemiblock* will produces a *right axis deviation* with right bundle branch block pattern. (Other causes of right axis deviation such as right ventricular hypertrophy and myocardial infarction should be excluded.) When all three fascicles are blocked, complete heart block and atrioventricular dissociation may result.[115]

BRUGADA SYNDROME

The Brugada syndrome is a special case in which a right bundle branch block is part of the ECG findings. The Brugada syndrome was first recognized (though not defined) in 1986 by Pedro and Josep Brugada when a 3-year-old boy from Poland presented with several episodes of syncope. His ECG showed ST-segment elevation in leads V_1 through V_3, and his sister had a similar clinical profile and ECG pattern but died at 2 years of age. Subsequently, the Brugada brothers described

several more patients who presented with the similar clinical and ECG pattern of ST-segment elevation and apparent right bundle branch block. Patients with Brugada syndrome are at risk for sudden death by ventricular tachycardia. The Brugada syndrome is linked to the *SCN5A* gene that encodes for the alpha subunit of the sodium channel. Several dozen mutations of the *SCN5A* gene cause the Brugada syndrome by failure of the sodium channel so that there is:

1. A shift in the voltage- and time-dependent sodium current activation, inactivation, or reactivation

2. Entry of the sodium current into an intermediate state of inactivation from which it recovers more slowly

3. Accelerated inactivation of the sodium current[159]

The appearance of the right bundle branch morphology, in part, may be due to early repolarization of the right ventricular epicardium rather than a conduction block in the right bundle branch.

The Brugada syndrome is 8–10 times more prevalent in males than in females, and the syndrome is more prevalent in Southeast Asia. Those patients who do not have sudden death may present with aborted sudden death and syncope. This group has the highest risk of recurrence (69%). The only proven treatment for Brugada syndrome is an AICD.

REFERENCES

1. Baine WB, Yu W, Weis KA. Trends and outcomes in the hospitalization of older Americans for cardiac conduction disorders or arrhythmias, 1991–1998. *J Am Geriatr Soc* 2001;49(6):763–770.

2. Upshaw CB Jr. Lower prevalence of intraventricular block in African-American patients compared with Caucasian patients: An electrocardiographic study II. *J Natl Med Assoc* 2003;95(9):818–824.

3. Littmann L, Symanski JD. Hemodynamic implications of left bundle branch block. *J Electrocardiol* 2000;33(Suppl): 115–121.

4. Wiberg TA, Richman HG, Gobel FL. The significance and prognosis of chronic bifascicular block. *Chest* 1977; 71(3):329–334.

5. Rossi L. Anatomopathology of the normal and abnormal AV conduction system. *Pacing Clin Electrophysiol* 1984;7(6 Pt 2):1101–1107.

6. Watanabe Y, Watanabe M. Impulse formation and conduction of excitation in the atrioventricular node. *J Cardiovasc Electrophysiol* 1994;5(5):517–531.

7. Meijler FL, Fisch C. Does the atrioventricular node conduct? *Br Heart J* 1989;61(4):309–315.

8. Narula OS. Atrioventricular block. In: Narula OS (ed.), *Cardiac Arrhythmias Electrophysiology, Diagnosis and Management.* Baltimore, MD: Williams & Wilkins, 1979, pp. 85–113.

9. Waller BF, Gering LE, Branyas NA, et al. Anatomy, histology, and pathology of the cardiac conduction system—Part V. *Clin Cardiol* 1993;16(7):565–569.

10. Davies MJ, Anderson RH, Becker AE. *The Conduction System of the Heart.* London: Butterworth & Co., 1983, pp. 1–336.

11. Waller BF, Gering LE, Branyas NA, et al. Anatomy, histology, and pathology of the cardiac conduction system—Part VI. *Clin Cardiol* 1993;16(8):623–628.

12. Nair CK, Runco V, Everson GT, et al. Conduction defects and mitral annulus calcification. *Br Heart J* 1980;44(2):162–167.

13. Teragaki M, Toda I, Sakamoto K, et al. Endomyocardial biopsy findings in patients with atrioventricular block in the absence of apparent heart disease. *Heart Vessels* 1999;14(4):170–176.

14. Ozawa T. Mitochondrial DNA mutations and age. *Ann N Y Acad Sci* 1998;854:128–154.

15. James TN, St Martin E, Willis PW 3rd, et al. Apoptosis as a possible cause of gradual development of complete heart block and fatal arrhythmias associated with absence of the AV node, sinus node, and internodal pathways.[see comment]. *Circulation* 1996;93(7):1424–1438.

16. Reisinger J, Dubrey SW, Lavalley M, et al. Electrophysiologic abnormalities in AL (primary) amyloidosis with cardiac involvement. *J Am Coll Cardiol* 1997;30(4):1046–1051.

17. Bharati S, Lev M. Pathology of atrioventricular block. In: Waller BF (ed.), *Symposium on Cardiac Morphology.* Philadelphia, PA: W. B. Saunders, 1984, pp. 741–751.

18. Weed CL, Kulander BG, Massarella JA, et al. Heart block in ankylosing spondylitis. *Arch Int Med* 1966;117(6):800–806.

19. Harris M. Rheumatoid heart disease with complete heart block. *J Clin Pathol* 1970;23(7):623–626.

20. Gallagher PJ, Gresham GA. Heart block with infected cardiac rheumatoid granulomas. *Br Heart J* 1973;35(1):110–112.

21. Ahern M, Lever J, Cosh J. Complete heart block in rheumatoid arthritis. *Ann Rheum Dis* 1982;41:319–324.

22. Sevy S, Kelly J, Ernst H. Fatal paroxysmal tachycardia associated with focal myocarditis of the Purkinje system in a 14-month-old girl. *J Pediatr* 1968;72(6):796–800.

23. Morales AR, Levy S, Davis J. Sarcoidosis and the heart. In: Sommers SC (ed.), *Pathology Annual.* New York: Appleton-Century-Crofts, 1974, pp. 138–144.

24. Waller BF. Clinicopathological correlations of the human cardiac conduction system. In: Zipes DP, Jalife J (eds.), *Cardiac Electrophysiology from Cell to Bedside.* Philadelphia, PA: W.B. Saunders, 1990, pp. 249–269.

25. Rossi L. *Histopathology of Cardiac Arrhythmias*, 2nd ed. Milan: Casa Editrice Ambrosiana, 1979, pp. 1–110.

26. Pauschinger M, Badorff C, Kuhl U, et al. Synkopebei AV-Block III(o). Nachweis von Virusgenom im Myokard. *Deutsche Medizinische Wochenschrift* 1998;123(48):1443–1446.

27. Siren MK, Julkunen H, Kaaja R, et al. Role of HLA in congenital heart block: Susceptibility alleles in children. *Lupus* 1999;8(1):60–67.

28. Cooley HM, Keech CL, Melny BJ, et al. Monozygotic twins discordant for congenital complete heart block. *Arthritis Rheum* 1997;40(2):381–384.

29. Borda E, Leiros CP, Bacman S, et al. Sjîgren autoantibodies modify neonatal cardiac function via M1 muscarinic acetylcholine receptor activation. *Intl J Cardiol* 1999;70(1):23–32.

30. Xiao GQ, Hu K, Boutjdir M. Direct inhibition of expressed cardiac l- and t-type calcium channels by igg from mothers whose children have congenital heart block. *Circulation* 2001;103(11):1599–1604.

31. Boutjdir M, Chen L, Zhang ZH, et al. Serum and immunoglobulin G from the mother of a child with congenital heart block induce conduction abnormalities and inhibit L-type calcium channels in a rat heart model. *Pediatr Res* 1998;44(1):11–19.

32. Eftekhari P, Salle L, Lezoualc'h F, et al. Anti-SSA/Ro52 autoantibodies blocking the cardiac 5-HT4 serotoninergic receptor could explain neonatal lupus congenital heart block. *Eur J Immunol* 2000;30(10):2782–2790.

33. Ristic AD, Maisch B. Cardiac rhythm and conduction disturbances: What is the role of autoimmune mechanisms? *Herz* 2000;25(3):181–188.

34. Li JM, Fan WS, Horsfall AC, et al. The expression of human endogenous retrovirus-3 in fetal cardiac tissue and antibodies in congenital heart block. *Clin Exp Immunol* 1996;104(3):388–393.

35. Uzun O, Gibbs JL. Progressive disease of the atrioventricular conduction axis in an infant of an anti-Ro positive mother. *Cardiol Young* 1999;9(2):192–193.

36. Probst V, Kyndt F, Potet F, et al. Haploinsufficiency in combination with aging causes SCN5A-linked hereditary Lenegre disease. *J Am Coll Cardiol* 2003;41(4):643–652.

37. Wang DW, Viswanathan PC, Balser JR, et al. Clinical, genetic, and biophysical characterization of SCN5A mutations associated with atrioventricular conduction block. *Circulation* 2002;105(3):341–346.

38. Sangwatanaroj S, Yanatasneejit P, Sunsaeewitayakul B, et al. Linkage analyses and SCN5A mutations screening in five sudden unexplained death syndrome (Lai-tai) families. *J Med Assoc Thai* 2002; 85(Suppl 1):S54–S61.

39. Rivolta I, Abriel H, Tateyama M, et al. Inherited Brugada and long QT-3 syndrome mutations of a single residue of the cardiac sodium channel confer distinct channel and clinical phenotypes. *J Biol Chem* 2001;276(33):30623–30630.

40. Kitaguchi T, Matsubara S, Sato M, et al. A missense mutation in the exon 8 of lamin A/C gene in a Japanese case of autosomal dominant limb-girdle muscular dystrophy and cardiac conduction block. *Neuromuscul Disord* 2001;11(6/7):542–546.

41. Jakobs PM, Hanson EL, Crispell KA, et al. Novel lamin A/C mutations in two families with dilated cardiomyopathy and conduction system disease. *J Cardiac Failure* 2001;7(3): 249–256.

42. Berul CI, Maguire CT, Aronovitz MJ, et al. DMPK dosage alterations result in atrioventricular conduction abnormalities in a mouse myotonic dystrophy model. *J Clin Invest* 1999;103(4):R1–R7.

43. Lee HC, Patel MK, Mistry DJ, et al. Abnormal Na channel gating in murine cardiac myocytes deficient in myotonic dystrophy protein kinase. *Physiol Genomics* 2003;12(2): 147–157.

44. Shirai N, Makita N, Sasaki K, et al. A mutant cardiac sodium channel with multiple biophysical defects associated with overlapping clinical features of Brugada syndrome and cardiac conduction disease. *Cardiovasc Res* 2002;53(2):348–354.

45. Bardien-Kruger S, Wulff H, Arieff Z, Brink P, et al. Characterisation of the human voltage-gated potassium channel gene, KCNA7, a candidate gene for inherited cardiac disorders, and its exclusion as cause of progressive familial heart block I (PFHBI). *Eur J Hum Genet* 2002;10(1):36–43.

46. Simon AM, Goodenough DA, Paul DL. Mice lacking connexin40 have cardiac conduction abnormalities characteristic of atrioventricular block and bundle branch block. *Curr Biol* 1998;8(5):295–298.

47. Hagendorff A, Schumacher B, Kirchhoff S, et al. Conduction disturbances and increased atrial vulnerability in Connexin40-deficient mice analyzed by transesophageal stimulation. *Circulation* 1999;99(11):1508–1515.

48. Miura M, Yamagishi H, Morikawa Y, et al. Congenital long QT syndrome and 2:1 atrioventricular block with a mutation of the SCN5A gene. *Pediatr Cardiol* 2003;24(1): 70–72.

49. Kyndt F, Probst V, Potel F, et al. Novel SCN5A mutation leading either to isolated cardiac conduction defect or Brugada syndrome in a large French family.[see comment]. *Circulation* 2001;104(25):3081–3086.

50. Wang JC, Lim SH, Teo WS, et al. Calcium channel blockers as first line treatment for broad complex tachycardia with right bundle branch block: ingenuity or folly? *Resuscitation* 2002;52(2):175–182.

51. Janse MJ, Wilde AA. Molecular mechanisms of arrhythmias. *Revista Portuguesa de Cardiologia* 1998;17(Suppl 2): II41–II46.

52. Arbustini E, Pilotto A, Repetto A, et al. Autosomal dominant dilated cardiomyopathy with atrioventricular block: A lamin A/C defect-related disease. *J Am Coll Cardiol* 2002;39(6):981–990.

53. Berul CI, Maguire CT, Gehrmann J, et al. Progressive atrioventricular conduction block in a mouse myotonic dystrophy model. *J Interv Card Electrophysiol* 2000;4(2): 351–358.

54. Ferrari F, Nascimento P, Jr., Vianna PT. Complete atrioventricular block during renal transplantation in a patient with Alport's syndrome: Case report. *Sao Paulo Med J* 2001;119(5):184–186.

55. Noda M, Yamaguchi H, Fujii H, et al. Spontaneous regression over a 16-year period of tachyarrhythmias to sick sinus syndrome and complete atrioventricular block in a young patient with Epstein's anomaly. *Pacing Clin Electrophysiol* 2001;24(7):1158–1160.

56. Katsanos KH, Elisaf M, Bairaktari E, et al. Severe hypomagnesemia and hypoparathyroidism in Kearns-Sayre syndrome. *Am J Nephrol* 2001;21(2):150–153.

57. Tsuchiya Y, Arahata K Emery-Dreifuss syndrome. *Curr Opin Neurol* 1997;10(5):421–425.

58. Doi Y, Toda G, Yano K. Sisters with atypical Fabry's disease with complete atrioventricular block. *Heart* 2003;89(1):e2.

59. Veinot JP, Johnston B. Cardiac sarcoidosis—an occult cause of sudden death: A case report and literature review. *J Forensic Sc* 1998;43(3):715–717.

60. Bergfeldt L. HLA-B27-associated cardiac disease.[see comment]. *Ann Intern Med* 1997;127(8 Pt 1):621–629.

61. Koehler U, Fus E, Grimm W, et al. Heart block in patients with obstructive sleep apnoea: Pathogenetic factors and effects of treatment. *Eur Respir J* 1998;11(2):434–439.

62. Leonelli FM, Dunn JK, Young JB, et al. Natural history, determinants, and clinical relevance of conduction abnormalities following orthotopic heart transplantation. *Am J Cardiol* 1996;77(1):47–51.

63. Barold SS, Hayes DL. Second-degree atrioventricular block: A reappraisal. *Mayo Clin Proc* 2001;76(1):44–57.

64. Medeiros A, Iturralde P, Millan F, et al. Bloqueo auriculoventricular completo durante el esfuerzo. *Archivos del Instituto de Cardiologia de Mexico* 1999;69(3):250–257.

65. Gill JS, Prasad K, Blaszyk K, et al. Initiating sequences in exercise induced idiopathic ventricular tachycardia of left bundle branch-like morphology. *Pacing Clin Electrophysiol* 1998;21(10):1873–1880.

66. Shimamoto T, Nakata Y, Sumiyoshi M, et al. Transient left bundle branch block induced by left-sided cardiac catheterization in patients without pre-existing conduction abnormalities. *Jpn Circ J* 1998;62(2):146–149.

67. Michaeli J, Bassan MM, Brezis M. Second degree type II and complete atrioventricular block due to hyperkalemia. *J Electrocardiol* 1986;19(4):393–396.

68. Tiberti G, Bana G, Bossi M. Complete atrioventricular block with unwidened QRS complex during hyperkalemia. *Pacing & Clinical Electrophysiology* 1998;21(7): 1480–1482.

69. Przybojewski JZ, Knott-Craig CJ. Hyperkalaemic complete heart block. A report of 2 unique cases and a review of the literature. *S Afr Med J* 1983;63(11): 413–420.

70. Lai KN, Swaminathan R, Pun CO, et al. Hemofiltration in digoxin overdose. *Arch Intern Med* 1986;146(6): 1219–1220.

71. Wenger TL, Butler VP, Jr., Haber E, et al. Treatment of 63 severely digitalis-toxic patients with digoxin-specific

antibody fragments. *J Am Coll Cardiol* 1985;5(5 Suppl A): 118A–123A.

72. Pritza DR, Bierman MH, Hammeke MD. Acute toxic effects of sustained-release verapamil in chronic renal failure. [see comment]. *Arch Intern Med* 1991;151(10): 2081–2084.

73. Kjeldsen SE, Syvertsen JO, Hedner T. Cardiac conduction with diltiazem and beta-blockade combined. A review and report on cases. *Blood Pressure* 1996;5(5):260–263.

74. Rosenmund A, Brand B, Straub PW. Hyperlactataemia, hyperkalemia and heart block in acute iron overload: The fatal role of the hepatic iron-incorporation rate in rats on ferric citrate infusions. *Eur J Clin Invest* 1988; 18(1):69–74.

75. Laurita KR, Chuck ET, Yang T, et al. Optical mapping reveals conduction slowing and impulse block in iron-overload cardiomyopathy. *J Lab Clin Med* 2003;142(2):83–89.

76. Littman L, Monroe MH, Svenson RH. Brugada-type electrocardiographic pattern induced by cocaine. *Mayo Clin Proc* 2000;75(8):845–849.

77. Asao Y, Matsumoto M, Wake M, et al. Transient complete left bundle branch block during epidural anesthesia with mepivacaine. *Masui* 1996;45(4):483–486.

78. Glauser J. Tricyclic antidepressant poisoning. *Cleve Clin J Med* 2000;67(10):704–706.

79. Lown B. Electrical reversion of cardiac arrhythmias. *Br Heart J* 1967;29(4):469–489.

80. Gregoratos G, Abrams J, Epstein AE, et al. ACC/AHA/ NASPE 2002 Guideline Update for Implantation of Cardiac Pacemakers and Antiarrhythmia Devices— summary article: A report of the American College of Cardiology/American Heart Association Task Force on Practice Guidelines (ACC/AHA/NASPE Committee to Update the 1998 Pacemaker Guidelines). *J Am Coll Cardiol* 2002;40(9):1703–1719.

81. Brignole M. Sick sinus syndrome. *Clin Geriatr Med* 2002;18(2):211–227.

82. Agruss NS, Rosin EY, Adolph RJ, et al. Significance of chronic sinus bradycardia in elderly people. *Circulation* 1972;46(5):924–930.

83. Belic N, Talano JV. Current concepts in sick sinus syndrome. II. ECG manifestation and diagnostic and therapeutic approaches. *Arch Intern Med* 1985;145(4):722–726.

84. Kantelip JP, Sage E, Duchene-Marullaz P. Findings on ambulatory electrocardiographic monitoring in subjects older than 80 years. *Am J Cardiol* 1986;57(6):398–401.

85. Molgaard H, Sorensen KE, Bjerregaard P. Minimal heart rates and longest pauses in healthy adult subjects on two occasions eight years apart. *Eur Heart J* 1989;10(8): 758–764.

86. Ferrer MI. The sick sinus syndrome in atrial disease. *JAMA* 1968;206(3):645–646.

87. Alpert MA, Flaker GC. Arrhythmias associated with sinus node dysfunction. Pathogenesis, recognition, and management. *JAMA* 1983;250(16):2160–2166.

88. Adan V, Crown LA. Diagnosis and treatment of sick sinus syndrome. *Am Fam Phys* 2003;67(8):1725–1732.

89. Lamas GA, Lee K, Sweeney M, et al. The mode selection trial (MOST) in sinus node dysfunction: Design, rationale, and baseline characteristics of the first 1000 patients. *Am Heart J* 2000;140(4):541–551.

90. Rodriguez RD, Schocken DD. Update on sick sinus syndrome, a cardiac disorder of aging. *Geriatrics* 1990; 45(1):26–30.

91. Brignole M, Menozzi C, Gianfranchi L, et al. Neurally mediated syncope detected by carotid sinus massage and head-up tilt test in sick sinus syndrome. *Am J Cardiol* 1991;68(10):1032–1036.

92. Brignole M, Menozzi C, Sartore B, et al. L'ipersensibilita senocarotidea cardioinibitrice nei soggetti con disfunzione sinusale sintomatica. *Giornale Italiano di Cardiologia* 1986;16(8):643–647.

93. Rubenstein JJ, Schulman CL, Yurchak PM, et al. Clinical spectrum of the sick sinus syndrome. *Circulation* 1972;46(1):5–13.

94. Sgarbossa EB, Pinski SL, Jaeger FJ, et al. Incidence and predictors of syncope in paced patients with sick sinus syndrome. *Pacing & Clinical Electrophysiology* 1992;15(11 Pt 2):2055–2060.

95. Shaw DB, Holman RR, Gowers JI. Survival in sinoatrial disorder (sick-sinus syndrome). *Br Med J* 1980; 280(6208): 139–141.

96. Bower PJ. Sick sinus syndrome. *Arch Intern Med* 1978; 138(1):133–137.

97. Wahls SA. Sick sinus syndrome. *Am Fam Phys* 1985; 31(3):117–124.

98. Bigger JT Jr., Reiffel JA. Sick sinus syndrome. *Ann Rev Med* 1979;30:91–118.

99. Colquhoun M. When should you suspect sick sinus syndrome? *Practitioner* 1999;243(1598):422–425.

100. Brignole M, Sartore B, Barra M, et al. Limiti della prova da sforzo nella diagnostica della malattia del nodo del seno. *Giornale Italiano di Cardiologia* 1984;14(12): 1045–1051.

101. Bashour TT. Classification of sinus node dysfunction. *Am Heart J* 1985;110(6):1251–1256.

102. Rokseth R, Hatle L. Prospective study on the occurrence and management of chronic sinoatrial disease, with follow-up. *Br Heart J* 1974;36(6):582–587.

103. Alboni P, Menozzi C, Brignole M, et al. Effects of permanent pacemaker and oral theophylline in sick sinus syndrome the THEOPACE study: A randomized controlled trial. *Circulation* 1997;96(1):260–266.

104. Sutton R, Kenny RA. The natural history of sick sinus syndrome. *Pacing & Clinical Electrophysiology* 1986; 9(6 Pt 2):1110–1114.

105. Andersen HR, Nielsen JC, Thomsen PE, et al. Long-term follow-up of patients from a randomised trial of atrial versus ventricular pacing for sick-sinus syndrome. [see comment]. *Lancet* 1997;350(9086):1210–1216.

106. Andersen HR, Thuesen L, Bagger JP, et al. Prospective randomised trial of atrial versus ventricular pacing in sick-sinus syndrome. [see comment]. *Lancet* 1994;344(8936): 1523–1528.

107. Connolly SJ, Kerr CR, Gent M, et al. Effects of physiologic pacing versus ventricular pacing on the risk of stroke and death due to cardiovascular causes. Canadian Trial of Physiologic Pacing Investigators. [see comment]. *N Engl J Med* 2000;342(19):1385–1391.

108. Lamas GA, Orav EJ, Stambler BS, et al. Quality of life and clinical outcomes in elderly patients treated with ventricular pacing as compared with dual-chamber pacing. Pacemaker Selection in the Elderly Investigators. [see comment]. *N Engl J Med* 1998;338(16):1097–1104.

109. Nielsen JC, Andersen HR, Thomsen PE, et al. Heart failure and echocardiographic changes during long-term follow-up of patients with sick sinus syndrome randomized to single-chamber atrial or ventricular pacing. *Circulation* 1998;97(10):987–995.

110. Stone JM, Bhakta RD, Lutgen J. Dual chamber sequential pacing management of sinus node dysfunction: Advantages over single-chamber pacing. *Am Heart J* 1982;104(6): 1319–1327.

111. Simon AB, Janz N. Symptomatic bradyarrhythmias in the adult: Natural history following ventricular pacemaker implantation. *Pacing & Clinical Electrophysiology* 1982; 5(3):372–383.

112. Barold SS. Atrioventricular block revisited. *Compr Ther* 2002;28(1):74–78.

113. Norris RM. Heart block in posterior and anterior myocardial infarction. *Br Heart J* 1969;31(3):352–356.

114. Bexton RS, Camm AJ. First degree atrioventricular block. *Eur Heart J* 1984;5(Suppl A):107–109.

115. Goldberger AL (ed.), *Atrioventricular Heart Block*. 6th ed. St. Louis, MO: Mosby, 1999, pp. 178–187.

116. Iliev II, Yamachika S, Muta K, et al. Preserving normal ventricular activation versus atrioventricular delay optimization during pacing: the role of intrinsic atrioventricular conduction and pacing rate. *Pacing & Clinical Electrophysiology* 2000;23(1):74–83.

117. Robles de Medina EO, Bernard R, Coumel P, et al. Definition of terms related to cardiac rhythm. The WHO/ICS Task Force. *Amn Heart J* 1978;95(6):796–806.

118. Surawicz B, Uhley H, Borun R, et al. The quest for optimal electrocardiography. Task force I: Standardization of terminology and interpretation. *Am J Cardiol* 1978;41(1): 130–145.

119. Massie B, Scheinman MM, Peters R, et al. Clinical and electrophysiologic findings in patients with paroxysmal slowing of the sinus rate and apparent Mobitz type II atrioventricular block. *Circulation* 1978;58(2):305–314.

120. Hayes DL, Barold SS, Camm AJ, et al. Evolving indications for permanent cardiac pacing: An appraisal of the 1998 American College of Cardiology/American Heart Association Guidelines. *Am J Cardiol* 1998;82(9): 1082–1086.

121. Getchell WS, Larsen GC, Morris CD, et al. Epidemiology of syncope in hospitalized patients. *J Gen Intern Med* 1999;14(11):677–687.

122. Goldberger AL (ed.), *Ventricular Conduction Disturbances: Bundle Branch Blocks*. 6th ed. St. Louis, MO: Mosby, 1999, pp. 68–80.

123. Massing GK, James TN. Anatomical configuration of the His bundle and bundle branches in the human heart. *Circulation* 1976;53(4):609–621.

124. Flowers NC. Left bundle branch block: A continuously evolving concept. *J Am Coll Cardiol* 1987;9(3):684–697.

125. Pruitt RD, Essex HE, Burchell BH. Studies on the spread of excitation through the ventricular myocardium. *Circulation* 1951;3:418–432.

126. DePasquale NP. Editorial: To pace or not to pace. *Ann Intern Med* 1974;81(3):395–396.

127. Lev M. The pathology of complete atrioventricular block. *Prog Cardiovasc Dis* 1964;6:317–326.

128. Frink RJ, James TN. Normal blood supply to the human His bundle and proximal bundle branches. *Circulation* 1973;47(1):8–18.

129. Upshaw CB Jr. Seeing through the maze of complete left bundle branch block. *J Med Assoc Ga* 1993;82(11):593–599.

130. Recke SH, Esperer HD, Eberlein U, et al. Assessment of left ventricular function from the electrocardiogram in left bundle branch block. *Int J Cardiol* 1989;24(3):297–304.

131. Hamby RI, Weissman RH, Prakash MN, et al. Left bundle branch block: A predictor of poor left ventricular function in coronary artery disease. *Am Heart J* 1983;106(3): 471–477.

132. Virtanen KS, Heikkila J, Kala R, et al. Chest pain and rate-dependent left bundle branch block in patients with normal coronary arteriograms. *Chest* 1982;81(3):326–331.

133. Kafka H, Burggraf GW. Exercise-induced left bundle branch block and chest discomfort without myocardial ischemia. *Am Jf Cardiol* 1984;54(6):676–677.

134. Perin E, Petersen F, Massumi A. Rate-related left bundle branch block as a cause of non-ischemic chest pain. *Cathet Cardiovasc Diagn* 1991;22(1):45–46.

135. Hertzeanu H, Aron L, Shiner RJ, et al. Exercise dependent complete left bundle branch block. *Eur Heart J* 1992;13(11):1447–1451.

136. Sgarbossa EB. Value of the ECG in suspected acute myocardial infarction with left bundle branch block. [see comment]. *J Electrocardiol* 2000;33(Suppl):87–92.

137. Delonca J, Camenzind E, Meier B, et al. Limits of thallium-201 exercise scintigraphy to detect coronary disease in patients with complete and permanent bundle branch block: A review of 134 cases. *Am Heart J* 1992;123(5):1201–1207.

138. DePuey EG, Guertler-Krawczynska E, Robbins WL. Thallium-201 SPECT in coronary artery disease patients with left bundle branch block. [see comment]. *J Nucl Med* 1988;29(9):1479–1485.

139. Vaduganathan P, He ZX, Raghavan C, et al. Detection of left anterior descending coronary artery stenosis in

patients with left bundle branch block: Exercise, adenosine or dobutamine imaging? *J Am Coll Cardiol* 1996;28(3):543–550.

140. Takeshita A, Basta LL, Kioschos JM. Effect of intermittent left bundle branch block on left ventricular performance. *Am J Med* 1974;56(2):251–255.

141. Grover M, Engler RL. Acute pulmonary edema induced by left bundle branch block. *Am J Cardiol* 1983;52(5): 648–649.

142. Littmann L, Goldberg JR. Apparent bigeminy and pulsus alternans in intermittent left bundle-branch block. *Clin Cardiol* 1999;22(7):490.

143. Bourassa MG, Boiteau GM, Allenstein BJ. Hemodynamic studies during intermittent left bundle branch block. *Am J Cardiol* 1962;10:792.

144. Xiao HB, Brecker SJ, Gibson DG. Effects of abnormal activation on the time course of the left ventricular pressure pulse in dilated cardiomyopathy. *Br Heart J* 1992;68(4):403–407.

145. Xiao HB, Lee CH, Gibson DG. Effect of left bundle branch block on diastolic function in dilated cardiomyopathy. *Br Heart J* 1991;66(6):443–447.

146. Talreja D, Gruver C, Sklenar J, et al. Efficient utilization of echocardiography for the assessment of left ventricular systolic function. [see comment]. *Am Heart J* 2000;139(3): 394–398.

147. Kulbertus HE. Electrocardiographic recognition of anterior infarction in left anterior fascicular block: A diagnostic challenge. *Chest* 1972;62(1):91–93.

148. Altieri P, Schaal SF. Inferior and anteroseptal myocardial infarction concealed by transient left anterior hemiblock. *J Electrocardiol* 1973;6(3):257–258.

149. Abinader EG, Naschitz J. Left anterior hemiblock modifying anteroseptal myocardial infarction. *Ir J Med Sci* 1978;147(3):97–102.

150. Khair GZ, Tristani FE, Brooks HL. Recognition of myocardial infarction complicated by left anterior hemiblock: A diagnostic dilemma. *J Electrocardiol* 1980; 13(1):93–98.

151. Agarwal AK, Venugopalan P. Right bundle branch block: Varying electrocardiographic patterns. Aetiological correlation, mechanisms and electrophysiology. *Int J Cardiol* 1999;71(1):33–39.

152. Okabe M, Fukuda K, Nakashima Y, et al. A quantitative histopathological study of right bundle branch block complicating acute anteroseptal myocardial infarction. *Br Heart J* 1991;65(6):317–321.

153. Gelband H, Waldo AL, Kaiser GA, et al. Etiology of right bundle-branch block in patients undergoing total correction of tetralogy of Fallot. *Circulation* 1971;44(6): 1022–1033.

154. Lev M. Anatomic basis for atrioventricular block. *Am J Med* 1964;37:742–752.

155. Lenegre J. Etiology and pathology of bilateral bundle branch block in relation to complete heart block. *Prog Cardiovasc Dis* 1964;6:406–510.

156. Rosenbaum MB, Elizari MV, Lazzari JO, et al. Intraventricular trifascicular blocks. The syndrome of right bundle branch block with intermittent left anterior and posterior hemiblock. *Am Heart J* 1969;78(3):306–317.

157. Dancy M, Leech G, Leatham A. Significance of complete right bundle-branch block when an isolated finding. An echocardiographic study. *Br Heart J* 1982;48(3):217–221.

158. Doi Y, Ogawa S, Hiroki T, et al. Right bundle branch block. Echocardiographic study with special reference to the site of block within the right bundle. *Jpn Heart J* 1990; 31(6):767–776.

159. Antzelevitch C, Brugada P, Brugada J, et al. Brugada syndrome: 1992–2002: A historical perspective. *J Am Coll Cardiol* 2003;41(10):1665–1671.

23

Pacemakers and Automatic Implantable Cardiac Defibrillators in the ED

Robert Wahl
Sridevi Pitta
Robert J. Zalenski

HIGH YIELD FACTS

- Pacemaker infections are potentially life threatening, with a mortality reported as high as 5%.
- The chest radiograph may identify the type of pacemaker or automatic implantable cardioverter-defibrillator (AICD).
- Bipolar pacemaker leads can produce very small depolarization spikes that may not be seen in all ECG leads.
- Defibrillation is not contraindicated when a pacemaker or AICD present, but it is preferred to be done with the lowest current possible, using the biphasic mode, with the pads in the anterior-posterior position, or the paddles at least 10 cm from the generator box.
- A magnet placed over the pacemaker will result in it pacing in a asynchronous mode, whereas if placed over the AICD, it will temporarily disable tachyarrhythmia intervention, but will have no effect on the pacing function.
- Three or more ICD discharges in a 24-hour period constitute a medical emergency.

INTRODUCTION

Emergency physicians will increasingly encounter clinical situations involving patients with cardiac devices, in particular, pacemakers and automatic ICDs. Transvenous pacing was first used clinically in 1960, and the first human implant of an ICD was in 1980. In the United States by the year 2000, approximately 600,000 patients had pacemakers and nearly 200,000 additional patients had ICDs.[1] Between 1990 and 2000, the number of patients with pacemakers increased by 22%, and the rate of implantation of ICDs increased 11-fold. An aging U.S. population, and newer indications for pacemakers and ICDs, make it certain that implantation of these devices will continue to increase. Clinical trials evaluating the benefits of cardiac device therapy in patients with atrial fibrillation, dilated and hypertrophic obstructive cardiomyopathy (HOCM), heart failure, and neurocardiogenic syncope may advance device applications beyond their primary use in sinus node dysfunction, carotid sinus hypersensitivity, and atrioventricular (AV) block. Although the function of the device itself may or may not be responsible for a patient seeking acute care, it is important for the emergency physician to have a working knowledge of cardiac devices to provide optimal patient care and to communicate effectively with consultants and treating physicians.[2–4]

Pacemaker Terminology

It is important to understand terminology that applies to pacemaker systems. Definitions of pertinent terms will be provided here.

Bipolar lead. A pacing lead with two electrical poles that are external from the pulse generator. The negative pole or cathode is the electrode at the extreme distal tip of the pacing lead, while the positive pole or anode is an annular electrode several millimeters proximal to the cathode. The cathode is the electrode through which the stimulating pulse is delivered. Relatively small spikes on the paced EGG characterize bipolar leads.

Unipolar lead. A pacing lead with a single electrical pole at the distal tip of the pacing lead (negative pole or cathode). The pulse generator case serves as the anode (positive pole). The cathode is the electrode through which the stimulating pulse is delivered.

Single chamber. A pacing mode with one electrode placed in a single cardiac chamber, atrium or ventricle.

Dual chamber. A pacing mode or pulse generator capable of pacing and/or sensing in both the atrium and the ventricle.

Biventricular pacing. A method of pacing with leads in one atrium and in each ventricle. The left ventricle is typically accessed transvenously through the coronary sinus and into an epicardial vein overlying the left ventricular (LV) free wall.

Pacemaker Components and Function

Pacemakers have the capability to receive and respond to electrical signals from the heart. There are two components to a pacemaker system, a lithium battery-powered pulse generator and one or more leads. The pulse generator is designed to deliver energy, known as the pacing stimulus, through the pacemaker leads to the electrode-cardiac tissue interface, where the polarization potential is propagated causing contraction of the chamber being paced. The pulse generator also has a sensing function, allowing it to analyze the patient's cardiac electrical activity and determine the appropriate time to deliver a paced beat. At the time of implantation, the pulse generator is programmed to deliver a sufficient amount of energy to depolarize only the intended target cardiac tissue, and not unintended tissues, such as the diaphragm or skeletal muscle. Additionally, the sensitivity is programmed to allow the pacemaker to optimally sense P waves and QRS complexes, and filter out other sources of electrical input, such as skeletal muscle potentials (myopotentials). Pulse generators have a lithium battery-powered source with a lifetime of 4–10 years, depending on the current drain.

The pacemaker leads are insulated flexible wires that conduct electrical signals between the pulse generator and the heart. The vascular system is most commonly accessed via the subclavian vein. In dual-chamber pacemaker systems, the atrial lead is typically positioned in the right atrial appendage, while the ventricular lead is positioned in the right ventricular apex. The lead tip is anchored into the endocardial surface with either passive fixation (tined tip) or active fixation (screw tip). Pacemaker leads are steroid-eluted to suppress inflammation of the cardiac tissue at the lead-myocardium interface. Leads can be unipolar or bipolar. Unipolar leads use the distal aspect of the lead in contact with the endocardial surface as the cathode and the pulse generator as the anode. Each bipolar lead functions as both the cathode (distally) and the anode (proximally), being separated by a few centimeters.

NASPE/BPEG Generic Pacemaker Code

In order to more effectively communicate information about pacemakers, a code was developed and published

in 1987 after being adopted by the North American Society of Pacing and Electrophysiology (NASPE) and the British Pacing and Electrophysiology Group (BPEG), and became known as the NASPE/BPEG Generic (NBG) Code for Antibradycardia Pacing. Beginning in April 2001, a revision of this code was undertaken to maintain compatibility with significant advances in pacing technology and practice, particularly the issue of multisite pacing. The revision sought to maintain simplicity for convenience of conversation, avoid confusion with the existing code, delete specifications no longer needed, and provide a means of representing the presence of multisite pacing. The Revised NBG Code for Antibradycardia Pacing uses letters to identify five positions, all of which are used exclusively to describe antibradycardia pacing. Position I indicates the chamber being paced, position II the chamber that is sensed, and position III the response to each instance of sensing, whether to trigger or inhibit subsequent pacing stimuli. Position IV indicates only whether an adaptive rate mechanism (rate modulation) is present (R) or absent (O). This position is unique in that it refers to the automatic adjustment of the pacing rate to compensate for an inadequate heart rate. Position V indicates the presence or absence of multisite pacing and where it occurs if present. Advances in pacing technology allow for pacing both atria, both ventricles, more than one pacing site in any single chamber, or any combination of these. In general, the first three positions are always used when describing a pacemaker. Positions IV and V are used to specify the presence of rate modulation and/or multisite pacing respectively, or to emphasize the absence of either function.

The Revised NASPE/BPEG Generic Code for Antibradycardia Pacing is shown in Table 23-1.

The following examples will illustrate conventional use of the pacemaker code, also called the mode code. An AAI (AAIO, AAIOO, *atrial demand*) pacemaker paces the atrium via a single lead and is inhibited by sensed spontaneous atrial depolarizations. There is no rate modulation or multisite pacing. A VOO (VOOO or VOOOO) pacer has a single lead into the ventricle that provides asynchronous (nondemand) ventricular pacing, i.e., without sensing, rate modulation, or multisite pacing. The heart will simply be paced at a programmed rate without regard for the patient's underlying rhythm. A VVIRV pacemaker (*ventricular demand* pacer) has ventricular pacing and sensing, is inhibited in response to a sensed spontaneous depolarization, has rate modulation capability, and multisite pacing with either biventricular pacing leads, or more than one pacing site within a single ventricle (Fig. 23-1).

Table 23-1. Revised NASPE/BPEG Generic Code for Antibradycardia Pacing

Position	I	II	III	IV	V
Category:	Chamber(s) paced	Chamber(s) sensed	Response to sensing	Rate modulation	Multisite pacing
	O = none A = atrium V = ventricle D = dual (A + V)	O = none A = atrium V = ventricle D = dual (A + V)	O = none T = triggered I = inhibited D = dual (T + I)	O = none R = rate modulation	O = none A = atrium V = ventricle D = dual (A + V)
Manufacturer's designation only	S = single (A or V)	S = single (A or V)			

The VDD (*atrial synchronous*) pacemaker essentially senses the atrium and paces the ventricle. It is inhibited by ventricular depolarization, either from a conducted P wave or a premature ventricular contraction. The DVI (*A-V sequential*) pacemaker paces both the atrium and ventricle in a patient with sinus node dysfunction and AV block. It does not sense the atrium, but senses the ventricle and is inhibited either by a conducted beat from the atrium or a premature ventricular contraction. Finally, a DDDRA pacemaker senses and paces from both the atrium and ventricle, can be inhibited or triggered based on the sensing function, with adaptive rate pacing and multisite

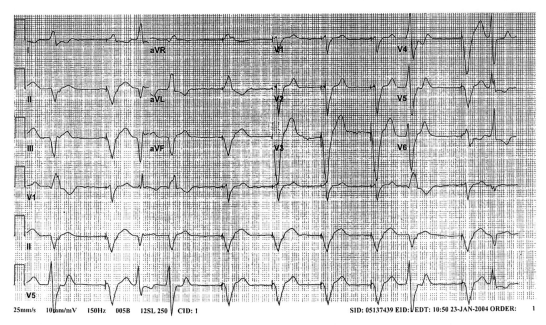

25mm/s   10μm/mV   150Hz   005B   12SL 250   CID: 1   SID: 05137439 EID:UEDT: 10:50 23-JAN-2004 ORDER: 1

Fig. 23-1. Ventricular demand pacemaker (VVI). A single pacemaker spike (marked by arrows) is followed by QRS complex, which is wide and resembles ventricular beat. There are some normal QRS complexes that suppress the pacemaker when they occur faster than the rate set for the pacemaker.

atrial pacing (i.e., biatrial pacing, more than one pacing site in a single atrium, or both features). It can operate in different modes depending on the patient's native rhythm.

INDICATIONS FOR CARDIAC PACEMAKERS AND ANTIARRHYMIC DEVICES

The American College of Cardiology, American Heart Association, and the North American Society for Pacing and Electrophysiology (ACC/AHA/NASPE) have established the indications for implantation of cardiac pacemakers and antiarrhythmia devices. Initial guidelines were established in 1980, and have since been revised and updated to incorporate new information from relevant clinical trials. The most recent guidelines update was published in *Circulation*, October 15, 2002, or can be found on the American College of Cardiology website *http://www.acc.org* under the menu item "clinical statements/guidelines."[5] The guidelines summarize indications for implantation of cardiac devices into three classes of recommendation. (See Table 23-2 for common class I indications.) See class table (p. i) for class and level of evidence definitions. Although a detailed listing of the indications for implantation of cardiac pacemakers and antiarrhythmia devices is beyond the scope of this chapter, listed below are the main section headings within the guidelines, under which class I, II, and III recommendations are listed and described. The sections listed include pacing for acquired AV block in adults, chronic bifascicular and trifascicular block, AV block associated with acute myocardial infarction (AMI), sinus node dysfunction, prevention and termination of tachyarrhythmias by pacing, hypersensitive carotid sinus and neurocardiogenic syncope,

Table 23-2. Common Class I Indications for Permanent Pacing (See Class Table for Class Recomendations and Level of Evidence Definitions): Modified from ACC/AHA/NASPE Guidelines

---

Acquired atrioventricular block
  Class I
Third-degree and advanced second-degree AV block at any anatomic level, associated with any one of the following conditions:
  a. Symptomatic bradycardia (Level of Evidence: C)
  b. Arrhythmias and other medical conditions that require drugs that result in symptomatic bradycardia (Level of Evidence: C)
  c. Documented periods of asystole ≥3.0 s or any escape rate <40 bpm in asymptomatic patients (Level of Evidence: B, C)

Atrioventricular block with acute myocardial infarction
  Class I
1. Persistent second-degree AV block in the His-Purkinje system with bilateral bundle branch block or third-degree AV block within or below the His-Purkinje system after AMI (Level of Evidence: B)
2. Transient advanced (second- or third-degree) infranodal AV block and associated bundle branch block (Level of Evidence: B)
3. Persistent and symptomatic second- or third-degree AV block (Level of Evidence: C)

Chronic bifascicular block and trifasicular block
  Class I
1. Intermittent third-degree AV block (Level of Evidence: B)
2. Type II second-degree AV block (Level of Evidence: B)
3. Alternating bundle branch block (Level of Evidence: C)

Sinus node dysfunction
  Class I
1. Symptomatic bradycardia, including frequent sinus pauses that produce symptoms (Level of Evidence: C)
2. Symptomatic chronotropic incompetence (Level of Evidence: C)

Source: Adapted from Gregoratos G, Abrams J, et al. *Circulation* 2002;106:2145–2161.

children, adolescents, and patients with congenital heart disease, and pacing in specific conditions, namely, HOCM, idiopathic dilated cardiomyopathy, and cardiac transplantation. Also included is a section with indications for ICD therapy.

The decision to initiate treatment with a cardiac device is based primarily on the presence of symptoms in relation to an arrhythmia or conduction abnormality. Sinus node dysfunction and AV block are currently the most frequent indications for pacing. However, indications for pacing therapy are expanding in consideration as a treatment option to improve patients' overall hemodynamic function. Newer and emerging indications for pacing include dilated cardiomyopathy with heart failure, neurocardiogenic syncope, hypertrophic cardiomyopathy, first-degree AV block, and prevention of atrial fibrillation.

Occasionally, clinical situations do not easily fit into these guidelines, and considerable clinical judgment and expertise is necessary to recommend the most beneficial treatment. However, these guidelines are widely endorsed. Emergency temporary pacing is indicated when a conduction abnormality is associated with severe hemodynamic compromise, and permanent pacing may not be indicated or readily available. Indications for temporary pacing are similar to permanent pacing, but also include transient conditions, such as medication effect.

The ICD has been primarily used to reduce mortality from sudden death. Current models of ICDs have antibradycardia and antitachycardia pacing programming, can deliver low-energy cardioversion and high-energy biphasic shocks, and have multiprogrammable capability. Many clinical trials have sought to investigate new applications and benefits of ICDs. For example, the Multicenter Automatic Defibrillator Implantation Trial (MADIT-II) evaluated ICD use in patients with heart failure, and has been included in the implantation guidelines as class IIa (weight of evidence/opinion is in favor of usefulness/efficacy) recommendation for ICD use.

Implantation Complications

Complications related to implantation of cardiac devices are related to the "pocket" housing the pulse generator, the leads or their vascular placement, or the electrode-myocardium interface (see Table 23-3).

Pocket Complications

The pulse generator is usually implanted in a prepectoral or subpectoral location within the anterior chest wall.

Table 23-3. Implantation Complications

Pocket complications
Pocket hematoma
Pocket infection
Wound dehiscence
Migration of generator

Lead placement complications
Pneumothorax
Hemothorax
Venous thrombosis
Lead endocarditis

Electrode-myocardium interface
Fibrosis
Lead migration
Lead penetration

This subcutaneous or submuscular pocket is a common location for potential complication secondary to permanent pacemaker implantation. Dissection of tissue planes during the formation of a suitable pocket can lead to localized bleeding and the development of a *pocket hematoma*. An arterial bleeder, or blood tracking along the pacemaker lead from its insertion into the vein can contribute to the hematoma formation. A hematoma of sufficient size to be palpable requires treatment, usually surgical exploration and correction of the underlying cause. Needle aspiration of a pocket hematoma may not completely evacuate the clot, potentially increasing the risk of infection. Also, the needle may violate the insulation covering the lead causing failure of the lead.

Pacemaker *pocket infection* should be viewed as a potentially life-threatening complication, and occurs in 0.5–5.1% of permanent pacemaker implantations.[6] The results of one metaanalysis suggest that systemic antibiotic prophylaxis at the time of implantation significantly reduces the incidence of serious infection complications from implantation of a permanent pacemaker.[7] The presence of pain, swelling, and redness at the pulse generator site should alert the clinician to the possibility of pocket infection. When pocket infection is present, onset of symptoms less than 6 weeks from the last procedure on the implantation site are more commonly due to *Staphylococcus aureus*, whereas those occurring longer than 6 weeks tend to be due to *Staphylococcus epidermidis*. Aggressive management with antistaphylococcal antibiotic coverage is indicated to prevent the serious sequelae of lead infection or pacemaker lead endocarditis. Definitive management requires complete removal (explantation) of the pacemaker, and subsequent reimplantation at a new site once the infection is eradicated.

Uncommonly, *wound dehiscence* can occur, exposing the pacemaker pocket and its contents to the environment. A pacemaker pocket that is too small, patient manipulation or trauma to the site, or pocket hematoma or infection may result in wound dehiscence. An attempt can be made to save the site by surgical debridement and reapproximation of the wound edges. However, if too far advanced, implantation at a new site on the opposite side may be necessary.

Occasionally, *migration* of the pulse generator away from its original site of implantation can occur. This does not generally cause a malfunction of the pacer. However, the pulse generator can migrate to a location that has less soft tissue protection, and may over time lead to erosion of the skin overlying the unit. Any evidence of infection should be treated and the pacemaker will need to be relocated to a new site.

Lead Placement Complications

Lead placement complications during implantation are related to the chosen method of vascular access. With the subclavian approach, *pneumothorax* is an uncommon complication dependent on operator experience and difficulty accessing the subclavian vein. The pneumothorax may be asymptomatic initially, and recognized only on follow-up chest x-ray. Clinically significant pneumothoraces (>10%) requiring chest tube insertion occur in about 0.8% of cases. The use of the cephalic cutdown technique for lead placement can virtually eliminate this complication. *Hemothorax* can result if the great vessels are traumatized during venous access. Proper technique by avoiding side-to-side movements of the insertion needle while trying to access the vein can minimize injury or laceration to the subclavian vein or artery. Patients with a hemothorax require a chest tube for management.

Venous thrombosis is a recognized complication of lead placement, and may be as high as 40%, although not all instances are clinically significant. Approximately 5% of cases are acutely symptomatic, and an estimated 2 patients per 1000 may develop a superior vena cava syndrome. Symptoms of arm swelling, engorgement of collateral veins on the arm, thorax, or abdomen, and potential swelling of the face with head and neck discomfort can result from thrombosis of the subclavian, cephalic, or superior vena cava. The diagnosis can be confirmed by ultrasound, and treatment initiated with anticoagulation therapy. Immediate lead removal is not usually required, but may be necessary if complications persist.

Infection related to the pacemaker system, including pocket infection, lead infection, and *pacemaker lead endocarditis* are serious and potentially life-threatening complications after pacemaker implantation.[8,9] Typical reported incidences of cardiac device infections vary from 0.13 to 7%. Emergency physicians must maintain a high index of suspicion and consider potential pacemaker lead infection in the appropriate clinical setting. Clinical signs of pocket infection include redness, warmth, pain, swelling, fluctuance, dehiscence, or skin erosion at the pacemaker insertion site. The presence of fever, chills, and systemic evidence of illness should alert the treating physician to the possibility of bacteremia. Clinical investigation should be undertaken to identify the presence of endocarditis, which carries an in-hospital mortality of 7% and overall mortality of 27% in spite of appropriate antibiotic treatment.

Patients with suspected cardiac device infection should have a CBC, ESR, C-reactive protein, blood cultures, and cultures obtained from the pocket site, especially if the site is red, swollen, or painful. Once cultures have been obtained, patients should be started on empiric antibiotics to cover *S. aureus* and *S. epidermidis*).[10] Transesophageal echocardiography is superior to transthoracic echocardiography in identifying vegetations along the pacemaker leads or heart valves and valvular destruction. Patients with identifiable vegetations require removal of the entirety of the cardiac device. Once the infection is eradicated, reimplantation of a pacemaker at a new site can be performed.

Complications at the Electrode-Myocardium Interface

Implantation complications can occur at the electrode-myocardium interface. Leads are attached to the endocardial surface of the heart in one of two ways, passively with tines grabbing onto the surface, or actively by screwing the lead into place. Over time, fibrosis develops at the attachment site, and can lead to problems with pacemaker function. At the time of implantation, the pacemaker is programmed to an optimal threshold voltage to provide optimal sensing and capture of electrical signals. Excessive fibrosis can decrease the ability of the pacemaker to sense a depolarization, and increase the output necessary to capture the myocardium. This can lead to undersensing and *exit block*, or failure of the pacemaker to capture and depolarize the heart muscle. The use of steroid-eluting electrodes has helped to reduce this degree of reaction at the electrode-myocardium interface.

Lead migration can occur, in which the lead tip may loosen and move from its original site of fixture (Fig. 23-2). If intermittent, it can lead to brief periods of failure to sense or capture. The lead may become affixed to another site and result in unintended pacing of the diaphragm (phrenic nerve stimulation), or pectoral muscle stimulation if the lead tip is retracted, such as in Twiddler syndrome. Leads can also *penetrate* into the myocardium, either at the time of implantation or due to migration of the lead tips. Penetration can also lead to undersensing or failure of the pacemaker to capture. Penetration can progress to complete *perforation* of the myocardium into the pericardial space, causing hemopericardium, which can lead to pericardial tamponade.

Twiddler Syndrome

The Twiddler syndrome is an infrequent cause of pacemaker failure.[11–14] It is characterized by physical manipulation and rotation of the pulse generator on its vertical axis within the pacemaker pocket. This results in

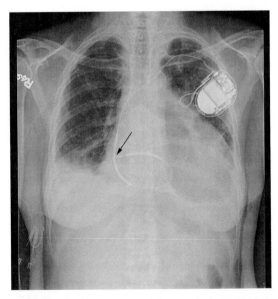

Fig. 23-2. Lead dislodgement. The ventricular lead tip is dislodged and arrow demonstrates the free end of lead. Normal placement of the distal tip should be in right ventricular apex.

winding or twisting of the leads around the pulse generator, thereby effectively shortening the leads, which can cause lead dislodgement and failure to capture. Pacemaker-dependent patients may present with symptoms of decreased cerebral perfusion, such as confusion, weakness, presyncope, or syncope. The patient may present with rhythmic muscular contractions of the chest wall, shoulder, or upper extremity due to stimulation of muscles by the displaced pacing lead. The electrocardiogram may show evidence of loss of capture, but may also show normal pacing function if the dislodgement occurs intermittently. A chest x-ray provides the diagnosis, and may show twisting or coiling of the pacemaker lead(s) around the pulse generator, possible lead fracture, displacement, or migration. Surgical treatment is necessary to correct this pacemaker complication. Twiddler syndrome has also been reported with ICDs.

Pacemaker Syndrome

The pacemaker syndrome most often occurs in patients with a single chamber ventricular pacemaker. This syndrome results from the loss of AV synchrony, which limits atrial assistance to preload and ultimately reduces cardiac output. Contributing factors may include neuro-humeral responses to the decreased cardiac output, retrograde conduction of the paced ventricular stimulus to the atrium (causing atrial contraction prematurely against closed valves or during ventricular systole), the presence of LV disease, or sinus rhythm. Symptoms can be vague and ambiguous, and include shortness of breath, a choking sensation, pulsations felt in the neck or abdomen, palpitations, dizziness, fatigue, anxiety, or confusion. Physical findings may suggest a reduced cardiac output (hypotension, tachycardia, diaphoresis, cool extremities, reduced urinary output) or fluid overload (jugular venous distention, rales, S_3 gallop, cannon A waves). Cannon A waves are prominent waves seen in the neck when the right atrium contracts against a closed tricuspid valve. An electrocardiogram may provide evidence of retrograde conduction during ventricular pacing and reveal a retrograde P wave in a symptomatic patient. It may also show rapid atrial pacing and AV block. The pacemaker syndrome can also occur in patients with a dual-chamber pacemaker. Failure of the atrial circuit can result in the pacemaker functioning solely as a ventricular pacemaker. Inappropriate mode switching from dual chamber to ventricular pacing in a patient in sinus rhythm can also lead to the development of pacemaker syndrome.

Treatment of pacemaker syndrome requires the restoration of adequate AV synchrony. The proper programming adjustments to the pacemaker depend on the cause of asynchrony, and may include altering the AV delay, turning off the activity mode, or reducing the lower limit below the sinus rhythm. Patients with single chamber ventricular pacemakers may also benefit from upgrading to a dual-chamber pacemaker.[15]

Evaluating the Pacemaker Patient

When a pacemaker patient presents to the emergency department, consideration should be given to the pacemaker system as a possible cause of the patient's symptomatology. At a minimum, a thorough history and physical examination, 12-lead electrocardiogram, and chest x-ray will help determine whether a malfunction of the pacemaker system exists.[16]

HISTORY

In order to properly assess the pacer type, the history must include information about the type of pacemaker implanted into the patient. Most patients carry an identification card listing the manufacturer, model number, and program code of the pacemaker. If the pacer manufacturer is known, toll free phone numbers exist to provide technical support. If this information is not available, a chest x-ray will show an identification number on the pulse generator, which can be matched with charts available from pacemaker manufacturers for identification. Other needed information includes the date of implantation, most recent pacemaker check, and contact information for the treating physician or cardiologist. The history of the patient's complaints should pay particular attention to signs and symptoms that may relate directly to the pacemaker system. Since most pacemakers are placed for sinoatrial dysfunction and AV block, this is likely to recur in patients with a malfunctioning pacemaker. Patients may complain of palpitations, weakness, lightheadedness, dizziness, presyncope or syncope, or difficulty breathing. Complaints of muscle twitching or hiccoughs may indicate voluntary muscle or diaphragmatic stimulation from displaced leads. Discomfort and swelling at the implantation site may indicate pocket hematoma or infection.

PHYSICAL EXAMINATION

The physical examination should document careful evaluation of the vital signs, level of alertness, car-

diopulmonary system, and the site of implantation. Evidence of decreased cardiac output, inadequate organ and tissue perfusion, cardiac ischemia, congestive failure, and local or systemic infection may indicate that the pacemaker system may be contributing to the symptoms. Hypotension, bradyarrhythmia, and decreased mentation can signify a return to sinoatrial dysfunction with resultant decreased cardiac output. This could be due to oversensing, lead failure, or generator output failure. Increased jugular venous distention, or the presence of cannon A waves can signify an exacerbation of underlying cardiac disease or heart failure, cardiac tamponade from lead perforation of the myocardium, or loss of AV synchrony (pacemaker syndrome). The presence of a new cardiac murmur may alert the physician to the possibility of pacemaker lead infection and associated endocarditis. Abnormal lung findings may suggest a primary pulmonary etiology; however, in one study, 45% of patients with pacemaker lead infection manifesting more that 6 weeks from the most recent pacemaker procedure had pulmonary symptoms suggestive of bronchitis or pneumonia. Auscultation of a cardiac friction rub may indicate lead penetration or perforation of the myocardium with subsequent development of pericarditis.

ASSESSMENT OF THE PACER'S FUNCTION

Patients should have their cardiac rhythm monitored continuously. However, the rhythm strip alone may not be sufficient to fully evaluate the pacemaker's function. Pacemaker spikes may not be seen in all leads, as bipolar electrode systems typically have smaller spikes than those from unipolar leads, and may not be readily visualized. The rate and rhythm on the 12-lead electrocardiogram should be identified. It is important to look for P waves, QRS complexes, and pacer spikes, and to note their interrelationships when assessing for sensing and capture. Electrocardiogram tracings in patients with a paced rhythm classically reveal a left bundle branch block (LBBB) pattern and left axis deviation, as the ventricular lead is most often located at the apex of the right ventricle (Fig. 23-3). Since cardiac depolarization does not occur through the normal conduction system in the paced patient, the QRS morphology will be widened. Depolarization is also occurring from the apex of the ventricle to the base, and from right to left across the septum, both opposite to the native depolarization process. The resulting tracing is similar to that when the left bundle branch is blocked. If a right bundle branch block pattern is identified in a paced

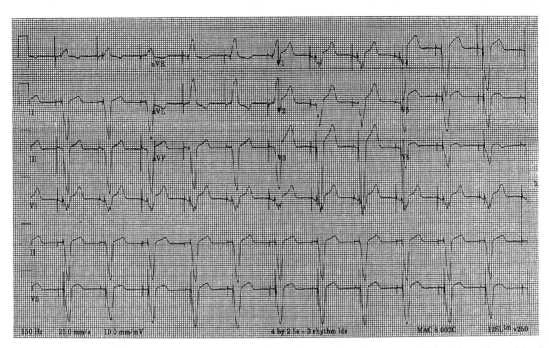

Fig. 23-3. Dual-chamber atrioventricular sequential pacing (DDD). Two pacemaker spikes are seen within each complex, atrial spike and a ventricular spike.

electrocardiogram, it may signify that the ventricular lead has perforated the septum or traversed a septal defect and come to lie in the left ventricle.

APPLICATION OF A MAGNET

Application of a proper magnet over the pulse generator of the pacemaker activates a reed switch, which disables the sensing function of the pacer and places it into an asynchronous or nondemand mode. As long as the magnet is held over the pulse generator, the pacer will continue to fire at a set rate, without regard to the patient's underlying cardiac rhythm. This allows the physician to determine that the pacer is generating output in a situation where no pacer spikes are identified on the initial 12-lead ECG. Pacer spikes will become visible with the application of the magnet as long as there is generator output. Once the magnet is removed, the pacer will revert to its programmed mode and function. It is important not to wave the magnet over the pulse generator, as a changing magnetic field may inhibit the function of older model pacemakers. The magnet may also be helpful to identify when a pacemaker battery is

nearing its end of life. Some pacers may pace at a reduced rate near the end of battery life, or they may begin asynchronous pacing.

CHEST X-RAY

As long as the patient is stable, a PA and lateral chest x-ray can provide evidence to diagnose lead dislodgement, lead fracture, disconnection from the pulse generator, and Twiddler syndrome, as well as to help identify the model of pacemaker when not known by the patient. Comparison with prior radiographs may indicate lead migration, penetration, or perforation.

LABORATORY STUDIES

Appropriate laboratory tests can provide necessary information about the underlying condition of the patient, which can affect pacemaker function. Metabolic derangements attributable to acidosis, hypoxemia, hypokalemia, hypothyroidism, and some antiarrhythmic drugs can alter the pacing threshold necessary for pacing to occur. Correction of these abnormalities can improve pacemaker function.

Interpretation of the Pacemaker Electrocardiogram

It is important for the treating physician to have an organized approach to the interpretation of the pacemaker electrocardiogram. In the emergency department, it is most important to determine that the ventricular lead has appropriate output, sensing, and capture.[4] Knowledge of the mode of pacing and an understanding of basic pacemaker parameters will assist the physician in this process of interpreting the paced electrocardiogram.[17]

The paced electrocardiogram will show pacer spikes, which are narrow perpendicular voltage deflections or "spikes" that are 0.5–2.0 ms in duration and 0.5–3.0 mV high. The presence of spikes indicates output from the pulse generator. The pacer spike is generally larger with unipolar lead pacing systems. In a pacemaker with bipolar leads, it is important to obtain a 12-lead ECG to detect the pacer spikes and not rely on cardiac monitor rhythm strips because the pacer spike can be small and difficult to detect.

Depending on the operating mode of the pacemaker, one or two pacer spikes will be seen with each P-QRS-T complex. The pacer spike will precede the P wave if the atrium is being paced, and it will precede the QRS complex if the ventricle is being paced. If both the atrium and the ventricle are being paced, two pacer spikes 100–250 ms apart will be seen, one preceding the P wave and one preceding the QRS complex. When the atrium is paced, the morphology of the P wave will depend on the location of the pacing electrode within the atrium. The closer it is to the sinoatrial node, the more similar the paced P wave will appear to a sinus P wave. The ventricular lead is most commonly placed within the right ventricle near its apex. As already discussed, this will give the paced QRS complex its classic LBBB pattern.

The lower rate limit interval (LRLI), expressed in milliseconds, corresponds to the lower rate limit of the pacemaker. It represents the longest time period the pacemaker will wait before pacing the ventricle, if no ventricular complexes are sensed. Given that there are 60,000 ms in 1 min, if the lower rate limit is 60 bpm, the LRLI is 1000 ms between beats, whereas a lower rate limit of 75 bpm would have an LRLI of 800 ms. The AV interval is similar to the PR interval on the surface electrocardiogram. The AV interval is the time, typically 100–250 ms duration, between a native sensed or paced P wave and the insertion of a ventricular pacing spike. The ventriculoatrial (VA) interval is the amount of time the pacemaker waits after the last ventricular spike to pace the atrium. The summation of the AV and VA intervals equals the LRLI. The LRLI is calculated by determining the time between two consecutive ventricular pacemaker spikes. The escape interval is the amount of time following a native QRS and the next pacemaker spike. An understanding of these parameters helps to assess the pacemaker for proper output, sensing, and capture.[18] Figure 23-4 is an algorithm designed to guide through the evaluation of the symptomatic patient with suspected malfunction of pacemaker.

Generator Output Failure

Identification and recognition of pacer spikes identifies that the pacemaker pulse generator is providing output. If no pacer spike is seen when one is expected, there may be a failure of the generator to output. There should be a pacer spike between two native QRS complexes occurring at a rate slower than the LRLI. If native beats are occurring at a rate below the LRLI and no pacer spikes are seen, generator output failure is occurring. This output failure may be continuous in the setting of lead fracture, lead disconnection, battery end of life, or some other component failure of the pulse generator. The output failure may be intermittent if oversensing is present.

Oversensing, defined as the failure of delivery of a pacemaker stimulus at the anticipated time according to the programmed escape interval or automatic interval, is a frequent cause of pacemaker pauses. In patients that are pacemaker dependent, oversensing can lead to significant problems with reduced cardiac output and syncope. Oversensing occurs when unintended or unwanted signals are sensed and inhibit the pacemaker from firing, and can occur when the sensitivity of the pacemaker is set too high. There are many sources of unwanted signals that can cause oversensing, such as voltages generated within the pacing system, physiologic voltages of the P wave and T wave, afterpotentials, skeletal muscle myopotentials, interference from distant electromagnetic fields, and possibly concealed ventricular extrasystoles. Whatever the cause, there will be pacemaker pauses, which may be intermittent or continuous. Application of a proper magnet will help diagnose oversensing by eliminating any arrhythmia due to the sensing function when the pacemaker converts to the asynchronous, or fixed-rate mode. It may also help diagnose lead fractures if there are pauses that are exact multiples of the automatic interval during asynchronous pacing. Oversensing can be alleviated by alterations in the programming of the pacemaker, such as reducing the sensitivity, decreasing the generator pulse width, or prolonging the refractory period after the pulse stimulus.[19]

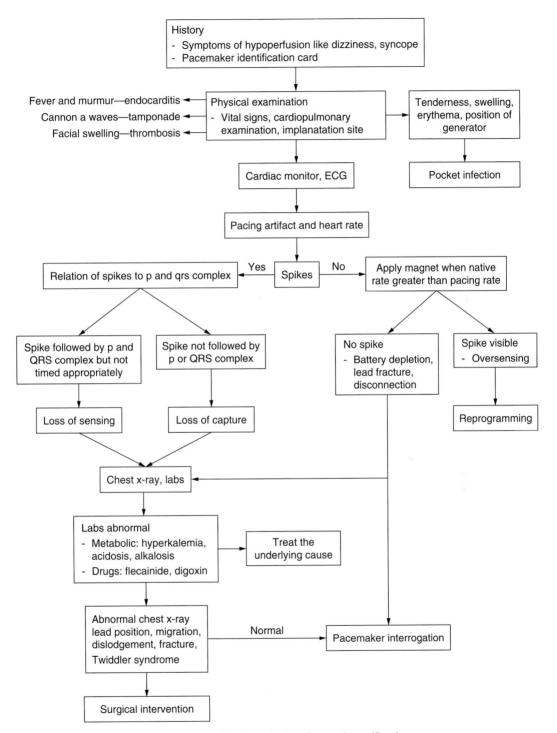

Fig. 23-4. Algorithm for evaluation of pacemaker malfunction.

Failure to Sense

Failure to sense or undersensing occurs when an electric signal is not recognized or sensed, and a pacing spike occurs earlier than would be expected (Fig. 23-5). In this instance, a pacer spike is preceded by a native QRS at an interval less than the LRLI. It creates a situation where there is competition between the patient's native rhythm and the pacemaker, and rarely causes an emergent problem. However, excessive stimulation in the atrium can lead to atrial fibrillation, and in injured (ischemic) ventricular myocardium, could cause ventricular tachycardia or fibrillation. Undersensing can occur as a result of scar tissue formation at the electrode-myocardium interface and inability to properly conduct the electrical signal to the lead tip. Not all undersensing is a true malfunction of the pacemaker, and may represent signals that are occurring during the pacemaker's refractory period or blanking period. The blanking period is an interval initiated by the delivery of an output pulse during which the sensing amplifier of the pulse generator is temporarily disabled. In dual-chamber pulse generators, the blanking period is intended to prevent the inappropriate detection of signals from the opposite chamber (crosstalk).

Failure to Capture

Failure to capture occurs when the pacemaker output does not depolarize the myocardium and produce a contraction. A pacing spike will be seen on the electrocardiogram, but there will not be any evidence of a depolarization (no P wave or QRS complex). For pacemaker-dependent patients, this can be a significant problem. This can be caused by scar tissue formation at the electrode-myocardium interface necessitating an increase in voltage to depolarize the tissue. Lead dislodgement is the most common reason for failure to capture. With active fixation lead tips, this is less of a complication than with passive lead fixation. Twiddler syndrome can be an uncommon cause of failure to capture. True fusion beats between a paced beat and a native beat verify evidence of capture. However, pseudofusion beats, where the pacing stimulus overlies the native complex and deforms it, but is not a true hybrid of the paced and native complexes, are evidence of failure to capture.

Individual pacemakers can operate in more that one mode. As an example, the DDD pacemaker (Fig. 23-3) may operate in the DVI, VDD, AAI, or VVI mode, even though it may be programmed to the DDD mode. For example, in the VDD mode (atrial synchronous pacer and atrial sensing, ventricular inhibited pacemaker [ASVIP]),

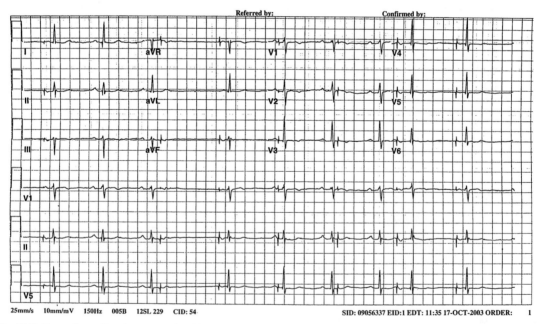

Fig. 23-5. Pacemaker malfunction-non-sensing. The arrows point to the spike, which follows normal QRS complex. The pacemaker has failed to sense the preceding native complexes.

the pacer functions by sensing the atrium and pacing the ventricle. It is inhibited by a ventricular depolarization, whether from a conducted P wave or a premature ventricular contraction. In the AAI mode, this pacer functions as the typical "atrial demand" pacemaker, which is inhibited whenever the patient's native P wave occurs.

In a patient with an unknown pacemaker type, careful scrutiny of the 12-lead electrocardiogram can provide clues to its mode of operation. The first step is to note the number of spikes on the electrocardiogram and their relationship to P waves and QRS complexes. If two consecutive pacer spikes are separated by 100–250 ms, the pacemaker is either a DVI or DDD pacemaker. The pacemaker is operating in the DVI (AV sequential) mode if there are always two spikes separated by approximately 200 ms, and both spikes show capture. The DVI mode of function paces both the atrium and ventricle, as required in a patient with both sinoatrial dysfunction and AV block; however, only the ventricle is sensed. The stimulus for pacing the ventricle is inhibited if a conducted atrial beat leads to a spontaneous ventricular depolarization or if there is a premature ventricular contraction. If somewhere else on the same tracing, there is only one spike preceded by a native P wave within 120–275 ms, the pacemaker is operating in the VDD mode. In this situation, the ventricle is paced if the programmed AV interval is exceeded. Any tracing that shows both DVI and VDD modes of pacing, must be a DDD pacemaker, because at various times, both the atrium and the ventricle are paced and sensed.

It is more of a challenge to determine the mode of pacing in a tracing when only one pacing spike is seen on the tracing. In this situation, it is necessary to determine the relationship amongst the P waves, pacing spike, and QRS complexes. If a native P wave precedes the spike by 120–275 ms, and either a paced QRS or nothing (noncapture) immediately follows the spike, and the spike-spike interval is relatively rapid (80–90/min), the pacer is likely operating in the VDD mode. This shows that the native atrial depolarization is sensed and followed by an attempt to pace the ventricle after the programmed AV interval. If there is no other area on the tracing showing a captured P wave following a spike, it is a VDD pacemaker. If there is evidence of captured P wave following a spike, it is a DDD pacemaker, because both the atrium and ventricle are being sensed and paced.

To identify the AAI mode, it is important to look for native P waves, and determine the interval to the next pacemaker spike. This interval will be relatively constant (within a few milliseconds), indicating a relationship between the native P waves and the pacer spike. There

will either be a paced P wave or nothing (noncapture) following the pacer spike. If the captured P wave conducts to the ventricles, a native QRS will follow the paced P wave by approximately 40 ms. If AV block is present, there will not be any QRS complex following the paced P waves. The native QRS complexes may or may not be related to the pacing spikes. If the PR interval is constant and there is 1:1 conduction, both the P waves and the QRS complexes will be related to the pacing spikes. If there is AV block or a varying PR interval, there will be a constant interval between the native P waves and the spikes, but not between the QRS complexes and the spikes.

Diagnosing Acute Myocardial Infarction in a Paced Electrocardiogram

Recognition of an AMI in a paced electrocardiogram is a significant challenge.[20] Uncomplicated ventricular pacing yields secondary repolarization changes that manifest as T waves of opposing polarity to that of the predominant QRS deflection. When pacing from the right ventricular apex, most leads on a surface 12-lead electrocardiogram show a predominantly negative deflection QRS complex followed by J point elevation of the ST segment and positive deflection T waves, which may be similar to those elicited by an injury pattern consistent with an AMI. Investigators from the GUSTO-I trial examined the value of the initial 12-lead electrocardiogram to diagnose AMI in ventricular-paced patients.[20] Admission 12-lead ECGs for a subset of paced patients with proven AMI were compared to a randomly selected external control group of right ventricular-paced patients with angiographically confirmed stable coronary disease. The following three criteria were identified to have acceptable specificity for the diagnosis of AMI. The only statistically significant finding was ST-segment elevation greater than or equal to 5 mm in leads with predominantly negative (discordant) QRS complexes. This finding yielded 53% sensitivity and 88% specificity for the diagnosis of AMI, with a P value of 0.025. Two other criteria had acceptable specificity to diagnose of AMI. ST-segment elevation greater than or equal to 1 mm in any lead with a predominantly positive (concordant) QRS complex (94% specificity) and ST-segment depression greater than or equal to 1 mm in leads V_1, V_2, or V_3 (82% specificity). In addition, comparison with a previous electrocardiogram may show superimposed ischemic changes alerting the physician to the diagnosis of AMI. It should be recognized that a paced ECG that does not meet these criteria does not exclude the presence of an AMI. The interpretation of the ECG should be used within the context of the clinical situation and in conjunction with other diagnostic criteria. These criteria, like those for diagnosing AMI with a LBBB are unlikely to be generalisable to unselected nonstudy patients. The ability to more rapidly diagnose AMI in the paced patient permits appropriate interventions and treatment to be offered in a timely manner.

Electromagnetic Interference

It is important to consider the effect of electromagnetic interference (EMI) from medical and environmental sources on cardiac devices.[21] The risk of EMI depends on the distance from the potential source of EMI, the oscillation frequency and field strength of the disturbing electromagnetic field, and technical specifications of the device, such as the programmed sensitivity or lead configuration (unipolar vs. bipolar). In pacemakers, EMI can result in oversensing, generation of tachyarrhythmias, and output failure due to detection of unwanted electromagnetic disturbances. In ICDs, EMI may lead to false arrhythmia detection, and may cause inappropriate antitachycardia pacing or internal shock delivery.

In the medical setting, exposure to various electromagnetic fields with magnetic resonance imaging (MRI) can effect device function. The most severe potential complication is "runaway" pacing at extremely high ventricular rates synchronized to the radiofrequency pulses during actual imaging. Theoretically, local heating of long conductive wires could cause thermal damage to adjacent myocardial tissue. In addition, activation of the reed switch in pacemakers will cause asynchronous pacing, and suspension of tachyarrhythmia detection can occur in ICDs.

Performing an MRI in a pacemaker patient can be concerning. Although there is little risk of magnetic forces and torque effecting pacemakers, these forces may affect ICDs. The metallic parts of pacemaker leads are composed of an alloy that is not ferromagnetic, and therefore should not become dislodged or move in response to a magnetic field. Despite this reassurance, the presence of a pacemaker is still a primary contraindication for MRI, with consideration of alternative imaging techniques. If MRI is deemed absolutely necessary, patients not dependent on the pacemaker can be programmed to a subthreshold output, or to the OOO mode. Pacemaker-dependent patients should be programmed to the asynchronous mode.

Electrosurgical techniques vary in the potential for EMI. In general, techniques that produce a current being passed through tissue have the potential to interact with implanted cardiac devices. The common electrosurgical modalities of electrocoagulation and electrocutting deliver current in a monopolar mode and involve passing current through tissue. Current begins at the active electrode on the instrument, travels through the body, and returns to the electrosurgical generator through a dispersing grounding pad. A bipolar configuration reduces potential for EMI because current flow is localized across the two poles of an instrument and doesn't pass far from the surgical site.

Radiation oncology patients undergoing radiation therapy are at risk for damage due to cumulative radiation exposure to the pulse generator. Ionizing therapeutic radiation acts on the silicone and silicone oxide insulators within the semiconductor components of the pulse generator. This can lead to random damage or complete failure to circuit components, or create electrical shorts that can result in premature battery depletion. Diagnostic radiology procedures pose no immediate or cumulative effects on pulse generators.

Cellular telephones have the potential to cause cardiac device malfunction, although EMI is unlikely to be significant at a distance of greater than 2 m. However, it is still recommended that mobile phones not be used in any areas where electronic devices are used in patient care.[22,23] Similarly, airport metal detectors are unlikely to produce clinically relevant interactions with pacemakers or ICDs due to their brief exposure time.[24]

Drug Effect on Pacemakers

Certain antiarrhythmic agents, such as beta-blockers, class 1a antidysrhythmics, and flecanide can alter the threshold potential at the tissue level. The tendency is to elevate the threshold, making it more difficult to depolarize the tissues. This is unlikely to be of clinical importance at therapeutic drug levels. However, flecanide-like drugs can cause pacemaker malfunction at therapeutic concentrations, most commonly failure to capture and failure to sense. Treatment may be aimed at lowering the threshold potential with isoproterenol, temporary external pacing, or sodium loading with either sodium bicarbonate or hypertonic saline for sodium channel blocking class 1a agents.

Trauma

Trauma remains an uncommon, but potentially life-threatening cause, of pacemaker complications or malfunction. Pacemaker-dependent patients with abrupt cessation of pacing may sustain cardiac arrest due to asystole, syncope due to a reduced cardiac output, or mental obtundation. Emergency intervention first with the application of transcutaneous pacing, and if unsuccessful at capture, the insertion of a transvenous pacemaker, may be necessary to stabilize the patient. Most commonly, dislodgement of a lead or lead fracture can occur secondary to a traumatic incident. Lead dislodgement and fracture can cause failure to sense and capture. A chest x-ray should provide evidence to support this diagnosis. Significant direct trauma to the chest overlying the pulse generator can rarely cause failure of the pulse generator or output failure, which can also lead to dire clinical circumstances. It is important for the emergency physician to methodically assess the function of the pacemaker system as a potential cause of these clinical findings, along with potential injuries sustained during the traumatic event. Trauma secondary to a shoulder harness in motor vehicle collisions or direct trauma by an object overlying the pulse generator can cause the development of a pocket hematoma, which may require surgical management to prevent the possibility of developing infection or abscess.

Cardiac Arrest and Defibrillation

Implementation of Advanced Cardiac Life Support protocols is not contraindicated in pacemaker patients. Cardiac arrhythmias such as ventricular fibrillation and tachycardia can cause malfunction of the pacemaker. Restoration of the patient's hemodynamic status is the top priority. Direct current cardioversion and defibrillation can cause damage to an implanted cardiac device depending on the amount of energy applied, the distance from the paddles or pads to the pulse generator, and characteristics of the device and leads. The minimum energy likely to be successful should be delivered to the patient. Defibrillation with a biphasic waveform, if available, is most energy efficient. The paddles or pads should be placed in the anterior-posterior location whenever possible, or insure a distance of 10 cm between the paddles or pads from the pulse generator in the standard infraclavicular-apical method. External defibrillation is a well-known cause of failure to capture, likely due to localized tissue changes at the electrode-myocardium interface. This is usually temporary, but may require replacement of a lead if persistent. All devices require postintervention interrogation and testing for proper function.

Evolving Indications for Pacemaker Therapy

New and evolving indications for pacemaker therapy have been investigated in numerous clinical trials over recent years. Patients with these clinical conditions may benefit from pacemaker therapy beyond simple rate control.

Congestive Heart Failure and Dilated Cardiomyopathy

Certain patients with congestive heart failure (CHF) and dilated cardiomyopathy may benefit from biventricular pacing, a mode of therapy known as resynchronization therapy. Patients with severe LV dysfunction and left-sided intraventricular conduction delay (LBBB pattern) exhibit a dyssynchronous pattern of LV activation. Clinical consequences of ventricular asynchrony include abnormal interventricular septal wall motion, reduction in diastolic filling times, and worsening of mitral regurgitation. Biventricular pacing induces a more coordinated and efficient LV contraction and reduces the degree of electromechanical asynchrony. The 2002 pacing implantation guidelines recommend biventricular pacing as a class IIa indication (weight of evidence/opinion is in favor of usefulness/ efficacy) for patients with medically refractory symptomatic NYHA class III or IV dilated or ischemic cardiomyopathy, QRS $\geq$130 ms, and an ejection fraction $\leq$35%. Benefits of resynchronization therapy include improved systolic blood pressure, pulse pressure, and LV ejection fraction.[25] Additionally, biventricular pacing reduces LV volume and end-diastolic diameter, mitral regurgitation, wedge pressure, and the degree of neurohumoral stimulation.[26,27]

Atrial Fibrillation

Pacemaker therapy may prevent atrial fibrillation in highrisk patients; however, the antiarrhythmic mechanism is not well understood. The Mode Selection Trial (MOST) and Canadian Trial of Physiologic Pacing (CTOPP) have shown a reduction in atrial fibrillation in patients with dualchamber pacers (physiologic pacing) versus ventricular pacemakers. An additional benefit may include a reduction in the need for antithrombotic therapy. Besides dualchamber pacing, dual-site right atrial pacing (high right atrium and coronary sinus ostium) and unconventional single site atrial pacing are also being investigated.

Neurocardiogenic Syncope

Because of the relatively benign course of the disease, and varying degrees of vasodilatation in addition to bradycardia that play a role in neurocardiogenic syncope, the value of pacemaker therapy to prevent syncope has been questioned. The pacemaker implantation guidelines recommend pacing carefully prescribed on the basis of tilt table testing as a class IIa indication. The role of pacemaker therapy for syncope will likely be limited to highly selected patients, such as those with frequent episodes of syncope, in the setting of poor quality-of-life, risk of injury, occupational hazard, and episodes with the absence of warning.[28]

Hypertrophic Obstructive Cardiomyopathy

The benefits of pacemaker therapy for patients with HOCM are unproven, and there may be a significant placebo effect of pacemaker therapy in this clinical condition. Although pacing appears to reduce the LV outflow gradient, it is unclear that this translates directly into clinical improvement. The pacemaker implantation guidelines list medically refractory symptomatic HOCM with significant resting (≥ 30 mmHg) or provoked (≥ 50 mmHg) LV outflow obstruction as a class IIb (usefulness/efficacy is less well established by evidence/opinion) recommendation. At this time, pacing for HOCM should be considered only in medication-refractory patients (especially the elderly) in whom surgical treatment with myomectomy is not feasible.

First-Degree AV Block

Prolongation of the PR interval results in suboptimal timing of atrial and ventricular systole. Synchrony of atrial and ventricular contractions optimizes cardiac output. A very prolonged PR interval disrupts AV synchrony, and can lead to a decrease or loss of the atrial kick, and produce symptoms similar to paced patients with pacemaker syndrome. This occurs when the atria try to contract while the tricuspid and mitral valves are closed and the ventricles are in systole. Pacemaker therapy attempts to restore a more physiologic AV interval to a range usually between 120 and 200 ms. In patients with a normal LV function, a dual-chamber pacemaker may suffice, while patients with poor LV function should be considered for biventricular pacing. The pacemaker implantation guidelines classify first- (or second-) degree AV block with symptoms similar to pacemaker syndrome as a class IIa recommendation.

Clinical Trials with Pacemakers

The specific modality of cardiac pacing that will benefit a patient will depend on the indication for pacing, whether to provide support for chronotropic insufficiency, or reduce cardiac asynchrony. As pacemaker systems have evolved with significant advances in technology, newer applications for pacemaker therapy have been investigated. Studies have been designed to evaluate the effects of pacing mode choice in patients with bradycardia (CTOPP, PASE), symptomatic sinus node dysfunction (MOST), and

AV block (UKPACE). Other areas of clinical investigation include potential benefits of pacemaker therapy in patients with atrial fibrillation, CHF, hypertrophic and dilated cardiomyopathy, syncope, and even sleep apnea syndrome.

In patients with bradycardia, the CTOPP study was a randomized-controlled trial of 2568 patients with a mean age of 73 years randomized to either ventricular pacing or physiologic pacing (atrial or dual chamber) at enrollment.[29] The primary endpoint was stroke or death due to cardiovascular causes, and secondary endpoints were overall mortality, development of atrial fibrillation, and hospitalization for heart failure. The perioperative complication rate was significantly higher with physiologic pacing (9.0% vs. 3.8%), and there was no difference in the primary endpoints of stroke or cardiovascular death rate (ventricular: 5.5% vs. physiologic: 4.9%). The annual rate of atrial fibrillation was significantly reduced in the physiologic pacing group (ventricular: 6.6% vs. physiologic: 5.3%, $P = 0.05$). In addition, the annual rate of progression of chronic atrial fibrillation was reduced in the physiologic pacing group (2.8% vs. 3.8% ventricular group, $P = 0.016$). The Pacemaker Selection in the Elderly (PASE) trial was a single blind randomized-controlled comparison of 407 patients with a mean age of 76 years, randomized to either the VVIR or DDDR pacing mode at enrollment. The primary endpoint was the health-related quality of life; the secondary endpoints were death from all causes, first nonfatal stroke or death, first hospitalization for heart failure, development of atrial fibrillation, or development of pacemaker syndrome. The results showed that the quality of life improved with both pacing modes when compared to baseline, but no difference was noted in quality of life between the two pacing modes. No difference was detected between the two pacing modes in any of the secondary outcomes. However, a 26% crossover rate from the VVIR to the DDDR mode was observed due to the development of pacemaker syndrome.

The MOST clinical trial evaluated pacing mode choice in patients with symptomatic sinus node dysfunction.[30] This was a single blind randomized trial of 2010 patients with a mean age of 74 years who received dual-chamber pacers and were randomized to the DDD or VVI pacing modes. The primary endpoint was death and nonfatal stroke, and multiple secondary endpoints included chronic atrial fibrillation and quality of life. There was no difference in the combined primary endpoint of death and nonfatal stroke (DDD: 21.5% vs. VVI: 23.0%, $P = 0.48$). However, there was a significant reduction in chronic atrial fibrillation in the dual-chamber pacing group (DDD: 15.2% vs. VVI: 26.7%, $P = <0.001$). The overall complication rate for pacemaker implantation was 4.8% at 30 days.

The United Kingdom Pacing and Cardiovascular Events (UKPACE) trial evaluated the effect of pacing mode choice in elderly patients with AV block.[31] This was a randomized-controlled trial of 2021 patients with a mean age of 80 years, who were randomized to VVI, VVIR, or DDDR pacing modes. The primary endpoint was all-cause mortality, and secondary endpoints were stroke, quality of life, and exercise tolerance. There was no difference in mortality among the pacing modes. However, there was an increase in stroke and transient ischemic attack (TIA) associated with dual-chamber pacing mode when compared with ventricular pacing.

Clinical trials evaluating the use of pacemaker therapy in patients with atrial fibrillation include Atrial Dynamic Overdrive Pacing Trial (ADOPT) and Effect of Atrial Pacing Therapies on Atrial Tachyarrhythmia Burden and Frequency (ATTEST). The ADOPT study evaluated the effects of atrial overdrive pacing algorithms in patients with paroxysmal atrial fibrillation.[32] This was a randomized-controlled trial of 319 patients with a mean age of 71 years, all of whom received pacemakers with atrial pacing capability including overdrive pacing, who were then randomized to having specialized atrial pacing algorithms turned on or off. Primary endpoints were symptomatic atrial fibrillation burden and adverse events, and secondary endpoints were the number of symptomatic atrial fibrillation episodes, hospitalizations, cardioversions, and quality of life. There was a significant reduction in atrial fibrillation burden at 1, 3, and 6 months in the "on" group, but no difference between the two groups in the number of atrial fibrillation episodes or hospitalizations. The ATTEST trial sought to evaluate the effectiveness of an atrial therapy device using preventative and antitachycardia pacing in patients with symptomatic atrial fibrillation. Patients were randomized to having atrial prevention or termination of the arrhythmia by any of three algorithms either turned on or off. In this study, there were no significant differences in either the frequency, burden, or symptomatic burden of atrial tachycardia or atrial fibrillation.

Cardiac resynchronization therapy (CRT), or biventricular pacing has emerged as a new form of pacemaker therapy in heart failure patients with intraventricular conduction delays or ventricular asynchrony. The Multicenter Insync Randomized Clinical Evaluation (MIRACLE) trial compared the effect of CRT versus no CRT on quality of life and functional capacity in patients with chronic heart failure and ventricular dysynchrony. There were 266 NYHA class III or IV patients randomized to CRT or no CRT. CRT was found to be safe, well tolerated, and improved quality of life, functional NYHA class, and exercise capacity. In addition, there was echocardio-graphic evidence of a significant decrease in the left ventricular end-diastolic diameter (LVEDD) and an increase in the left ventricular ejection fraction (LVEF).[33–35] The Pacing Therapies for Congestive Heart Failure (PATH-CHF) trial evaluated LV versus biventricular pacing as the best method for CRT for heart failure patients in a single blind randomized crossover trial.[36,37] Overall, clinical effects of optimal univentricular pacing and biventricular pacing were similar, and were associated with significant improvements in oxygen uptake, 6-min walk distance, quality of life, and NYHA functional class when compared to baseline.[26]

Automatic Implantable Cardioverter-Defibrillators

The introduction of the automatic ICD into clinical practice in the 1980s has had a significant impact on the treatment of patients at high risk for sudden cardiac death. ICDs are multiprogrammable devices capable of delivering high-energy defibrillation shocks, antitachycardia pacing, low-energy (cardioversion) shocks for ventricular tachycardia, and antibradycardia pacing. The devices can be interrogated and reprogrammed noninvasively. The ICD generator contains the electronic circuitry, power source, and memory capability. Battery life varies from 5 to 9 years, depending mainly on the frequency of shock delivery. Advances in technology have reduced the size of the ICD generator such that ICDs leads can be implanted transvenously via the subclavian or cephalic route in the same manner as pacemakers, with the generator in a subcutaneous or submuscular pocket of the anterior chest wall. Thus, complications due to implantation are similar to those for pacemakers, and are managed similarly, and are detailed above. Pocket complications include hematoma, infection, dehiscence, erosion, and migration. Lead complications include pneumothorax, hemothorax, infection, and venous thrombosis.

A right ventricular lead is used for sensing and pacing. The lead also contains a coil that delivers a shock between the coil and the case of the generator, or to a second coil in the lead located in the vicinity of the superior vena cava. Two coils in the same lead help improve defibrillation efficiency. Dual-chamber ICDs have a second lead placed in the right atrium, which allows for better discrimination between ventricular and supraventricular tachyarrhythmias. Once implantation is completed, the unit is tested intraoperatively to determine proper pacing and sensing thresholds, and reliable detection and termination of ventricular fibrillation. Maximal output for an ICD can be between 26 and 38 J according to the model. ICDs recognize ventricular tachyarrhythmias based on programmable rate and duration criteria. Other criteria, such as "sudden onset" help discriminate between sinus tachycardia and ventricular tachycardia, while "rate stability" criteria are useful to distinguish rapid atrial fibrillation from ventricular tachycardia.

Identification cards similar to that for a pacemaker provides information regarding the manufacturer, generator model, lead system, therapy options, and a 24-hour emergency contact telephone number. If the card is unavailable, a chest x-ray will reveal a radiopaque marker identifying the unit. If emergency deactivation of the ICD is necessary, a magnet placed on top of all ICD models will temporarily disable tachyarrhythmia intervention, and will have no effect on pacing function.

Electromagnetic radiation can also interfere with ICD function, leading to inhibition of antibradycardia pacing, inadvertent delivery of shocks or antitachycardia pacing, reversion to temporary asynchronous pacing, resetting of programmed parameters, and damage to the generator or tissues interfacing with the leads. Electrocautery procedures can be performed as long as the tachyarrhythmia detection is deactivated prior to the procedure and reestablished immediately following the procedure. An ICD remains a strong contraindication for MRI studies.

ICDs can malfunction in much the same way as pacers. Shortly after implantation, failure to capture is usually due to lead dislodgement or perforation. "Make-break" signals caused by lead fracture, or faulty connections, can cause pacing inhibition accompanied by spurious shocks. In symptomatic patients, with pacing pauses or bradycardia, temporary pacing may be necessary. However, the ICD should be deactivated first to prevent double or triple counting of pacing artifacts and QRS complexes, which can trigger spurious shocks. Patients can present with sustained VT or VF without ICD intervention. Failure of arrhythmia detection can be due to an intrinsic rate below the programmed cutoff, or exhaustion of programmed therapies. The ICD patient in cardiac arrest should receive standard cardiopulmonary resuscitation. Paddle position should be anterior-posterior when possible.

Multiple ICD shocks in a short period of time (≥ 3 discharges in ≤ 24 hours) constitute a medical emergency. They may result from recurrent ventricular arrhythmias (*ventricular electrical storm*), supraventricular arrhythmias, or ICD system malfunctions. Multiple shocks can result in substantial battery depletion. It is necessary to determine the cause of multiple shocks, and consultation with a cardiac electrophysiologist is usually necessary for definitive therapy. The ICD may be functioning appropriately to try to terminate recurrent ventricular tachyarrhythmias. Antiarrhythmic drugs may increase defibrillation energy requirements.

Patients experiencing multiple shocks should be taken care of in a setting where advanced cardiac resuscitation is immediately available, and they may require sedation with a benzodiazepine. A 12-lead electrocardiogram should be obtained for clues to other causes, such as electrolyte abnormality, drug toxicity, or myocardial ischemia. Intravenous antiarrhythmic drugs may be necessary to treat arrhythmias. Shocks triggered by atrial tachyarrhythmias require AV-nodal blockade, with calcium-channel blockers and beta-blockers.

ICD system infection closely parallels that with pacers, with *S. aureus* more common with infections of less than 6 weeks duration, and *S. epidermidis* for chronic infections greater than 6 weeks duration.[38] In general, the entire ICD system will need to be removed.

Clinical Trials Involving ICDs

Automatic ICDs were first introduced for the treatment of sudden cardiac death and have proven survival benefit in at-risk patients. The recurrence rate of sudden cardiac death has decreased from approximately 30% to 1–2% per year in high-risk sudden cardiac death survivors.[39] Clinical trials with ICD devices began in the 1990s. Six prospective randomized clinical trials supporting the benefit of ICD in primary (prevention of a first life-threatening arrhythmia) and secondary (prevention of life-threatening arrhythmia in survivors of cardiac arrest) prevention of sudden cardiac death are CASH, AVID, and CIDS (primary prevention), and MADIT-I, MADIT-II, and MUSTT (secondary prevention). These trials have shown a relative risk reduction of 31–55% in the primary prevention trials, and 20–41% relative risk reduction in total mortality with ICD therapy in secondary prevention.

The Cardiac Arrest Survival in Hamburg (CASH) trial was a prospective, multicenter, randomized study that assigned 288 survivors of cardiac arrest due to documented ventricular arrhythmias to an ICD or antiarrhythmic drugs (amiodarone, metoprolol, or propafenone). The primary endpoint was all-cause mortality, while sudden death and recurrence of cardiac arrest were secondary endpoints. The propafenone group was discontinued early due to an increased mortality rate. After a mean follow-up of 57 months, there was a nonsignificant 23% relative reduction in all-cause mortality in patients receiving an ICD compared to those treated with amiodarone or metoprolol (36.4% vs. 44.4%, $P = 0.08$).[40]

The Canadian Implantable Defibrillator Study (CIDS), another prospective, multicenter, randomized trial assigned 659 patients resuscitated from VT, VF, or unmonitored syncope deemed to be secondary to arrhythmia, to amiodarone, or an ICD. The primary endpoint was all-cause mortality, and the secondary endpoint was arrhythmic death. After a 5-year follow-up, the total mortality with the ICD was not significantly reduced compared to amiodarone (8.3% vs. 10.2% per year, P = 0.142), and there was a nonsignificant reduction in arrhythmic death (3% vs. 4.5% per year, P = 0.094). A 20% relative risk reduction occurred in all-cause mortality and a 33% reduction occurred in arrhythmic mortality with ICD therapy compared with amiodarone; this reduction did not reach statistical significance. Further analysis showed patients in the highest risk quartile, who had ≥2 risk factors (age ≥70, LVEF ≤35%, and NYHA class III or IV), had a significant reduction of death from the ICD compared to amiodarone (14.4% vs. 30%).[41]

The Antiarrhythmic Drug Versus Defibrillator (AVID) trial enrolled 1016 patients who were resuscitated from near-fatal VF, or who had undergone cardioversion from sustained VT and had either syncope or other serious cardiac symptoms and an LVEF ≤40%. The unadjusted survival for the ICD versus drug groups were 89% versus 82% at 1 year, 82% versus 75% at 2 years, and 75% versus 65% at 3 years (P <0.02).[42]

The MADIT-I trial, a prospective, multicenter, randomized trial enrolled 196 patients with a prior MI, unsustained VT, and LV dysfunction (LVEF <35%), who underwent electrophysiologic study risk stratification, and randomly assigned to amiodarone or an ICD. The primary endpoint was death from any cause, and the secondary endpoint was cardiac death. The Safety & Monitoring Committee terminated the study prematurely because of the survival benefit noted with the ICD compared to conventional therapy. After 27-month follow-up, there were significant reductions in the incidence of overall mortality with a hazard ratio for overall mortality, 0.46 (95% confidence interval, 0.26–0.82; P = 0.009). The conclusion was that in patients with a prior MI, asymptomatic unsustained VT, an LVEF ≤35%, and inducible VT or VF that are not suppressible during electrophysiologic studies, a prophylactic ICD reduces mortality rates.[43]

The MADIT-II trial prospectively randomized 1232 patients with AMI more than 30 days prior to enrollment (and more than 3 months if bypass surgery was performed) and LV dysfunction (LVEF ≤30%) without prior EPS risk stratification to ICD plus conventional medical therapy versus conventional medical therapy alone. The primary endpoint was death from any cause,

and there were multiple secondary endpoints. The study was prematurely terminated after an average follow-up of 20 months because the ICD significantly reduced all-cause mortality by 30%; 14.2% versus 19.8% for conventional therapy, hazard ratio 0.65 (95% confidence interval 0.51–0.93). They concluded that in patients with a prior MI and advanced LV dysfunction, prophylactic ICD therapy improves survival when compared to conventional therapy alone.[44,45]

The Multicenter UnSustained Tachycardia Trial (MUSTT) investigated 704 patients to see if electrophysiologically guided antiarrhythmic therapy with an ICD in patients with coronary artery disease, a LVEF of less than 40%, and asymptomatic, unsustained VT, would reduce the risk of sudden death over similar patients without antiarrhythmic therapy. The primary endpoint was cardiac arrest or death from arrhythmia. They concluded that electrophysiologically guided antiarrhythmic therapy with implantable defibrillators, but not with antiarrhythmic drugs, reduces the risk of sudden death in high-risk patients with coronary disease (25% with antiarrhythmic therapy vs. 32% without antiarrhythmic therapy), relative risk, 0.73 (95% confidence interval, 0.53–0.99), representing a reduction in risk of 27%.[46]

CONCLUSION

The use of pacemakers and AICDs will only expand in the United States due to the aging of the populations and the expanding indications for these devices. The emergency physician must be conversant with the indications, complications, and potential malfunctions of pacemakers and AICDs. The algorithm (Fig. 23-4) is designed to walk the emergency physician through the process of evaluating a patient in the ED with symptoms possibly caused by malfunctions or complications due to a permanent pacemaker. A firm understanding of the indications and operations of pacemakers, and the systematic assessment of potential malfunctions raises the likelihood of a successful outcome.

REFERENCES

1. Maisel WH, Sweeney MO, Stevenson WG, et al. Recalls and safety alerts involving pacemakers and implantable cardioverter-defibrillator generators. *JAMA* 2001;286:793–799.
2. Cardall TY, Chan TC, Brady WJ, et al. Permanent cardiac pacemakers: Issues relevant to the emergency physician, part I. *J Emerg Med* 1999;17:479–489.
3. Cardall TY, Brady WJ, Chan TC, et al. Permanent cardiac pacemakers: Issues relevant to the emergency physician, part II, *J Emerg Med* 1999;17:697–709.

4. Harper RJ, Brady WJ, Perron AD, et al. The paced electrocardiogram: Issues for the emergency physician. *Am J Emerg Med* 2001;19:551–560.

5. Gregoratos G, Abrams J, Epstein AE, et al. ACC/AHA/NASPE 2002 guideline update for implantation of cardiac pacemakers and antiarrhythmia devices: Summary article: A report of the American College of Cardiology/American Heart Association Task Force on Practice Guidelines (ACC/AHA/NASPE Committee to Update the 1998 Pacemaker Guidelines). *Circulation* 2002;106:2145–2161.

6. Jara FM, Toledo-Pereyra L, Lewis JW Jr., Magilligan DJ Jr. The infected pacemaker pocket. *J Thorac Cardiovasc Surg* 1979;78:298–300.

7. Da Costa A, Kirkorian G, Cucherat M, et al. Antibiotic prophylaxis for permanent pacemaker implantation: A metaanalysis. *Circulation* 1998;97:1796–1801.

8. Dumont E, Camus C, Victor F, et al. Suspected pacemaker or defibrillator transvenous lead infection. Prospective assessment of a TEE-guided therapeutic strategy. *Eur Heart J* 2003;24:1779–1787.

9. Klug D, Lacroix D, Savoye C, et al. Systemic infection related to endocarditis on pacemaker leads: Clinical presentation and management. *Circulation* 1997;95:2098–2107.

10. Chamis AL, Peterson GE, Cabell CH, et al. Staphylococcus aureus bacteremia in patients with permanent pacemakers or implantable cardioverter-defibrillators. *Circulation* 2001;104:1029–1033.

11. Newland GM, Janz TG. Pacemaker-twiddler's syndrome: A rare cause of lead displacement and pacemaker malfunction. *Ann Emerg Med* 1994;23:136–138.

12. Veltri EP, Mower MM, Reid PR. Twiddler's syndrome: A new twist. *Pacing Clin Electrophysiol* 1984;7:1004–1009.

13. Fahraeus T, Hoijer CJ. Early pacemaker twiddler syndrome. *Europace* 2003;5:279–281.

14. Young KR, Bailey WM. Twiddler's syndrome: An unusual cause of pacemaker malfunction. *J La State Med Soc* 2002;154:152–153.

15. Van Orden Wallace CJ. Diagnosing and treating pacemaker syndrome. *Crit Care Nurse* 2001;21:24–31, 35;quiz 36–37.

16. Sarko JA, Tiffany BR. Cardiac pacemakers: Evaluation and management of malfunctions. *Am J Emerg Med* 2000;18:435–440.

17. Garson A Jr. Stepwise approach to the unknown pacemaker ECG. *Am Heart J* 1990;119:924–941.

18. Hayes DL, Vlietstra RE. Pacemaker malfunction. *Ann Intern Med* 1993;119:828–835.

19. Barold SS, Falkoff MD, Ong LS, et al. Oversensing by single-chamber pacemakers: Mechanisms, diagnosis, and treatment. *Cardiol Clin* 1985;3:565–585.

20. Sgarbossa EB, Pinski SL, Gates KB, et al. Early electrocardiographic diagnosis of acute myocardial infarction in the presence of ventricular paced rhythm. GUSTO-I investigators. *Am J Cardiol* 1996;77:423–424.

21. Pinski SL, Trohman RG. Interference in implanted cardiac devices, part II. *Pacing Clin Electrophysiol* 2002;25:1496–1509.

22. Klein AA, Djaiani GN. Mobile phones in the hospital—past, present and future. *Anaesthesia* 2003;58:353–357.

23. Chiladakis JA, Davlouros P, Agelopoulos G, et al. In-vivo testing of digital cellular telephones in patients with implantable cardioverter-defibrillators. *Eur Heart J* 2001;22:1337–1342.

24. Kolb C, Schmieder S, Lehmann G, et al. Do airport metal detectors interfere with implantable pacemakers or cardioverter-defibrillators? *J Am Coll Cardiol* 2003;41:2054–2059.

25. Cazeau S, Leclercq C, Lavergne T, et al. Effects of multisite biventricular pacing in patients with heart failure and intraventricular conduction delay. *N Engl J Med* 2001;344:873–880.

26. Boehmer JP. Device therapy for heart failure. *Am J Cardiol* 2003;91:53D–59D.

27. Haywood G. Biventricular pacing in heart failure: Update on results from clinical trials. *Curr Control Trials Cardiovasc Med* 2001;2:292–297.

28. Connolly SJ, Sheldon R, Thorpe KE, et al. Pacemaker therapy for prevention of syncope in patients with recurrent severe vasovagal syncope: Second Vasovagal Pacemaker Study (VPS II): A randomized trial. *JAMA* 2003;289:2224–2229.

29. Connolly SJ, Kerr CR, Gent M, et al. Effects of physiologic pacing versus ventricular pacing on the risk of stroke and death due to cardiovascular causes. Canadian Trial of Physiologic Pacing Investigators. *N Engl J Med* 2000;342:1385–1391.

30. Lamas GA, Lee KL, Sweeney MO, et al. Ventricular pacing or dual-chamber pacing for sinus-node dysfunction. *N Engl J Med* 2002;346:1854–1862.

31. Toff WD, Skehan JD, De Bono DP, et al. The United Kingdom pacing and cardiovascular events (UKPACE) trial. United Kingdom Pacing and Cardiovascular Events. *Heart* 1997;78:221–223.

32. Carlson MD, Ip J, Messenger J, et al. A new pacemaker algorithm for the treatment of atrial fibrillation: Results of the Atrial Dynamic Overdrive Pacing Trial (ADOPT). *J Am Coll Cardiol* 2003;42:627–633.

33. Abraham WT, Hayes DL, Fisher WG, et al. Cardiac resynchronization in chronic heart failure. *Circulation* 2003;108:2596–2603.

34. St John Sutton MG, Plappert T, Abraham WT, et al. Effect of cardiac resynchronization therapy on left ventricular size and function in chronic heart failure. *Circulation* 2003;107:1985–1990.

35. Abraham WT, Fisher WG, Smith AL, et al. Cardiac resynchronization in chronic heart failure. *N Engl J Med* 2002;346:1845–1853.

36. Achilli A, Sassara M, Ficili S, et al. Long-term effectiveness of cardiac resynchronization therapy in patients with refractory heart failure and "narrow" QRS. *J Am Coll Cardiol* 2003;42:2117–2124.

37. Auricchio A, Stellbrink C, Butter C, et al. Clinical efficacy of cardiac resynchronization therapy using left ventricular pacing in heart failure patients stratified by severity of ventricular conduction delay. *J Am Coll Cardiol* 2003;42:2109–2116.

38. Chua JD, Wilkoff BL, Lee I, et al. Diagnosis and management of infections involving implantable electrophysiologic cardiac devices. *Ann Intern Med* 2000;133:604–608.

39. Akhtar M, Jazayeri M, Sra J, et al. Implantable cardioverter defibrillator for prevention of sudden cardiac death in patients with ventricular tachycardia and ventricular fibrillation: ICD therapy in sudden cardiac death. *Pacing Clin Electrophysiol* 1993;16:511–518.

40. Kuck KH, Cappato R, Siebels J, et al. Randomized comparison of antiarrhythmic drug therapy with implantable defibrillators in patients resuscitated from cardiac arrest: The Cardiac Arrest Study Hamburg (CASH). *Circulation* 2000;102:748–754.

41. Connolly SJ, Gent M, Roberts RS, et al. Canadian implantable defibrillator study (CIDS): A randomized trial of the implantable cardioverter defibrillator against amiodarone. *Circulation* 2000;101:1297–1302.

42. A comparison of antiarrhythmic-drug therapy with implantable defibrillators in patients resuscitated from near-fatal ventricular arrhythmias. The Antiarrhythmics versus Implantable Defibrillators (AVID) Investigators. *N Engl J Med* 1997;337:1576–1583.

43. Moss AJ, Hall WJ, Cannom DS, et al. Improved survival with an implanted defibrillator in patients with coronary disease at high risk for ventricular arrhythmia. Multicenter Automatic Defibrillator Implantation Trial Investigators. *N Engl J Med* 1996;335:1933–1940.

44. Moss AJ. MADIT-II and its implications. *Eur Heart J* 2003;24:16–18.

45. Moss AJ, Zareba W, Hall WJ, et al. Prophylactic implantation of a defibrillator in patients with myocardial infarction and reduced ejection fraction. *N Engl J Med* 2002;346:877–883.

46. Buxton AE, Lee KL, Fisher JD, et al. A randomized study of the prevention of sudden death in patients with coronary artery disease. Multicenter Unsustained Tachycardia Trial Investigators. *N Engl J Med* 1999;341:1882–1890.

24

AEDs and EMS Defibrillation

Thomas E. Collins, Jr.

HIGH YIELD FACTS

- After sudden cardiac death, the probability of successful resuscitation declines by 10% per minute.
- Early defibrillation programs have had a significant impact on survival from out-of-hospital sudden cardiac arrest.
- Automated external defibrillators (AEDs) are remarkably simple to use; on average, untrained sixth grade students took only 23 s longer to defibrillate than the trained emergency medical technicians (EMTs).
- In nearly 3500 cardiac arrests treated with an AED, there was a 99.9% specificity for correct AED usage.
- With the introduction of the first prehospital biphasic AED in 1996, the industry is now migrating to almost entirely biphasic waveform technology.

INTRODUCTION

While there are many strategies to promote early defibrillation, the development and implementation of AEDs in public safety agencies, businesses, and community life has permanently changed the response to out-of-hospital sudden cardiac death. With over 300,000 sudden cardiac deaths from coronary disease each year, the AED has made significant impact on cardiac arrest survival.[1] Traditional emergency medical service (EMS) response to victims in sudden cardiac arrest has typically resulted in survival rates of no more than 5% since the introduction of cardiopulmonary resuscitation (CPR) and advanced life-support techniques. With AED early defibrillation programs, communities are demonstrating important improvements in sudden cardiac arrest survival. White et al., reported in Rochester, Minnesota that patients received

earlier defibrillation and had higher survival rates to discharge when treated by AED-equipped police officers.[2] The Public Access Defibrillation (PAD-1) Trial is one of the most comprehensive AED trials to date that evaluates the impact of PAD programs. In this study, Ornato et al., placed more than 1600 AEDs in 24 communities in the United States and Canada and trained over 20,000 volunteers in CPR or CPR/AED techniques. Results of the trial showed significant increased survival from sudden cardiac arrest for CPR emergency response plans that include an AED.[3]

The majority of patients who suffer out-of-hospital sudden cardiac arrest are initially in ventricular tachycardia (VT). This degenerates into ventricular fibrillation (VF) in the first few minutes after the arrest. Early defibrillation can terminate the VF and increases the likelihood of survival.[4] It is estimated that the likelihood of successful defibrillation decreases by 10% for every minute after a victim collapses. If an early defibrillation program is going to be successful, a rapid response is crucial.

The "Chain of Survival" concept stresses the importance of early defibrillation as a crucial link, distinct from early advanced life support. This emphasizes the importance of a community approach to sudden cardiac death using AEDs, outside of public safety agencies when possible. A successful early defibrillation program hinges on a prepared community with AED access and training in both CPR and AED use.

INDICATIONS AND USE

AEDs are indicated for early defibrillation in patients suffering from sudden cardiac arrest. Response algorithms indicate that an AED should be placed on a victim of sudden collapse without a pulse. Once turned on, the AED will prompt the rescuer to attach the defibrillation pads. The AED will analyze the underlying rhythm and recommend defibrillation if VF or VT are present. Alternatively, if VF/VT are not detected, then the AED will recommend a period of CPR followed by a repeat waveform analysis.

INTEGRATION WITH EMS

AEDs are a vital resource in sudden cardiac arrest survival and should be integrated into the community EMS system. This includes notifying EMS agencies when an AED has been placed at a location. Therefore, in communities with computer-aided dispatch (CAD) systems, information about AED location can be given to a caller seeking emergency help. Additionally, many EMS agencies will assist with AED training, oversight questions, and may even resupply defibrillation pads when the AED is used. Communities and businesses may want to consult their local EMS agencies in the purchasing process, as some AED equipment can seamlessly integrate monitoring/defibrillation pads and data into the advanced life support (ALS) monitors that are used by paramedics. Finally, EMS may assist in reviewing the AED usage summary and providing feedback to community providers.

Design and Ease of Use

AEDs are designed to be simple to use, lightweight, and very portable. As an indication of their simplicity, trained EMTs were compared to untrained sixth grade students in a mock cardiac arrest scenario. On average, the untrained sixth grade students took only 23 s longer to defibrillate than the trained EMTs.[5] While training in AED use is recommended, these devices are simple enough that even untrained users are likely to apply the device correctly (Fig. 24-1).

AEDs have designs that reflect their intended use. Police and fire department first responders need devices that are rugged and will withstand years of movement while stored on vehicles. They may also have expanded battery configurations to allow more frequent usage. Defibrillators placed in malls, stadiums, and offices will be subject to less daily stress and can therefore be smaller.

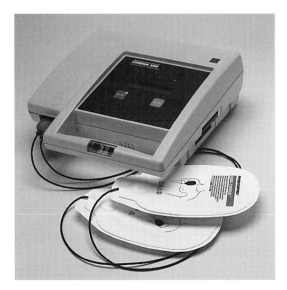

Fig. 24-1. LifePak 500 automated external defibrillator. (Source: Courtesy of Medtronic Inc., Redmond, Washington.)

There are three basic designs that allow appropriate tailoring to the setting that the AED will be used:

- AEDs intended for use by public safety forces are usually more rugged and slightly heavier, due to the need to withstand the movement of the emergency vehicle and more frequent use.

- AEDs intended for PAD programs are typically mounted in one location, so they can be less rugged, smaller, and lighter. PAD AEDs may elect to use the more rugged public safety design.

- AEDs intended for use in hospitals can be the standard AED or may have more monitoring capabilities and be convertible to manual defibrillators/external pacemakers once properly trained personnel arrive. The conversion of an AED to manual defibrillator may involve insertion of a key, or simply turning a control switch on the device.

AEDs should be equipped with the tools necessary to aid in pad placement and with ventilation. These typically include gauze for drying diaphoretic skin, razor for shaving excess hair, and a mouth-to-mouth ventilation mask with one-way valve. Most AEDs either have voice or picture prompts to assist the rescuer in using the device and integrating CPR with AED use.

Arrhythmia analysis algorithms have proven very adept at correctly detecting shockable VF/VT rhythms. MacDonald et al. reviewed nearly 3500 cardiac arrests treated with an AED and found a 99.9% specificity for AED usage.[6] This helps to support the PAD advocacy programs that AEDs are simple to use, and the likelihood of harming a victim of sudden cardiac arrest is extremely low.

ENERGY DELIVERY AND WAVEFORMS

Over the last decade, the science of cardiology has embraced the benefit of biphasic waveforms for energy delivery during defibrillation. Automatic internal cardiac defibrillators (AICD) now exclusively use biphasic waveform technology. EMS has many traditions, one of which is the use of stacked shocks (200 J–300 J–360 J) delivered in a monophasic waveform. With the introduction of the first prehospital biphasic AED in 1996, the industry is gradually migrating to almost entirely biphasic waveform technology. Biphasic waveforms offer multiple advantages. Biphasic waveforms require lower energy settings and allow AED manufacturers to use smaller batteries and capacitors. Not only is this directly reflected in cost savings, but smaller and cheaper AEDs make PAD programs more feasible.[7] The 2000 American Heart

Association Guidelines state that biphasic waveform defibrillation with shocks of 200 J or less is safe and has the equivalent or higher efficacy for termination of VF compared with higher energy escalating monophasic shocks.[8] The optimized response to cardiac arrest (ORCA) trial demonstrated greater defibrillation success rates using 150 J biphasic defibrillation compared to standard higher energy monophasic shocks.[9]

Countershock with a biphasic waveform has theoretic advantages that translate into a lower defibrillation threshold (less energy required for successful defibrillation) and reduced postcountershock myocardial dysfunction. Evidence to date suggests that nonprogressive impedance-adjusted low-energy (150 J three times) biphasic countershock is safe and clinically effective.[10]

EARLY DEFIBRILLATION STRATEGIES

With the advent of AEDs, the traditional paramedic-defibrillator response has evolved to incorporate multiple strategies and providers with the ultimate goal of delivery of rapid defibrillation. It is important to understand the multiple aspects of EMS when discussing best early defibrillation strategies. EMS as a whole can impact survival from cardiac arrest and time to defibrillation at multiple levels. Even before an event occurs, EMS agencies work to train the lay public in CPR and AED techniques. Automatic vehicle location systems using global positioning system (GPS) technologies allow dispatchers to track the exact locations of ambulances, helping to dispatch the closest available ambulance.

Paramedic Only Response

The paramedic only response relies on ALS ambulances and in some cases, fire engines, to respond to all cardiac arrests. While this is the traditional EMS response in urban areas, few communities have adequate resources to assure the rapid response in the 4–6 min that would allow early defibrillation to be successful. Rural fire/EMS agencies are challenged by larger coverage areas and have a longer response interval. Urban areas face traffic congestion and "vertical response" times that delay defibrillation. Alternatively, some suburban fire/EMS agencies may have geographically small coverage areas and the paramedic only defibrillation program may be adequate.

First Responder Response

Many communities are using police and fire department resources as first responders to medical emergencies

including cardiac arrest. These rescuers can have training that includes the following:

- CPR/AED
- First responder
- EMT
- Paramedic

First responder programs use existing rapid response resources (police, fire personnel) to respond to cardiac arrest and begin CPR and AED use while the ALS ambulance is still responding. Communities should analyze response times for police, fire, and EMS vehicles to ascertain if equipping first responders with AEDs can aid delivery of defibrillation in the critical early minutes after sudden cardiac arrest.

Public Access Defibrillation

With the heightened emphasis on rapid defibrillation in the first few minutes following sudden cardiac arrest, EMS and first responder response needs to be supplemented wherever possible. PAD programs place AEDs in locations that have a reasonable chance of benefiting a victim of sudden cardiac arrest. Special consideration should be made for any barriers that may limit an adequate paramedic or AED first responder rapid response. These include:

- Congested areas where EMS response may be limited by traffic
- Rural areas where EMS coverage is limited and response times may be longer
- Buildings where EMS needs to use multiple stairs or elevators and the additional "vertical" response after EMS arrives on scene may further delay rapid defibrillation
- Factories or settings in which there may be a significant distance between where EMS arrives and the physical location of the patient

Specific locations in which PAD programs should be considered include:

- Shopping malls
- Sports venues
- Community centers
- Gyms/fitness centers
- Airports

- Skilled nursing and assisted living facilities
- Office buildings and factories
- Apartment buildings, especially those with high proportion of older occupants

A successful PAD program extends beyond the AED itself. Staff and/or residents should be trained in CPR and AED usage. A quality monitoring program should be in place to review AED usage, and most states require the authorization of a physician medical director prior to purchasing the AED.

SPECIAL CONSIDERATIONS IN AED PLACEMENT

Airlines

Based on Federal Aviation Administration (FAA) guidelines, most major U.S. airlines have placed AEDs in their aircraft to supplement the basic medical kit. Prior to AED placement, an in-flight sudden cardiac arrest was almost always fatal. Since the medical response to in-flight sudden cardiac arrest is dependent on the basic training of the flight attendants and the possibility of on-board medical providers, the AED is crucial. Airlines that have used AEDs have reported very good rates of successful defibrillation and survival to hospital discharge largely due to rapid application after cardiac arrest.[11,12]

Schools/Pediatric Use

Although the frequency of sudden cardiac arrest in children is much lower than adults, VF and VT do occur in children and these patients may benefit from rapid defibrillation. The International Liaison Committee on Resuscitation has updated recommendations on AED use in children to include that AEDs may be used in children 1–8 years of age who have no signs of circulation.[13]

Since current AED models are designed and programmed for optimal use in adults, most would deliver excessive amounts of energy during standard defibrillation. Some manufacturers have developed pediatric defibrillation pads and cable systems that will reduce energy delivered to the pediatric cardiac arrest patient by the AED, allowing more appropriate doses in the 50–75 J range. In selecting AEDs for a school-based PAD program, one should select a model with the capacity for use with children.

AEDs can now be found in schools with increasing frequency. Although there are relatively few sudden cardiac arrest in children, they are typically unexpected and almost always tragic. In many cases, VF/VT are caused by long

Q-T syndrome, hypertrophic cardiomyopathy, congenital aortic stenosis, coronary artery abnormalities, myocarditis, or aortic dissection.[14]

VF/VT can also be precipitated from a direct blunt force to the chest known as commotio cordis. Although traditionally associated with competitive sports, the U.S. Commotio Cordis Registry has noted that nearly 40% of sudden cardiac arrests occurred during daily activities such as playing at home or in the schoolyard, or during recreational sports.[15] The mechanism of VF/VT induction in these cases is the confluence of a direct blunt force over the heart and precise timing of the force hitting during the vulnerable phase of repolarization prior to the peak of the T wave.

Placement of an AED should be considered in schools under the following circumstances:

- Children or adults known to be at risk of sudden cardiac arrest, especially children with congenital heart disease, known arrhythmias, long Q-T syndrome, or heart transplants
- Schools that have a significant number of adults on school grounds, to include sporting events, community meetings, and school volunteers
- Schoolyards and ball fields that are used for recreational sports for adults or children

Controversies in early Defibrillation

Traditionally, defibrillation is attempted immediately after the arrival of the AED or manual defibrillator. There is increasing evidence that a brief period of CPR prior to the defibrillation attempt may improve patient outcomes. In a study conducted in Norway, patients were randomized to receive immediate defibrillation or 3 min of CPR prior to defibrillation.[16] In emergency calls where the response times were greater than 5 min, there was a statistically significant improvement in survival to hospital discharge and 1-year survival rates for patients who received 3 min of CPR prior to defibrillation. Seattle, Washington reported similar improvements in survival using a protocol that provided 90 s of predefibrillation CPR when response intervals were greater than 4 min.[17,18] Several swine studies have demonstrated that precountershock CPR improves successful defibrillation after prolonged arrest and highlights the importance of rapid defibrillation after cessation of CPR.[19]

Callaway et al., reported using the scaling exponent, a VF waveform analysis, as a predictor for successful defibrillation.[20] As time progresses after collapse from VT or VF, the VF waveform deteriorates, the scaling exponent changes as well. In the future, the scaling exponent may be a useful tool for predicting which patients will respond to immediate defibrillation and which would benefit from predefibrillation CPR.

HOSPITAL-BASED EARLY DEFIBRILLATION PROGRAMS

Many hospitals are incorporating AEDs in the internal code response system. A patient found in cardiac arrest can have an AED placed, and if indicated, defibrillated rapidly by personnel who may not have had formal ACLS training. Many hospitals are purchasing monitor/defibrillators that have an AED mode for use by the initial code response personnel. Once advanced cardiac life support (ACLS) trained personnel arrive, these monitors can be converted to manual mode for standard use.

TRAINING

As mentioned earlier, AEDs are simple to use and fairly intuitive. The American Heart Association, the American Red Cross, and several other organizations offer formal AED training programs. Courses typically last 4–8 hours in length and most include basic CPR instruction in the program.

Many schools are adopting CPR and AED training curriculum during the high school years. These programs can be taught by school teachers who have undergone AED instructor training or in many cases, are partnering with the local fire and EMS agencies to provide instruction.

LEGISLATION AND LIABILITY

There are a number of federal laws that address AEDs in the workplace. The Airline Passenger Safety Act of 1998, along with rules from the FAA, now requires airlines to have appropriately stocked medical kits, including AEDs.[22] The Cardiac Arrest Survival Act (CASA) of 2000, directs the Department of Health and Human Services to establish guidelines for placing AEDs in federal buildings.[21] These guidelines include recommendations for training, maintenance, oversight, and coordination with local EMS. CASA strengthens liability protection afforded under Good Samaritan laws for organizations that purchase or individuals that use AEDs in a voluntary setting. Persons who have a specific duty to respond to medical emergencies (physicians, nurses, paramedics, public safety first responders) do not have the same type of protection due to their duty to treat.

States laws regarding AEDs are very diverse with regard to who needs to authorize the AED, what (if any) training is recommended, and what additional conditions of use (training, oversight, quality assurance) are required. AED manufacturers should be able to provide an updated summary of state requirements when an organization or business is considering its purchase.

There are liability discussions involving AEDs that center around two questions.

- What liability does a business incur by not having an AED?
- What liability exists if a business or organization has an AED but uses it improperly?

Several actions taken against airlines, a theme park, and health clubs support the trend that having an early defibrillation program using AEDs reduces an organization's risk of liability.[23] Some initial fears of improper use of an AED leading to negligence claims have not proven themselves due to the simplicity of use and difficulty to misuse the device.

ADVOCACY

Early defibrillation programs uniquely bring together partners in the fight against sudden cardiac arrest. Physicians, public health officials, EMS agencies, business and community leaders engage cooperatively in the goal of reducing death. Each partner should realize their role in being vocal advocates for lifestyles and work styles that promote good cardiovascular health, training, and supporting knowledge of CPR and AED use in the public setting and the workplace. Additional advocacy may be needed to ensure that public safety agencies are adequately staffed and equipped to provide rapid ALS support.

SUMMARY

Early defibrillation programs have had a significant impact on survival from out-of-hospital sudden cardiac arrest. The effects of the AED not only include the delivery of the intended shock, but also have increased the public's awareness of the quick action needed in saving a life. AEDs have demonstrated excellent results in determining when a shock is needed and designs continue to become even more rescuer friendly. Although the AED may never be as common as the fire extinguisher, the technology continues to evolve to make the devices smaller, less expensive, and easier to use. As more research is focused on the crucial first minutes after sudden cardiac arrest, the AED will hopefully become commonplace in the hands of rescuers.

REFERENCES

1. American Heart Association. *Heart Disease and Stroke Statistics—2004 Update.* Dallas, TX: American Heart Association.
2. White RD, Asplin BR, Bugliosi TF, et al. High discharge survival rate after out-of-hospital ventricular fibrillation with rapid defibrillation by police and paramedics. *Ann Emerg Med* 1996;28:480.
3. American Heart Association, Press Release November 11, 2003. Dallas, TX: American Heart Association.
4. American Heart Association. The International Liaison Committee on Resuscitation. Guidelines 2000 for cardiopulmonary resuscitation and emergency cardiovascular care. *Circulation* 2000;102(Suppl):I160.
5. Gundry JW, Comess KA, DeRook FA, et al. Comparison of naive sixth-grade children with trained professionals in the use of an automated external defibrillator. *Circulation* 1999;100:1703.
6. MacDonald RD, Swanson JM, Mottley JL, et al. Performance and error analysis of automated external defibrillator use in the out-of-hospital setting. *Ann Emerg Med* 2001;38:262.
7. Bardy GH, Marchlinski FE, Sharma AD, et al. Multicenter comparison of truncated biphasic shocks and standard damped sine wave monophasic shocks for transthoracic ventricular defibrillation. *Circulation* 1996;94:2507.
8. Atkins DL, Bossaert LL, Hazinski MF, et al. Automated external defibrillation/public access defibrillation. *Ann Emerg Med* 2001;37:S60.
9. Schneider T, Martens PR, Paschen H, et al. Multicenter, randomized, controlled trial of 150-J biphasic shocks compared with 200- to 360-J monophasic shocks in the resuscitation of out-of-hospital cardiac arrest victims. *Circulation* 2000;102:1780.
10. Cummins RO, Hazinski MF, Kerber RE. Low-energy biphasic waveform defibrillation: Evidence-based review applied to emergency cardiovascular care guidelines: A statement for healthcare professionals from the American Heart Association Committee on Emergency Cardiovascular Care and the Subcommittees on Basic Life Support, Advanced Cardiac Life Support, and Pediatric Resuscitation. *Circulation* 1998;97:1654.
11. Page RL, Joglar JA, Kowal RC, et al. Use of automated external defibrillators by a U.S. airline. *N Engl J Med* 2000;343:1210.
12. Groeneveld PW, Kwong JL, Liu Y, et al. Cost-effectiveness of automated external defibrillators on airlines. *JAMA* 2001;286:1482.
13. Samson RA, Berg RA, Bingham R. Use of automated external defibrillators for children: An update—An Advisory Statement from the Pediatric Advanced Life Support Task Force, International Liaison Committee on Resuscitation. *Pediatrics* 2003;112:163.
14. Liberthson RR. Sudden death from cardiac causes in children and young adults. *N Engl J Med* 1996;334:1039.
15. Maron BJ, Gohman TE, Kyle SB, et al. Clinical profile and spectrum of commotio cordis. *JAMA* 2002;287:1142.
16. Wik L, Hansen TB, Fylling F, et al. Delaying defibrillation to give basic cardiopulmonary resuscitation to patients with out-of-hospital ventricular fibrillation: A randomized trial. *JAMA* 2003;289:1389.
17. Cobb LA, Fahrenbruch CE, Walsh TR, et al. Influence of cardiopulmonary resuscitation prior to defibrillation in patients with out-of-hospital ventricular fibrillation. *JAMA* 1999;281:1182.
18. Berg RA, Hilwig RW, Kern KB, et al. Precountershock cardiopulmonary resuscitation improves ventricular fibrillation median frequency and myocardial readiness for successful defibrillation from prolonged ventricular fibrillation: A randomized, controlled swine study. *Ann Emerg Med* 2002;40:563.
19. Berg RA, Hilwig RW, Kern KB, et al. Automated external defibrillation versus manual defibrillation for prolonged ventricular fibrillation: Lethal delays of chest compressions before and after countershocks. *Ann Emerg Med* 2003;42:458.
20. Callaway CW, Sherman LD, Mosesso VN, et al. Scaling exponent predicts defibrillation success for out-of-hospital ventricular fibrillation cardiac arrest. *Circulation* 2001;103:1656.
21. *Proceedings from the 106th Congress of the United States of America.* Public Law No: 106–505, full text available from the Library of Congress, Washington, DC. Available at: http://thomas.loc.gov.
22. *Proceedings from the 105th Congress of the United States of America.* Public Law No: 105–170, full text available from the Library of Congress, Washington, DC. Available at: http://thomas.loc.gov.
23. Lazar RA. Liability no barrier. AED programs can reduce legal risk. *JEMS* 2002;27(Suppl. 6).

PART IV

25

Demographics and Economics

Deborah B. Diercks

HIGH YIELD FACTS

- Heart failure is a disease reaching epidemic proportion in the United States.
- Heart failure is the leading cause of hospitalization in patients over the age of 65.
- In the United States, the incidence of heart failure is increasing.
- Heart failure exerts a high economic cost to the health care system with over $22 billion spent in 2002.

INTRODUCTION

Heart failure is a disease reaching epidemic proportion in the United States. It is a progressive disorder that often begins with asymptomatic dysfunction. The American Heart Association (AHA) reports that the prevalence of patients with heart failure exceeded 5 million in 2002, with an incidence of 550,000 new cases a year.[1] The new AHA practice guidelines divide this disorder into four stages, two of which are asymptomatic, which may result in the number of patients with heart failure being underestimated.[2] The magnitude of the heart failure problem is evident in the high rate of mortality, morbidity, and cost.[3] As the population ages, the human and economic expense will further increase. Patients who develop heart failure have a markedly decreased quality of life and physical functioning, and approximately 50% of patients will die within 5 years of their diagnosis.[4] The rate of hospitalization for heart failure increased 165% from 1979 to 2000.[1] In addition, heart failure is the single most common cause for hospital admission in patients aged >65 years. To fully understand this epidemic, the impact of comorbid illnesses, patient demographics, and cost need to be explored.

Heart failure is predominately a disease of the elderly. The rapid increase in the incidence of heart failure can be attributed to the increase in patients over the age of 65. Data from the Framingham Heart Study report that incidence of heart failure rises from less than 2 per 1000 patient-years in those less than 60 years old, then approximately 10 per 1000 patient-years in those aged 70–79 years, to 25 per 1000 patient-years when age is greater than 80[4] (Fig. 25-1).

CORMORBIDITIES

To understand the impact that comorbidities have on heart failure it is essential to view heart failure as a disease process that results from a large number of pathologic events. Heart failure results from many of the disease processes that are common in the elderly, such as hypertension and ischemic heart disease (Fig. 25-2). Gender also appears to play a role in the comorbidities associated with heart failure. Women with heart failure tend to be older, have associated diabetes mellitus, and hypertension, and more frequently have preserved ventricular function.[5] In a large study of self-reported heart failure patients, obese patients and former or current smokers had a high prevalence of heart failure. Hypertension and coronary artery disease are major comorbid factors, with 30% heart failure patients having both hypertension and coronary artery disease.[6]

In addition, age-related abnormalities in artery compliance can result in left ventricular hypertrophy and diastolic heart failure. Diastolic heart failure is defined as having signs and symptoms of heart failure, but with preserved left ventricular function as defined as an ejection fraction greater than 40%. Reports have shown that diastolic heart failure accounts for almost 50% of the heart failure patients older than 70, while it only is present in 8% of those less than 65.[7] Although diastolic heart failure patients have a lower rate of mortality than systolic heart failure patients, the large number of hospitalizations in patients older than 65 years of age results in diastolic heart failure accounting for more deaths.

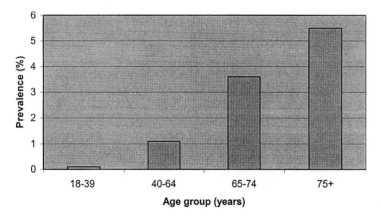

Fig. 25-1. Prevalence of self-reported heart failure. (Source: Adapted from Ni, H. Prevalence of self-reported heart failure among US adults: Results from the 1999 National Health Interview Survey. *Am Heart J* 2003;146:121–128.)

The pathologic processes leading to the development of heart failure often speed the progression of the disease process and impact treatment options. As previously mentioned hypertension is a major factor in the development of heart failure, through its association with increased risk of ischemic heart disease, the development of after-load-induced cardiomyopathy, and impairment of diastolic dysfunction.[5] This is especially evident in Blacks. Unfortunately, therapeutic responses to current treatment options have been found to be less pronounced in this patient population.[8]

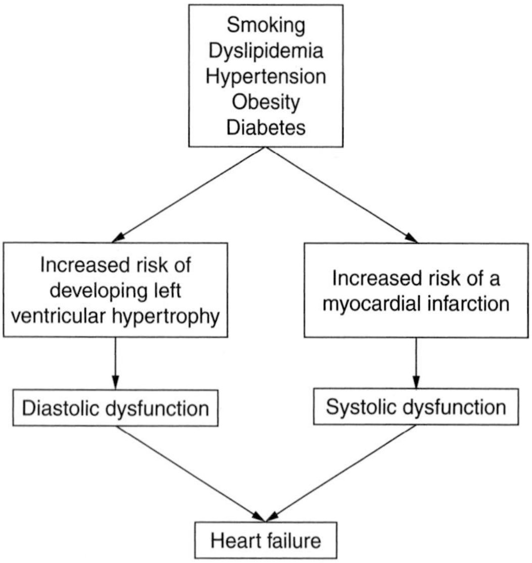

Ischemic heart disease also features prominently as a cause of heart failure. In most of the major heart failure trials, over 50% of the patients have a history of ischemic heart disease. Coronary artery disease leads to heart failure through multiple mechanisms, including myocardial infarction.[5] Additionally, transient ischemia may result in episodic dysfunction even in the presence of normal resting ventricular function.

Hyperlipidemia has been shown to be present in up to 26% of patients enrolled in intervention trials of chronic heart failure,[5] and another risk factor for the development of heart failure is obesity. Obesity increases the risk of heart failure through increased left ventricular mass, and obese patients often have a high chronic cardiac workload due to the amount of blood volume needed to supply the peripheral tissue. This increased workload results in increased left ventricular mass though an increase in non-muscular tissue. This increased mass is associated with left ventricular hypertrophy, which in turn leads to varying degrees of systolic and diastolic dysfunction.[9]

Diabetes is a common comorbidity in heart failure. Diabetics are at increased risk for cardiovascular disease, and in the Framingham study there was an increased rate of heart failure and coronary artery disease in diabetic patients. This difference was especially noticed in women.[12] Diabetics not only are at increased risk of developing heart failure, but have worse symptoms for their degree of systolic dysfunction and higher mortality than nondiabetics.[5,10,11] In a 10-year longitudinal study, diabetes was associated with a twofold increase in heart failure in men, and a fourfold increase in women. This risk persisted after adjustment for age, coronary artery disease, and hypertension.[12] Diabetes may be related to heart failure

Fig. 25-2. Schematic relationship between comorbidities and the progression to heart failure. (Source: Adapted from Krum H, Gilbert RE. Demographics and concomitant disorders in heart failure. *Lancet* 2003;362:147–158.)

through three mechanisms: associated comorbidities, ischemic heart disease, and diabetic cardiomyopathy. Common comorbidities often associated with diabetes include those often characterized as the metabolic syndrome.[13] These include obesity, hyperlipidemia, hypertension, hypercoagulability, and inflammation.[14] Despite this relationship of associated risk factors, studies have shown the glycemic control is an independent risk factor for the development of heart failure even after adjusting for age, gender, obesity, and blood pressure.[15] Heart failure symptoms in diabetics may also be related to increased rate of cardiomyopathy. It has been proposed that diabetic cardiomyopathy is a result of abnormalities in microangiography, myocardial fibrosis, and metabolic factors. In addition, the deposition of advanced glycation end products may increase left ventricular stiffness and lead to diastolic dysfunction.[16,17]

COSTS

Heart failure results in significant cost to the health care system. One study reported approximately half of the patients with heart failure were hospitalized, 53% visited an emergency department, and 50% had over 10 visits to their doctor in a 12-month period.[6] Of the patients who present to the emergency department with acute decompensation of congestive heart failure approximately 80% are admitted to the hospital.[18,19] Additionally, the rate of recidivism in heart failure patients is high. The rate of hospitalization following an index visit is approximately 50–100%[21] by 6 months. In fact, in 1998 $3.7 billion were paid to Medicare beneficiaries for heart failure. This high expenditure of Medicare dollars is derived from heart failure being the most common cause in hospitalizations in patients aged >65 years.[1,20]

In 2002, costs related to heart failure are estimated to consist of $22.2 billion in direct costs and $24.3 billion in indirect costs.[1] Unfortunately heart failure care is costly, with the average U.S. hospital losing $1288 for each hospital admission.[22] A study that evaluated the impact of comorbidity on the cost of heart failure care demonstrated that the costs of treating heart failure remain high, and 1-year follow-up costs exceed those of initial hospitalization by 50%.[23] Costs increased with each comorbidity, especially diabetes and renal failure. In this study, approximately one-third were rehospitalized, and this percentage increased with additional comorbidity. Although initial length of stay did not vary with added comorbidity, the total length of stay (including initial and follow-up hospitalization) increased from 9.9 days with no comorbidity to 15.2 days with all comorbidities.[23]

Payments of the elderly are structured on the diagnosis-related group (DRG) system, and thus payment is based on diagnosis. The main source of a hospital's cost in heart failure is therefore related to the length of stay. A length of stay greater than 5 days is about the point at which hospitals begin to lose money.[22] The complexity of the patients with heart failure and the associated comorbidities makes addressing the length of stay issue a challenge.

Unresolved Issues

Will the epidemic of heart failure be controlled as treatment improves? Current statistics report that heart failure accounts for 250,000 deaths a year.[1] However, the Framingham study reports a decline in adjusted mortality after the onset of heart failure in the last decade.[4] This suggests that although the number of patients who die from heart failure may increase, due to the aging of the population, the prognosis for the individual patient is improving. This may be due to the increased use of therapeutic agents such as beta-blockers and angiotensin converting enzyme inhibitors.[23]

Will improved outpatient management of heart failure patients decrease health care costs? Recently emphasis has been placed on the team approach to the management of the chronic heart failure patient. This system incorporates discharge planning and multispecialty outpatient care. Studies that have evaluated this approach have reported improved patient outcome with decreased emergency department visits.[24,25] As this approach becomes more commonplace, the health care burden of the heart failure patient may be reduced.

REFERENCES

1. American Heart Association. *Heart Disease and Stroke Statistics—2003 Update.* Dallas, TX.: American Heart Association, 2003.
2. Hunt Sa, Baker DW, Chin MH, et al. ACC/AHA guidelines for the evaluation and management of chronic heart failure in the adult: Executive summary. A report of the American College/American Heart Association Task Force on Practice Guidelines (Committee to revise the 1995 Guidelines for the Evaluation and Management of Heart Failure). *J Am Coll Cardiol* 2001;38:2101–2113.
3. Baker DW, Einstadter D, Thomas C, et al. Mortality trends for 23,505 Medicare patients hospitalized with heart failure in Northeast Ohio, 1991 to 1997. *Am Heart J* 2003;146(2): 258–64.
4. Ho KKL, Finsky JL, Kannel WB, et al. The epidemiology of heart failure: The Framingham study. *J Am Coll Cardiol* 1993;22:6A–13A.

5. Krum H, Gilbert RE. Demographics and concomitant disorders in heart failure. *Lancet* 2003;362:147–158.

6. Ni H. Prevalence of self-reported heart failure among US adults: Results from the 1999 National Health Interview survey. *Am Heart J* 2003;146:121–128.

7. Senni M, Tribouilloy CM, Rodeheffer RJ, et al. Congestive heart failure in the community: A study of all incident cases in Olmsted County, Minnesota, in 1991. *Circulation* 1998;98:2282–2289.

8. Carson P, Ziesche S, Johnson G, et al. Racial differences in response to therapy for heart failure: Analysis vasodilator-heart failure trials. *J Cardiol Failure* 1999;5:178–187.

9. Contaldo F, Pasanisi F, Finelli C, et al. Obesity, heart failure, and sudden death. *Nutr Metab Cardiovasc Dis* 2002; 12:190–197.

10. Stone PH, Muller JE, Hartwell T, et al. The effect of diabetes mellitus on prognosis and serial left ventricular function after acute myocardial infarction: Contribution of both coronary disease and diastolic left ventricular dysfunction to the adverse prognosis: The MILIS study. *J Am Coll Cardiol* 1989;14:49–57.

11. Gustafsson I, Hildebrandt P, Seibaek M, et al. Long-term prognosis of diabetic patients with myocardial infarction; relation to antidiabetic treatment regimen: The TRACE Study. *Eur Heart J* 2000;21:1937–1943.

12. Kannel WB, Hjortand M, Catelli WP. Role of diabetes in congestive heart failure. *Am J Cardiol* 1974;34:29–34.

13. Bauters C, Lamblin N, McFadden EP, et al. Influence of diabetes mellitus on heart failure risk and outcome. *Cardiovasc Diabetol* 2003;3:1–16.

14. Tarnow L, Rossing P, Gal MA, et al. Prevalence of arterial hypertension in diabetic patients before and after JNC-V *Diabetic Care* 1994;17:1247–1251.

15. Iribarren C, Karter AJ, Go AS, et al. Glycemic control and heart failure among adult patients with diabetes. *Circulation* 2001;106:2668–2673.

16. Standl E, Schnell O. A new look at the heart in diabetes mellitus: Form ailing to failing. *Diabetologia* 2000; 43:1455–1469.

17. Brownies M, Cerarri A, Vlassara H. Advanced glycosylation end products in tissue and the biochemical basis of diabetic complications. *N Engl J Med* 1988;318:1315–1321.

18. Graff L, Orledg J, Radford MJ, et al. Correlation of the Agency for Health Care Policy and Research congestive heart failure admission guideline with mortality: Peer review organization voluntary hospital association initiative to decrease events (PROVIDE) for congestive heart failure. *Ann Emerg Med* 1999;34:429–437.

19. Centers for Medicare and Medicaid Services. Available at: http/www.cms.gov. Accessed August 19, 2002.

20. National 2001 Medicare Benchmark for Economics for U.S. Hospitals for DRG-127 (MedPar data).

21. Peacock WF, Remer EE, Aponte JH, et al. Effective observation unit treatment of decompensated heart failure. *Congest Heart Fail* 2002;8(2):68–73.

22. Weintraub WS, Kawabata H, Tran M, et al. Influence of co-morbidity on cost of care for heart failure. *Am J Cardiol* 2003;91:1011–1016.

23. Ansari M, Massie BM. Heart failure: How big is the problem? Who are the patients? What does the future hold? *Am Heart J* 2003;146:1–4.

24. Stewart S, Marley JE, Horowitz JD. Effects of a multidisciplinary, home-based intervention on planned readmissions and survival among patients with chronic congestive heart failure: A randomized controlled trial. *Lancet* 1999;354: 1007–1083.

25. Rich MW, Beckham V, Wittenburg C, et al. A multidisciplinary intervention to prevent the readmission of elderly patients with congestive heart failure. *N Engl J Med* 1995; 333:1190–1195.

26

Prognosis and Pathophysiology

Deborah B. Diercks

HIGH YIELD FACTS

> - Heart failure results from an index event that elicits activation of neurohormonal pathways.
> - Activation of these pathways is the result of hemodynamic alterations or threats to arterial pressure.
> - Neurohormonal activation of the renin-angiotensin-aldosterone-system (RAAS), adrenergic system, endothelin, and vasopressin results in vasoconstriction, fluid retention, and cardiac remodeling.
> - The natriuretic peptide system and kinin system are counter-regulatory neurohormones and cause vasodilatation, diuresis, and prevent fibrosis.
> - Levels of the neurohormones and the physiologic consequences of neurohormonal activation are significant predictors of morbidity and mortality in heart failure patients.

HEART FAILURE PROGNOSIS

The ability to risk stratify patients and identify those at risk for poor outcomes has been challenging. Recent studies have shown that simple risk stratification models can be useful in identifying high-risk patients. Lee et al. derived and validated a risk score using data available at the initial presentation to identify patients at high risk for 30-day and 1-year mortality. This score used a combination of points based on age, initial respiratory rates, blood pressure, renal function, hematocrit, and past medical history.[1] In addition to these models, multiple tools can independently be used to risk stratify patients. Information obtained from the history, physical examination, laboratory testing, and the electrocardiogram can be easily be used to identify a high-risk group of patients.

Although a significant predictor of risk, documentation of left ventricular (LV) ejection fraction may not be available in the acute decompensation setting and therefore not useful to the emergency practitioner. This review will discuss data that are available to the practitioner in the acute setting.

The only neurohormone measurement that currently has clinical relevance to the practicing clinician is the B-type natriuretic peptide (BNP) level. Levels of BNP have been shown to correlate with ejection fraction, morbidity, and heart failure classification, and BNP levels have been shown to predict future cardiac events. In a 6-month follow-up of 325 patients who presented to the ED with dyspnea and had BNP levels drawn, BNP was a good predictor of the combined endpoint of death, hospital admission with a cardiac diagnosis, or repeat ED visits for heart failure (HF).[2] The cumulative probability of a HF event within 6 months was 51% in the 67 patients with a BNP level greater than 480 pg/mL, compared with 2.5% in the 205 patients with BNP values less than 230 pg/mL. For BNP levels greater than 230 pg/mL, the relative risk (RR) of cardiac death within 6 months was 37.9, and the RR for HF death was 24.1. BNP has also been shown to predict sudden death, and death from pump failure, over 3 years of follow-up.[3]

There are multiple readily available historic and diagnostic tests that can be used by the practicing physician for rapid risk stratification of the heart failure patient. In addition to BNP levels, abnormalities of sodium, renal function, and hematocrit, can be predictors of adverse outcomes. Hyponatremia has been shown to correlate with long-term prognosis for cardiac-related death.[4] In addition, the ratio of serum to urinary sodium correlated with plasma renin activity, and therefore prognosis. Neurohormonally mediated renal effects, that result in a decline in the glomerular filtration rate (GFR), increase the number and severity of patients with chronic heart failure at 1 year.[5] A simple assessment of abnormal renal function, as measured by blood urea nitrogen is a strong predictor of death.[1]

Electrocardiographic findings can also be used to risk stratify patients with congestive heart failure. Evaluation of conduction defects can predict mortality. Up to 20% of patients with heart failure have a QRS in excess of 120 ms, which is indicative of abnormal ventricular contraction. The QRS duration appears to be associated with depressed ejection fraction. In a study of patients with chronic heart failure, a QRS greater than 150 ms was associated with 60% rate of death at 5 years, compared to 35% of those patients with QRS less than 150 ms. The increased risk of mortality associated with QRS prolongation may identify a group of patients who would benefit from biventricular pacing.[6] The presence of a left bundle branch block has also been shown to be an independent predictor of death at 1 year, although this risk was not observed in patients with a right bundle branch block. Electrocardiographic signs of LV hypertrophy are also predictors of poor outcome.

The physical examination can also provide useful information of risk stratification. The presence of systemic hypotension in patients presenting with acute pulmonary edema is predictive of mortality. It appears that, in acute decompensation, a hypertensive response may be protective although the exact mechanism of this is unknown.[1] Clinical assessment of a patient's hemodynamic status can also be used for risk stratification. In a study by Nohria et al., patients were classified by assessment into four profiles: A, no evidence of poor perfusion or congestion (warm-dry); B, congestion with good perfusion (wet-dry); C, congestion and hypoperfusion (wet-cold); and D, hypoperfusion without congestion (dry-cold). Patients were followed for the endpoints of death and urgent transplantation at 1 year. Patients in profile B and C had an increased risk of death or urgent transplantation after adjusting for other comorbidities and heart failure classification.[7] The combination of clinical examination and easily available laboratory tests can provide the treating physician with important risk stratification information.

HF PATHOPHYSIOLOGY

Introduction

Heart failure occurs when the ventricles are unable to generate sufficient pressure during contraction or when high pressures are required to fill the ventricles. It usually is the result of an index event, such as myocardial infarction, which results in impaired cardiac function and vascular congestion. Over the last 20 years, there has been an increased understanding of the pathophysiology of congestive heart failure. This coincides with a dramatic increase in the incidence of congestive heart failure that has paralleled the rise in elderly population. The earlier hypothesis that progression of heart failure was based on impaired contractility and pump dysfunction has evolved into the current understanding of the importance of the neurohormonal role in heart failure.[8] Although impaired contractility and pump dysfunction are important to understanding and treatment of acute decompensated heart failure, chronic progression of heart failure is now thought to be integrally linked to neurohormonal events and pathologic reflexes. Heart failure, like most clinical syndromes, is the end result of a cascade of events. LV remodeling encompasses numerous mechanisms, such as cell death, collagen break down, and myocyte hypertrophy, and is a result of the neurohormonal response that occurs in heart failure.

Activation of neurohormonal pathways are adaptive in the short term to maintain blood pressure but can promote the progression of heart failure through LV remodeling when long-term activation occurs. According to the neurohormonal concept, an index event occurs resulting in the activation of neurohormones and cytokines, which then cause the development and progression of LV remodeling resulting in the clinical syndrome of heart failure.[8] As heart failure progresses there is an increase in vasoconstrictive substances and a decline in counter-regulatory effects of endogenous vasodilators, such as nitric oxide, bradykinin (BK), and the natriuretic peptides. The most notable neuroendocrine systems are the RAAS and sympathetic adrenergic system.

The clinical syndrome of heart failure has been divided into two separate classes based on the ejection fraction. A normal ejection fraction is 60%. If the patient has an ejection fraction of less than 40%, systolic heart failure is diagnosed. Diastolic heart failure, also termed preserved systolic function (PSF), is defined as signs and symptoms of heart failure in patients with relatively normal LV function (e.g., ejection fraction greater than 40%). Studies have shown that 50% of elderly patients who present with symptoms of heart failure have preserved LV systolic function.[9] This diagnosis appears to be most prevalent in elderly females with hypertension and coronary artery disease.[9] Heart failure with PSF may be difficult to diagnose, since a large number of patients with presumed diastolic dysfunction have other medical comorbidities. A recent study reported that elderly patients with diastolic heart failure had pathophysiologic abnormalities similar to patients with systolic heart failure. Results of this study suggest that the underlying pathophysiology of both systolic and diastolic heart failure may be similar, and neurohormonal therapies may be beneficial in both populations.[9]

This chapter will review the pathophysiologic processes that are responsible for the development and progression of heart failure. The majority of this chapter will focus on the neurohormonal pathways that are activated in heart failure, as these processes are relevant in both systolic and diastolic heart failure.

Index Event

Patients often go through a period of latent or asymptomatic heart failure prior to presentation; therefore, it is often difficult to determine the etiology of their disease.[10] However, in many patients there is an index event that results in congestive heart failure. Events such as myocardial infarction that results in loss of contractile tissue, myocarditis, the development of systolic hypertension, valvular insufficiency and a volume overload state, or genetic myocardial dysfunction, can result in heart failure[8] (Fig. 26-1). Coronary artery disease leads to heart failure through multiple mechanisms. Myocardial infarction can lead to regional contractile dysfunction, myocyte hypertrophy, apoptosis, and deposition of extracellular matrix.[11] In addition, transient ischemia may result in episodic dysfunction even in the presence of normal resting ventricular function.[11]

In many cases, we do not know the etiology of the heart failure. Its development is often a slow process, and may be multifactorial. Disorders affecting extracardiac organs, such as hyperthyroidism and severe chronic obstructive lung disease, can also cause heart failure. In the United States, most cases of heart failure are the result of coronary artery disease or a combination of hypertension, LV hypertrophy, and diabetes.[11] The common pathway from any index event is the response that the heart takes to maintain effective blood circulation and protective blood flow to vital organs.[8]

At the cellular level there is often an inflammatory component after the initial index event, this can lead to hypertrophy of myocytes and apoptosis. In situations in which the index event results in a more chronic fluid overloaded state, such as mitral regurgitation, there is elongation of the cardiac myocytes. Although in the initial phase elongation and resulting heart chamber dilation may maintain stroke volume, in time this leads to further impaired systolic function. In patients with excessive afterload, myocyte hypertrophy also occurs and is associated with increased cellular thickness. In these

situations, the common factor is the resulting ventricular remodeling.

An index event can result in acute decompensation in a patient with chronic heart failure. Patients with previously diagnosed heart failure can have acute exacerbations as a result of conditions such as myocardial ischemia, arrhythmias, worsening renal function, and natural progression of this chronic disease.[8] Other situations, such as poorly controlled hypertension, dietary noncompliance, and medication noncompliance can also result in worsening heart failure symptoms.

Renin-Angiotensin-Aldosterone-System

Since activation of neurohormonal pathways is a result of mechanoreceptors that sense alterations in arterial pressure, this process is present in patients with both high output failure, such as thyrotoxicosis, and low output states as in cardiac ischemia. As cardiac output declines, there is activation of the renin-angiotensin system. This results in arteriolar constriction, which increases blood pressure and thus maintains the GFR, in part by angiotensin-II and sympathetic nervous system activity.[12] The RAAS system is cascade of neurohormonal release that is initiated by the release of renin from the kidney. Renin cleaves angiotensinogen, which is produced primarily in the liver. Angiotensin-II results from the conversion of angiotensinogen to angiotensin-I, which is then cleared by angiotensin-converting enzyme (ACE).[12]

In heart failure nonrenin production also exists for angiotensin-II. These pathways are predominantly in the vascular endothelium and are activated by stretch. Nonrenin production of angiotensin-II plays an important role in the resistance to treatment with ACE inhibitors.[13] Angiotensin-II commences its physiologic cascade by activation of two

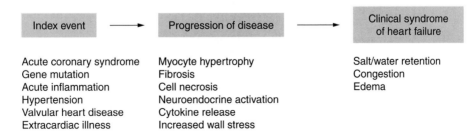

Fig. 26-1. Working hypothesis of heart failure. (Source: Adapted from Francis GS. Pathophysiology of chronic heart failure. *Am J Med* 2001;110(Suppl 7A):37S–46S.)

receptors, angiotensin type 1 (AT1) and angiotensin type 2 (AT2), see Fig. 26-2. Activation of the AT1 receptor mediates the deleterious hemodynamic actions, endocrine, and mitogenic effects of angiotensin-II noted in heart failure.[14] In the kidney the activation of the AT1 receptor results in constriction of the afferent and efferent arterioles, and while this reduces overall renal blood flow, it may augment the GFR. The decline in the renal blood flow and the direct effect of angiotensin-II on the renal tubules results in impaired sodium and water excretion. In addition to these effects on the kidney, activation of the AT1 receptor induces cellular proliferation and tissue remodeling. The activation of AT1 also leads to increased prothrombotic effects and increased atherosclerosis in the coronary arteries as a result of activation of inflammatory cytokines.[14] Activation of the AT2 receptor triggers BK, nitric oxide, and cyclic GMP cascades, which appear to antagonize the activation of the AT1 receptor.[15] Angiotensin-II, in addition to being a potent vasoconstrictor, causes the reabsorption of sodium in the renal tubules, and stimulates the adrenal cortex to secrete aldosterone.

Aldosterone further promotes the absorption of sodium in exchange for potassium in the renal tubes. In congestive heart failure, its secretion is stimulated by angiotensin-II,

elevated potassium concentrations, catecholamines, endothelins, and vasopressin. Unlike angiotensin-II, which promotes sodium absorption in the proximal renal tubules, aldosterone acts on the distal cortical collecting duct to further prevent sodium reabsorption.[12] Aldosterone causes a reduction in endothelial nitric oxide, which reduces arterial compliance and results in endothelial dysfunction. Increased sympathetic activity and decreased parasympathetic activity have also been attributed to aldosterone. The increase in sympathetic activity is attributed to the blocking of catecholamine reuptake by aldosterone. These alterations in sympathetic activity can result in a proarrhythmic state that can lead to sudden cardiac death.[14] In addition, aldosterone-induced increases in myocardial hypertrophy, fibrosis, and apoptosis (programmed myocellular necrosis) result in increased ventricular stiffness which can lead to LV dysfunction and worsening heart failure.[12] Activation of the RAAS therefore results in a number of pathologic consequences that lead to the progression of heart failure by attempting to restore adequate renal perfusion, which can result in salt and water retention, and by facilitating cardiac myocyte growth, therefore promoting LV remodeling[12] (Table 26-1).

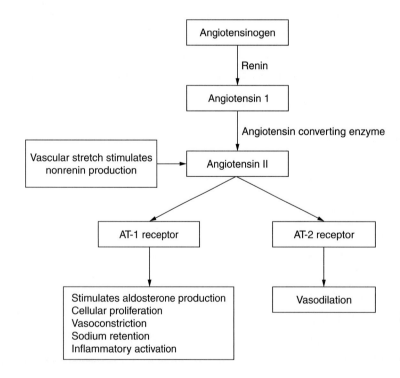

Fig. 26-2. RAAS system. (Source: Adapted from Brewster UC, Setaro JF, Perazella MA. The renin-angiotensin-aldosterone system: Cardiorenal effects and implications for renal and cardiovascular disease states. *Am J Med Sci* 2003;326:15–24.)

Table 26-1. Aldosterone

Renal effects
Sodium retention
Potassium/magnesium loss
Vasoconstriction

Vascular effects
Vasoconstriction
Cellular hypertrophy

Myocardial effects
Induces hypertrophy
Increased fibrosis
Apoptosis
Stimulates arrhythmia by blocking norepinephrine uptake

Neurohormonal effects
Stimulates norepinephrine release

Adrenergic Nervous System

In patients with congestive heart failure, the immediate response to beta-adrenergic system activation, increased heart rate, and contractility are beneficial. A fall in cardiac output results in increased sympathetic activity. This results in increased heart rate and force of ventricular contraction via beta-receptor activation, and peripheral vasoconstriction from alpha-receptor activation. However, prolonged stimulation of these receptors results in beta-adrenergic desensitization. This is a function of reduced beta-1-receptor density and uncoupling of beta-2 receptors downstream, and results in a decreased arterial baroreceptor reflex control of heart rate in patients with heart failure.[16] In addition, there is a decreased inotropic response through alteration in calcium-mediated contractile proteins and leads to a decline in cardiac output, and thus worsening of congestive heart failure. These factors ultimately result in alteration in calcium transport across the sarcoplasmic reticulum, as well as the release of calcium to maintain contractility.[17] It is unknown if these adrenergic signal abnormalities are an adaptive response to overstimulation or maladaptive change that depresses contractility and drives heart failure progression. These effects on the adrenergic system result in upregulation of central and peripheral chemoreceptors, which have been shown to contribute to the development of central sleep apnea that occurs in one-third of all heart failure patients.[18]

The release of norepinephrine, an effector of the adrenergic nervous system, contributes to the progression of heart failure by many different mechanisms. Plasma norepinephrine level correlates with the severity of heart failure and also the long-term prognosis. Studies have shown that the release of norepinephrine is associated with increased pulmonary artery pressure and pulmonary wedge pressure, which lead to the hypothesis that there is a link between cardiopulmonary baroreceptors and efferent cardiac sympathetic activity.[19] The elevation of norepinephrine results in both local and systemic effects, such as direct myocardial toxicity, sodium and water retention, peripheral vasoconstriction, induction of apoptosis, activation of the RAAS, and the stimulation of arrhythmias.[20] The presence of chronically elevated norepinephrine, along with tumor necrosis factor (TNF) and inflammatory cytokines, leads to an increased nitric oxide production that can result in cellular proliferation and apoptosis[20] (Table 26-2).

Inflammatory Markers and Cytokines

Recent studies have suggested that the myocardial stunning that occurs in sepsis is similar to the process that occurs in heart failure. The myocardial effects of sepsis have three characteristics similar to congestive heart failure: activation of inflammatory mediators, reversible myocardial depression, and beta-adrenergic desensitization. The reversible myocardial depression can be attributed to nitric oxide production. Although the exact role that nitric oxide plays in heart failure is incompletely understood, it appears to have negative inotropic properties by increasing intracellular cycle guanosine monophosphate and further reducing sensitivity to beta-adrenergic stimulation.[21]

Table 26-2. Adrenergic Neurohormonal System

Renal effects
Vasoconstriction
Sodium/water retention

Vascular effects
Vasoconstriction
Endothelial dysfunction

Myocardial effects
Receptor desensitization
Apoptosis
Increased fibrosis

Neurohormonal effects
Stimulates angiotensin-II, aldosterone, vasopressin
    production

TNF is a proinflammatory cytokine that plays a pivotal role in host responses to injury and infection. TNF has been detected in patients with heart failure and has shown to correlate with clinical severity.[21] It reduces vascular smooth muscle tone and myocardial contractility. The decline in contractility is mediated by nitric oxide. TNF has also been shown to induce myocyte apoptosis, which can lead to LV dysfunction. Early expression of TNF may diminish cardiac contractility through altered calcium homeostasis and modifications of the beta-adrenergic receptor-G-protein-adenylyl cyclase coupling that are reversible. However, chronic stimulation results in apoptosis and remodeling through matrix metalloprotease processes leading to permanent damage.[22]

Endothelin

Other vasoactive systems such as endothelin and arginine vasopressin also play a role in congestive heart failure. Endothelin-1 is an endogenous vasoconstrictor.[23] It is produced by the vascular endothelium in response to alterations in vascular tone. Its effects are mediated through endothelin-A and endothelin-B receptors in the vascular smooth muscle, which leads to increased calcium concentrations. Activation of endothelin-B receptors causes vasodilation through nitric oxide and prostacyclin release. In addition, the endothelin-B receptors in the lung are the major pathway of clearance. In heart failure, there appears to be an upregulation of endothelin-A receptors and a downregulation of endothelin-B receptors.[23] Factors that influence endothelin expression are vascular stretch, epinephrine, angiotensin-II, thrombin, and inflammatory cytokines. In heart failure, the pulmonary vascular bed seems to be the main source of circulating endothelin.[24] Vasoconstrictive effects of endothelin are evident in the renal vasculature and result in reduced renal plasma blood flow, GFR, and sodium excretion.[25] Its vasoconstrictive properties contribute to the increased vascular resistance of heart failure. It is also associated with the growth of both the cardiac myocytes and the interstitial matrix, therefore promoting the LV remodeling process of heart failure[25] (Table 26-3). The effect of endothelin-receptor antagonism as a treatment for heart failure is currently being researched.

Vasopressin

Arginine vasopressin, thru its actions in the kidney, promotes sodium retention. Like endothelin it has also been shown to increase systemic vascular resistance. Binding of vasopressin to two distinct receptors (V1a and V2) results in body fluid regulation, vascular tone regulation, and cardiac contractility. The V1a receptors are

Table 26-3. Endothelin

Renal effects
Sodium retention
Vasoconstriction
Vascular effects
Vasoconstriction
Myocardial effects
Hypertrophy
Fibrosis
Neurohormonal effects
Stimulates renin release
Stimulates aldosterone release

located on the vascular smooth muscle and cardiac myocytes. Activation of this receptor, as result of increased vasopressin release stimulated by a reduction in pressure detected through baroreceptors, stimulates arteriole constriction. In addition, there are V1a receptors on platelets and lymphocytes that result in platelet aggregation and coagulation factor release.[26] In response to alterations in plasma tonicity, vasopressin is secreted from the posterior pituitary. Vasopressin then binds to the V2 receptor, which stimulates the production of cyclic 3,5-adenosine phosphate that activates protein kinase A. Protein kinase A activation results in the synthesis of aquaporin-2 water channel proteins. These channels allow free water to be reabsorbed in the collecting duct.

Therefore, the activation of the V1a and V2 receptors increases systemic vascular resistance, increases collecting duct permeability, and increases water reabsorption.[26] Vasopressin is elevated in patients with chronic heart failure, especially in patients with hyponatremia. In patients with heart failure, the stimulation of the baroreceptors as a result in the decrease in arterial pressure seems to outweigh the reduction that these patients have in osmolality, which would normally decrease vasopressin release. An increase in the number of aquaporin-2 water channels in the collecting duct also leads to free water retention and therefore hyponatremia in heart failure patients (Table 26-4).

Vasopressin release can also stimulate protein synthesis and cellular growth, leading to myocyte hypertrophy. Activation of the V1a receptor leads to activation of protein kinase C. Protein kinase C causes hypertrophic growth through secondary gene activation.[27] In addition to the direct effect on myocyte hypertrophy, vasopressin augments the renal and hemodynamic effects of norepinephrine and

Table 26-4. Vasopressin

Renal effects
Increased free water reabsorbtion

Vascular effects
Vasoconstriction

Myocardial effects
Increased fibrosis
Hypertrophy

Neurohormonal effects
Potentiates effects of angiotensin-II and norepinephrine

Table 26-5. Natriuretic Peptides

Renal effects
Promotes diuresis
Promotes natriuresis

Vascular effects
Vasodilates veins
Vasodilates arteries

Myocardial effects
Dilates coronary arteries, Lusitropy (causes cardiac relaxation)

Neurohormonal effects
Decreases aldosterone production
Decreases endothelin production

angiotensin, which further propagate the clinical syndrome of congestive heart failure. Therefore, through direct effects and synergistic interactions with other neurohormones, increased vasopressin leads to fluid retention, vasoconstriction, and myocyte hypertrophy.

Natriuretic Peptides

Natriuretic peptides are released from the atria (atrial natriuretic peptide [ANP]) and ventricles (BNP) in response to atrial and ventricular stress. ANP and BNP levels increase in a response to either volume expansion or pressure overload of the heart. Although ANP and BNP have similar physiologic properties, the secretion and turnover of the mRNA and BNP is faster, which in part accounts for its increased clinical utility. There are three main receptors for the natriuretic peptides. These receptors are found in target tissues and are members of the receptor guanylyl cyclase family. Activation of two of these receptors results in the production of cyclic guanosine monophosphate (cGMP), which mediates most of the physiologic properties of ANP and BNP. The third (type C) receptor is thought to be responsible for clearance of the natriuretic peptides.[28] Natriuretic peptides regulate the permeability of vascular system, cellular growth, cellular proliferation, and cardiac hypertrophy.[28] These mechanisms are the result of increased production of cGMP that in turn activates cGMP-dependent protein kinases (PKG). This interaction and stimulation of PKG acts as an antagonist to the myocyte growth that occurs during heart failure.[29]

The natriuretic peptides therefore act in a counter-regulatory fashion to the detrimental neurohormonal activation of the RAAS, adrenergic nervous system, and endothelin. Natriuretic peptides cause efferent renal arterial constriction, but afferent arterial dilation, which promotes increased diuresis and sodium excretion. In addition, the natriuretic peptides inhibit aldosterone and renin secretion and serve as physiologic antagonist to angiotensin-II. They promote vascular relaxation and blood pressure reduction by reducing sympathetic tone, and decreasing synthesis of catecholamines and endothelin-1.[20] Release of ANP and BNP may delay systemic and renal arterial vasoconstriction, venoconstriction, and sodium retention, therefore balancing the activation of the RAAS.[12] Through the increased production of cGMP, the natriuretic peptides decrease the activation of plasminogen activator-1 which induces the prothrombotic state of heart failure. However, in acute decompensated heart failure the release of stored natriuretic peptides and production of the peptides is insufficient to balance the vasoconstriction and fluid retention of the RAAS (Table 26-5).

BRADYKININ

Bradykinin is a hormone, which exerts pathophysiologic as well as pronounced beneficial physiologic effects, mainly by stimulation of BK B(2) receptors. Stimulation of BK B(2) receptors is not only implicated in the pathogenesis of inflammation, pain, and tissue injury, but also in powerful cardioprotective mechanisms. These are mainly triggered by the synthesis and release of the vasorelaxant, antihypertrophic and antiatherosclerotic endothelial mediators, nitric oxide, prostaglandins, and tissue-type plasminogen activator, by ischemic preconditioning and by an increase in insulin sensitivity.[29] It appears that in patients with LV hypertrophy and fluid overload there is an increase in BK B(2) receptors. Since the ACE is responsible to the degradation of BK, some of the benefits of the treatment with an ACE inhibitor are related to the elevation of BK levels.[30]

SUMMARY

The pathophysiology of heart failure is complex. Often it is difficult to identify the index event that leads to heart failure. Current concepts of heart failure pathophysiology not only include understanding the implications of hemodynamic derangements, but neurohormonal and inflammatory processes. The development of heart failure is caused by a paradoxical activation of neurohormonal regulatory systems that result in sodium retention, vascular remodeling, and vascular constriction. The regulatory neurohormonal systems that initially are activated as a stabilizing effort after an initial assault, chronically become maladaptive and result in LV remodeling and increased circulatory congestion. This neurohormonal activation acts as a positive feedback loop with the deleterious activation of the RAAS, adrenergic nervous system, increased production of endothelin and vasopressin, and activation of inflammatory proteins. The natriuretic systems act as a regulatory force to this feedback loop by inhibiting the cardiac effects of these hormones, inducing vasodilation and diuresis, and inhibiting the secretion of endothelin and angiotensin-II. Unfortunately, in patients with decompensated heart failure this regulatory system is overrun. This may be due to the downregulation of natriuretic peptide receptors, increased degradation of the natriuretic peptides, alteration of the natriuretic peptide itself, or decreased delivery to the colleting duct.[20] It is understanding the significance of the RAAS, sympathetic nervous system, natriuretic peptide system, and the inflammatory system that have led to improvements in therapy for these patients.

UNRESOLVED ISSUES

How will the knowledge of nuerohormonal activation of heart failure affect treatment? Current recommendations for the management of heart failure patients include the use of ACE inhibitors, aldosterone antagonist, and beta-blockers. Synthetic BNP, nesiritide, has been shown to be useful in the treatment of patients with acute and chronic heart failure. Trials are underway to determine the effect of vasopressin and endothelin antagonist.

What treatment options for acute decompensated heart failure should be performed due to the presence of poor prognostic indicators? Treatment of patients with acute decompensated heart failure is based on the patient's presentation and few studies have delineated appropriate interventions. In fact, despite numerous guidelines for a wide range of various medical conditions, no major medical society has promoted an acute decompensated heart failure treatment algorithm. Treatment today is still based on the response to individual clinical symptoms and is based on estimates of perfusion status and level of congestion. Elevations of BNP, although correlated well with prognosis, are more useful in the diagnostic phase of the evaluation of heart failure patient. There has been no E.D. study that has guided pharmacologic therapy based on BNP levels.

Can predictors of poor prognosis be used to guide triage decisions? Lee et al. recently published a risk stratification protocol for patients with acute decompensated heart failure. The stratification tool identifies patients based on risk for adverse events. Although a tool such as this can identify patients at risk for adverse events, disposition decisions in the emergency department setting are often based on symptomotology and available resources. In fact, the treatments used to manage these acute decompensated patients may guide the disposition decisions as much as clinician preference. For example, a patient on a nitroglycerin infusion is required to be admitted to the intensive care unit in some institutions. Unfortunately, there are no studies that have used prognostic indicators to guide treatment.

REFERENCES

1. Lee DS, Austin PC, Rouleau, et al. Predicting mortality among patients hospitalized for heart failure: Derivation and validation of a clinical model. *JAMA* 2003;290:2581–2587.
2. Harrison A, Morrison LK, Krishnaswamy P, et al. B-type natriuretic peptide predicts future cardiac events in patients presenting to the emergency department with dyspnea. *Ann Emerg Med* 2002;39(2):131–138.
3. Berger R, Huelsman M, Strecker K, et al. B-type natriuretic peptide predicts sudden death in patients with chronic heart failure. *Circulation* 2002;105(20):2392–2397.
4. Brophy JM, Deslauriers G, Rouleau JL. Long-term prognosis of patients presenting to the emergency room with decompensated congestive heart failure. *Can J Cardiol* 1994;10(5):543–547.
5. Hillege HL, van Gilst WH, van Veldhuisen DJ, et al. Accelerated decline and prognostic impact of renal function after myocardial infarction and the benefits of ACE inhibition: The CATS randomized trial. *Eur Heart J* 2003;24(5):412–420.
6. Kearney MT, Zaman A, Eckberg DL, et al. Cardiac size, autonomic function, and 5-year follow-up of chronic heart failure patients with severe prolongation of ventricular activity. *J Card Fail* 2003;9:93–99.

7. Nohria A, Tsang SW, Fang JC, et al. Clinical assessment identifies hemodynamic profiles that predict outcomes in patients admitted with heart failure. *J Am Coll Cardiol* 2003;41:1797–1804.

8. Francis GS, Tang WH. Pathophysiology of congestive heart failure. *Rev Cardiovasc Med* 2003;4:S14–S20.

9. Kitzman DW, Little WC, Brubaker PH, et al. Pathophysiological characterization of isolated diastolic heart failure in comparison to systolic heart failure. *JAMA* 2002;288:2144–2150.

10. Vasan RS, Larson MG, Benjamin EJ, et al. Left ventricular dilatation and the risk of congestive heart failure in people without myocardial infarction. *N Engl J Med* 1997;336:1350–1355.

11. Krum H, Gilbert RE. Demographics and concomitant disorders in heart failure. *Lancet* 2003;362:147–155.

12. Weber KT. Aldosterone in congestive heart failure. *N Engl J Med* 2001;345:1689–1697.

13. Wier MR, Dzau VJ. The renin-angiotensin-aldosterone system: A specific target for hypertension management. *Am J Hypertens* 1999;45:403–410.

14. Brewster UC, Setaro JF, Perazella MA. The renin-angiotensin-aldosterone system: Cardiorenal effects and implications for renal and cardiovascular disease states. *Am J Med Sci* 2003;326:15–24.

15. Wood AJJ. Angiotensin receptors and their antagonist. *N Engl J Med* 1996;16:1649–1654.

16. Floras JS. Sympathetic activation in human heart failure; diverse mechanisms, therapeutic opportunities. *Acta Physiol Scand* 2003;177:391–398.

17. Houser SR, Margulies KB. Is depressed myocyte contractility centrally involved in heart failure? *Circ Res* 2003;92:350–358.

18. Mansfield, D, Kaye DM, LaRocca HB, et al. Raised sympathetic nerve activity in heart failure and central sleep apnea is due to heart failure severity. *Circulation* 2003;107:1396–1400.

19. Esler M, Lambert G, Rocca B, et al. Sympathetic nerve activity and neurotransmitter release in humans: Translation from pathophysiology into clinical practice. *Acta Physiol Scand* 2003;177:275–284.

20. Schrier RW, Abraham WT. Hormones and hemodynamics in heart failure. *N Engl J Med* 1999;341:577–585.

21. Pugh PJ, Jones RD, Jones TH, et al. Heart failure as an inflammatory condition: Potential role for androgens as immune modulators. *Eur J Heart Fail* 2002;4:673–680.

22. Fledman AM, Kadokami T, Higuichi Y, et al. The role of anticytokine therapy in heart failure: Recent lessons from perclinical and clinical trials? *Med Clin North Am* 2003;87:419–440.

23. Boerrigter G, Burnett JC. Endothelin in neurohormonal activation in heart failure. *Coron Artery Dis* 2003;14:495–500.

24. Spieker LE, Luscher TF. Will endothelin receptor antagonist have a role in heart failure. *Med Clin North Am* 2003;87:459–474.

25. Luscher TF, Enseleit F, Pacher R, et al. Hemodynamic and neurohumoral effects of selective endothelin A (ET(A)) receptor blockade in chronic heart failure: The Heart Failure ET(A) Receptor Blockade Trial (HEAT). *Circulation* 2002;106:2666–2672.

26. Lee CR, Watkins ML, Patterson JH, et al. Vasopressin: A new target for the treatment of heart failure. *Am Heart J* 2003;146(1):9–18.

27. Nakanura Y, Haneda T, Osaki J, et al. Hypertrophic growth of cultured neonatal rat heart cells mediated by vasopressin V1a receptor. *Eur J Pharmacol* 2000;391:39–48.

28. Silberbach M, Roberts CT. Natriuretic peptide signaling; molecular, and cellular pathways to growth regulation. *Cell Signal* 2001;13:221–231.

29. Holtwick R, van Eickels M, Skryabin BV, et al. Pressure-independent cardiac hypertrophy in mice with cardiomyocyte-restricted inactivation of the atrial natriuretic peptide receptor guanylyl cyclase-A. *J Clin Invest* 2003;111:1399–1407.

30. Kofi T, Onishi K, Dahi K, et al. Addition of angiotensin II receptor antagonist to an ACE inhibitor in heart failure improves cardiovascular function by a bradykinin-mediated mechanism. *J Cardiovasc Pharmacol* 2003;41:632–639.

27

Diagnosis of Heart Failure

Alan B. Storrow
Chong Meng Seet

HIGH YIELD FACTS

- Dyspnea, especially on exertion, is the most common symptom of heart failure (HF) and is due in part to raised pulmonary venous and capillary pressures.

- The presence of jugular venous distention (JVD) and a third heart sound carries a particularly poor prognosis.

- There may be a lag in radiographic development of HF by several hours, and similarly, with clinical improvement radiographic resolution may take a few days.

- Brain or b-type natriuretic peptide (BNP) is most useful when it is normal because it has great predictive value in excluding HF.

- Confounders to BNP interpretation include that as creatinine clearance worsens the cut point for maximum diagnostic accuracy increases, and that right ventricular strain secondary to a pulmonary embolus will cause a 300–400 pg/mL rise in BNP.

- BNP and N-terminal pro-BNP (NT-BNP) do not give similar numerical results, although BNP and NT-BNP have been validated against left ventricular ejection fraction (LVEF) and have both been found to have similar test characteristics.

- Because only the kidney clears NT-BNP, it would be expected that renal disease would have a much greater impact on interpretation of NT-BNP results than BNP results.

INTRODUCTION

The high prevalence, increasing incidence, poor prognosis, and staggering health care burden of HF highlight the importance of accurate diagnosis in the emergency department (ED). Approximately 2% of the population, and up to 10% in the elderly, are affected with HF,[1] and 20 million additional persons are likely to become symptomatic in 1–5 years.[2]

Both hospitalization and the number of HF-related deaths are rising[3]; it is reportedly the leading diagnosis requiring inpatient care for those >65 years of age.[2] Despite advances in detection and treatment, prognosis after detection is appalling.[4–7] Establishing an accurate diagnosis early in the natural history not only facilitates current acute treatment, but also may assist with delays in subsequent chronic clinical progression.

Unfortunately, the undifferentiated nature of patients and wide presentation spectrum of HF can make the ED diagnosis a distinct challenge. While acute decompensation of HF accounts for the major cause of ED presentation, a first time diagnosis (HF of new onset) is common. Emergency physicians must be proficient at combining a complex of historical, examination, and laboratory factors in evaluation of patients with signs and symptoms of potential HF. While identification of HF is largely a bedside diagnosis, additional tests such as chest radiography and blood testing add to confirmation or exclusion.

DEFINITION

HF can be defined as the pathophysiologic state in which, at normal filling pressures, the heart is unable to pump sufficient blood to meet the metabolic needs of the body. Systemic perfusion may, however, be maintained by compensatory mechanisms but this will result in elevated filling pressure. HF can be classified in various ways such as systolic or diastolic, left- or right-sided, acute or chronic, and high or low output.

HF is not a specific disease entity but a broad clinical syndrome with many different etiologies (Table 27-1). In 1972, data from the Framingham study showed that hypertension was the most likely cause of HF,[8] but in recent decades, coronary artery disease has become most common.[9–12] This could be due to earlier diagnosis and better treatment of hypertension as well as the recognition that coronary artery disease is the more likely cause of HF in patients with both conditions. The etiology of HF may also vary with different populations. In developed countries, HF is usually due to coronary artery disease and hypertension, while in poorer countries HF may be more likely due to rheumatic valvular disease and nutritional deficiency state (e.g., thiamine deficiency).

In assessing a patient with HF, besides looking for the etiology, one must also search for precipitating causes

Table 27-1. Etiology of Heart Failure

Coronary artery disease
Valvular dysfunction (mitral or aortic/stenosis or
  regurgitation)
  Rheumatic heart disease
  Papillary muscle dysfunction
  Rupture of chordae tendinea
  Malfunction of prosthetic valve
Infective endocarditis
Cardiomyopathy
  Idiopathic dilated
  Hypertrophic
  Restrictive (e.g., hemochromatosis, amyloidosis,
    sarcoidosis)
Systemic hypertension
Myocarditis
  Viral
Chagas disease
  Radiation
  Autoimmune
Toxins
  Alcohol
  Adriamycin, doxorubicin
  Cocaine
Pericardial disorders
  Constrictive pericarditis
  Pericardial tamponade
Atrial myxoma
High-output states
  Anemia
  Thyrotoxicosis
Pregnancy
Arteriovenous fistula
Thiamine deficiency
  Paget disease

Table 27-2. Precipitating Causes of Heart Failure

Myocardial infarction or ischemia
Excessive dietary salt or fluid intake
Arrhythmias
  Atrial fibrillation/flutter
  Ventricular tachyarrhythmias
  Bradyarrhythmias
Uncontrolled hypertension
Noncompliance with heart failure medication
Negative inotropic drugs
  Beta-blockers
  Calcium-channel blockers
  Antiarrhythmic agents
Systemic infection
Pulmonary embolism
Acute valvular dysfunction
High-output states
  Anemia
  Hyperthyroidism
  Pregnancy

TRADITIONAL EVALUATION

Risk Factors

Risk factors for HF have been reported in various prospective cohort studies.[14–17] They include coronary heart disease, hypertension, diabetes, valvular heart disease, left ventricular hypertrophy, old age, male sex, and obesity. Data from the National Health and Nutrition Examination Survey III (NHANES III) have further identified smoking, physical inactivity, and lesser education as risk factors for HF.[18]

History

Symptoms of HF can be divided into those due to left- or right-sided HF. Left-sided HF gives rise to symptoms such as dyspnea, orthopnea, paroxysmal nocturnal dyspnea (PND), nocturia, feeling of fatigue, and altered mental state. Right-sided HF, on the other hand, usually results in gastrointestinal complaints such as anorexia, nausea, right upper abdominal pain, abdominal bloating, and peripheral edema.

Dyspnea

Dyspnea, especially on exertion, is the most common symptom of HF. It may be defined as an uncomfortable awareness of breathing, and, when it occurs at rest or at a level of activity where it is not expected, it is abnormal.

(Table 27-2). Patients with HF may be asymptomatic or mildly symptomatic due to compensatory mechanisms. However, in the presence of precipitating factors, they may decompensate and become more symptomatic. Without correcting the precipitating cause of the HF, treatment is often inadequate and ineffective. A substudy of a large, prospective trial[13] suggested that the most common precipitants of HF were noncompliance with salt restriction (22%), pulmonary infections (15%), or arrhythmias (13%).

Considering both the etiologies of HF and the precipitants of acute decompensation, emergency physicians evaluating patients with potential HF must focus on risk factors, history, physical examination, and ancillary tests.

Dyspnea is due, in part, to raised pulmonary venous and capillary pressures occurring as a result of failure of the left side of the heart. The rise in pulmonary venous pressure causes a shift of fluid into the interstitium of the lungs resulting in compression of the airways and alveoli. This increases the work of breathing, resulting in dyspnea. It usually increases in severity as the HF progresses and can be quantified by asking the patient how many steps or stairs he or she can take before they begin to feel breathless. Unfortunately, the complete mechanism of dyspnea, especially exertional dyspnea, is not well understood; it is likely due to other reasons beyond increased pulmonary capillary wedge pressure and decreased cardiac output.[19–22] An increase in respiratory rate (commonly >16 breaths/min) usually accompanies dyspnea and may be a sign of acute decompensation in a patient with known HF. Unfortunately, dyspnea is a nonspecific symptom and may occur with a wide variety of pulmonary, cardiac, chest wall, or even neurologic disorders.[23]

Orthopnea and Paroxysmal Nocturnal Dyspnea

Orthopnea and PND are other manifestations of HF due to pulmonary congestion. Orthopnea refers to breathlessness that occurs when lying flat and is relieved by sitting upright. It occurs as a result of the redistribution of water from the dependent parts of the body, such as the lower limbs, to the lungs in the recumbent position. It can be quantified by asking the patient how many pillows he or she requires in order to feel comfortable when sleeping. PND is another consequence of the redistribution of water from the dependent parts of the body to the lungs in the recumbent position. PND refers to severe breathlessness waking the patient up a few hours after he or she had fallen asleep and can be quite frightening to the patient. It is often associated with coughing.

Other Symptoms of Heart Failure

The patient with HF often complains of fatigue. This is due to the decreased cardiac output with consequent decreased skeletal muscle perfusion. The decreased oxygen supply to the skeletal muscles give rise to the feeling of fatigue, which progressively gets worse as the HF increases in severity. Like dyspnea, the complete mechanism of fatigue is uncertain and may be associated with abnormalities of skeletal muscle and other noncardiac problems such as anemia.

Another consequence of the redistribution of water in the recumbent position is nocturia. This refers to the increased frequency of urination at night, and is due to

increased renal perfusion in the recumbent position. In severe HF, decreased cardiac output causes a decrease in cerebral perfusion, which can result in an altered mental state. This happens more frequently in the elderly, and the patient may be confused and have difficulty remembering or concentrating.

Right-sided HF increases systemic venous pressure giving rise to gastrointestinal symptoms such as anorexia, nausea, right upper abdominal pain, and abdominal bloating. The increased systemic venous pressure also causes peripheral edema resulting in swelling of the dependent parts of the body such as the lower extremities and sacral region.

Physical Examination

Although limited in many respects, a thorough physical examination is important in the evaluation of the ED patient with potential HF. Findings may assist the physician in determining the cause and severity of the syndrome. An experienced caregiver may sense the severity shortly after meeting and observing the patient.

The patient is usually tachypreic, often with labored breathing, and may insist on sitting in an upright position. Tachycardia is usually present due to the increased sympathetic drive. The increased sympathetic drive also causes peripheral vasoconstriction resulting in cold, clammy, and pale extremities.

Rales (or crackles) are often present in both lungs as a result of the pulmonary congestion. They are usually inspiratory and extend upward from the lung bases, depending on the severity of the HF. Wheezing may be present due to bronchoconstriction from the surrounding edema (cardiac asthma). The lung bases may be dull to percussion due to presence of pleural effusion.

Auscultation in the ED is difficult, but may reveal some diagnostic information. A gallop rhythm, due to the presence of a third heart sound, may be heard. The third heart sound is due to decreased compliance of the left ventricle and is most commonly present in patients with volume overload and tachycardia. It is not particularly sensitive for left ventricular dysfunction,[24] but, when detected, is specific for elevated left ventricular pressure,[25] low ejection fraction,[26] and worse outcomes.[27–29] In severe cases, pulsus alternans may be present. This unusual finding refers to alternate strong and weak cardiac contractions detected by feeling the peripheral pulse; it is virtually diagnostic of severe advanced HF and often present in the terminally ill.[30]

Raised systemic venous pressure, due to right HF, results in JVD, peripheral edema, liver engorgement, and ascites. JVD assessment is likely the most important physical examination sign for estimating volume status. The patient should be observed, if possible, while at 45 degrees, and from the right side. The presence of JVD and a third heart sound carries a particularly poor prognosis.[26] Peripheral edema accumulates in dependent parts of the body and is usually present in the feet, ankles, and pretibial region of the legs in ambulatory patients. In bedridden patients, edema is usually found at the sacral regions. Ascites is due to both transudation of fluid into the peritoneal cavity, as well as elevation of pressure in the hepatic veins. Engorgement of the liver results in hepatomegaly, tenderness of the liver to palpation, hepatic pulsations. JVD may occur on compression of the liver, especially in patients with mild HF, a phenomenon referred to as the hepatojugular reflex (HJR).

Ancillary Tests

The ED evaluation of patients with potential new onset or acute decompensation of chronic HF is assisted by numerous ancillary tests. Definitive diagnosis is provided by right-heart catheterization. However, this is an invasive procedure and is not done in the ED, and rarely for diagnostic purposes only. HF can be diagnosed indirectly by measuring the ejection fraction by means of echocardiography or radionuclide scanning. Echocardiography also allows the chamber size, wall motions, and valvular functions to be assessed. Radionuclide scanning can also assess areas of hypokinesia and akinesia. However, these tests are not immediately available in the ED setting.

While ED history and examination findings can suggest an increased likelihood of HF, objective tools improve diagnostic accuracy. Foremost among these are chest radiography, electrocardiography, and selected blood tests.

Chest Radiography

The chest radiograph initially shows upper lobe diversion as the pulmonary blood redistributes to the upper portion of the lungs. With further increase in the pulmonary capillary wedge pressure, fluid starts to accumulate in the interstitial spaces, resulting in Kerley B lines. In the final stages, fluid accumulates in the alveoli, resulting in the classic perihilar butterfly infiltrates. On the x-ray, the cardiac shadow is often enlarged (cardiothoracic ratio of more than 50%) and there may be presence of unilateral (more often on the right side) or bilateral pleural effusions. Unfortunately, 20% of cardiomegaly seen on echocardiography is missed on chest radiography,[31] the cardiothoracic ratio is poor in predicting left ventricular dysfunction,[32] and pulmonary congestion

can be minimal or absent even with significantly elevated pulmonary artery wedge pressures.[33]

While radiographic findings of pulmonary congestion may precede the presence of rales, the changes sometimes do not correlate well with the patient's clinical condition. There may be a lag in radiographic development of HF by several hours, and, similarly, with clinical improvement radiographic resolution may take a few days.

Electrocardiography

The electrocardiogram (ECG) is not helpful in diagnosing HF, although it frequently shows abnormalities. Evidence of ischemia, acute myocardial infarction, or sustained arrhythmias may help establish a precipitating cause. Atrial fibrillation develops in around one-third of patients with HF,[34] is a frequent cause of decompensation,[35,36] and represents a worse prognosis than in those who maintain sinus rhythm.[37] Intraventricular conduction delays are present in up to 25% of patients with HF, and are also a prognostic marker of adverse outcome.[7] In chronic HF, the ECG often shows evidence of chamber hypertrophy, Q waves from old myocardial infarction, dysrhythmias, or conduction defects.

Blood Testing

Most blood tests, except for the natriuretic peptides, are not helpful for establishing a diagnosis of HF. However, it is recommended that in new-onset HF, and acute decompensation of chronic HF, that these patients undergo some routine testing.

Serum sodium and potassium may be altered due to activation of the renin-angiotensin-aldosterone-system (RAAS), as well as by diuretic treatment. Hyponatremia has shown correlation with worse prognosis, as has worsening renal function. A complete blood count may reveal support for underlying infection or anemia; both may serve as a precipitating cause. Arterial blood gases are helpful in assessing the acid-base and gas exchange status of patients with severe HF. They may show metabolic acidosis (from lactate accumulation due to inadequate perfusion of tissues), hypoxemia, and respiratory acidosis.

Clinical Scoring Scales

Sole reliance on the aforementioned tools to distinguish between cardiac and noncardiac causes of dyspnea is often challenging. While signs and symptoms of fluid overload raise the suspicion of HF, their lack of sensitivity makes them poor screening tools.[38] The frequent limitations of this information have been extensively reported.[24,31–33,38–46] As a result, tools such as the Framingham criteria[6,47] and

Boston criteria[48] have been used to assist in the diagnosis of HF. The Framingham criteria (Table 27-3) uses major and minor clinical findings to establish a diagnosis of HF, while the Boston criteria (Table 27-4) uses a point system, such that a higher score is associated with a greater possibility of HF. Unfortunately, point scoring systems completely miss patients with asymptomatic HF, which is why the American Heart Association scoring system identifies asymptomatic patients with significant risk factors as in the initial stages of HF.

DIAGNOSTIC ADVANCEMENTS—THE NATRIURETIC PEPTIDES

It has been known for about 50 years that the heart is a cardiorespiratory and an endocrine organ. Hemodynamic changes and neurohormonal activation are caused by left ventricular dysfunction. The sympathetic nervous system, RAAS, and endothelin pathway are activated to maintain blood pressure, improve perfusion, and increase chronotropy (heart rate) and inotropy (strength of contraction). It is well known, however, that prolonged activation of these systems may lead to deleterious effects such as hypertrophy, fibrosis and apoptosis (programmed cell death).

The natriuretic peptides represent a counter-regulatory system. They unload the failing heart through diuresis, natriuresis, and vasodilation by suppressing the RAAS and endothelin. These peptides are secreted in response

Table 27-3. Framingham Criteria*

Major Criteria	Minor Criteria
Paroxysmal nocturnal dyspnea	Ankle edema
	Night cough
Orthopnea	Dyspnea on exertion
Neck-vein distention	Hepatomegaly
Rales	Pleural effusion
Cardiomegaly	Vital capacity
Acute pulmonary edema	decreased 50%
Maximum	HR >120/min
S₃ gallop	
Increased venous pressure >16 cm of water	
Circulation time ≥25 s	
Hepatojugular reflux	
Major or minor criteria†	

*Diagnosis of heart failure with two major, or one major and two minor criteria are required.
†Weight loss ≥4.5 kg in 5 days in response to treatment.

Table 27-4. Boston Criteria for Diagnosing Heart Failure*

History	
Dyspnea at rest	4
Orthopnea	4
Paroxysmal nocturnal dyspnea	3
Dyspnea while walking	2
Dyspnea while climbing stairs	1
Chest x-ray	
Alveolar pulmonary edema	4
Interstitial pulmonary edema	3
Bilateral pleural effusions	3
Cardiothoracic ratio >0.5	3
Kerley A lines	2
Physical examination	
HR 91–110 bpm	1
HR >110 bpm	2
JVD >6 cm H₂	2
JVD and edema or hepatomegaly	3
Basilar rales	1

*Diagnosis of heart failure—definite (score 8–12 points), possible (score 5–7 points), and unlikely (score ≤4 points). HR, heart rate; JVD, jugular venous distention.

to hemodynamic stress, with higher stress resulting in higher levels of secretion.

The natriuretic peptides are promising markers of myocardial dysfunction and HF. In 1956, electron microscopy was used to demonstrate granules present in the atria that were absent in the ventricle.[49] Henry and Pearce observed an increase in urine flow when a balloon was inflated in the atrium of a dog.[50] Influenced by these initial investigations, subsequent studies have identified three natriuretic peptides: atrial natriuretic peptide (ANP, predominantly secreted from atrial myocardium), brain or b-type natriuretic peptide (BNP, predominantly secreted from ventricular myocardium), c-type natriuretic peptide (CNP, predominantly secreted from vascular endothelium) (Fig. 27-1), and d-type natriuretic peptide (DNP, predominantly secreted by the kidney).

Of these peptides, BNP has received the most study. BNP is released under conditions of increased myocardial pressure and stretching, and possesses vasodilatory and natriuretic properties. It is released as a prohormone and on secretion from the myocyte, is cleaved into the biologically active BNP (32 amino acids in length) and the biologically inactive NT-BNP (76 amino acids) (Fig. 27-2). BNP is primarily removed by natriuretic peptide receptors with a small amount of renal clearance, while the kidney primarily clears NT-BNP (Table 27-5).

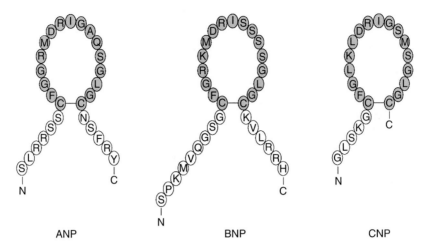

Fig. 27-1. Biochemical structure of the natriuretic peptides.

BNP and NT-BNP assays have generally proven superior in diagnostic accuracy and clinical performance as prognostic markers than ANP, or its precursor NT-ANP.[51] BNP and NT-BNP have both received attention as markers useful for the diagnosis or exclusion of HF in ED patients. Furthermore, the Task Force of the European Society of Cardiology for the Diagnosis and Treatment of Chronic HF has recommended that a cardiac natriuretic hormone assay be included in the initial evaluation of HF.[52]

BNP

The Breathing Not Properly Multinational Study confirmed findings from pilot studies that BNP was useful as a diagnostic marker in patients presenting to the ED with undifferentiated dyspnea[53] (Fig. 27-3). A BNP value less than 100 pg/mL frequently excludes HF as a cause of dyspnea (sensitivity = 90%, specificity = 76%, negative predictive value, NPV = 89%), while a patient with a BNP value over 400 pg/mL is highly likely to have HF.[54] However, there were a small percentage of patients with a history of HF but "no acute exacerbation" that did have BNP values over 100 pg/mL. An intermediate BNP (100–400 pg/mL) needs to be interpreted in the context of the patient's clinical evaluation and have been termed "grey zone" values (Fig. 27-4). In this population, a BNP value of >100 pg/mL was more accurate (83%) than the commonly used Framingham criteria (73%).

While BNP is helpful at levels <100 and >400 pg/mL, there are some other confounders when using the test. The cutoff levels mentioned above for patients with normal creatinine clearance do not apply to patients with renal insufficiency. In a separate analysis of the BNP study, it was found that as creatinine clearance worsened the cutoff point for maximum diagnostic accuracy increased as well.[55] For example, patients with noncardiac dyspnea

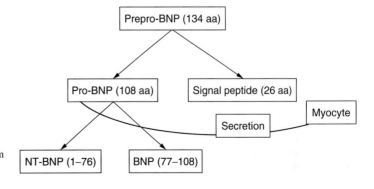

Fig. 27-2. Secretion of NT-BNP and BNP from the myocyte.

Table 27-5. Characteristics of BNP and NT-BNP

Characteristic	BNP	NT-BNP
Size	32 AA	76 AA
Half-life	20 min	60–90 min
Stability	Up to 4 h at room temperature	Up to 6 h at room temperature
Clearance	Natriuretic peptide receptor-C (NPR-C) endopeptidase, kidney	Kidney

and moderately reduced renal function (estimated GFR = 30–59 mL/min/1.73 m^2) had a mean BNP level over 200 pg/mL (Fig. 27-5). However, nearly 90% of subjects with a BNP value of ≥500 pg/mL had HF regardless of the severity of renal insufficiency. In addition, right ventricular strain secondary to a pulmonary embolus will cause a 300–400 pg/mL rise in BNP.[56,57] Knowledge of a patient's compensated "dry weight" BNP would be useful during an acute decompensation, similar to baseline peak flows in an asthmatic with an acute asthma exacerbation (Fig. 27-6).

The BNP study also demonstrated that those patients with diastolic dysfunction had significant elevations in BNP, compared with those patients without HF; the median BNP was 413 pg/mL in diastolic dysfunction and 821 pg/mL in systolic dysfunction.[58]

Age and gender also appear to have an influence on BNP levels. Redfield and colleagues evaluated 2042 randomly selected residents of Olmstead County, Minnesota and found that in the normal subgroup of patients ($n = 767$) that BNP values were significantly higher in women compared with men ($P < 0.001$) and that BNP values increased with age within each gender.[59]

Because BNP is increased during increases in ventricular wall stretch, it tends to correlate with symptoms of HF, especially dyspnea. There is a high degree of correlation with the New York Heart Association functional class, a classification schema based on the extent of patient's disability (Fig. 27-7).

Finally, there has been a report of BNP levels <100 pg/mL, despite the clinical presentation of decompensated HF.[60] When this occurs, these patients tended to be female, morbidly obese, and have a higher rate of atrial fibrillation. Because one of BNP's metabolic pathways includes degradation by neutral endopeptidase, which may be present in elevated levels in the morbidly obese, it has been hypothesized that this contributes to the relatively lower BNP concentration in these patients.

BNP Summary

BNP is most useful when it is normal because it has great predictive value in excluding HF. With a high sensitivity and negative predictive value at a cutoff of 100 pg/mL, it is highly unlikely that subjects with BNPs ≤100 pg/mL have HF. Above 400 pg/mL, it is highly likely the patient suffers from decompensated HF. However, a minority of

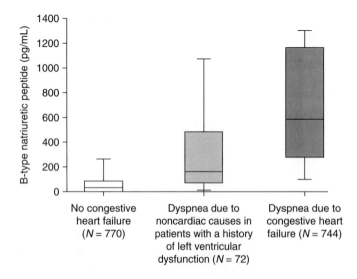

Fig. 27-3. Data from the BNP Multinational Study. Box plots showing median levels of BNP in the three groups of ED patients. Boxes show interquartile range and bars represent highest and lowest values. (Source: Reprinted with permission from Maisel AS, Krishnaswamy P, Nowak RM, et al. Rapid measurement of B-type natriuretic peptide in the emergency diagnosis of heart failure. *N Engl J Med* 2002;347(3):161–167.)

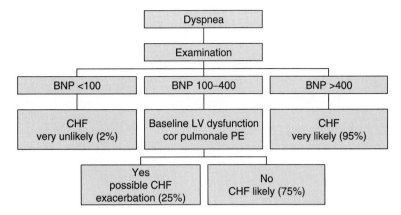

Fig. 27-4. General BNP decision tree.

patients will have "baseline" or "dry weight" BNP values well above this level. In the area of 100–400 pg/mL, BNP requires clinical correlation because of the effect of age, sex, and other disease processes.

NT-BNP

While it has not been validated to the extent of BNP, especially in the ED setting of undifferentiated dyspnea, recent studies of NT-BNP have confirmed earlier findings that it is an accurate marker of left ventricular dys-

function.[61-63] BNP and NT-BNP correlated well with each other ($r^2 = 0.94$) and were predictive of New York Heart Association functional class and ejection fraction in ambulatory patients. NT-BNP proved to be a strong marker of reduced systolic function (EF < 40%) in a cohort of 2193 patients admitted to a general hospital. Those patients with reduced systolic function were detected at a sensitivity of 78%, specificity of 76%, NPV of 96%, and positive predictive value (PPV) of 30%. These findings were similar to earlier studies performed with BNP.[64] One would expect overall lower diagnostic test

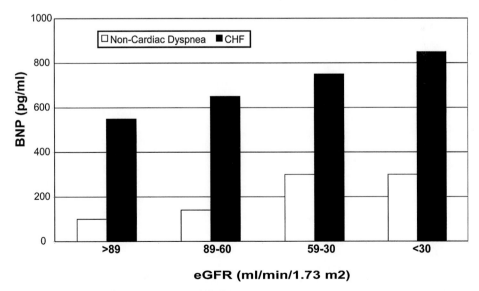

Fig. 27-5. Mean BNP values by kidney function and final diagnosis of HF or noncardiac dyspnea. (Source: Reprinted with permission from McCullough PA, Duc P, Omland T, et al. B-type natriuretic peptide and renal function in the diagnosis of heart failure: An analysis from the Breathing Not Properly Multinational Study. *Am J Kidney Dis* 2003;41(3):571–579.)

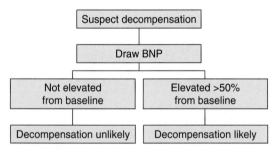

Fig. 27-6. BNP decision tree in a patient with known baseline (dry weight) values.

characteristics when an assay is compared solely to LVEF because there is a large cohort of patients with diastolic dysfunction that would have elevated NT-BNP values but have normal LVEF. This study also found that both serum creatinine and age added significant information when predicting a reduced LVEF.

In 415 ambulatory patients with possible HF, NT-BNP increased as EF worsened (Table 27-3).[65] It was less helpful in patients with diastolic dysfunction, especially those with only mild relaxation abnormalities. Interestingly, while NT-BNP was helpful in those subjects where the examining cardiologist felt there was a "strong" (NT-BNP = 227 pmol/L) or "no" (NT-BNP = 66 pmol/L) suspicion of HF, it was not

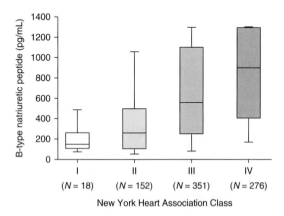

Fig. 27-7. Box plots showing median levels of b-type natriuretic peptide among patients in each of the four New York Heart Association Classifications. Boxes show interquartile ranges, and I bars represent highest and lowest values. (Source: Reprinted with permission from Maisel AS, Krishnaswamy P, Nowak RM, et al. Rapid measurement of B-type natriuretic peptide in the emergency diagnosis of heart failure. *N Engl J Med* 2002;347(3):161–167.)

helpful in the group with "moderate" clinical suspicion of HF (mean NT-BNP = 85 pmol/L vs. 73 pmol/L in normal subjects). This clinical scenario may be similar to the "intermediate" level seen with the BNP assay (100–400 pg/mL) where clinical suspicion combined with BNP levels may be most helpful. While those with creatinine >130 µmol/L had a significantly elevated NT-BNP compared to those with normal creatinine (NT-BNP = 173 pmol/L vs. 81 pmol/L, $P < 0.0001$), multiple logistic regression revealed no correlation between creatinine and NT-BNP. Similar to previous studies, after multiple logistic regression, age >75 years predicted an increased NT-BNP. The age-dependence of the NT-BNP assay was also seen in a study of 243 consecutive healthy subjects with no history of cardiovascular illness or HF risk factors. The authors suggested the normal NT-BNP cutoff for subjects <50 years should be 100 pg/mL and the normal cutoff for subjects >50 years should be 200 pg/mL.

NT-BNP and BNP Summary

It is challenging to compare studies of BNP and NT-BNP due to differing populations, study designs, gold standards, clinical settings, and immunoassays. However, BNP and NT-BNP have been validated against LVEF and have both been found to have similar test characteristics. While BNP increases with age and sex, NT-BNP seems to do so at a much greater degree. A number of studies have found age-appropriate cutoffs for NT-BNP, and one of the commercially available assays suggests two cutoffs based on age (age <75 normal cutoff = 125 pg/mL, age ≥75 normal cutoff = 450 pg/mL). Both BNP and NT-BNP are elevated in patients with renal insufficiency even though they may have no clinical or echocardiographic evidence of HF. While BNP's relationship to creatinine clearance has been well defined (>90% chance of HF when BNP > 500 pg/mL), the relationship with NT-BNP is less well delineated. Because only the kidney clears NT-BNP it would be expected that renal disease would have a much greater impact on interpretation of NT-BNP results than BNP results. Finally, both BNP[53] and NT-BNP have been confirmed in an ED population using hospital discharge diagnosis of HF as the gold standard (capturing both systolic and diastolic dysfunction).

SUMMARY

Emergency physicians must be proficient at combining a complex of historical, examination, and laboratory factors in evaluation of patients with potential HF. While there are limitations to traditional signs and symptoms in the diagnosis of HF, attention to this condition as a broad clinical syndrome with many acute precipitants and risk factors will assist in this challenge.

The natriuretic hormones BNP and NT-BNP have proven utility in the evaluation of undifferentiated ED patients with dyspnea, and are particularly useful in excluding the presence of HF in individual patients. These findings represent the rationale for choosing such an assay as part of the initial ED work-up of possible HF.

REFERENCES

1. Association AH. *Heart and Stroke Statistical Update*, 2001.
2. Graves EJ, Gillum BS. 1994 summary: National Hospital Discharge Survey. *Adv Data* 1996;(278):1–12.
3. Hoes AW, Mosterd A, Grobbee DE. An epidemic of heart failure? Recent evidence from Europe. *Eur Heart J* 1998; 19(Suppl L):L2–L9.
4. Mosterd A, Cost B, Hoes AW, et al. The prognosis of heart failure in the general population: The Rotterdam Study. *Eur Heart J* 2001;22(15):1318–1327.
5. Cowie MR, Wood DA, Coats AJ, et al. Survival of patients with a new diagnosis of heart failure: A population based study. *Heart* 2000;83(5):505–510.
6. Ho KK, Anderson KM, Kannel WB, et al. Survival after the onset of congestive heart failure in Framingham Heart Study subjects. *Circulation* 1993;88(1):107–115.
7. Senni M, Tribouilloy CM, Rodeheffer RJ, et al. Congestive heart failure in the community: A study of all incident cases in Olmsted County, Minnesota, in 1991. *Circulation* 1998; 98(21):2282–2289.
8. Kannel WB, Castelli WP, McNamara PM, et al. Role of blood pressure in the development of congestive heart failure. The Framingham study. *N Engl J Med* 1972;287(16):781–787.
9. Kannel WB, Ho K, Thom T. Changing epidemiological features of cardiac failure. *Br Heart J* 1994;72(2 Suppl): S3–S9.
10. Fox KF, Cowie MR, Wood DA, et al. Coronary artery disease as the cause of incident heart failure in the population. *Eur Heart J* 2001;22(3):228–236.
11. Massie BM, Shah NB. Evolving trends in the epidemiologic factors of heart failure: Rationale for preventive strategies and comprehensive disease management. *Am Heart J* 1997;133(6):703–712.
12. Gheorghiade M, Bonow RO. Chronic heart failure in the United States: A manifestation of coronary artery disease. *Circulation* 1998;97(3):282–289.
13. Tsuyuki RT, McKelvie RS, Arnold JM, et al. Acute precipitants of congestive heart failure exacerbations. *Arch Intern Med* 2001;161(19):2337–2342.
14. Kannel WB, D'Agostino RB, Silbershatz H, et al. Profile for estimating risk of heart failure. *Arch Intern Med* 1999; 159(11):1197–1204.
15. Levy D, Larson MG, Vasan RS, et al. The progression from hypertension to congestive heart failure. *JAMA* 1996; 275(20):1557–1562.
16. Chen YT, Vaccarino V, Williams CS, et al. Risk factors for heart failure in the elderly: A prospective community-based study. *Am J Med* 1999;106(6):605–612.
17. Chae CU, Pfeffer MA, Glynn RJ, et al. Increased pulse pressure and risk of heart failure in the elderly. *JAMA* 1999;281(7):634–639.
18. He J, Ogden LG, Bazzano LA, et al. Risk factors for congestive heart failure in US men and women: NHANES I epidemiologic follow-up study. *Arch Intern Med* 2001;161(7):996–1002.
19. Francis GS, Goldsmith SR, Cohn JN. Relationship of exercise capacity to resting left ventricular performance and basal plasma norepinephrine levels in patients with congestive heart failure. *Am Heart J* 1982;104(4 Pt 1):725–731.
20. Franciosa JA, Ziesche S, Wilen M. Functional capacity of patients with chronic left ventricular failure. Relationship of bicycle exercise performance to clinical and hemodynamic characterization. *Am J Med* 1979;67(3):460–466.
21. Franciosa JA, Park M, Levine TB. Lack of correlation between exercise capacity and indexes of resting left ventricular performance in heart failure. *Am J Cardiol* 1981;47(1):33–39.
22. Benge W, Litchfield RL, Marcus ML. Exercise capacity in patients with severe left ventricular dysfunction. *Circulation* 1980;61(5):955–959.
23. Wasserman K. Dyspnea on exertion. Is it the heart or the lungs? *JAMA* 1982;248(16):2039–2043.
24. Davie AP, Francis CM, Caruana L, et al. Assessing diagnosis in heart failure: Which features are any use? *QJM* 1997;90(5):335–339.
25. Patel R, Bushnell DL, Sobotka PA. Implications of an audible third heart sound in evaluating cardiac function. *West J Med* 1993;158(6):606–609.
26. Drazner MH, Rame JE, Stevenson LW, et al. Prognostic importance of elevated jugular venous pressure and a third heart sound in patients with heart failure. *N Engl J Med* 2001;345(8):574–581.
27. Rame JE, Dries DL, Drazner MH. The prognostic value of the physical examination in patients with chronic heart failure. *Congest Heart Fail* 2003;9(3):170–175, 178.
28. Glover DR, Littler WA. Factors influencing survival and mode of death in severe chronic ischaemic cardiac failure. *Br Heart J* 1987;57(2):125–132.
29. Spodick D, Quarry V. Prevalence of the fourth heart sound by phonocardiography in the absence of cardiac disease. *Am Heart J* 1974;87(1):11–14.
30. Lee YC, Sutton FJ. Pulsus alternans in patients with congestive cardiomyopathy. *Circulation* 1982;65(7):1533–1534.
31. Kono T, Suwa M, Hanada H, et al. Clinical significance of normal cardiac silhouette in dilated cardiomyopathy—evaluation based upon echocardiography and magnetic resonance imaging. *Jpn Circ J* 1992;56(4):359–365.
32. Clark AL, Coats AJ. Unreliability of cardiothoracic ratio as a marker of left ventricular impairment: Comparison with radionuclide ventriculography and echocardiography. *Postgrad Med J* 2000;76(895):289–291.
33. Mahdyoon H, Klein R, Eyler W, et al. Radiographic pulmonary congestion in end-stage congestive heart failure. *Am J Cardiol* 1989;63(9):625–627.

34. Middlekauff HR, Stevenson WG, Stevenson LW. Prognostic significance of atrial fibrillation in advanced heart failure. A study of 390 patients. *Circulation* 1991;84(1):40–48.

35. De Ferrari GM, Tavazzi L. The role of arrhythmias in the progression of heart failure. *Eur J Heart Fail* 1999;1(1):35–40.

36. Opasich C, Febo O, Riccardi PG, et al. Concomitant factors of decompensation in chronic heart failure. *Am J Cardiol* 1996;78(3):354–357.

37. Mathew J, Hunsberger S, Fleg J, et al. Incidence, predictive factors, and prognostic significance of supraventricular tachyarrhythmias in congestive heart failure. *Chest* 2000; 118(4):914–922.

38. Stevenson LW, Perloff JK. The limited reliability of physical signs for estimating hemodynamics in chronic heart failure. *JAMA* 1989;261(6):884–888.

39. Badgett RG, Lucey CR, Mulrow CD. Can the clinical examination diagnose left-sided heart failure in adults? *JAMA* 1997;277(21):1712–1719.

40. Zema MJ. Diagnosing heart failure by the Valsalva maneuver: Isn't It finally time? *Chest* 1999;116(4):851–853.

41. Zema MJ, Masters AP, Margouleff D. Dyspnea: The heart or the lungs? Differentiation at bedside by use of the simple Valsalva maneuver. *Chest* 1984;85(1):59–64.

42. Zema MJ, Restivo B, Sos T, et al. Left ventricular dysfunction—bedside Valsalva maneuver. *Br Heart J* 1980;44(5):560–569.

43. Rihal CS, Davis KB, Kennedy JW, et al. The utility of clinical, electrocardiographic, and roentgenographic variables in the prediction of left ventricular function. *Am J Cardiol* 1995; 75(4):220–223.

44. Silver MT, Rose GA, Paul SD, et al. A clinical rule to predict preserved left ventricular ejection fraction in patients after myocardial infarction. *Ann Intern Med* 1994;121(10):750–756.

45. Packer M, Cohn JN. Consensus recommendations for the management of chronic heart failure. *Am J Cardiol* 1997; 83(Suppl 1):A-38A.

46. Bales AC, Sorrentino MJ. Causes of congestive heart failure. Prompt diagnosis may affect prognosis. *Postgrad Med* 1997;101(1):44–49, 54–56.

47. McKee PA, Castelli WP, McNamara PM, et al. The natural history of congestive heart failure: The Framingham study. *N Engl J Med* 1971;285(26):1441–1446.

48. Mosterd A, Deckers JW, Hoes AW, et al. Classification of heart failure in population based research: An assessment of six heart failure scores. *Eur J Epidemiol* 1997;13(5):491–502.

49. Kisch B. Electron microscopy of the atrium of the heart. *Exp Med Surg* 1956;14:99–112.

50. Henry JP, Pearce JW. The possible role of cardiac stretch receptors in the induction of changes in urine flow. *J Physiol* 1956;131:572–594.

51. Clerico A, Emdin M. Diagnostic accuracy and prognostic relevance of the measurement of cardiac natriuretic peptides: A review. *Clin Chem* 2004;50(1):33–50.

52. Remme WJ, Swedberg K. Guidelines for the diagnosis and treatment of chronic heart failure. *Eur Heart J* 2001; 22(17):1527–1560.

53. Maisel AS, Krishnaswamy P, Nowak RM, et al. Rapid measurement of B-type natriuretic peptide in the emergency diagnosis of heart failure. *N Engl J Med* 2002;347(3): 161–167.

54. Maisel A. B-type natriuretic peptide measurements in diagnosing congestive heart failure in the dyspneic emergency department patient. *Rev Cardiovasc Med* 2002;3(Suppl 4): S10–S17.

55. McCullough PA, Duc P, Omland T, et al. B-type natriuretic peptide and renal function in the diagnosis of heart failure: An analysis from the Breathing Not Properly Multinational Study. *Am J Kidney Dis* 2003;41(3):571–579.

56. Kucher N, Printzen G, Goldhaber SZ. Prognostic role of brain natriuretic peptide in acute pulmonary embolism. *Circulation* 2003;107(20):2545–2547.

57. ten Wolde M, Tulevski II, Mulder JW, et al. Brain natriuretic peptide as a predictor of adverse outcome in patients with pulmonary embolism. *Circulation* 2003;107(16):2082–2084.

58. Maisel AS, McCord J, Nowak RM, et al. Bedside B-Type natriuretic peptide in the emergency diagnosis of heart failure with reduced or preserved ejection fraction. Results from the Breathing Not Properly Multinational Study. *J Am Coll Cardiol* 2003;41(11):2010–2017.

59. Redfield MM, Rodeheffer RJ, Jacobsen SJ, et al. Plasma brain natriuretic peptide concentration: Impact of age and gender. *J Am Coll Cardiol* 2002;40(5):976–982.

60. Tang WHW, Girod JP, Lee MJ, et al. Plasma B-type natriuretic peptide levels in ambulatory patients with established chronic symptomatic systolic HF. *Circulation* 2003;108:2964–2966.

61. Groenning BA, Nilsson JC, Sondergaard L, et al. Detection of left ventricular enlargement and impaired systolic function with plasma N-terminal pro brain natriuretic peptide concentrations. *Am Heart J* 2002;143(5):923–929.

62. Hammerer-Lercher A, Puschendorf B, Mair J. Cardiac natriuretic peptides: New laboratory parameters in heart failure patients. *Clin Lab* 2001;47(5/6):265–277.

63. McDonagh TA, Robb SD, Murdoch DR, et al. Biochemical detection of left-ventricular systolic dysfunction. *Lancet* 1998;351(9095):9–13.

64. Dao Q, Krishnaswamy P, Kazanegra R, et al. Utility of B-type natriuretic peptide in the diagnosis of congestive heart failure in an urgent-care setting. *J Am Coll Cardiol* 2001;37(2):379–385.

65. Alehagen U, Lindstedt G, Eriksson H, et al. Utility of the amino-terminal fragment of pro-brain natriuretic peptide in plasma for the evaluation of cardiac dysfunction in elderly patients in primary health care. *Clin Chem* 2003;49(8): 1337–1346.

28

Heart Failure Management in the Emergency Department

Douglas S. Ander

HIGH YIELD FACTS

- Recognition that heart failure (HF) is a neurohormonal disease.
- Therapeutic plans should be established based on a bedside assessment of hemodynamic parameters.
- Vasodilators in combination with loop diuretics are the primary treatment choices for the fluid overloaded patient.
- Nesiritide significantly improves filling pressures and blocks the neurohormonal derangements of HF.
- Inotropic and pressor support should be limited to patients with evidence of hypoperfusion.
- Common medications used in the treatment of chronic HF include diuretics, digoxin, nitrates, angiotensin-converting enzyme (ACE) inhibitors, beta-blockers, and spironolactone.

INTRODUCTION

Heart failure is a common diagnosis facing approximately 4,900,000 people. Over the past three decades we have seen a significant rise in the number of hospital discharges for HF[1] and since the majority of admitted patients enter through the emergency department (ED), proper initial management is important. Treatment instituted by the emergency physician can have a significant impact on the patient's short-term prognosis and hospital course. The overall goal in the ED is to reduce filling pressures and provide symptomatic improvement.

HF is a clinical spectrum and not a specific diagnosis. Patients will have a wide variety of presentations.

Patients may present to the ED with minimal symptoms such as mild dyspnea or weight gain. Conversely, they may present with evidence of significant fluid overload. Independent of their fluid status the same patient may present to the ED with adequate perfusion or evidence of shock. Some physicians use the term congestive HF for every patient presenting to the ED with abnormal cardiac function. However, not all patients presenting to the ED with a diagnosis of HF will have clinical evidence of fluid overload. Consequently, the term "congestive" does not adequately define the possible range of presentations to the ED.

Recognition that HF patients may fall into different categories allows the clinician to tailor treatment based on their initial assessment of the hemodynamic parameters. Using components of the history and physical examination, and potentially bioimpedance hemodynamic monitoring, the clinician can develop a treatment plan individualized to that patient. Diuretics, vasodilators, ACE inhibitors (ACEI), noninvasive ventilation, and new agents such as the natriuretic peptides can be customized to the patient's hemodynamic and symptomatic needs. The fact that HF is a neurohormonal process and not only a hemodynamic problem is important in considering the therapeutic interventions. Certain agents (e.g., inotropes) historically felt to be efficacious in the treatment of HF may be deleterious. Furthermore, newer agents that address both the neurohormonal and hemodynamic aspects of HF may provide added benefit to the patient.

The emergency physician plays a key role in the initial evaluation and management of HF patients. With the improved outpatient treatment of HF, the aging of America, and growing ED volumes, the importance of the emergency physician in HF management is apparent. The emergency physician needs to have a firm understanding of the hemodynamic classifications of acute exacerbations of HF and an evidence-based medicine approach to its treatment in the ED. This chapter will provide the emergency physician with an understanding of the principles of HF management in the ED. Each agent or therapeutic intervention will be reviewed in detail including a review of published trials. The role of each modality within the overall ED management of HF will be explained. Additionally, the role played by several outpatient medications will be reviewed. Although the emergency physician will most likely not be using medications such as beta-blockers, spironolactone, and angiotensin receptor blockers, they should be aware of their indications, the literature supporting their use, and any potential impact on ED care. Finally, there will be a brief review of several emerging medications designed to counteract the adverse neurohormonal processes seen in HF.

INITIAL STABILIZATION

There are several required steps during the first few minutes of a patient's arrival to the ED with dyspnea and presumed HF. The first is initial stabilization of the clinical condition. This is followed by an evaluation that includes laboratories, radiographs, and a search for reversible causes including ischemia and arrhythmias, all while considering any available advanced directives by the patient. Finally, treatment is instituted based on an assessment of the hemodynamic status.

Patients presenting to the ED with a presumed exacerbation of HF require an initial assessment and stabilization. Impending respiratory failure should be treated with supplemental oxygen. Although controversial in the HF patient, noninvasive ventilation is sometimes used in an attempt to forestall intubation. Patients who are unable to control their airway, cannot tolerate noninvasive ventilation or worsen despite these measures should be considered for endotracheal intubation.

When HF is considered the most likely etiology of the patient's symptoms, the initial workup should include establishment of intravenous access, a history and physical examination, assessment of the degree of fluid overload and perfusion, evaluation of oxygenation, assessment of the cardiac rhythm, the performance of a 12-lead electrocardiogram, and chest x-ray. Blood should be drawn for a complete blood cell count, electrolytes, either b-type natriuretic peptide (BNP) or N-terminal pro-BNP levels, and cardiac markers.

Because of the chronic and terminal nature of HF, if possible, advance directives should be discussed with the patient or family, especially if the patient is in extremis. This information will help direct the management plan established by the emergency physician.

Precipitants of the HF exacerbation should be investigated by the emergency physician (Table 28-1). The identifiable reversible causes should be treated in conjunction with treatment of the HF. Unfortunately, in one study the authors could not identify a precipitant in 40% of the HF presentations.[2] Patient-related factors, such as noncompliance with medication and diet, should be addressed during the ED and hospital course. Poor compliance has ranged in several studies as the precipitant of the acute exacerbation from 21 to 41.9%.[2,3] Patient and family education cannot be underestimated. Several out-

patient studies have investigated the impact of education, and although these are not ED studies it is intuitive that increased education might result in an improvement in compliance.[4–6] Since smoking cessation in HF patients provides a mortality reduction equal to that of medical therapy, counseling on the importance of terminating this habit is important. Finally, the indication that smoking cessation counseling was provided during an inpatient hospitalization is currently required by the joint commission on hospital accreditation.

Cardiac ischemia is a leading cause of HF and a common cause of acute exacerbations.[7] The emergency physician should attempt to diagnose and treat acute ischemia. Cardiac arrhythmias have been associated with a worse prognosis in HF.[8] In the acute care setting cardiac arrhythmias (e.g., atrial fibrillation, ventricular arrhythmias) and conduction abnormalities can precipitate an exacerbation. Treatment should be focused on the hemodynamic effects and not correction of every arrhythmia. Patients with chronic HF are at significant risk for ventricular arrhythmias, and the risk of sudden cardiac death increases proportionally to the degree of left ventricular dysfunction. Therefore, drugs that potentiate arrhythmia (e.g., dobutamine[9]) are discouraged in the treatment of HF.

Table 28-1. Precipitants of Heart Failure Exacerbations

Noncompliance
  Medications
  Diet
Ischemic events
  Acute myocardial infarction
  Cardiac ischemia
Uncontrolled hypertension
Valvular disease
Cardiac arrhythmias
  Atrial fibrillation with a rapid ventricular response
  Ventricular tachycardia
  Bradycardia
  Conduction abnormalities
Noncardiac events
  Pulmonary embolus
  Anemia
  Systemic infection
  Thyroid disorders
  Stress
  Drugs and alcohol
Adverse effects of medications
Undefined factors

PRINCIPLES OF TREATMENT

The classic picture of HF, characterized by acute pulmonary edema, frothing at the mouth, and cyanosis is only one possible extreme of ED HF presentation. While some present with respiratory distress, others may have mild symptomatic dyspnea, and still others complain only of fatigue.

In order to properly treat HF, it is important to accurately classify patients across this spectrum of disease. The American College of Cardiology and American Heart Association have developed guidelines that divide cardiac dysfunction into three clinical entities: (1) acute cardiogenic pulmonary edema, (2) cardiogenic shock, and (3) acute decompensation of chronic left HF.[10] Describing HF using these terms might be useful when trying to communicate with a cardiologist or internist, but they do not indicate what therapeutic interventions will be helpful to manage the patient in the ED.

A more useful approach to categorizing HF in the ED is to use a hemodynamic classification system (Fig. 28-1). Based on the initial history and physical, patients can be placed into a hemodynamic category and then appropriate therapy can be selected. Fluid overload can be assessed by the presence or absence of dyspnea, orthopnea, pulmonary rales, elevated jugular venous pressure, a third heart sound, and hepatomegaly. Perfusion can be estimated by evaluating for the presence or absence of fatigue, nausea, symptomatic hypotension, and cool extremities (Table 28-2).

When using these signs and symptoms to predict hemodynamic status the emergency physician must realize that history and physical suffers from inherent inaccuracies and low interrater reliability.[11] Diagnostic assessment using these indicators is usually made by an aggregate of findings, and supplemented with diagnostic testing to improve the accuracy. Because of the limitations of current technology available in the ED, the clinical assessment provides the best estimate of a patient's hemodynamic status.

Most patients presenting with HF will be fluid overloaded and have adequate perfusion, i.e., "wet and warm." These patients will benefit from diuretics and vasodilatation. The fluid overloaded patient could also present with diminished perfusion, termed "wet and cold," representing increased filling pressures and poor cardiac output, and increased systemic vascular resistance (SVR). Those with elevated SVR will require vasodilation. Those with symptomatic hypotension and diminished SVR may require inotropic support. The least common presentation is the patient that has been overdiuresed and has evidence of hypoperfusion,

		Congestion at rest	
		No	Yes
Low perfusion at rest	No	Warm and dry (a) (compensated) CO normal, PCWP normal	Warm and wet (b) CO normal, ↑PCWP
	Yes	Cold and dry (d) (euvolemic HF) ↓CO, ↓ to normal PCWP	Cold and wet (c) (CHF) ↓CO, ↑PCWP Normal SVR ⇔ ↑SVR

Fig. 28-1. Bedside assessment of hemodynamic status and corresponding therapeutic intervention. (a) Well compensated. If symptomatic typically require minor adjustments in medications and follow-up. (b) Fluid overloaded and well perfused. Vasodilators and diuretics are the treatment modalities. (c) Diminished perfusion and fluid overloaded. For those with elevated SVR, vasodilators and diuretics should improve symptoms for symptomatic hypotension, consider addition of a pressor agent. (d) Poor perfusion and dry. Typically require a fluid bolus. Addition of inotropic support and pressors for patients unresponsive to the initial bolus. (Source: Stevenson LW, Tailored Therapy to hemodynamic goals for advanced heart failure. *Eur J. Heart Failure* 1999;1:251–257.)

Table 28-2. Clinical Bedside Assessment of Heart Failure

Evidence of congestion
Dyspnea
Orthopnea
Paroxysmal nocturnal dyspnea
Jugular venous distention
Hepatojugular reflex
Third heart sound
Edema
Hepatomegaly
Rales

Evidence of diminished perfusion
Fatigue
Nausea
Narrow pulse pressure
Cool extremities
Symptomatic hypotension

---

known as "cold and dry." This patient may require an approach that incorporates the use of a fluid bolus and the addition of both pressors and inotropic support.

To maximize forward flow and cardiac output, HF patients are best served by lower blood pressures, and will commonly tolerate systolic blood pressures in the 80–90 mmHg range. As long as they are asymptomatic, continue to mentate, and have appropriate urine output, therapy directed at raising the blood pressure is unnecessary and may be counterproductive. In these cases, the addition of a pressor may worsen the hemodynamic status by adding undo afterload on the failing heart.

The above referenced hemodynamic classification system provides the emergency physician with a framework for the initial assessment and treatment of the ED HF patient. Unfortunately, these are imprecise measures. Therefore, initial treatment is guided by an estimate of the current hemodynamic status and is adjusted, depending on the initial response to the therapeutic interventions. Until more accurate diagnostic modalities are available, the emergency physician should use the framework presented in this section to develop his/her therapeutic plan.

THERAPEUTIC STRATEGIES—DIURETICS

Patients presenting with evidence of fluid overload, the "wet" patient, will benefit by the use of a diuretic. Loop diuretics promote diuresis by the inhibiting renal sodium reabsorption into the loops of Henle. The resultant volume reduction causes a decrease in filling pressures and pulmonary congestion. This provides the patient with symptomatic improvement. Furosemide is the most commonly used IV and oral loop diuretic. Peak diuretic effect is typically seen within 30 min of administration.

Some controversy exists regarding the physiologic effects of furosemide. One study noted that in the first 5–15 min after administration of furosemide there was a decrease in filling pressures and preload which preceded the increase in urine output. Subsequent studies have revealed an initial rise in filling pressures and SVR, prior to a fall in filling pressures that was associated with diuresis.[12,13] By increasing renin, norepinephrine, and vasopressin levels,[12] furosemide also has adverse neurohormonal effects in the HF patient. Interestingly, Kraus et al. have demonstrated that adding high-dose nitrates and ACEIs to furosemide blunted the initial rise in filling pressures.[13]

The usual starting dose of furosemide is 20–80 mg intravenously. A patient with no previous exposure to furosemide may have adequate response to lower doses. If a patient is currently on furosemide, using their current daily oral dose as an intravenous bolus is a good starting point. Doses should be titrated based on urine output and creatinine. If no response is seen within 30 min the initial dose can be doubled. The effect of furosemide can be augmented with the administration of metolazone (2.5–5.0 mg) 20 min prior to the loop diuretic.[14,15] Treatment with diuretics may lead to hypokalemia and hypomagnesemia; therefore, monitoring and treatment of electrolyte abnormalities are critical when using diuretics in HF management. Despite some of the potential adverse hemodynamic and neurohormonal effects of loop diuretics, the ultimate diuresis, reduction in filling pressures, and symptomatic improvement seen with furosemide administration makes it a commonly used drug for the fluid overloaded patient.

THERAPEUTIC STRATEGIES: VASOACTIVE AGENTS

Historically, ED treatment of acute decompensated HF has centered on the relief of congestion by the use of diuretics. Despite the deleterious effect of diuretics on the neurohormonal axis in HF patients, they provide relatively rapid relief of congestion, and represent routine ED management. Recent data have suggested value in adding vasoactive agents in the treatment of acute decompensated HF.[16] The ADHERE registry is a large database of patients hospitalized with decompensated HF. When the outcomes of 46,599 patients were analyzed based on if they received a vasoactive agent in the ED (mean time to therapy 1.1 hour), compared to receiving vasoactives as an inpatient (average time to treatment was 22 hours after admission), those receiving ED treatment had significantly ($P = 0.0001$) shorter ICU and hospital length of stay, fewer invasive procedures, and lower mortality. This analysis excluded patients with concurrent myocardial infarction or systolic blood pressure less than 90 mmHg, and vasoactive therapy was defined as any of the following: nesiritide, nitroglycerin (NTG), nitroprusside (NTP), dobutamine, dopamine, or milrinone. Although retrospective registry data, this study suggests that there is value of early aggressive treatment in the management of decompensated HF.

THERAPEUTIC STRATEGIES—VASODILATORS

Vasodilators-Natriuretic Peptides

The "cold and wet," and selected "wet and warm" patient may benefit from vasodilatation. Nesiritide (Scios, Sunnyvale, CA) is an IV form of human BNP and provides a combination of neurohormonal and hemodynamic effects that are beneficial in the initial management of HF. Neurohormonal effects include improved sodium and water excretion, and decreased endothelin, norepinephrine, aldosterone, renin, and angiotensin levels.[17] Hemodynamic effects include decreasing filling pressures and SVR, and an increase in cardiac output, without an increase in heart rate.[17–19]

Several trials have studied the effects of nesiritide on inpatients with HF. Colucci et al. reported a dose-dependent decrease in filling pressures and improved symptoms.[20] The Vasodilation in the Management of Acute HF trial, compared the addition of intravenous nesiritide or intravenous NTG to standard HF therapy.[21] Nesiritide, administered as a 2 μg/kg bolus, followed by a maintenance infusion of 0.01 μg/kg/min resulted in decreased filling pressures and improvement in dyspnea compared to standard therapy.

With the increased use of observation units for the treatment of HF, the use of nesiritide in this environment has been studied in the Prospective Randomized Outcomes Study of Acutely Decompensated Congestive HF Treated Initially in Outpatients with Natrecor (PROACTION) trial. In this randomized, double-blind placebo-controlled pilot study of 250 patients, the nesiritide group had similar rates of adverse events as compared to standard therapy. In the month after treatment, the nesiritide group was hospi-

talized an average of 2.5 days, compared to 6.5 days in the standard therapy cohort.[22]

Although no large scale trials exists using nesiritide, the fact that it has comparable or slightly better hemodynamic attributes than NTG, does not require titration, has no associated tachycardia, no tachyphylaxis, is nonarrythmogenic, and attenuates the neurohormonal derangements of HF, suggests an important role in the treatment of decompensated HF.

There are limited cost analysis data available; however, several published abstracts suggest that nesiritide reduces length of ICU stay in decompensated HF.[23,24] Future work should prospectively elucidate how to best use the medication in a cost-effective manner.

Vasodilators-Nitrates

The patient with fluid overload and poor to reasonable perfusion, considered along the continuum of "cold and wet," to "warm and wet," can be successfully treated with a reduction in preload and decreased ventricular workload. NTG achieves the reduction in filling pressures by dilation of the venous system.[16] At higher doses there is dilation of the arterial system causing decreased left ventricular work. NTG also dilates epicardial coronary arteries increasing collateral blood flow.[25] Some evidence exists that high doses of nitrates result in better outcomes, with decreased need for mechanical ventilation and fewer myocardial infarctions.[26,27] In patients requiring urgent preload reduction, NTG can be administered sublingually either as a spray or pill (0.4 mg) at 1 min interval. This can be done effectively before institution of intravenous access. This may be followed by transdermal NTG paste (1–2 in.) if the patient is perfusing adequately to permit absorption. If continued reductions in preload and afterload are required, a NTG drip may be started and titrated to effect. Dosing can start at 10–20 μg/min and titrated quickly, every 3–5 min or faster, as needed. Doses can reach 200–300 μg/min to achieve the desired effect. If further afterload reduction is needed, nitroprusside must be considered. Adverse effects of nitrates include headache, sinus tachycardia, tachyphylaxis, and hypotension. Despite a minimal number of prospective trials, nitrates with diuretics form the basis behind the treatment of the fluid overloaded patients.

Vasodilators-Nitroprusside (NTP)

Some patients with extreme elevations of SVR require additional afterload reduction beyond NTG. NTP can be added to those patients who require further afterload reduction. NTP is a potent vasodilator that relaxes both arteriolar and venous smooth muscle.[28] The decrease in preload and afterload results in augmentation of cardiac output and stroke volume. An intravenous infusion starts at 0.1–0.2 µg/kg/min and can be increased every 5 min. Dangerous hypotension can occur precipitously mandating continuous blood pressure monitoring. Other adverse effects include the hypothesized "coronary steal" syndrome (possible with all vasodilators). The coronary steal syndrome is postulated to occur in patients with a fixed coronary lesion that becomes flow limiting when there is a generalized vasodilated state throughout the vascular bed. Patients with renal failure are at risk for thiocyanate toxicity with prolonged treatment with NTP. If absolutely required in the renal failure population, there may be some benefit from addition of hydroxycobalamin. Finally, a reflex tachycardia secondary to NTP-induced vasodilation, may adversely effect myocardial oxygen consumption.

THERAPEUTIC STRATEGIES—FLUIDS

Patients with poor perfusion and who have been overdiuresed, the "cold and dry" cohort, present a treatment dilemma for the emergency physician. These patients typically report an increased use of diuretics. They can be recognized by symptoms of increased fatigue, nausea, cool extremities, and hypotension without any evidence of fluid overload. Although counterintuitive to the treatment of HF, these patients may benefit from a fluid bolus of 250–500 cc of isotonic fluid. This should be done cautiously with frequent reassessment of response and the patient's fluid status.

Therapeutic Strategies—Inotropic/Pressor Support

In the "cold and wet" cohort, patients with poor perfusion, inadequate blood pressure (usually a systolic less than 85 mmHg), and signs of fluid overload, inotropic support is sometimes indicated.

If cardiogenic shock is present, a mixed catecholamine agonist such as dopamine may be added to the regimen. The definition of cardiogenic shock implies evidence of poor perfusion, and is independent of a specific blood pressure. Many NYHA class IV patients often have systolic blood pressures in the 90s and tolerate the 80s quite well, and the addition of a pressor may worsen their HF. Intraaortic balloon pump placement may also be considered as a bridge to cardiac transplantation.

The ultimate goal of HF management is improvement of the neurohormonal and hemodynamic milieu. Addition of inotropic and pressor agents while sometimes necessary

may ultimately have deleterious effects. Several studies have shown increased ventricular ectopy without a mortality or length of stay improvement with the use of inotropic support.

Therapeutic Strategies—ACE Inhibitors

The renin-angiotensin-aldosterone-system (RAAS) plays an important role in the neurohormonal derangements of HF. Activation of the RAAS, while initially beneficial, leads to many of the adverse hemodynamic consequences of HF. Elevated levels of angiotensin and aldosterone contribute to the adverse hemodynamics in HF by increasing SVR and causing sodium retention, and are directly associated with HF mortality. Interruption of the RAAS forms the basis of all treatments demonstrated to reduce mortality in chronic HF.

The ability of ACEIs to relax both arterial resistance and venous vessels, and lower impedance to LV ejection provide the patient with a hemodynamic advantage. Their ability to block the neurohormonal derangements of HF provides the theoretical advantage in the treatment of HF exacerbations in the ED. Patients with asymptomatic LV dysfunction and chronic HF derive a mortality reduction from therapy with ACEI.[29,30] Several studies of severe chronic HF demonstrate dramatic improvements in hemodynamics immediately after administration of an ACEI.[31–33] This hemodynamic data suggest a potential ED role for the acute administration of ACEIs.

Some preliminary evidence exists supporting the ED use of ACEI for HF.[34,35] In a small prospective, randomized, double-blind, placebo-controlled trial of 48 patients, Hamilton et al. evaluated the role of sublingual captopril for acute pulmonary edema. They measured HF severity using a composite of four parameters: patient reported dyspnea, physician judgment of respiratory distress, diaphoresis, and level of bed elevation tolerance. Using this composite score they demonstrated that sublingual captopril results in better scores during the first 40 min of therapy.[35] In addition, there was a trend toward less intubation in the captopril group (9%) versus the placebo group (20%) with a 95% CI of –8 to 31%.

ACEIs can be administered as captopril 25 mg by mouth or sublingually. Oral captopril has an onset of action within 15–30 min. Sublingual captopril significantly decreases pulmonary capillary wedge pressure after 10 min.[36] Care must be taken if the patient's systolic blood pressure is less than 90 mmHg. Use in these patients may result in hypotension, decreased cardiac perfusion, and decreased glomerular filtration, which may lead to an increase in serum creatinine.

Despite the lack of definitive, large scale trials, some centers advocate the use ACEIs as a routine component of their therapeutic regimen.[37] Based on known, hemodynamic data, one ED study, and its neurohormonal effects, addition of ACEIs in patients with high SVR is enticing. However, because there are no large placebo-controlled trials using ACEIs in the ED, they cannot be recommended as a standard of care.

Therapeutic Strategies—Respiratory Considerations

All patients presenting with HF should receive supplemental oxygen. Those with respiratory distress and dyspnea will typically respond to aggressive medical management. Failure of medical management and worsening respiratory status may lead to endotracheal intubation. Two controversial noninvasive ventilatory techniques are: continuous positive airway pressure (CPAP) and bilevel positive airway pressure (BiPAP), and these are reviewed in Chap. 29.

Therapeutic Strategies—On the Horizon

Endothelins

Endothelin, a peptide with significant vasoconstrictor effects, is synthesized by endothelial and smooth muscle cells. Endothelin (ET-1) has predominantly vascular effects through activation of specific ET_A and ET_B receptors on vascular smooth muscle cells. Its major effects are vasoconstriction and cell proliferation. In the normal state, ET-1 contributes to basal vascular tone. In addition, ET-1 influences myocardial contractility and sodium excretion. The vasoconstriction from ET-1 is independent of vasoconstriction seen with activation of the other neurohormonal systems. ET-1 is elevated in patients with chronic HF and high levels predict a worse prognosis.[38–41] Preliminary studies revealed some improvement in cardiac hemodynamics with the administration of the endothelin antagonists bosentan or tezosentan,[42–47] although subsequent clinical studies have not shown any improvement with the addition of endothelin antagonists to standard therapy for acute exacerbations of HF.[48–52]

ARGININE VASOPRESSIN ANTAGONISTS

Arginine vasopressin (AVP) is a powerful vasoconstrictor and promotes water reabsorption in the kidneys. Elevated levels of AVP have been reported in chronic HF. Early trials of V_1 receptor antagonists have demonstrated a favorable hemodynamic response and an increase in urine output.[53]

NEUTRAL ENDOPEPTIDASE/ACE INHIBITORS

Neutral endopeptidase (NEP) is an enzyme present in the heart, blood vessels, and kidneys that degrades atrial natriuretide peptide (ANP), BNP, angiotensin II, and endothelin. Inhibition of NEP results in increased concentrations of ANP and BNP, potentially beneficial in patients with HF. Unfortunately, initial trials of a combination agent containing NEP and ACEI demonstrated no difference in mortality when compared to enalapril.[54]

MANAGEMENT OF CHRONIC MEDICATIONS

Chronic HF is treated as an outpatient with a variety of different medications. The emergency physician will rarely prescribe a patient one of these medications but should be aware of the rationale behind their use and how they may affect clinical practice.

ANGIOTENSIN II RECEPTOR BLOCKERS

Angiotensin II receptor blockers (ARBs) therapeutic effects are secondary to their ability to block the angiotensin receptor. Normally, stimulation of the subtype 1 receptor by angiotensin II causes arterial vasoconstriction, aldosterone release, and LV remodeling. Patients who have failed ACEIs due to a severe cough or angioedema are considered for ARB therapy. ARBs have efficacy that is similar to ACEIs but not superior,[55] and they are not considered first-line agents for chronic HF.

Aldosterone

Aldosterone levels increase in chronic HF due to stimulation by angiotensin II and decreased hepatic clearance. The Randomized Aldactone Evaluation Study evaluated the use of the aldosterone blocker spironolactone in patients with NYHA III or IV HF, demonstrated a 30% reduction in mortality and hospitalizations.[56] Hyperkalemia is a potential side effect of spironolactone and addition of the medication should be avoided in patients with renal insufficiency or hyperkalemia.

The eplerenone postacute myocardial infarction HF efficacy and survival study examined the role of aldosterone blockade in patients with LV dysfunction.[57] Patients receiving eplerenone had a reduction in mortality, hospitalizations, stroke, arrhythmias, and HF.

Beta-Blockers

Activation of the sympathetic system in chronic HF has long-term detrimental effects on the cardiovascular system. Use of beta-blockers to counteract these harmful effects has been demonstrated to decrease mortality and hospitalizations.[58–60] Patients presenting to the ED with an exacerbation of HF and who are currently being treated with beta-blocker pose a dilemma for the emergency physician. Abrupt interruption of the beta-blockers may worsen the patient's symptoms. If the patient is admitted to the hospital, the physicians may decide to temporarily halt the beta-blocker, or continue but at a reduced dose. If the patient is stable to the point that discharge from the ED is considered, then they are encouraged to continue the beta-blocker.

MEDICATIONS TO AVOID

Nonsteroidal Anti-inflammatory Drugs

Patients already treated with ACEIs are at increased risk of an acute decompensation when they are started on a nonsteroidal anti-inflammatory drugs (NSAID) therapy.[61,62] Normally, prostaglandins act as renal arteriole vasodilators. However in certain at-risk populations, loss of vasodilation related to the interaction between NSAIDs and ACEIs can result in a reduction in renal perfusion and an increase in SVR. This effect, and the greatest risks, are seen during the first several days of NSAID use. NSAIDs should be avoided in patients with HF, in particular those being treated with ACEIs or those with renal insufficiency.

Calcium-Channel Blockers

Calcium-channel blockers are not recommended as vasodilator therapy for HF.[63] Patients should be preferentially treated both in the outpatient setting with increased doses of ACEIs and beta-blockers. In patients who require rate control, and who have failed other first-line alternative medications, amlodipine may be considered.

REFERENCES

1. Association AH. *2003 Heart and Stroke Statistical Update.* Dallas, TX: American Heart Association, 2003.
2. Opasich C, Rapezzi C, Lucci D, et al. Precipitating factors and decision-making processes of short-term worsening heart failure despite "optimal" treatment (from the IN-CHF Registry). *Am J Cardiol* 2001;88(4):382–387.
3. Michalsen A, Konig G, Thimme W. Preventable causative factors leading to hospital admission with decompensated heart failure. [see comment]. *Heart* 1998;80(5):437–441.
4. Philbin EF. Comprehensive multidisciplinary programs for the management of patients with congestive heart failure. [see comment]. *J Gen Intern Med* 1999;14(2): 130–135.
5. Rich MW, Beckham V, Wittenberg C, et al. A multidisciplinary intervention to prevent the readmission of elderly patients with congestive heart failure. [see comment]. *N Engl J Med* 1995;333(18):1190–1195.
6. West JA, Miller NH, Parker KM, et al. A comprehensive management system for heart failure improves clinical outcomes and reduces medical resource utilization. *Am J Cardiol* 1997;79(1):58–63.
7. Goldberger JJ, Peled HB, Stroh JA, et al. Prognostic factors in acute pulmonary edema. *Arch Intern Med* 1986;146(3): 489–493.
8. Dries DL, Exner DV, Gersh BJ, et al. Atrial fibrillation is associated with an increased risk for mortality and heart failure progression in patients with asymptomatic and symptomatic left ventricular systolic dysfunction: A retrospective analysis of the SOLVD trials. Studies of left ventricular dysfunction. *J Am Coll Cardiol* 1998;32(3):695–703.
9. Burger AJ, Horton DP, LeJemtel T, et al. Effect of nesiritide (B-type natriuretic peptide) and dobutamine on ventricular arrhythmias in the treatment of patients with acutely decompensated congestive heart failure: The PRECEDENT study. *Am Heart J* 2002;144(6):1102–1108.
10. Anonymous. Guidelines for the evaluation and management of heart failure. Report of the American College of Cardiology/American Heart Association Task Force on Practice Guidelines (Committee on Evaluation and Management of Heart Failure). *J Am Coll Cardiol* 1995; 26(5):1376–1398.
11. Badgett RG, Lucey CR, Mulrow CD. Can the clinical examination diagnose left-sided heart failure in adults? [see comment]. *JAMA* 1997;277(21):1712–1719.
12. Francis GS, Siegel RM, Goldsmith SR, et al. Acute vasoconstrictor response to intravenous furosemide in patients with chronic congestive heart failure. Activation of the neurohumoral axis. *Ann Intern Med* 1985;103(1):1–6.
13. Kraus PA, Lipman J, Becker PJ. Acute preload effects of furosemide. *Chest* 1990;98(1):124–128.
14. Peacock WF, Freda B. The clinical challenge of heart failure: Comprehensive, evidence-based management of the hospitalized patient with acute myocardial decompensation-diagnosis, risk stratification, and outcome effective treatment. *Emerg Med Rep* 2002;23:1–13.
15. Channer KS, McLean KA, Lawson-Matthew P, et al. Combination diuretic treatment in severe heart failure: A randomised controlled trial. *Br Heart J* 1994;71(2):146–150.
16. Peacock WF, Emerman CL, Costanzo MR, et al. Early initiation of intravenous therapy improves heart failure outcomes: An analysis from the ADHERE registry database. *Ann Emerg Med* 2003;42(4):S26.
17. Abraham WT, Lowes BD, Ferguson DA, et al. Systemic hemodynamic, neurohormonal, and renal effects of a steady-state infusion of human brain natriuretic peptide in

patients with hemodynamically decompensated heart failure. *J Card Fail* 1998;4(1):37–44.

18. Marcus LS, Hart D, Packer M, et al. Hemodynamic and renal excretory effects of human brain natriuretic peptide infusion in patients with congestive heart failure. A double-blind, placebo-controlled, randomized crossover trial. *Circulation* 1996;94(12):3184–3189.

19. Hobbs RE, Miller LW, Bott-Silverman C, et al. Hemodynamic effects of a single intravenous injection of synthetic human brain natriuretic peptide in patients with heart failure secondary to ischemic or idiopathic dilated cardiomyopathy. *Am J Cardiol* 1996;78(8):896–901.

20. Colucci WS, Elkayam U, Horton DP, et al. Intravenous nesiritide, a natriuretic peptide, in the treatment of decompensated congestive heart failure. Nesiritide Study Group. *N Engl J Med* 2000;343(4):246–253.

21. Publication Committee for the VI. Intravenous nesiritide vs nitroglycerin for treatment of decompensated congestive heart failure: A randomized controlled trial. *JAMA* 2002; 287(12):1531–1540.

22. Peacock WF, Emerman C, on behalf of the PROACTION Study Group. Safety and efficacy of nesiritide in the treatment of decompensated heart failure in observation patients. *J Am Coll Cardiol* 2003;4(6), Suppl A:336A.

23. Chang R, Elatre WA, Heywood JT. Effect of nesiritide on length of hospital stay in decompensated heart failure. *J Am Coll Cardiol* 2003;41(S6):161A.

24. Lenz TL, Foral PA, Malesker MA, et al. Impact of nesiritide on health care resource utilization & complications in patients with decompensated heart failure. *Pharmacotherapy* 2004;24(9):1137–46.

25. Cohen MC DJ, Sonnenblick EH, Kirk ES. The effects of nitroglycerin on coronary collaterals and myocardial contractility. *J Clin Invest* 1973;52:2836–2847.

26. Cotter G, Metzkor E, Kaluski E, et al. Randomised trial of high-dose isosorbide dinitrate plus low-dose furosemide versus high-dose furosemide plus low-dose isosorbide dinitrate in severe pulmonary oedema. *Lancet* 1998; 351(9100):389–393.

27. Sharon A, Shpirer I, Kaluski E, et al. High-dose intravenous isosorbide-dinitrate is safer and better than Bi-PAP ventilation combined with conventional treatment for severe pulmonary edema. [see comment]. *J Am Coll Cardiol* 2000;36(3):832–837.

28. Rossen RM, Alderman EL, Harrison DC. Circulatory response to vasodilator therapy in congestive cardiomyopathy. *Br Heart J* 1976;38(7):695–700.

29. Anonymous. Effects of enalapril on mortality in severe congestive heart failure. Results of the Cooperative North Scandinavian Enalapril Survival Study (CONSENSUS). The CONSENSUS Trial Study Group. *N Engl J Med* 1987;316(23):1429–1435.

30. Anonymous. Effects of enalapril on survival in patients with reduced left ventricular ejection fractions and congestive heart failure. The SOLVD Investigators. *N Engl J Med* 1991;325(5):293–302.

31. Haude M, Erbel R, Meyer J. Sublingual administration of captopril versus nitroglycerin in patients with severe congestive heart failure. *Int J Cardiol* 1990;27:351–359.

32. Powers ER, Stone J, Reison DS, et al. The effect of captopril on renal, coronary, and systemic hemodynamics in patients with severe congestive heart failure. *Am Heart J* 1982;104:1203–1210.

33. Kubo SH, Laragh JH, Prida XE, et al. Immediate converting enzyme inhibition with intravenous enalapril in chronic congestive heart failure. *Am J Cardiol* 1985;55:122–126.

34. Annane D, Bellissant E, Pussard E, et al. Placebo-controlled, randomized, double-blind study of intravenous enalaprilat efficacy and safety in acute cardiogenic pulmonary edema. *Circulation* 1996;94(6):1316–1324.

35. Hamilton RJ CW, Gallagher EJ. Rapid improvement of acute pulmonary edema with sublingual captopril. *Acad Emerg Med* 1996;3:205–212.

36. Barnett JC ZK, Touchon RC. Sublingual captopril in the treatment of acute heart failure. *Curr Ther Res* 1991;49(2): 274–281.

37. Sacchetti A, Ramoska E, Moakes ME, et al. Effect of ED management on ICU use in acute pulmonary edema. *Am J Emerg Med* 1999;17(6):571–574.

38. McMurray JJ, Ray SG, Abdullah I, et al. Plasma endothelin in chronic heart failure. *Circulation* 1992;85(4):1374–1379.

39. Wei CM, Lerman A, Rodeheffer RJ, et al. Endothelin in human congestive heart failure. *Circulation* 1994; 89(4):1580–1586.

40. Pacher R, Stanek B, Hulsmann M, et al. Prognostic impact of big endothelin-1 plasma concentrations compared with invasive hemodynamic evaluation in severe heart failure. *J Am Coll Cardiol* 1996;27(3):633–641.

41. Pousset F, Isnard R, Lechat P, et al. Prognostic value of plasma endothelin-1 in patients with chronic heart failure. *Eur Heart J* 1997;18(2):254–258.

42. Sutsch G, Bertel O, Kiowski W. Acute and short-term effects of the nonpeptide endothelin-1 receptor antagonist bosentan in humans. *Cardiovasc Drugs Ther* 1997;10(6):717–725.

43. Sutsch G, Kiowski W, Yan XW, et al. Short-term oral endothelin-receptor antagonist therapy in conventionally treated patients with symptomatic severe chronic heart failure. *Circulation* 1998;98(21):2262–2268.

44. Kiowski W, Sutsch G, Hunziker P, et al. Evidence for endothelin-1-mediated vasoconstriction in severe chronic heart failure. *Lancet* 1995;346(8977):732–736.

45. Torre-Amione G, Young JB, Durand J, et al. Hemodynamic effects of tezosentan, an intravenous dual endothelin receptor antagonist, in patients with class III to IV congestive heart failure. *Circulation* 2001;103(7):973–980.

46. Cotter G, Kiowski W, Kaluski E, et al. Tezosentan (an intravenous endothelin receptor A/B antagonist) reduces peripheral resistance and increases cardiac power therefore preventing a steep decrease in blood pressure in patients with congestive heart failure. *Eur J Heart Fail* 2001;3(4):457–461.

47. Schalcher C, Cotter G, Reisin L, et al. The dual endothelin receptor antagonist tezosentan acutely improves hemodynamic

parameters in patients with advanced heart failure. *Am Heart J* 2001;142(2):340–349.

48. O'Connor CM, Gattis WA, Adams KF Jr., et al. Tezosentan in patients with acute heart failure and acute coronary syndromes: Results of the Randomized Intravenous TeZosentan Study (RITZ-4). [see comment]. *J Am Coll Cardiol* 2003; 41(9):1452–1457.

49. Kaluski E, Kobrin I, Zimlichman R, et al. RITZ-5: Randomized intravenous TeZosentan (an endothelin-A/B antagonist) for the treatment of pulmonary edema: A prospective, multicenter, double-blind, placebo-controlled study. *J Am Coll Cardiol* 2003;41(2):204–210.

50. Coletta AP, Cleland JG. Clinical trials update: Highlights of the scientific sessions of the XXIII Congress of the European Society of Cardiology—WARIS II, ESCAMI, PAFAC, RITZ-1 and TIME. *Eur J Heart Fail* 2001;3(6):747–750.

51. Louis A, Cleland JG, Crabbe S, et al. Clinical Trials Update: CAPRICORN, COPERNICUS, MIRACLE, STAF, RITZ-2, RECOVER and RENAISSANCE and cachexia and cholesterol in heart failure. Highlights of the Scientific Sessions of the American College of Cardiology, 2001. [Review] [22 refs]. *Eur J Heart Fail* 2001;3(3):381–387.

52. Packer M. Effects of the endothelin receptor antagonist bosentan on the morbidity and mortality in patients with chronic heart failure. Results of the ENABLE 1 and 2 trial program. Paper presented at Congress of the American College of Cardiology, Late Breaking Clinical Trials, 2002.

53. Udelson JE, Smith WB, Hendrix GH, et al. Acute hemodynamic effects of conivaptan, a dual V(1A) and V(2) vasopressin receptor antagonist, in patients with advanced heart failure. *Circulation* 2001;104(20):2417–2423.

54. Packer M, Califf RM, Konstam MA, et al. Comparison of omapatrilat and enalapril in patients with chronic heart failure: The Omapatrilat Versus Enalapril Randomized Trial of Utility in Reducing Events (OVERTURE). [see comment]. *Circulation* 2002;106(8):920–926.

55. Pitt B, Poole-Wilson PA, Segal R, et al. Effect of losartan compared with captopril on mortality in patients with symptomatic heart failure: Randomised trial—the Losartan Heart Failure Survival Study ELITE II. [see comment]. *Lancet* 2000;355(9215):1582–1587.

56. Pitt B, Zannad F, Remme WJ, et al. The effect of spironolactone on morbidity and mortality in patients with severe heart failure. Randomized Aldactone Evaluation Study Investigators. [see comment]. *N Engl J Med* 1999; 341(10):709–717.

57. Pitt B, Remme W, Zannad F, et al. Eplerenone, a selective aldosterone blocker, in patients with left ventricular dysfunction after myocardial infarction. [see comment] [erratum appears in *N Engl J Med* 2003;348(22):2271]. *N Engl J Med* 2003;348(14):1309–1321.

58. Packer M, Colucci WS, Sackner-Bernstein JD, et al. Double-blind, placebo-controlled study of the effects of carvedilol in patients with moderate to severe heart failure. The PRECISE Trial. Prospective Randomized Evaluation of Carvedilol on Symptoms and Exercise. [see comment]. *Circulation* 1996;94(11):2793–2799.

59. Anonymous. The Cardiac Insufficiency Bisoprolol Study II (CIBIS-II): A randomised trial. [see comment]. *Lancet* 1999;353(9146):9–13.

60. Anonymous. Effect of metoprolol CR/XL in chronic heart failure: Metoprolol CR/XL Randomised Intervention Trial in Congestive Heart Failure (MERIT-HF) [see comment]. *Lancet* 1999;353(9169):2001–2007.

61. Hall D, Zeitler H, Rudolph W. Counteraction of the vasodilator effects of enalapril by aspirin in severe heart failure. *J Am Coll Cardiol* 1992;20(7):1549–1555.

62. Garcia Rodriguez LA, Hernandez-Diaz S. Nonsteroidal anti-inflammatory drugs as a trigger of clinical heart failure. *Epidemiology* 2003;14(2):240–246.

63. Betkowski AS, Hauptman PJ. Update on recent clinical trials in congestive heart failure. [Review] [85 refs]. *Curr Opin Cardiol* 2000;15(4):293–303.

29

Acute Pulmonary Edema

Charles L. Emerman

HIGH YIELD FACTS

- Pulmonary edema can occur from a variety of causes.
- The treatment of pulmonary edema varies depending on whether it is due to cardiogenic or noncardiogenic causes.
- Noninvasive ventilation is an option for selected patients with respiratory failure.
- Inotropic therapy is associated with short- and long-term adverse outcomes.
- Nesiritide has rapid onset of action without the development of tolerance.
- Nitroglycerin use requires much higher doses than typically used for antianginal effect.
- Clusters of patients with noncardiogenic pulmonary edema may raise the suspicion of exposure to industrial agents of bioterrorism agents.

INTRODUCTION

A patient presenting with acute pulmonary edema can present in a variety of manners. The occurrence of "flash" pulmonary edema can be a dramatic occasion with patients presenting with diaphoresis and acute respiratory distress. Fortunately, only a minority of patients present in this manner. Most patients presenting to the emergency department with pulmonary edema, particularly those with pulmonary edema due to heart failure have a slow onset of symptoms. This chapter will focus primarily on cardiogenic pulmonary edema although other forms of pulmonary edema will also be discussed.

PATHOPHYSIOLOGY

There is normally a balance between the accumulation and removal of extravascular fluid in the lungs. Driving fluid

into the lung interstitium are the hydrostatic vascular pressure and the osmotic pressure within the interstitium of the lung. Forcing fluid back out of the lung interstitium are the hydrostatic pressures within the interstitium and the osmotic pressure within the blood vessels. The balance between these is called Starling forces.[1] The barrier between the pulmonary vessels and the interstitium is generally resistant to the flow of fluid from the vessels to the lung. Diseases or conditions, which alter the membrane permeability, can also lead to pulmonary edema. As would be expected from the physiologic description, there are several ways in which pulmonary fluid can accumulate. This would include situations in which the hydrostatic pressures within the blood vessels are increased, such as may occur with heart failure, situations in which there is a change in the balance of osmotic pressure between the two sides of the vascular membrane, or conditions that affect membrane permeability.

Extravascular pulmonary fluid can accumulate in several spaces. A small amount of fluid can accumulate in the interstitial space itself. A greater amount of fluid can accumulate in the space that surrounds the bronchi and pulmonary vessels. The appearance of this fluid in the bronchovascular space in what is visible radiographically as Kerley B-lines. Finally, fluid can leak out of these compartments and appear as pleural effusions.

CLINICAL FEATURES

The primary complaint of patients with pulmonary edema is dyspnea. Patients with pulmonary edema may complain of dyspnea at rest, dyspnea under exertion, or, particularly in the case of patients with heart failure, paroxysmal nocturnal dyspnea. A variety of other complaints may be expressed depending on the etiology of acute pulmonary edema. The patient may notice that they are wheezing. Patients with cardiac disease may have weight gain, fatigue, chest discomfort that may or may not be related to ischemia, cough, clear sputum production, abdominal bloating, and peripheral edema among other symptoms. Patients with noncardiogenic edema may have symptoms again relating to their underlying disease process, for example, fever in the case of a patient with non-cardiogenic pulmonary edema due to sepsis. The physical examination will depend on the underlying etiology of pulmonary edema. Those patients with pulmonary edema due to ventricular dysfunction or fluid overload may have increased jugular venous pressure, Cheyne-stokes respirations, cardiac murmurs or gallop rhythm, a displaced point of maximum cardiac impulse, an irregular heart beat from atrial fibrillation or other arrhythmias, hepatosplenomegaly, ascites or peripheral edema. The lung examination may show inspiratory crackles, rales, wheezing, or decreased breath sounds. The physical findings of pleural effusions include decreased breath sounds or dullness to percussion. The above signs and symptoms are not specific for pulmonary edema and can be a reflection of other disease processes. Studies conducted in patients with chronic heart failure have found that the signs and symptoms typically associated with that process have limited sensitivity and specificity.[2]

The chest radiograph is used as part of the diagnostic process for patients with acute pulmonary edema. Typically, the chest radiograph is examined for signs of interstitial or extrapulmonary fluid. This may include increases in the interlobular spaces, perivascular cuffing, Kerley B-lines, pleural effusions, or fluid in the fissures. Pulmonary edema that is cardiac in origin may also have signs that include cardiomegaly, redistribution of pulmonary venous distribution and enlargement of vascular pedicles. The chest radiograph can at times be difficult to interpret. Previous work has demonstrated that other techniques such as bioimpedance may demonstrate an increase in pulmonary fluid even when the radiograph is not interpreted as showing pulmonary edema. Prior studies have shown that up to 20% of the time bioimpedance may detect pulmonary edema in the presence of a chest radiograph, which has not been read as indicating this process.[3] Bioimpedance works by detecting changes in the resistance across a number of chest electrodes. When combined with ECG information, bioimpedance computers can provide additional information about cardiac stroke volume, systemic vascular resistance, and ejection fraction. These techniques however have not been widely adopted.

DIFFERENTIAL DIAGNOSIS

Similar clinical and radiographic patterns can occur from diseases other than those that primarily cause pulmonary edema. Patients with pneumonia can have patterns that include interstitial fluid and pleural effusions. Patients can have pulmonary hemorrhage from a variety of reasons including trauma and coagulopathies. Pleural effusions can occur with neoplasms, connective tissue disorders and, as reactive effusions for patients with primary abdominal disorders such as pancreatitis, or with drug reactions. Pleural effusions with enlargement of the hilar vessels can occur with pulmonary embolus, tumors, tuberculosis, and sarcoidosis. An interstitial edema pattern can occur from primary fluid overload such as may occur in patients with renal failure, a variety of pneumonias, connective tissue disorders, mediastinal masses, and other idiopathic pulmonary disorders.

DIAGNOSTIC TESTING

The electrocardiogram may sometimes be helpful in identifying the cause of acute pulmonary edema. In particular, the ECG should be examined for signs of right or left atrial enlargement, left ventricular hypertrophy, and signs of ischemic cardiovascular diseases including acute ischemia, acute infarction, or evidence suggesting a prior myocardial infarction. The arterial blood gas may show varying degrees of hypoxemia. Because of the occurrence of expiratory airflow limitation, patients may have hypercarbia with or without acidosis. The complete blood count may reflect the underlying disease process although the findings will be nonspecific. Patients may have anemia due to chronic disease, renal failure, or other etiologies. The white count may be elevated in patients with sepsis although that pattern is not always consistent. The white blood count may also be elevated as a nonspecific stress reaction. Similarly, the serum electrolytes may be reflective of an underlying disease process such as renal failure with an elevated blood urea nitrogen (BUN) and creatinine, hyponatremia that can occur from congestive heart failure, pneumonia, or other etiologies, and low serum bicarbonate which may be a manifestation of shock. The assessment of cardiac markers of ischemia can be indicated in patients with risk of coronary artery events. Cardiac markers have been found to be elevated in 5–10% of patients presenting to the emergency department with decompensated heart failure.[4] The troponin however can be elevated in the absence of coronary artery occlusion in patients with heart failure or renal failure.

Acute pulmonary edema can have a variety of effects on lung mechanics. The increased vascular congestion that occurs with decompensated heart failure or renal failure can lead to an increase in gas defusing times. Interstitial edema can lead to impairment in expiratory flow and a ventilation-perfusion mismatch. Additionally, the increase in interstitial fluid can lead to problems with lung compliance and a decrease in total lung volumes. The clinical manifestations of these processes are an increase of work of breathing, wheezing, and a perception of chest tightness by the patient.

MANAGEMENT

Most patients with pulmonary edema are treated initially with oxygen. The administration of oxygen can help to relieve the patient's sense of dyspnea and may have beneficial effects on pulmonary mechanics. Patients with mild distress may be adequately treated with oxygen provided by nasal cannula, guided by the results of pulse oximetry or arterial blood gas analysis. Patients with underlying severe chronic obstructive pulmonary disease (COPD) may have an increase in hypercarbia with resultant acidosis. Oxygen administration should be conducted cautiously in these patients by using a controlled flow device such as a Venturi mask. Although it had been previously thought that patients with COPD developed hypercarbia due to a decrease in ventilatory drive, subsequent studies have shown that this is not the case.[5] Patients with COPD who develop hypercarbia with oxygen administration generally do so because of the Haldane effect with the release of carbon dioxide in the pulmonary vasculature on exposure to high concentrations of oxygen. In addition, the normally linear carbon dioxide dissociation curve is altered in COPD patients. Patients with increased distress may require even higher concentrations of oxygen using a nonrebreather mask.

Patients in severe distress may require mechanical ventilation. There are two primary means of accomplishing this including noninvasive ventilation and intubation. Noninvasive ventilation has been demonstrated to be an effective means of stabilizing appropriately selected patients. Patients treated with noninvasive ventilation have shown a decrease in morbidity rate with a decreased length of stay in the intensive care unit.[6,7] Approximately two-thirds of all patients treated with noninvasive ventilation for respiratory failure, including pulmonary edema, can avoid intubation.

Patients must be carefully selected for noninvasive ventilation. The appropriate patients must be awake and able to cooperate with instructions. Patients with anatomic facial disorders may not be able to be fitted with an appropriate mask. Patients who are obtunded, apneic, or near respiratory arrest, are not suitable for noninvasive ventilation. The performance of noninvasive ventilation requires a commitment of time by a physician, nurse, or respiratory therapist who can instruct the patient, adjust the controls, and monitor for successful implementation of this technique. Two forms of noninvasive ventilation are available, continuous positive airway pressure (CPAP) or bilevel positive airway pressure (BiPAP). Each of these techniques has been used successfully for the management of pulmonary edema. There is little evidence suggesting that one technique is superior to the other although there have been some smaller studies which have suggested a superiority to CPAP over BiPAP. The use of CPAP is associated with a 26% decrease in the need for intubation in cardiogenic pulmonary edema.[7]

Both CPAP and BiPAP can decrease cardiac filling pressures, which is beneficial for patients with fluid overload.[8] At the same time, patients who are dependent on preload for maintaining cardiac output can have a drop in blood pressure with initiation of either of these techniques. This may include patients with right ventricular infarction.

BiPAP also has beneficial hemodynamic effects on patients with heart failure. It may lead to a more rapid improvement in symptoms over CPAP.[9] In comparison of the hemodynamic effects of BiPAP versus CPAP, BiPAP was better tolerated than CPAP using settings of 10 cm of water for CPAP with the BiPAP settings at 8–12 cm for inspiratory positive airway pressure (iPAP) and 10–15 cm for expiratory positive airway pressure (ePAP). The improvement in oxygenation was higher for patients receiving BiPAP than for those receiving CPAP. The decrease in mean pulmonary capillary wedge pressure was greater for patients with BiPAP compared to CPAP.[8] A study of BiPAP in patients with acute respiratory failure from a variety of causes including pulmonary edema, showed a lower incidence of complications and a shorter stay in the intensive care unit.[10] A few studies have suggested that BiPAP may not be beneficial for patients with acute pulmonary edema. An older study found a higher incidence of myocardial infarction in patients treated with BiPAP as compared to patients treated with intermittent boluses of intravenous nitroglycerin.[11] More recent studies comparing CPAP versus BiPAP for patients with acute pulmonary edema have found no increase in the incidence of myocardial infarction between the two groups with equal efficacy.[12,13] Similarly, CPAP has been studied in patients with acute cardiogenic pulmonary edema. Typically, patients receive CPAP with 10 cm of water. Using this technique many patients have an improvement in oxygenation, a decrease in hypocarbia, and a trend toward fewer requirements for intubation. A metaanalysis of similar studies found a 26% reduction in the risk of intubation using CPAP.[7]

Patients who fail noninvasive ventilation or those who are not appropriate for trials of noninvasive ventilation may require intubation. Intubation under these circumstances can be facilitated through the use of a variety of medications. These would include sedating agents such as morphine or a benzodiazepine. Alternatively, patients can be treated with barbiturates such as thiopental, that have the advantage of lowering blood pressure, or other agents such as etomidate which do not have a similar effect on blood pressure. These may be followed by the use of paralytic agents such as succinylcholine or vecuronium. Previous work has suggested that intubation using a combination of medications, which include a paralytic, may have a lower complication rate compared to intubation without drug facilitation.[14] Once intubated, patients should be provided with adequate oxygenation. In the case of patients with acute pulmonary edema, the addition of positive end-expiratory pressure, typically 10 cm of water, may decrease ventricular filling pressures and improve the clearance of pulmonary water.

Morphine

Acute pulmonary edema due to fluid overload or heart failure is typically treated with a combination of agents leading to diuresis, a decrease in pulmonary artery pressure, and an improvement in cardiac output. Morphine sulfate has been used for many decades for the treatment of pulmonary edema. Morphine has only modest hemodynamic effects and the amount of venodilation that occurs is a relatively minimal.[15,16] Morphine will help to relieve some patients' symptoms of dyspnea. In a retrospective analysis–, however, the use of morphine was associated with an increased incidence of intubation. When used, morphine sulfate should be administered in small increments, typically 2–4 mg at a time, monitoring the patient for further respiratory distress or obtundation. Because of the risk of confusion with other abbreviations, orders for morphine should be spelled out rather than using the common abbreviations of MS or MSO_4.

Diuretics

Most patients with acute cardiogenic pulmonary edema receive diuretics. Intravenous diuretics can help to temporize while other agents are being prepared. Typically, patients are given an intravenous bolus of a diuretic such as furosemide, starting with the patients' total outpatient daily dose. For patients who have not previously been on furosemide a typical dose is 20–40 mg. Patients who are going to respond to diuretics will usually do so promptly. If there has not been the initiation of an adequate diuresis within 30 min then the diuretic can be repeated, usually doubling the dose of diuretics up to a total of furosemide 360 mg. Other diuretics can be used, typically bumetanide in doses of 1–2 mg. Again, the patient should be monitored for the initiation of adequate diuresis. Patients with renal insufficiency or heart failure may be relatively resistant to diuretics. Further, even a single dose of diuretics in the setting of renal insufficiency or heart failure can precipitate a drop in glomerular filtration rate.[17] Patients with renal insufficiency receiving repeated doses of diuretics may have a blunted response with a decrease in urine output over

time. This is true with intermittent and continuous administration of diuretics although the effect is somewhat less with continuous infusion of diuretics.[18]

Inotropes

The use of inotropic therapy for patients with decompensated heart failure has been reexamined in light of several recent studies. The PRECEDENT Trial showed an increase in ventricular ectopy and the occurrence of ventricular tachycardia when patients were given dobutamine as compared to patients given nesiritide.[19] Further, there was a long-term adverse effect. Those patients given dobutamine had a greater 6-month mortality rate compared to those patients getting nesiritide.[20] The OPTIME Study was a comparison of the routine use of milrinone for patients receiving otherwise standard therapy for heart failure.[21] This did not demonstrate an improvement in hospital length of stay for those patients given milrinone. There was an increase in the adverse event rate, primarily driven by symptomatic hypotension. There was also an increase in the incidence of myocardial infarction, atrial fibrillation, and the mortality rate although these did not reach statistical significance. Inotropic therapy may be necessary for patients with shock states. The adverse effects of milrinone are more pronounced in patients with ischemic cardiomyopathy.[22] In this setting, the dose of inotrope used should be that which is necessary to maintain cerebral and renal function. Milrinone may be beneficial for patients with shock who are also on outpatient beta-blockers.

Vasodilators

There are three primary vasodilators that are used for patients with acute pulmonary edema. Nitroprusside is a potent arterial and venous dilator. Nitroprusside can substantially reduce patients' blood pressure to the extent that patients require very frequent blood pressure monitoring and frequently invasive hemodynamic monitoring in order to safely titrate the doses of this drug. Patients with renal insufficiency can develop cyanide or thiocyanate toxicity as can patients receiving prolonged administration of nitroprusside. Patients receiving nitroprusside can develop methemoglobinemia as can patients receiving nitroglycerin. The initiation of nitroprusside should be started at 10 μg/min with increases in 5–10 μg/min increments every 5 min until clinical endpoints or hemodynamic monitoring endpoints are achieved.

Nitroglycerin has been used for a number of years for acute cardiogenic pulmonary edema. The doses of nitroglycerin, which are needed to achieve adequate drops in pulmonary capillary wedge pressure, are much higher than those used for antianginal effects. Therapy can be initiated with topical nitroglycerin, typically 1–2 inches, although there has not been significant investigation into its effects in this setting. A randomized comparison of milrinone and nitroglycerin found that patients receiving milrinone were more likely to achieve hemodynamic goals than nitroglycerin-treated patients and that the time to achieve these hemodynamic goals was less for the milrinone-treated patients than the nitroglycerin-treated patients.[23] In that study it took almost 1 hour for the nitroglycerin-treated patients to achieve hemodynamic goals. In patients with chronic congestive heart failure, high-dose transdermal nitroglycerin leads to a drop in pulmonary capillary wedge pressure and right atrial pressure that begins about 1 hour after the initiation of therapy. Patients develop tolerance to this effect, which lasts for at most 24 hours.[24] In patients with heart failure and coronary artery disease, intravenous administration of nitroglycerin is associated with an initial fall in pulmonary wedge pressure followed by an increase, which begins at 12 hours.[25] Data from the VMAC Trial, which compared nitroglycerin with nesiritide, found that the onset of action of nesiritide was earlier than that for nitroglycerin.[26] After 2 hours the drop in wedge pressure with nitroglycerin matched that of nesiritide; however, there was the early onset of tolerance to nitroglycerin. Patients treated with nitroglycerin required increasing doses of the drug and in spite of these increases, the wedge pressure began to increase after 2 hours.[27] The use of vasodilating agents including nitroprusside, nitroglycerin, and nesiritide may be contraindicated in patients who are dependent on preload. This will include patients with constrictive paracarditis, hypertrophic obstructive cardiomyopathy, and significant aortic stenosis.

Nesiritide is a member of the natriuretic peptide class of agents. In addition to being a balanced vasodilator, nesiritide has beneficial effects on neurohormonal activation leading to a decrease in plasma aldosterone and norepinephrine.[28] Nesiritide is associated with an early fall in pulmonary capillary wedge pressure, typically occurring within 15 min of administration. There has been no demonstration of tolerance to the effects of nesiritide. Compared to nitroglycerin, nesiritide causes a more rapid decrease in pulmonary capillary wedge pressure, pulmonary artery pressure, and a greater improvement in patient symptoms. Nesiritide has been used safely in patients with renal insufficiency and no adjustment in doses is needed for patients with renal insufficiency.[29] The drug is typically initiated in doses of 2 µg/min as a bolus followed by 0.01 µg/kg/min as an infusion based on the patients' actual body weight. If symptomatic hypotension occurs then the drip is temporarily discontinued. A small proportion of patients may require an infusion of a small volume of crystalloid.

Treatment Summary

Patients with cardiogenic pulmonary edema can present with varied severity from mild distress to fulminant pulmonary edema. Patients with significant distress should be treated with the administration of oxygen as described above, diuretics for patients with volume overload or cardiogenic pulmonary edema, and consideration for vasodilators. Those patients who should be treated with vasodilators, in the absence of contraindications, include those with renal insufficiency, depressed ejection fraction, significant pulmonary edema, those who are hypertensive on presentation, and those without a brisk response to an initial dose of diuretics. Analysis of heart failure registries has indicated that the initiation of vasodilator therapy in general and nesiritide therapy specifically in the emergency department leads to a better outcome than delayed initiation on the inpatient unit.[30,31] The early initiation of vasodilating agents such as nesiritide is associated with a decreased hospital length of stay, decreased stay in the ICU, and lower overall mortality rate.

Noncardiogenic Pulmonary Edema

Patients with noncardiogenic pulmonary edema are initially treated with oxygen with evaluation for the need for noninvasive ventilation. Unless these patients have increased cardiac filling pressures or evidence of cardiogenic edema, they are generally not treated with vasodilators or diuretics. In patients with adequate filling pressures, CPAP or BiPAP can help to improve oxygenation. Caution should be taken to avoid precipitating hypotension.

Therapy is otherwise directed at the underlying cause of noncardiogenic pulmonary edema. Patients may require treatment for sepsis, connective tissue disorders, or toxic exposure. A variety of other agents have been investigated for use in this setting including corticosteroids, prostaglandin E_1, antiendotoxin antibodies, surfactant, and pentoxifylline. Corticosteroids have been extensively investigated in this setting. Although they have been thought to lead to a benefit in patients with acute lung injury, there has been some renewed interest in this therapy.[31] The therapy of noncardiogenic pulmonary edema is generally supportive.

Noncardiogenic pulmonary edema is a common outcome of exposure to many bioterrorism agents. The diagnosis of exposure to a deliberately released or accidental industrial exposure may be suggested by the appearance of clusters of patients with acute noncardiogenic pulmonary edema. Phosgene is used in the manufacture of plastics and pesticides. During World War I, it was used as a chemical warfare agent and goes by the military designation, "CG." With acute exposure patients can have significant early respiratory symptoms. There may also be a delayed response with the appearance after 48 hours of either cardiogenic or nonardiogenic edema. Chlorine is used in a variety of manufacturing processes. Acute exposure can cause the rapid progression of pulmonary symptoms as can exposure to various cyanogen compounds. Ricin is associated with the onset of symptoms within hours of exposure. Pulmonary edema typically occurs within 1 day. Anthrax, usually associated with a hemorrhagic pneumonitis and mediastinitis can also cause pulmonary edema. There are a variety of biologic and chemical agents which can lead to acute pulmonary edema. Identification of unusual presentations or clusters of cases may be the clues to diagnosis.

UNRESOLVED ISSUES

- Are there criteria to select patients to receive one form of noninvasive ventilation over another?
- Are there survival benefits of using nesiritide over nitroglycerin?
- Is there a role for steroids in noncardiogenic pulmonary edema?

REFERENCES

1. Sibbald W, Anderson R, Holliday R. Pathogenesis of pulmonary edema associated with the adult respiratory distress syndrome. *Can Med Assoc J* 1979;120(4):445–450.
2. Stevenson LW, Perloff JK. The limited reliability of physical signs for estimating hemodynamics in chronic heart failure. *JAMA* 1989;261(6):884–888.
3. Peacock WF, IV, Albert NM, Kies P, et al. Bioimpedence monitoring for detecting pulmonary fluid in heart failure: Equal to chest radiography. *Congest Heart Fail* 2000; 6:86–89.
4. Peacock WF, Emerman CL, Doleh M, Civic K, Butt S. A Retrospective Review. The Incidence of non-ST segment elevation MI in Emergency Department patients presenting with decompensated heart failure. *Congest Heart Fail* 2003;9(6):303–308.
5. Hanson CW, 3rd, Marshall BE, Frasch HF, et al. Causes of hypercarbia with oxygen therapy in patients with chronic obstructive pulmonary disease. *Crit Care Med* 1996;24:23–28.
6. Poponick JM, Renston JP, Bennett RP, et al. Use of a ventilatory support system (BiPAP) for acute respiratory failure in the Emergency Department. *Chest* 1999;116:166–171.
7. Pang D, Keenan SP, Cook DJ, et al. The effect of positive pressure airway support on mortality and the need for intubation in cardiogenic pulmonary edema. *Chest* 1998;114(4):1185–1192.
8. Philip-Joet FF, Paganelli FF, Dutau HL, et al. Hemodynamic effects of bilevel nasal positive airway pressure ventilation in patients with heart failure. *Respiration* 1999;66(2):136–143.
9. Mehta S, Jay GD, Woolard RH, et al. Randomized, prospective trial of bilevel versus continuous positive airway pressure in acute pulmonary edema. *Crit Care Med* 1997;25(4):620–628.
10. Antonelli M, Conti G, Rocco M, et al. A comparison of non-invasive positive-pressure ventilation and conventional mechanical ventilation in patients with acute respiratory failure. *N Engl J Med* 1998;339:429–435.
11. Sharon A, Shpirer I, Kaluski E, et al. High-dose intravenous isosorbide-dinitrate is safer and better than Bi-PAP ventilation combined with conventional treatment for severe pulmonary edema. *J Am Coll Cardiol* 2000;36(3): 832–837.
12. Cross AM, Cameron P, Kierce M, et al. Non-invasive ventilation in acute respiratory failure: A randomized comparison of continuous positive airway pressure and bi-level positive airway pressure. *Emerg Med J* 2003;20(4):531.
13. Levitt M. A prospective, randomized trial of BiPAP in severe acute congestive heart failure. *J Emerg Med* 2001; 21(4):363–369.
14. Poponick JEA, Emerman C. Efficacy of rapid sequence intubations in medical patients in the emergency department. *Chest* 1996;110(suppl 4):151S.
15. Timmis AD, Rothman MT, Henderson MA, et al. Haemodynamic effects of intravenous morphine in patients with acute myocardial infarction complicated by severe left ventricular failure. *Br Med J* 1980;280(6219):980–982.
16. Sacchetti A, Ramoska E, Moakes ME, et al. Effect of ED management on ICU use in acute pulmonary edema. *Am J Emerg Med* 1999;17(6):571–574.
17. Gottlieb SS, Skettino SL, Wolff A, et al. Effects of BG9719 (CVT-124), an A_1-adenosine receptor antagonist, and furosemide on glomerular filtration rate and natriuresis in patients with congestive heart failure. *J Am Coll Cardiol* 2000;35(1):56–59.
18. Rudy DW, Voelker JR, Greene PK, et al. Loop diuretics for chronic renal insufficiency: A continuous infusion is more efficacious than bolus therapy. *Ann Intern Med* 1991;115(5): 360–366.
19. Burger AJ, Horton DP, LeJemtel T, et al. Effect of nesiritide (B-natriuretic peptide) and dobutamine ventricular arrhythmias in the treatment of patients with acutely decompensated congestive heart failure: The PRECEDENT study. *Am Heart J* 2002;144(6):1102–1108.
20. Silver MA, Horton DP, Ghali JK, et al. Effect of nesiritide versus dobutamine on short-term outcomes in the treatment

of patients with acutely decompensated heart failure. *J Am Coll Cardiol* 2002;39(5):798–803.

21. Cuffe MS, Califf RM, Adams KF, JR, et al. Short-term intravenous milrinone for acute exacerbation of chronic heart failure: A randomized controlled trial. *JAMA* 2002;287(12):1541–1547.

22. Felker GM, Benza RL, Chandler AB, et al. Heart failure etiology and response to milrinone in decompensated heart failure: Results from the OPTIME-CHF study. *J Am Coll Cardiol* 2003;41(6):997–1003.

23. Loh E, Elkayam U, Cody R, et al. A randomized multicenter study comparing the efficacy and safety of intravenous milrinone and intravenous nitroglycerin in patients with advanced heart failure. *J Card Fail* 2001;7(2):114–121.

24. Roth A, Kulick D, Freidenberger L, et al. Early tolerance to hemodynamic effects of high dose transdermal nitroglycerin in responders with severe chronic heart failure. *J Am Coll Cardiol* 1987;9(4):858–864.

25. Elkayam U, Kulick D, McIntosh N, et al. Incidence of early tolerance to hemodynamic effects of continuous infusion of nitroglycerin in patients with coronary artery disease and heart failure. *Circulation* 1987;76(3):577–584.

26. Publication Committee for the VMAC Investigators (Vasodilatation in the Management of Acute CHF). Intravenous nesiritide vs nitroglycerin for treatment of decompensated congestive heart failure: A randomized controlled trial. *JAMA* 2002;287(12):1531–1540.

27. Elkayam U, Akhter MW, Singh H, et al. Comparison of effects on left ventricular filling pressure of intravenous nesiritide and high-dose nitroglycerin in patients with decompensated heart failure. *Am J Cardiol* 2004;93(2):237–240.

28. Colucci WS, Elkayam U, Horton DP, et al. Intravenous nesiritide, a natriuretic peptide, in the treatment of decompensated congestive heart failure. Nesiritide Study Group. *N Engl J Med* 2000; 343(4):246–253.

29. Butler J, Emerman C, Peacock WF, et al. The efficacy and safety of B-type natriuretic peptide (nesiritide) patients with renal insufficiency and acutely decompensated congestive heart failure. *Nephrol Dial Transplant* 2004;19(2):391–399.

30. Emerman C, Costango M, Berkowitz REA. Early initiation of IV vasoactive therapy improves heart failure outcomes: An analysis from the ADHERE registry database. *Ann Emerg Med* 2003;42, in press.

31. Chadda K, Annane D. The use of corticosteroids in severe sepsis and acute respiratory distress syndrome. *Ann Med* 2002;34(7/8):582–589.

30

Emergency Department Observation Unit Management of Heart Failure

W. Frank Peacock IV

HIGH YIELD FACTS

- The Observation Unit (OU) can provide a venue for heart failure (HF) care in appropriately selected patients where length of hospitalization is decreased, 30-day revisits decline, and hospital costs are lowered.

- Because of an increased risk of mortality, patients with positive cardiac markers, systolic BP <115 mmHg, blood urea nitrogen (BUN) >43 mg/dL, or creatinine >2.75 mg/dL may not be optimal OU candidates.

- Parameters associated with successful OU management are systolic BP >160 mmHg and BUN <30 mg/dL.

- Disposition from the OU requires that the patient be able to ambulate, have stable vital signs, have had coexisting precipitants of HF exacerbation excluded, and have the appropriate resources to be able to manage his/her disease.

INTRODUCTION

In the last 20 years, the impact of HF has markedly increased. Hospitalizations for acute decompensated HF (ADHF) have risen by more than 150%, now exceeding 1 million each year,[1] but the mortality is unchanged. Worse, older patients suffer disproportionally, and much of the entire planet currently faces an aging demographic profile. Therefore, the impact of HF will only grow. Clearly new treatment and novel strategies are needed. OU HF management has recently been suggested as an alternative to hospitalization for the care of the HF patient.

HF is best characterized as a disease of revisits, and is commonly termed a "merry-go-round" because of frequent exacerbations and hospital readmissions. However, it is more accurately described as a clinical roller coaster. This is because its rhythm of improvement and deterioration is superimposed on a trend of a steadily deteriorating clinical course. The impact of this recidivism is clearly demonstrated in the emergency department (ED), where only 21% of ED HF patients represent a de novo presentation. Most ED HF patients present because of an acute exacerbation of a previously established HF diagnosis.

When examining ED HF management, historically 80% of all ED ADHF was admitted to an in-patient floor, where it is considered a diagnostic-related group (DRG) admission. These hospitalizations then last for several days. This was not unreasonable: ED HF visits result from either severe disease, or the consequence of a poor social situation, both of which are difficult to manage in the busy ED. However, with the advent and general availability of chest pain centers, there became an available alternative to in-patient care of the HF patient. By using the cardiovascular expertise of the chest pain unit, out-patient HF management has become a viable strategy.

ECONOMICS

Since HF is predominately a disease of the elderly, and the Centers for Medicare and Medicaid Studies (CMS) is the primary health insurer of Americans older than 65 years, CMS is the primary financial provider for 80% of all HF patients. This creates the unique situation where the majority of patients are insured. However since reimbursement arises from a single payer, the rules of CMS therefore dictate HF management strategy.

The CMS considers patients admitted for HF to be in a DRG. DRG 127 (HF) has a tremendous impact. It is the most common cause of hospitalization in patients older than 65, and the most common secondary discharge diagnosis. Of all diseases, DRG 127 is the single most expensive diagnosis for CMS, costing more than the combination of breast and lung cancers.

Because of the rules of CMS, there are three main drivers with regard to HF management. These are length of hospitalization, revisit frequency, and intensity of service. When a patient is admitted to a hospital and receives a DRG diagnosis, the facility receives a regionally standardized sum of money from CMS. The amount is independent of the actual cost of care for any specific patient, but represents a predetermined amount based on the diagnosis. The difference between CMS reimbursement and the actual cost to care for a specific patient represents the institution's profit margin. Since one of the most important determinants of cost is the length of hospitalization, this system prompts the institution to aggressively manage HF, with the goal of expeditious discharge, so that actual patient care costs are less than reimbursement.

Unfortunately, if the average length of stay to care for an ADHF patient is excessive, the result is financial loss for the hospital. For DRG 127, the break-even point occurs at approximately 5 days. Ultimately, this mandates a hospital maintain an average length of stay near 4 days. This is required to insure that the profit margin is sufficient to cover the costs of those HF patients with prolonged hospitalizations. Most facilities are unable to accomplish this; the average U.S. hospital loses $1288 per ADHF admission.

The second economic driver of HF management is revisit frequency. If the only economic incentive was length of stay, undue discharge pressure could potentially adversely impact patient care. Consequently, a second penalty is designed to prevent premature discharge that could result in rapid rehospitalization. After an index hospitalization, rehospitalization for the same DRG within 30 days may be considered as part of the first visit. Although CMS may refuse to provide additional reimbursement for readmissions within 30 days, this does not seem to be uniformly applied throughout the United States.

The final economic pressures are the actual resources required for managing ADHF. This represents the actual cost of care, and is proportional to the intensity of service provided. For example, compared to the OU, ICU hospitalization has markedly higher overhead costs and rapidly depletes the DRG award. Ultimately, while diagnostic and therapeutic interventions contribute to the cost of ADHF care, the predominate determinates of an institution's costs are the average length of stay, revisit frequency, and the intensity of service.

AMBULATORY PATIENT CLASSIFICATION

On April 1, 2002, CMS approved an ambulatory patient classification (APC) code for the outpatient management of HF in the ED OU. By this definition, the ED OU is defined as an outpatient environment, which provides the option of management without hospitalization. It also allows a reimbursement mechanism independent of the DRG revisit penalty. Not only economically advantageous to the institution, the option of a short intensive therapeutic management opportunity provides access to a low-cost venue to improve the quality of life of the HF patient.

Interestingly, by the definition of observation established by CMS, OU therapy does not have to occur in a specialized unit. For the purposes of reimbursement, the OU is a virtual location and therapy may occur in any unit throughout the hospital, as long as the patient is discharged with 48 hours of admission. However, despite billing rules that do not mandate a geographically defined location, a specialized OU with dedicated staff provides consistency of service and has the greatest potential for improved clinical outcomes.

The OU provides an environment where patients may receive care for up to 48 hours. However, since reimbursement from CMS ceases at 24 hours, most units plan for disposition by that time. Because of these criteria, the OU should not accept all HF patients. Nursing:patient ratios are usually in the range of 1:3–1:5. Therefore, HF patients admitted to an OU environment must be less critical than those requiring more intensive in-patient services. Ultimately, the OU cohort represents a subcategory of lower acuity HF patients. The advantage to the hospital is that a 24-hour OU stay results in treatment costs that are significantly lower than in-patient hospitalization costs. Thus, by decreasing overhead and providing care independent of the DRG revisit rule, the OU provides a twofold benefit.

An important corollary to the above billing structure is that billing codes may be changed, based on a patient's response to therapy, but only in the upward direction. What this means in practice is that while codes may be changed from an APC to a DRG without penalty, the converse is not true. Therefore, if a patient is admitted as an APC but is subsequently found to require a longer term of therapy than anticipated at presentation, this can be converted to a DRG admission. However, if a patient admitted as a DRG is able to leave at 24 hours, no down grading of the code is allowed. While it may initially seem advantageous to code all patients as DRG, to increase the profit margin, this is not a successful long-term strategy, as DRG payments are indexed over time to estimated costs. Consequently, a short average length of stay will ultimately result in a decrease in future DRG payments.

In addition to the care of the routine ED HF patient, the OU is able to provide for HF patients with specific difficulties complicating their outpatient management. For example, ejection fraction (EF) measurement is a standard for HF diagnosis and treatment,[2] and is required by the Joint Commission for Hospital Accreditation. EF measurement is difficult in a busy ED, and can be challenging after discharge in the nonambulatory elderly (e.g., nursing home patient) after leaving the hospital. Similar limitations occur with the multiple outpatient visits required for initiation and optimization of HF medication. In the OU, EF can be measured and medication dosing adjusted in a controlled environment. OU management which focuses on a comprehensive care approach can provide benefits to many patients, especially to those in difficult social situations.

OU CANDIDATE SELECTION: RISK STRATIFICATION

When a dedicated OU is available, candidates are selected based on the physician's impression that there will be sufficient clinical improvement, such that discharge is feasible within 24 hours. A number of situations should preclude OU admission in preference to in-patient therapy, these include patients whose clinical state suggests that decongestion will require in excess of 24 hours, if there are unstable hemodynamics or airway issues, and when there are coexistent morbidities complicating ADHF. As a corollary, patients needing IV medication that requires frequent titration, or IV infusions of agents to control arrhythmia will exceed the nursing capabilities of the OU.

Unfortunately, there are very little data to help guide the practitioner in selecting the optimal OU candidate. Data presented at the 2003 Society of Chest Pain Centers and Providers annual meeting indicated that emergency physicians are able to intuitively identify, based on clinical grounds, a cohort of patients of which 75% will be successfully discharged within 24 hours. In that analysis, the remaining 25% required in-patient hospitalization after OU management, and were subsequently hospitalized and converted to a DRG diagnosis.

Two other studies have specifically examined predictors of OU management success. Burkarhdt et al., in a study of 385 OU patients, noted that those with a BUN exceeding 30 mg/dL had an increased risk of OU therapy failure, defined as the requirement for admission after 24 hours of therapy.[3] Diercks et al. in examining low-risk predictors in 499 patients, found that a normal troponin or an initial BP greater than 160 mmHg, were associated with a length of stay less than 24 hours and no readmissions within the subsequent 30 days.[4]

An alternative approach to selection of OU candidates is to exclude those patients with high-risk features. Many studies have examined predictors of adverse events in HF. These include hyponatremia, anemia, the presence of a prolonged electrocardiographic QRS, low EF, an unchanging BNP level after treatment, and others. Unfortunately, the correlation between these findings and acute adverse events is poorly studied in the OU environment. While many of these parameters are associated with adverse events in the HF population, this may be on a time scale measured in years and consequently is of little help for ED decision-making.

Of greatest use are predictors associated with adverse outcomes that are available during the ED presentation. One analysis of over 80,000 hospitalized acutely decompensated HF patients, found a markedly increased mortality risk if the creatinine exceeded 2.75 mg/dL, the BUN was greater than 43 mg/dL, or the systolic BP was lower than 115 mmHg. Each parameter was associated with an increased in-hospital mortality, and if all three occurred simultaneously, the associated mortality was 22%. Comparatively, the absence of all three was associated with a mortality rate of only 2%.[5]

Finally, while not a study specifically evaluating the OU candidates, Lee et al. reported on a 30-day mortality prediction tool, validated in about 4000 patients,[6] that may be used to help screen for appropriate OU candidates. By this method, points are totaled, and if less than 70, 30-day mortality is less than 1% (see Table 30-1).

Table 30-1. 30 Day Mortality Prediction[6]; if Total <70 Points, 30 Day Mortality <1%

Variable	Score
Age (years)	Add age
Respiratory rate (breaths per minute)	Add rate (min 20, max 45)
Systolic BP (mmHg)	Subtract points <90 = −30, 90 − 99 = −35, 100 − 119 = −40, 120 − 139 = −45, 140 − 159 = −50, 160 − 179 = −55, >180 = −60
BUN (mg/dL)	Add level (max = 60 mg/dL)
Sodium (meq/L)	Add 10 if <136 meq/L
Cerebrovascular disease	Add 10
Chronic obstructive pulmonary disease	Add 10
Cancer	Add 15
Dementia	Add 20
Hepatic cirrhosis	Add 25

ROLE OF THE ED IN OU HF MANAGEMENT

Successful OU HF care begins in the ED, where two issues must be effectively managed. First, the diagnosis of HF must be correct, and second, appropriate therapy must be initiated expeditiously. An accurate diagnosis is critical, since inappropriate or inadequate treatment can result in increased adverse outcomes. However, because the easily available diagnostic tools (i.e., history, physical, ECG, and x-ray) are nonspecific and insensitive, diagnosing HF can be difficult. In fact, in the Breathing Not Proper study[7] of over 1500 patients, the correct diagnosis was found in only 81.5% of ED ADHF patients. The most accurate diagnosis they reported occurred when results from history, physical, and b-type natriuretic peptide (BNP) measurement in combination were considered. The presence of an elevated BNP, when coupled with a clinical impression of ADHF, may help select appropriate OU ADHF candidates. Since this assay has a negative predictive value that usually exceeds 90%, and a positive predictive value of 70–95%,[8] a negative BNP should suggest an alternative diagnosis for the patient's symptoms, and alternative therapeutic strategy sought.

The second important task for optimal HF management is to institute early and aggressive therapy. Delays in therapy are directly related to worse outcomes. In ADHF, mortality, hospitalization length of stay, and ICU length of stay, are directly related to the time until vasoactive HF treatment is initiated.[9]

OU PROTOCOL MANAGEMENT

When considering acutely decompensated HF that presents to an ED, it is unlikely that a few hours of therapy will be adequate to allow discharge. The most common rate-limiting event in the treatment of HF is relief of circulatory and pulmonary congestion. Consequently, the OU offers a unique opportunity for a longer term of therapy, which may prevent the necessity of an in-patient hospitalization.

In in-patient HF care, it has been shown that a multidisciplinary intervention program decreases 90-day readmissions, improves the quality of life, and decreases cost.[10–12] It is therefore reasonable to expect similar results would be obtained in the OU. Although a HF management protocol is not mandatory, it insures that the various interdisciplinary HF management goals are attained. Because HF therapy is a complicated task, standardized treatment insures that the many various details required for treatment occur in a timely fashion.

HF therapy requires the successful interplay of many different specialties, the use of individualized drug titration regimens, and the consideration of unique patient factors (e.g., education and compliance issues). This is challenging in the busy ED. Clearly defined management pathways have been published that demonstrate improved clinical and financial outcomes in the OU and outpatient environment. Consequently, we suggest protocol-driven management for the OU HF patient, and have validated our previously published[13] OU HF protocol. Tables 30-2 and 30-3 describe entry and exclusion criteria for the HF OU, and Table 30-4 is the protocol for patient care.

In a 10-month before and after study of 154 OU HF patients, comparing uncontrolled emergency physician management to protocol-driven care, we found that protocol managed patients had markedly improved outcomes. Patients managed with a HF protocol had a 44% lower rate of 90-day HF revisits ($P = 0.000$), and 36% fewer 90-day HF readmissions ($P = 0.007$). This occurred despite a 9% increase in OU discharge rates ($P = 0.008$), and a 10% decrease in hospital admissions ($P = 0.008$).

Although approximately 75% of appropriately selected OU HF patients will be decongested to the point that discharge is reasonable after a 1-day OU treatment algorithm, the remaining 25% will require longer therapy for the relief of their congestion. Even in this population of "OU failures," OU treatment provides clinical benefit. The total length of hospitalization in patients failing OU therapy and requiring in-patient therapy, inclusive of the OU admission time, was decreased from a mean 4.5–3.0 days ($P = 0.08$) by the use of an OU HF management protocol.[13]

Table 30-2. Suggested OU HF Protocol Entry Guidelines[*]

A. History
   Orthopnea, exertional dyspnea, paroxysmal nocturnal dyspnea, shortness of breath at rest, leg or abdominal edema, or weight gain
B. Examination
   Jugular venous distention or abdominal jugular reflux, S_3/S_4, rales, edema
C. Chest x-ray
   Cardiomegaly, pulmonary vascular congestion, Kerley B-lines, pulmonary edema, pleural effusion
D. Lab
   BNP >100 pg/mL

[*]Must have at least one from each category.

Table 30-3. OU HF Protocol Exclusion Criteria*

1. Unstable vital signs (despite ED therapy); blood pressure >220/120 mmHg, RR >25 bpm, HR >130 bpm, temperature >38.5°C
2. ECG or serum markers diagnostic of myocardial ischemia or infarction
3. Unstable airway, or nasal cannula oxygen requirement >4 L/min for SaO_2 >90%
4. Clinical scenario suggests cardiogenic shock, or with signs of end-organ hypoperfusion
5. Require continuous vasoactive medication (e.g., nitroglycerin), other than nesiritide
6. Clinically significant cardiac arrhythmia
7. Acute mental status abnormality
8. Severe electrolyte imbalances
9. Chronic renal failure requiring dialysis
10. Peak flow <50% of predicted, with wheezing
11. CXR with pulmonary infiltrates

*These criteria are meant to discourage entry by patients not likely to benefit from an aggressive diuresis and vasodilation management protocol.

Table 30-4. Summary of OU HF Management Protocol

Nursing-driven standard orders
Diuretic and neurohormonal antagonism (ACEI or nesiritide) algorithms

Aggressive fluid management monitoring
Admission weights
Strict recording of input and output
Fluid restriction
Low Na^+ diet

Diagnostic testing
K^+ and Mg^{2+} standing orders for measurement and dosing
Myocardial ischemia/infarction rule out by ECG and serum markers
Myocardial function and anatomy defined by echocardiography

Patient education
Educational movie
Personalized educational material
Nursing and physician bedside teaching
Dietetics consultations
Smoking cessation education

Discharge planning
Social work, visiting nurse consultation
HF specialist consultation

Finally, protocol-driven OU management results in institutional cost changes. Patients treated in an OU represent the "least sick" of the total hospital HF population. If they are then removed from the population of hospitalized HF patients, the remaining in-patient HF cohort will have a higher acuity of illness. In one study that estimated acuity by tracking of the rate invasive procedures (pulmonary artery catheterization, arterial pressure monitoring, endotracheal intubation, and so forth), the in-patient HF population had an 11% increase in invasive procedures by the initiation of an OU HF management protocol.[14]

Implementation of a HF pathway does require the investment of increased nursing resources in the OU. Reported in 1997 dollars, an OU pathway resulted in an additional cost of $81 per patient. However, this was offset by a net savings, predominantly from the result of readmission avoidance, of an annualized $89,321.[14]

HF pathways should incorporate proven, previously published, research-based HF treatment guidelines.[2] In this manner much of the results are not the effect of unique therapy, but result from attention to the details of HF management and education. Before protocol implementation, ED and OU staff education is needed. In our system, nurses attended a 4-hour class on acute HF management strategies and the use of medication algorithms. This includes teaching regarding an aggressive approach to the clinical assessment, patient education, and guidelines for when physician communication should occur. Having a specific OU (as opposed to a virtual unit) near the ED where physicians are available on a 24 × 7 basis, and having a dedicated nursing staff, can maximize the impact of educational efforts, and provide the greatest opportunity for optimal outcomes.

In HF patients, multiple revisits to the hospital are common.[2,11] The most common causes are medication and dietary noncompliance.[10–12,15] Since frequent hospitalization results in the deterioration of their quality of life, strategies proven to decrease admissions have the potential to improve the lifestyle of HF patients. Education of the symptomatic patient, in the form of nurse bedside teaching and by real time multidisciplinary consultation, may leverage an "educable moment" in the patient's disease course. Education while symptomatic may have greater impact on a successful lifestyle change than at other times in the patient's disease course.

SPECIFIC THERAPIES

Diuretics

Obtaining pulmonary decongestion is the rate-limiting step in OU HF patients. Therefore, initial therapy is directed at its relief with IV diuretics. Recommended dosing strategies are to administer the daily dose of furosemide (or its equivalent) as an IV bolus, to a maximum of 180 mg. If not currently on a diuretic, 40 mg of furosemide is usually adequate. Urine output and serum electrolytes are monitored to track diuresis volume, and to screen for treatment-induced hypokalemia. If target urine outputs are not met, the diuretic dose may be doubled and repeated at 2 hours. Adequate output should exceed 500 cc within 2 hours, unless the creatinine is >2.5 mg/dL, then 2-hour urine output goals are halved. Failure to meet output goals within 4 hours suggests in-patient hospitalization may be needed. Loop diuretics can prevent hospitalization and provide symptomatic relief. They are indicated for all patients with congestive findings, but not as monotherapy at discharge, since they have no effect on mortality.[2]

While historically the mainstay of HF therapy, aggressive diuresis is recognized to result in adverse renal effects. The effects of loop diuretics result in the negative consequences of stimulating the renin-angiotensin-aldosterone axis,[16] increasing vascular tone, and causing sodium and water retention. Although providing short-term benefit by decreasing congestion, it is hypothesized that by these unopposed mechanisms loop diuretics actually result in increased adverse outcomes chronically. Consequently, concurrent neurohormonal antagonism during diuresis is advocated to ameliorate the consequences of these pathologic neurohormonal reflexes.

NESIRITIDE

Nesiritide is biochemically identical to endogenous BNP. By providing hemodynamic and clinical benefits from the combination of vasodilation, natriuresis, and neurohormonal antagonism, it is an effective IV medication for decompensated HF therapy. Nesiritide improves dyspnea and hemodynamics more rapidly, and to a greater extent,[17] without the need for Swan-Ganz catheterization, than nitroglycerin.

While in general, hemodynamically active IV medications (nitroprusside, nitroglycerin, and inotropes) are discouraged for use in the OU, nesiritide has been demonstrated to be safe and effective. The Prospective Randomized Outcomes study of Acutely decompensated CHF Treated Initially as Outpatients with Nesiritide (PROACTION) Trial[18] was a blinded, randomized, placebo-controlled evaluation of standardized protocol-driven OU therapy with or without nesiritide in 237 patients. With respect to overall complications, there was no difference in adverse events or mortality between the control and nesiritide cohorts. After 3 hours, three nesiritide patients developed symptomatic hypotension that resolved without adverse sequelae, after drug termination.

With regard to efficacy, the use of nesiritide had a beneficial effect on readmissions during the following 30-day period. Those who received nesiritide during their OU stay had a 21% decrease in 30-day HF readmissions, as compared to standard therapy. Those with the most advanced disease (NYHA III and IV) had greater benefit, demonstrated by a 29% decrease in their 30-day readmission rate ($P = 0.057$). Finally, if OU treatment failed, and hospital admission was required, the 30-day readmission rate declined by 57% if on nesiritide. If an OU management failure patient did require rehospitalization within 30 days, there was a 45% decrease in their second admission length of stay if they had received nesiritide at their first visit.

During the month after the OU treatment, the total time spent in the hospital was 6.5 days if they had received standard therapy. This compared to 2.5 total in-hospital days in the subsequent month if their OU therapy had included nesiritide ($P = 0.032$). A financial analysis examining the total cost of therapy with either nesiritide or standard therapy found there was no difference between either strategies. Therefore, nesiritide use in the OU seems to improve revisit strategy, without adding to overall cost.

ANGIOTENSIN-CONVERTING ENZYME INHIBITORS

Vasodilators provide both symptomatic improvement and mortality reduction in HF,[19,20] but only if they antagonize the renin-angiotensin-aldosterone axis. This is not a class effect. Vasodilators without neurohormonal antagonism features, provide much less mortality benefit.[21] Angiotensin-converting enzyme inhibitors (ACEI), with both the effects of vasodilation and neurohormonal antagonism, represent a group of medications with a mortality reduction benefit of such magnitude that nearly all HF patients deserve a therapeutic trial. One hour after the initiation of furosemide, an ACEI may be initiated, unless the patient is on nesiritide (which has intrinsic neurohormonal antagonist activity). Contraindications to ACEI use include prior allergy, hyperkalemia, azotemia (creatinine >3 mg/dL), hypotension, or orthostatic dizziness. Blood pressure should be closely monitored following the initiation of an ACEI. All patients with systolic HF, and without contraindication, should be discharged on an ACEI.[2] Because of a higher cost, and less data demonstrating mortality reduction as compared to ACEIs, angiotensin receptor blockers (ARBs) are only used if there is significant intolerance or an ACEI contraindication exists.

VASODILATORS

There are three commonly used vasodilators for the treatment of decompensated HF: nitroprusside, nitroglycerin, and nesiritide. Nitroprusside induces excessive hemodynamic lability for safe use in the OU. Nitroglycerin induces rapid tachyphylaxis and the subsequent necessity for frequent dose adjustment (and each adjustment inducing a short period of potential hemodynamic instability) exceeds the nursing staff ratios for safe OU use. Patients requiring either nitroprusside, or nitroglycerin, should be considered to have a severity of illness that exceeds the OU objectives.

DIGOXIN

Digoxin prevents hospitalizations, but does not alter mortality. It is recommended for left ventricular (LV) systolic dysfunction and rate control in atrial fibrillation. Toxicity manifestations are cardiac arrhythmia (heart block, ectopy, or reentrant rhythms), gastrointestinal symptoms, or neurologic complaints (e.g., visual disturbances and confusion). While the measurement of serum levels can diagnose toxicity if >2.0 ng/mL, toxicity can occur at lower levels with hypokalemia or hypomagnesemia. Digoxin can be considered at a dose of 0.125–0.250 mg daily.[2]

BETA-BLOCKERS

Starting a Beta-blocker. Using beta-blockers in HF results in a profound mortality reduction, such that they are recommended in all HF patients.[22] However, because recommendations suggest that they should only be started in the decongested hemodynamically stable patient, their early OU use is contraindicated. Consequently, many patients are discharged home from the hospital without the initiation of a beta-blocker. Recent quality improvement data indicate that when this occurs, the outpatient initiation of beta-blockers is poor. In an intervention designed to improve the use of beta-blockers in HF patients, Fonorow initiated beta-blockers on hospital discharge. He found that patients started on beta-blockers at their discharge home, were much more likely to be on this life-saving therapy 1 month later, compared to those who were discharged without initiation.

Continuing a beta-blocker. Patients presenting with ADHF already taking a beta-blocker, represent a difficult management controversy, because abruptly stopping it may worsen already tenous hemodynamics. Therefore,

recommended therapy[2] is to continue administration of the beta-blocker, but at one dosing level lower than the patient's maintenance dose. Alternatively, some will give inotropes as a bridge to hemodynamic stability, while contintuing the beta-blocker. Importantly, if patients are at this stage of their disease, they are not ideal OU candidates.

ALDOSTERONE ANTAGONISTS

The aldosterone antagonist spironolactone decreases the relative risk of mortality in end-stage HF. Patients should receive 12.5–25 mg qd, in addition to their routine medications. Spironolactone is not recommended if the creatinine exceeds 2.5 mg/dL or the potassium is greater than 5.0 meq/L. If on spironolactone as an outpatient, it should be continued in the OU.

LABORATORY AND MONITORING

Aggressive diuresis commonly results in electrolyte and hemodynamic perturbations. Therefore, continuous ECG and oxygen saturation monitoring are indicated. Several other parameters also require close observation, and include the patient's initial weight, accurate urine output measurement, and fluid intake from all sources.

Because myocardial ischemia may precipitate HF, cardiac markers and ECGs are indicated. In an analysis of 67,924 ADHF patients, 6.2% had a positive troponin. Those with a positive troponin had a marked increase in acute adverse events, including higher rates of coronary artery bypass grafting, intraaortic balloon counterpulsation, mechanical ventilation, cardioversion, longer hospitalizations, longer ICU stays, and increased in-hospital mortality (8.0% vs. 2.7%, $P < 0.0001$).

Serum electrolytes should be monitored in a frequency based on urine output and clinical status. Any significant changes in HR, cardiac rhythm, or the new onset of conduction disturbances should prompt the performance of an ECG and electrolyte.

Potassium Administration

Potassium supplementation is commonly required, due to aggressive diuresis. However, if loop diuretics are used in concert with nesiritide, replacement needs are less. Potassium supplementation should be administered, either orally or intravenously, to maintain a K^+ of 4.0–5.0 meq/dL. If the creatinine exceeds 1.5 mg/dL, individualized therapy is needed. If the creatinine is below 1.5 mg/dL, the following guide can be used as a standing order:

a. If K^+ is <3.9 meq/dL, give 20 meq potassium PO × one dose.
b. If K^+ is <3.2 meq/dL, give 20 meq potassium IV and 40 meq PO × one dose.

Magnesium

Magnesium is an important cofactor for myocardial contractile function. It may be deficient in the HF patient, especially if chronic loop diuretic therapy has been required. Magnesium may be orally administered as 140 mg magnesium oxide, or if severely deficient it can be given IV as magnesium sulfate.

ECHOCARDIOGRAM

The echocardiogram is the gold standard for defining myocardial function. It is indicated in those without known systolic dysfunction, unless the EF has been defined within the prior year. Usually unnecessary in the ED, it can be obtained in the OU to assist in determining discharge treatment strategies.

DISCHARGE PLANNING

Discharge from the OU entails coordination of a multi-medication regimen including diuretics, digoxin, ACEI (or ARBs), possibly spironolactone, and beta-blockers. Optimally, medications are adjusted to meet target-dosing recommendations. Close consultation with the physician who will ultimately manage the outpatient course is necessary to provide optimum outcomes.

An aggressive management protocol can anticipate the discharge of 75% of HF patients admitted to the OU. Discharge planning is critical in HF. An outpatient multi-disciplinary team approach has been shown to improve HF outcome by decreasing revisit rates, lowering in-patient length of stay, and reducing hospital costs. One recent metaanalysis of 29 studies found a significantly decreased mortality by the use of a multidisciplinary team disease management approach.[23] The team approach should provide the option of consultations with social workers, dietitians, cardiologists, and advance practice nurses.

HF is a chronic condition with significant recidivism. Because noncompliance is the cause of 50% of HF rehospitalizations,[10] patient education is a critical facet in the OU. In fact, the new Joint Commission on Hospital Accreditation (JCAHO) guidelines require patient education. The four indicators required by the JCAHO are as follows:

1. At least 1 measurement of EF
2. Documentation of patient education
3. Documentation of smoking cessation counseling
4. One ACEI trial attempt

Suggested guidelines for discharge from the OU are noted in Table 30-5. Disposition from the OU is dependent on the improvement of dyspnea, decreasing congestion without long suffering orthostasis, and an adequate discharge environment. If these goals are unmet, hospitalization or assisted living facility placement should be considered. In-patient management should be considered in those with symptomatic end-stage HF, when there are severe coexisting disease(s), when additional workup is required, or if an intervention that cannot be performed on an outpatient basis is needed.

In appropriately selected HF patients, approximately 25% will require in-patient hospitalization after a 24-hour OU admission. This does not represent a failure of OU treatment. In an analysis of patients requiring continued in-patient therapy after an OU admission, the total length of stay was lowered by 24 hours (inclusive of the OU time) in those who had been admitted through the OU.[13] Thus, the OU represents an alternative to in-patient admission, which when coupled with aggressive 24-hour therapy, improves both patient and hospital outcomes.

Table 30-5. OU HF Discharge Guidelines*

1. Patient reports subjective improvement
2. If normally ambulatory, able to do so without significant orthostasis
3. Resting HR <100 bpm, systolic BP >80 mmHg
4. Total urine output >1 L, and urine output exceeds 30 cc/h (or >0.5 cc/kg/h)
5. Room air O_2 saturation >90% (unless on home O_2)
6. No ischemic-type chest pain
7. No ECG or cardiac marker evidence of myocardial ischemia/infarction
8. No new clinically significant arrhythmia
9. Normal electrolyte profile without increasing azotemia

*Patients not meeting all of the guidelines should be considered for in-patient treatment (except as appropriate in the end-stage palliative care cohort).

REFERENCES

1. American Heart Association. *Heart and Stroke Statistical Update*, 2001.
2. Packer M, Cohn JN. Consensus recommendations for the management of chronic heart failure. *Am J Cardiol* 1999; 83:2A,1A–38A.
3. Burkarhdt J, Peacock WF, Emerman C. Elevation in blood urea nitrogen predicts a lower discharge rate from the observation unit. *Ann Emerg Med* 2004;44(4):S99.
4. Diercks D, Peacock WF, Kirk D, et al. Identification of emergency department patients with decompensated heart failure at low risk for adverse events and prolonged hospitalization. *J Card Fail* 2004;10(4):S118.
5. Fonarow GC, Abraham WT, Adams K. Risk stratification for in-hospital mortality in heart failure using classification and regression tree (CART) methodology: Analysis of 33,046 patients in ADHERE. *Circulation* 2003;108:IV-693.
6. Lee DS, Austin PC, Rouleau JL, et al. Predicting mortality among patients hospitalized for heart failure: Derivation and validation of a clinical model *JAMA* 2003;290(19):2581–2587.
7. Maisel A, Krishnaswamy P, Nowak RM, et al. Rapid measurement of B-type natriuretic peptide in the emergency diagnosis of heart failure. *N Engl J Med* 2002;347(3):161–167.
8. Peacock WF. The B-type natriuretic peptide assay: A rapid test for heart failure. *Cleve Clin J Med* 2002;69(3):243–251.
9. Peacock WF, Emerman CL, Costanzo MR, et al. Early initiation of intravenous therapy Improves Heart Failure Outcomes: An Analysis from the ADHERE Registry Database. *Ann Emerg Med* 2003;42(4):S26.
10. Rich MW, Beckham V, Wittenberg C, et al. A multidisciplinary intervention to prevent the readmission of elderly patients with congestive heart failure. *N Engl J Med* 1995;333:1190–1195.
11. Rich MW, Vinson JM, Sperry JC, et al. Prevention of readmission in elderly patients with congestive heart failure. *J Gen Int Med* 1993;8:585–590.
12. Vinson JM, Rich MW, Sperry JC, et al. Early readmission of elderly patients with congestive heart failure. *JAGS* 1990;38:1290–1295.
13. Peacock WF 4th, Remer EE, Aponte J, et al. Effective observation unit treatment of decompensated heart failure. *Congest Heart Fail* 2002;8(2):68–73.
14. Albert NM, Peacock WF. Patient outcome and costs after implementation of an acute heart failure management program in an emergency department observation unit. *J Internat Soc Heart Lung Transplant* 1999;18(1):92.
15. Krumholz HM, Parent EM, Tu N, et al. Readmission after hospitalization for congestive heart failure among Medicare beneficiaries. *Arch Intern Med* 1997;157:99–104.
16. Bayliss J, Norell M, Canepa-Anson R, et al. Untreated heart failure: Clinical and neuroendocrine effects of introducing diuretics. *Br Heart J* 1987;57:17–22.
17. Publication Committee for the VMAC Investigators (Vasodilatation in the Management of Acute CHF). Intravenous nesiritide vs nitroglycerin for treatment of decompensated congestive heart failure: A randomized controlled trial. *JAMA* 2002;287(12):1531–1540.
18. Peacock WF, Emerman CE, Young J, on behalf of the PROACTION study group. Safety and efficacy of nesiritide for the treatment of decompensated heart failure in emergency department observation unit patients. *J Am Coll Cardiol* 2003;4(6):Suppl A, 336A.
19. The SOLVD Investigators. Effect of enalapril on mortality and the development of heart failure in asymptomatic patients with reduced left ventricular ejection fractions. *N Engl J Med* 1992;327(10):685–691.
20. The SOLVD Investigators. Effect of enalapril on survival in patients with reduced left ventricular ejection fractions and congestive heart failure. *N Engl J Med* 1991;325(5): 293–302.
21. Califf RM, Adams KF, McKenna WJ, et al. A randomized controlled trial of epoprostenol therapy for severe congestive heart failure: The Flolan International Randomized Survival Trial (FIRST). *Am Heart J* 1997;134(1):44–54.
22. Hjalmarson A, Goldstein S, Fagerberg B, et al. Effects of controlled release metoprolol on total mortality, hospitalization, and well being in patients with heart failure. The metoprolol randomized intervention trial in congestive heart failure (MERIT-HF). *JAMA* 2000;283:1295–1302.
23. McAlister FA, Stewart S, Ferrua S, et al. Multidisciplinary strategies for the management of heart failure patients at high risk for admission: A systematic review of randomized trials. *J Am Coll Cardiol* 2004;44(4):810–819.

31

Mechanical and Invasive Management of Heart Failure

Sean P. Collins

HIGH YIELD FACTS

- While the goal of an intraaortic balloon pump (IABP) is to support coronary artery perfusion, a ventricular assist device (VAD) supports the entire pulmonary and systemic circulation.
- Altered physiology of the transplanted heart renders atropine and digoxin ineffective, while adenosine has significantly more potent effects.
- Infection remains the most common cause of morbidity and mortality in the transplant patient.
- While outcomes from cardiac reduction therapy appear promising for ischemic cardiomyopathy (ICM) patients, these results have not been duplicated in patients with dilated cardiomyopathy (DCM).

INTRODUCTION

Patients with New York Heart Association (NYHA) functional class IV heart failure (HF) have a reported 1-year mortality of 33–37%.[1] Standard medical and surgical therapies benefit only a small percentage of these patients. Cardiac transplantation is an alternative for those class IV patients refractory to medical therapy. The registry for the International Society for Heart Transplantation in 1999 listed a cumulative total of 48,541 cardiac transplantations, performed in 304 transplant centers.[2] Unfortunately, while the incidence of HF continues to increase, the number of transplants has steadily decreased in the last few years.[2] As a result, alternatives to transplantation have been explored.

Mechanical circulatory devices were initially developed as short-term therapy for HF patients as a bridge to cardiac transplant, or to support postoperative patients

with postcardiotomy cardiogenic shock. However, with the increasing demand for heart transplantation (4000 patients on the heart transplant waiting list in October 1998) and decreasing number of surgeries, most centers experience a 10–20% mortality of patients on the waiting list.[3] As a result, mechanical circulatory support (MCS) has also been evaluated as a long-term alternative to orthotopic cardiac transplantation.

ASSISTED MECHANICAL CIRCULATION

Mechanical circulatory support benefits three distinct populations of HF patients (Table 31-1). The first group is those with "reversible" ventricular dysfunction after a myocardial infarction or open-heart surgery. Two to six percent of patients who undergo an open-heart operation develop postcardiotomy cardiogenic shock.[4] MCS allows the majority of these patients to be weaned from cardiopulmonary bypass (CPB).[5] The second group is those on the cardiac transplant waiting list with hemodynamic instability where it is used as a means to "bridge" the patient to transplantation. Finally, although controversial, patients with end-stage HF refractory to standard medical therapy may benefit from a permanent form of mechanical support, thus avoiding the need for transplantation.

History of MCS

The first clinical use of CPB was performed by Gibbon in 1953, during successful correction of an atrial septal defect.[6] Although subsequent uses of Gibbon's device proved unsuccessful, it encouraged further research in this area. Debakey and colleagues investigated the use of MCS in assisting patients who had undergone cardiotomy. They supported a patient for 10 days, after which the device was removed and the patient survived for a prolonged period of time.[7] Research performed over the same time period by Moulopoulos and colleagues resulted in the introduction of the IABP.[8] The IABP was first used clinically in a patient with cardiogenic shock in 1967.[9] In 1964, the National Heart and Lung Institute established its Artificial Heart Program, which spurred interest into development of permanent VADs. Over the next two decades, total artificial hearts (TAH) were implanted into humans to serve as permanent cardiac replacements and as bridges to permanent cardiac transplant. However, the results from these trials were not as promising as hoped for; the 1-year survival rate was only 37%, and many of the implantations were complicated by infection (36%) and embolic events (9%).[10] Because TAH implantation was not as successful as originally desired, research

Table 31-1. Patients Likely to Benefit from MCS

Reversible acute ventricular dysfunction
    Acute myocardial infarction
    Postcardiotomy
Hemodynamically unstable end-stage heart failure as a
bridge to transplant
End-stage heart failure as a permanent means of
mechanical support

efforts turned toward producing a long-term implantable
left ventricular assist device (LVAD). Initially used to treat
postcardiotomy shock, LVADs have also been investigated as a bridge to transplantation, as well as indefinite
circulatory support.

INTRAAORTIC BALLOON PUMP

Indications

The most common uses of IABP are in subjects with cardiogenic shock, either in association with an acute
myocardial infarction (AMI) or after open-heart surgery
(Table 31-2).[11] It can also be used preoperatively in those
patients with severe left ventricular dysfunction (LVD).
The situation where the emergency physician (EP) is most
likely to encounter the need for an IABP is the patient
with cardiogenic shock as a result of either an AMI or

Table 31-2. IABP Indications and Contraindications

Emergent indications
Cardiogenic shock
    Secondary to AMI
    Postcardiotomy
AMI complications
    Mitral regurgitation
    Ventricular septal defect

Contraindications
Absolute contraindications
    Aortic valve insufficiency
    Aortic dissection
Relative contraindications
    Femoral artery insertion
        Abdominal aortic aneurysm
        Severe aortic or femoral arterial disease
    Percutaneous insertion
        Recent ipsilateral groin incision
        Morbid obesity

decompensated HF. After pharmacologic support has
been maximized, the next step may be to initiate IABP
therapy in an effort to augment myocardial perfusion.
Clinical trials have shown the use of IABPs improves
short-term survival, postthrombolytic patency rates, and
may reduce stroke mortality after AMI.[12]

Design and Function

The IABP is inserted via Seldinger technique, either via
the common femoral artery (most common) or subclavian
artery, into the descending thoracic aorta just distal to the
left subclavian artery.[8] The dilator and sheath are inserted
together, with the dilator being removed, and the IABP
inserted into the introducer sheath. Subjects need to be
anticoagulated while on the device with the sheath in
place. An alternative "sheathless" technique allows
insertion of an IABP in the nonanticoagulated patient.
This technique avoids the use of the large dilator and
sheath assembly, minimizing obstruction to blood flow.
Once in place, the intraaortic balloon is set to inflate at the
dicrotic notch of the arterial pressure waveform, resulting
in balloon expansion during diastole. This diastolic rise in
aortic pressure augments coronary artery blood flow,
improving myocardial oxygen supply. Additional hemodynamic benefits occur by balloon deflation during ventricular contraction. This results in afterload reduction,
and a slight increase in systemic perfusion. The overall
net results of IABP use are a decrease in myocardial
oxygen consumption and a slight increase in systemic
perfusion (Table 31-3).[11]

Complications

The complication rate for IABP use ranges from 5 to
47%.[13,14] Major complications, such as limb ischemia and
aortic injury, occur less frequently (4–17%) than minor
complications; e.g., bleeding at the insertion site and
wound infection (7–42%).[15] Other complications that need
to be considered include hemorrhagic and ischemic stroke.
Limb ischemia requires removal of the IABP and possibly
femoral artery exploration. Leg ischemia is eliminated
with transthoracic IAB insertion. However, transient
ischemic attack, cerebrovascular accident, and mediastinitis can occur with insertion at the ascending aorta.

Summary

Though infrequent, the most common indication for
IABP use in the emergency department (ED) would be
the patient who remains in cardiogenic shock despite
maximum pharmacologic therapy. IABP can sustain

Table 31-3. Characteristics of Types of MCS

Device	Indications	Myocardial Effects	Systemic Effects	Complications	Lifestyle
IABP	Cardiogenic shock (secondary to ACS or ADHF)	Significant increase in coronary artery perfusion	Slight increase in systemic perfusion	1. Aortic injury 2. Ischemic/ hemorrhagic stroke 3. Limb ischemia	1. Anticoagulation 2. Must remain hospitalized
VAD	1. Cardiogenic shock (secondary to ACS or postcardiotomy) 2. Bridge to transplant 3. Permanent form of CV support	Negligible	Complete support of pulmonary and/or systemic circulation	1. Bleeding 2. Thromboembolic complications 3. Infection	1. Anticoagulation 2. May undergo rehabilitation and return to work
TAH	End-stage heart failure patients as a bridge to transplant or as a permanent form of support	Completely replaced myocardial circulation	Complete support of pulmonary and systemic circulation	1. Infection 2. Thromboembolism	1. Anticoagulation 2. May undergo rehabilitation and return to work

coronary artery perfusion and augment a small amount of peripheral circulation in an acutely failing ventricle.

VENTRICULAR ASSIST DEVICES

Indications

The original indication for a VAD was postcardiotomy cardiogenic shock in the subgroup of patients who were unable to be separated from CPB despite the use of an IABP.[11] However, the indications for VAD insertion have now extended to several other clinical situations: (1) as a bridge to transplantation in hemodynamically unstable HF patients; (2) hemodynamically unstable AMI patients in an effort to stabilize them as they await emergency revascularization. This can decrease mortality from 80%, to as low as 25–40%[16–18]; (3) as a permanent form of recovery in those awaiting transplantation. In some, ventricular recovery occurs to such a degree that the VAD can be removed and transplantation avoided.[19,20]

Design and Function

Unlike the IABP, which primarily supports the coronary circulation, VADs are designed to completely unload the

ventricle, thereby improving oxygen delivery to the systemic circulation (Table 31-1). There are both right and left ventricular VADs.[11] A right ventricular VAD withdraws blood from the right atrium and returns it to the main pulmonary artery, while a left ventricular VAD withdraws blood from the left atrium and returns it to the ascending aorta. In addition to supporting the periphery and unloading the ventricle, there are indications that mechanical unloading changes the structural and functional properties of the failing heart.[21] Myocytes decrease in cell volume, length, width, and length-to-thickness ratio.[22] There is also a reversal in apoptosis (programmed cell death) secondary to mechanical unloading.[23] Assist device implantation is also associated with increased contraction and reduced relaxation in isolated cardiomyocytes.[24] Unlike an IABP, which commits the patient to hospitalization until explantation, patients with VADs are mobilized early, placed in cardiac rehabilitation, and some even return to work and can be managed on an outpatient basis.[25]

Complications

Hemorrhage is seen in 14–50% of VAD recipients and is more common in patients who receive a VAD for postsurgical cardiogenic shock than in those who receive a VAD as a bridge to transplant.[19,26,20,27] Conversely, thrombus formation in the VAD, as a result of inadequate anticoagulation (target INR 2.5-3.0), can result in thromboembolic events. Though many VADs will have evidence of thrombus at explantation, there is often no associated clinical evidence of thromboembolism.[20] Infection occurs in up to 59% of VAD patients, but device-related infection occurs in a much smaller percentage.[19,20,26] The overall incidence of infection decreases with earlier chest tube removal, ambulation, and removal of indwelling lines and catheters.[20]

Summary

Ventricular assist devices are being used with increasing frequency as a bridge to transplant, and to rescue the acutely decompensated HF patient. With increased use of VADs in the ambulatory end-stage HF patient, EPs need to know the potential complications seen in these patients as they may present to the ED for acute evaluation.

TOTAL ARTIFICIAL HEART

Indications

With selection criteria similar to the VAD, the TAH is used as a bridge to transplantation, as well as a permanent form of circulatory support, in end-stage HF patients. A registry report covering the first 20 years of artificial heart transplants indicated that the majority (221/226, 98%) of the TAH transplants are performed as a bridge to transplant.[10] Under an FDA-approved protocol, four patients received the TAH as a permanent form of support. One patient lived 620 days, but all four patients had major complications from infection and thromboembolism.[28,29] The electrical TAH may ultimately prove to be a more compatible permanent TAH, but until a lightweight battery with a long cycle life is perfected, patients will have to rely on an external power source.[30]

Design and Function

The TAH is a biventricular device that is implanted orthotopically (in the patient's pericardium) while simultaneously removing the native heart. There are 11 different types of TAHs that have been implanted worldwide.[10] The devices are able to supplant the native ventricles and support the entire pulmonary and systemic circulation. All of the TAHs use similar design characteristics. The prosthetic ventricles contain flexible blood sacs that are compressed by air pulses generated by a bedside unit. A complex control system modifies cardiac output using

the Starling mechanism, such that an increase in preload results in increased ventricular filling and increased cardiac output.[11]

Complications

Similar to the VAD, the most frequent complications are related to infection, bleeding, and thrombosis (in the patient who is inadequately anticoagulated). Infectious complications appear to be the biggest obstacle preventing the use of TAH as a permanent form of circulatory support in the end-stage HF patient. In the first cohort of patients undergoing long-term use of a TAH, the major limiting factor was driveline infection, related to *Pseudomonas* and *Staphylococcal* species.[29]

Summary

The TAH can be used as a temporary form of support in the end-stage HF patient. However, unlike the VAD, its use as a long-term solution has not been as successful. As a result, those patients who experience hemodynamic instability while awaiting cardiac transplant are more likely to receive a VAD instead of a TAH.

PERMANENT SURGICAL THERAPY FOR HEART FAILURE

Heart Transplant

Background

The most definitive therapy for end-stage HF patients is cardiac transplantation. First performed by Christian Barnard at Groote Schuur Hospital in Cape Town, South Africa in December 1967,[31] there have now been over 33,000 transplantations worldwide as of 6/30/2001.[32] Shortly after the first transplant, there was a surge in the number of transplants performed worldwide. However, the 1-year survival was only 15%, and interest in transplantation declined in the 1970s.[33] However, better patient selection,[34] improved antirejection therapy, the development of the endomyocardial biopsy,[35] and a better understanding of posttransplant infection during the last decade, have all contributed to the subsequent improvement in posttransplantation mortality rates.

Indications

The majority of heart transplants are undertaken for ischemic heart disease and cardiomyopathy. The selection process is fairly complex and includes criteria based on ejection fraction, peak exercise oxygen consumption, age, and coexisting diseases. There is also a fairly robust list of contraindications that consider coexisting diseases, age, social, and psychiatric factors. Once subjects fulfill inclusion/exclusion criteria, they are then prioritized and placed on a waiting list based on their current clinical state. The highest priority patient is status 1A. These patients by definition must be inpatients with one of the following: (1) on some form of MCS; (2) mechanically ventilated; (3) continuous high-dose inotropic support; (4) life expectancy <7 days without transplant.[33]

Physiology and Cardiovascular Drugs in the Transplant Recipient

The transplanted heart is initially denervated, but there is evidence for partial return of both parasympathetic and sympathetic function within the first year.[33,36] Furthermore, it has been shown that adrenergic receptors of the cardiac conduction system do not depend on autonomic innervation to function normally.[37] These properties are important when considering baseline physiology, as well as pharmacologic effects in the transplant patient. For example, the incomplete reinnervation of the parasympathetic nervous system is responsible for a higher resting heart rate. Secondly, the transplanted heart's response to exercise is less than a native, healthy heart, but is adequate for most activities. The clinical impact of these effects is that the blunted heart rate response can result in orthostatic hypotension.[38,39]

Important for the EP is that, while incomplete cardiac innervation blunts the heart's ability to respond to physiologic responses, it enhances the body's responses to circulating epinephrine. Two studies of transplant patients found the responses to dobutamine and isoproterenol were greater in transplant patients than in normal controls.[40,41] Consequently, norepinephrine, which acts via intact adrenergic receptors, is helpful in hypotensive emergencies.[42] This may be beneficial when the hypotensive, acutely ill transplant patient is in need of vasopressors or inotropes (Table 31-4). Atropine works by a parasympa-

tholytic mechanism. Because the parasympathetic system is only partially reinnervated in the transplant patient, atropine will not increase the heart rate in bradycardia.[43]

Adenosine acts by blocking both the sinoatrial (SA) and atrioventricular (AV) nodes. In the transplant patient, there is an increased sensitivity of the donor SA and AV nodes. This can result in potentiation of the bradyarrhythmic effect of atropine at both of these sites.[44] As a result, a reduced dose of atropine should be used in the transplant patient. Digoxin acts on the SA and AV nodes through the autonomic nervous system. Therefore, digoxin has little effect in transplanted hearts when used as an AV-nodal blocking agent in atrial fibrillation/flutter with a rapid ventricular response.[45]

Care of the Posttransplant Patient

The EP may encounter transplant patients regarding a number of long-term care issues. Rejection, infection, and posttransplantation drug side effects may all lead to significant complications resulting in ED presentation. Having an understanding of the complications unique to postcardiac transplant patients is important for proper ED work-up, treatment, and disposition.

Rejection

Rejection can be divided into three types, based on time after transplantation. *Hyperacute rejection* occurs immediately after implantation and is the result of preformed anti-HLA antibodies. This is almost uniformly fatal unless the patient can be retransplanted in a timely manner. *Acute rejection*, a cell-mediated process, is experienced by virtually every transplant patient to some degree during the first transplant year. The Cardiac Transplant Research Database reported that the incidence of acute rejection peaked at 1 month after transplantation and then rapidly decreased.[46] Though most episodes of rejection

Table 31-4. Effects of Cardiac Drugs in the Transplant Patient

Drug	Effect on the Transplant Patient
Dobutamine	Increased cardiac output and heart rate
Isoproterenol	Increased cardiac output and heart rate; helpful in symptomatic bradycardia
Norepinephrine	Increased heart rate and cardiac output
Adenosine	Augmented bradyarrhythmic effect–a reduced dose is suggested
Atropine	No parasympatholytic effect—not helpful in bradycardia
Digoxin	Little effect as an AV- or SA-nodal blocking agent in supraventricular arrhythmias

are asymptomatic (detected only by endomyocardial biopsy), occasionally symptoms can occur. Arrhythmias, fatigue, and eventually dyspnea can occur.[47] The cornerstone of treatment for acute rejection includes high-dose intravenous steroids.[33] *Chronic rejection* is thought to be a result of graft atherosclerosis. Important to the ED, because of denervation, typical anginal symptoms are not reported by transplant patients. Therefore, the transplant patient with an acute coronary syndrome often presents with HF secondary to silent myocardial infarction, or sudden death.

Detection of Rejection

The gold standard for detection of myocardial rejection is the endomyocardial biopsy. Indications for biopsy include signs and symptoms of rejection (as indicated above) or routine surveillance. A typical rejection surveillance schedule includes weekly biopsies for the first month, with biopsy intervals progressively lengthening to every 6 months for the remainder of the transplant patient's life. Performed usually via the right internal jugular vein, the endomyocardial biopsy provides direct histologic evidence of myocardial damage. Patients may present to the ED with complications after endomyocardial biopsy including pneumothoraces, arrhythmias, myocardial perforation, or tricuspid regurgitation due to valve disruption.[33] Other noninvasive methods of graft rejection have been investigated. Measurement of cardiac troponin T has been shown to correlate with histologic findings on endomyocardial biopsy prior to clinical symptoms occurring.[48] Radionuclide scanning with technetium 99m-labeled annexin V has been shown to concentrate at sites of apoptosis and correlate with acute rejection in animal studies.[49]

Immunosuppressive Drugs and Complications

Immunosuppressive drugs focus on reducing the T-cell response to the transplanted heart (Table 31-5). Corticosteroids are one of the most common immunosuppressive agents used in transplant patients. They work by reducing the transcription of many genes involved in inflammation and immunity.[50] Common side effects include osteoporosis, peptic ulcer disease, adrenal gland suppression, and diabetes. Cyclosporin acts to limit the development of cytotoxic T lymphocytes. A number of toxicities are associated with cyclosporine, including renal insufficiency (40–70% of patients), hepatotoxicity, and neurotoxic effects such as paresthesias and seizures.[33] Tacrolimus (FK-506) has effects similar to cyclosporine, resulting in decreased development of cytotoxic T lymphocytes. Its biggest limiting side effect is renal toxicity and hyperkalemia, but neurotoxicity and hyperglycemia are also encountered. Because of its severe nephrotoxicity it is not used simultaneously with cyclosporine.[33] Azathioprine blocks proliferation of replicating lymphocytes. The major side effect of this agent is bone marrow suppression. OKT3 is a monoclonal antibody directed against the CD3 antigen and causes T-cell lysis. Its major side effect is "cytokine release syndrome" which develops 30–60 min after administration. This is manifested as a continuum from a flu-like illness to severe, life-threatening hypotension.

Infection

Infectious complications remain the most common cause of morbidity and mortality. In an analysis of 8620 patients

Table 31-5. Immunosuppressive Drugs—Mechanism of Action and Toxicity

Immunosuppressive Agent	Mechanism of Action	Side Effects
Corticosteroids	Decrease production of cytotoxic T lymphocytes	Osteoporosis, peptic ulcer disease, adrenal gland suppression, diabetes
Cyclosporin	Decreased cytotoxic T-lymphocyte production	Nephrotoxicity, hepatotoxicity, and neurotoxicity
Tacrolimus (FK-506)	Decreased cytotoxic T-lymphocyte development	Nephrotoxicity (hyperkalemia)*, neurotoxicity, and hyperglycemia
Azathioprine	Decreased lymphocyte proliferation	Bone marrow suppression
OKT3	T-cell lysis	Cytokine release syndrome

*Not to be used concurrently with cyclosporin.

who underwent cardiac transplantation from the early 1990s, about half suffered acute infection at 6 months, and over 60% at 1 year.[51] A separate analysis at Stanford University of 620 cardiac transplants revealed that infection was second only to rejection as the cause of early deaths, and was the most common cause of late deaths. The infectious events were split fairly evenly between bacterial (43.6%) and viral (41.7%), with a minority of the cases caused by fungi (10.2%).[52] Infections can be broken down into early and late categories. Early infection occurs within 1 month of transplantation. This is often manifested as nosocomial pneumonia by agents such as *Legionella, Staphylococcus epidermidis, Pseudomonas aeruginosa*, or *Klebsiella*.[33] Late infection is often caused by opportunistic infection as a result of chronic immunosuppression. Cytomegalovirus (CMV) infection is the most frequent viral infection in transplant patients, with an incidence between 73 and 100%.[53] CMV infection is characterized by both mild disease (fever, malaise, nausea) and severe disease, including pneumonitis (50% mortality), hepatitis, and leukopenia. While far less frequent than viral and bacterial infections, fungal infection (*Pneumocystis carinii, Candida, Aspergillus*) are more serious and lethal, and tend to be less responsive to therapy.[33]

Summary

Survival after cardiac transplant has improved significantly over the last couple of decades. Transplant recipients are often able to resume many of their normal daily activities. As a result, EPs are likely to encounter cardiac transplant recipients on a much more frequent basis. These patients have altered physiologic response to cardiovascular pharmacologic therapy, may suffer a number of toxic side effects from their immunosuppressive regimen, and are at increased risk for life-threatening opportunistic infections. Their work-up, treatment, and disposition should occur simultaneously with cardiology consultation.

LEFT VENTRICULECTOMY

Background

Left ventricular reconstruction aims to reduce wall stress and improve cardiac function in two disease processes. Patients with both DCM and ICM have ventricles that are either globally enlarged (DCM) or focally enlarged (ICM). Wall tension is governed by the law of Laplace: wall tension = (intraventricular pressure × left ventricular radius)/2 × wall thickness. A reduction in ventricular radius via surgical reconstruction results in a direct reduction of wall tension. Improving wall stress reduces myocardial oxygen consumption and improves myocardial efficiency.[54]

Indications and Surgical Results

There are two primary indications for ventricular reconstruction. The first indication is subjects suffering from symptomatic ICM refractory to maximal medical management. They undergo resection of the noncontractile wall and septum resulting in a reconstructed ventricle with reduced volume and dilation. Dor et al. studied a cohort of 781 ventricular restoration patients with mean left ventricular ejection fraction (LVEF) of $17 \pm 3\%$. Hospital mortality was 19.3%, but 1-year follow-up revealed a maintained improvement in LVEF ($39 \pm 11\%$). Late mortality at 5 years was 10%.[55] Similar results have been seen at The Cleveland Clinic, where 129 patients had a modified left ventriculectomy performed. Two-year survival rates were 82.5 and 98% in the akinetic and dyskinetic groups, respectively.[54] Unfortunately, the success of ventricular reconstruction for ICM has not been translated to patients with DCM. First performed by Batista, the partial left ventriculectomy (PLV) is performed in patients with DCM to reduce wall tension by reducing ventricular radius.[56] Results from several studies show a 2-year survival rate between 55 and 68%.[57–59] The disparity in outcomes may be related to the underlying disease processes in the two cohorts of patients (ICM vs. DCM) as well as proper patient selection. Future studies of surgical reconstruction in DCM will address these issues.

Summary

Left ventricular reconstruction aims to reduce wall tension by reducing the size of the ventricle. Ventricular reconstruction has been highly successful for patients with ICM, but less so for those with DCM.

ALTERNATIVE SURGICAL THERAPIES

Dynamic Cardiomyoplasty

Dynamic cardiomyoplasty uses the latissimus dorsi muscle as a wrap around the heart, with a pacer implanted that conditions the muscle into a slow, fatigue-resistant pump.[54] There are three proposed mechanisms for benefit from this device: (1) a girdling effect, providing passive diastolic restraint to the myocardium preventing further dilation and remodeling; (2) muscular support through the additive "wrapping" effect leading to reduced left ventricular free wall stress; (3) systolic contraction augmentation.[60] Survival rates at 1-year are 68–78%, with better survival rates in those with NYHA class III (compared with class IV) HF prior to surgery.[61,62]

Synthetic Cardiomyoplasty Devices

The success of using the latissimus dorsi has been extended to synthetic devices that also aim to reduce wall stress and augment systolic function. The *Acorn* wrap is an elastic mesh sheet that wraps around both the left and right ventricle. Early clinical human studies, where the device was placed at the time of coronary artery bypass graft (CABG), have demonstrated improvement in cardiac diameter while simultaneously improving HF symptoms.[63] Another device with similar features, the *Myosplint*, demonstrated an acute reduction in left ventricular volumes in humans similar to that seen in previous animal studies.[64]

FUTURE DIRECTIONS

Future therapies may impact treatment of HF by replacing infarcted myocardium with viable tissue. This could occur via autologous transfer of myoblasts (satellite cells originated from skeletal muscle), fetal cardiomyocytes, autologous heart cells, cells derived from bone marrow stem cells, and smooth muscle cells. It is then expected that these cells will differentiate into functional myocardium, replacing nonfunctional areas, and augmenting cardiac contractility and compliance. Experimental studies in animals have demonstrated recovery of myocardial contractility and compliance. Human studies are currently underway.[65]

UNRESOLVED ISSUES

- The use of the VAD and TAH as long-term solutions for those awaiting permanent cardiac transplant continues to be studied.

- The role of cardiac reduction surgery in patients with DCM will be determined by results of future clinical trials.

- With better understanding of the genetic basis for HF, gene therapy may have a progressively increasing role in chronic HF management in the next decade.

REFERENCES

1. Adams KF Jr., Zannad F. Clinical definition and epidemiology of advanced heart failure. *Am Heart J* 1998;135 (6 Pt 2 Su):S204–S215.
2. Hosenpud J, Bennett L, Keck BM. The registry of the International Society of Heart and Lung Transplantation: Sixteenth official report-1999. *J Heart Lung Transplant* 1999;18:611.
3. Miller LW. Listing criteria for cardiac transplantation: Results of an American Society of Transplant Physicians-National Institutes of Health conference. *Transplantation* 1998;66(7):947–951.
4. Pae WE Jr., Miller CA, Matthews Y, et al. Ventricular assist devices for postcardiotomy cardiogenic shock. A combined registry experience. *J Thorac Cardiovasc Surg* 1992;104(3): 541–552; discussion 552–553.
5. Mehta SM, Aufiero TX, Pae WE, Jr., et al. Results of mechanical ventricular assistance for the treatment of post cardiotomy cardiogenic shock. *Asaio J* 1996;42(3):211–218.
6. Gibbon JH Jr. Application of a mechanical heart and lung apparatus to cardiac surgery. *Minn Med* 1954;37(3):171–185; passim.
7. DeBakey ME. Left ventricular bypass pump for cardiac assistance. Clinical experience. *Am J Cardiol* 1971;27(1):3–11.
8. Moulopoulos SD, Topaz SR, Kolff WJ. Extracorporeal assistance to the circulation and intraaortic balloon pumping. *Trans Am Soc Artif Intern Organs* 1962;8:85–89.
9. Kantrowitz A, Tjonneland S, Freed PS, et al. Initial clinical experience with intraaortic balloon pumping in cardiogenic shock. *JAMA* 1968;203(2):113–118.
10. Johnson KE, Liska MB, Joyce LD, et al. Registry report. Use of total artificial hearts: Summary of world experience, 1969–1991. *Asaio J* 1992;38(3):M486–M492.
11. Richenbacher WE, Pierce WS. Treatment of heart failure: Assisted circulation. In: Braunwald E (ed.), *Heart Disease*. Philadelphia, PA: W.B. Saunders, 2001, 600–612.
12. Scheidt S, Wilner G, Mueller H, et al. Intra-aortic balloon counterpulsation in cardiogenic shock. Report of a cooperative clinical trial. *N Engl J Med* 1973;288(19): 979–984.
13. Makhoul RG, Cole CW, McCann RL. Vascular complications of the intra-aortic balloon pump: An analysis of 436 patients. *Am Surg* 1993;59(9):564–568.
14. Eltchaninoff H, Dimas AP, Whitlow PL. Complications associated with percutaneous placement and use of intraaortic balloon counterpulsation. *Am J Cardiol* 1993;71(4):328–332.
15. Richenbacher WE, Pierce WS. Management of complications of intraaortic balloon counterpulsation. In: Walderson JA, Orringer MB (eds.), *Complications in Cardiothoracic Surgery*. St. Louis, MO: Mosby-Year Book, 1991, p. 97.
16. Moritz A, Wolner E. Circulatory support with shock due to acute myocardial infarction. *Ann Thorac Surg* 1993; 55(1):238–244.
17. Chen JM, DeRose JJ, Slater JP, et al. Improved survival rates support left ventricular assist device implantation early after myocardial infarction. *J Am Coll Cardiol* 1999;33(7): 1903–1908.
18. Oaks TE, Pae WE, Jr., Miller CA, et al. Combined registry for the clinical use of mechanical ventricular assist pumps and the total artificial heart in conjunction with heart transplantation: Fifth Official Report—1990. *J Heart Lung Transplant* 1991;10(5 Pt 1):621–625.

19. Sun BC, Catanese KA, Spanier TB, et al. 100 long-term implantable left ventricular assist devices: The Columbia Presbyterian interim experience. *Ann Thorac Surg* 1999; 68(2):688–694.

20. McBride LR, Naunheim KS, Fiore AC, et al. Clinical experience with 111 thoratec ventricular assist devices. *Ann Thorac Surg* 1999;67(5):1233–1238; discussion 8–9.

21. Razeghi P, Mukhopadhyah M, Myers TJ, et al. Myocardial tumor necrosis factor-alpha expression does not correlate with clinical indices of heart failure in patients on left ventricular assist device support. *Ann Thorac Surg* 2001;72(6): 2044–2050.

22. Zafeiridis A, Jeevanandam V, Houser SR, et al. Regression of cellular hypertrophy after left ventricular assist device support. *Circulation* 1998;98(7):656–662.

23. Uray IP, Connelly JH, Frazier O, et al. Altered expression of tyrosine kinase receptors Her2/neu and GP130 following left ventricular assist device (LVAD) placement in patients with heart failure. *J Heart Lung Transplant* 2001;20(2):210.

24. Dipla K, Mattiello JA, Jeevanandam V, et al. Myocyte recovery after mechanical circulatory support in humans with end-stage heart failure. *Circulation* 1998;97(23):2316–2322.

25. Morales DL, Catanese KA, Helman DN, et al. Six-year experience of caring for forty-four patients with a left ventricular assist device at home: Safe, economical, necessary. *J Thorac Cardiovasc Surg* 2000;119(2):251–259.

26. McCarthy PM, Smedira NO, Vargo RL, et al. One hundred patients with the HeartMate left ventricular assist device: Evolving concepts and technology. *J Thorac Cardiovasc Surg* 1998;115(4):904–912.

27. Mehta SM, Aufiero TX, Pae WE, Jr., et al. Combined registry for the clinical use of mechanical ventricular assist pumps and the total artificial heart in conjunction with heart transplantation: Sixth official report—1994. *J Heart Lung Transplant* 1995;14(3):585–593.

28. DeVries WC. The permanent artificial heart. Four case reports. *JAMA* 1988;259(6):849–859.

29. Kunin CM, Dobbins JJ, Melo JC, et al. Infectious complications in four long-term recipients of the Jarvik-7 artificial heart. *JAMA* 1988;259(6):860–864.

30. MacLean GK, Aiken PA, Adams WA, et al. Comparison of rechargeable lithium and nickel/cadmium battery cells for implantable circulatory support devices. *Artif Organs* 1994;18(4):331–334.

31. Barnard CN. The operation. A human cardiac transplant: An interim report of a successful operation performed at Groote Schuur Hospital, Cape Town. *S Afr Med J* 1967; 41(48):1271–1274.

32. Bennett LE, Keck BM, Hertz MI, et al. Worldwide thoracic organ transplantation: A report from the UNOS/ISHLT international registry for thoracic organ transplantation. *Clin Transpl* 2001:25–40.

33. Miniati DN, Robbins RC, Reitz BA. Heart and heart-lung transplantation. In: Braunwald E (ed.), *Heart Disease: A Textbook of Cardiovascular Medicine*. Philadelphia, PA: W.B. Saunders, 2001, Vol. 1, Chapter 20, pp. 615–631.

34. Griepp RB, Stinson EB, Dong E, Jr., et al. Determinants of operative risk in human heart transplantation. *Am J Surg* 1971;122(2):192–197.

35. Caves PK, Billingham ME, Schulz WP, et al. Transvenous biopsy from canine orthotopic heart allografts. *Am Heart J* 1973;85(4):525–530.

36. Wesche J, Orning O, Eriksen M, et al. Electrophysiological evidence of reinnervation of the transplanted human heart. *Cardiology* 1998;89(1):73–75.

37. Mason JW, Stinson EB, Harrison DC. Autonomic nervous system and arrhythmias: Studies in the transplanted denervated human heart. *Cardiology* 1976;61(1):75–87.

38. Verani MS, George SE, Leon CA, et al. Systolic and diastolic ventricular performance at rest and during exercise in heart transplant recipients. *J Heart Transplant* 1988;7(2):145–151.

39. Scherrer U, Vissing SF, Morgan BJ, et al. Cyclosporine-induced sympathetic activation and hypertension after heart transplantation. *N Engl J Med* 1990;323(11): 693–699.

40. Borow KM, Neumann A, Arensman FW, et al. Cardiac and peripheral vascular responses to adrenoceptor stimulation and blockade after cardiac transplantation. *J Am Coll Cardiol* 1989;14(5):1229–1238.

41. Yusuf S, Theodoropoulos S, Mathias CJ, et al. Increased sensitivity of the denervated transplanted human heart to isoprenaline both before and after beta-adrenergic blockade. *Circulation* 1987;75(4):696–704.

42. Wagoner LE. Management of the cardiac transplant recipient: Roles of the transplant cardiologist and primary care physician. *Am J Med Sci* 1997;314(3):173–184.

43. Leachman RD, Cokkinos DV, Cabrera R, et al. Response of the transplanted, denervated human heart to cardiovascular drugs. *Am J Cardiol* 1971;27(3):272–276.

44. Ellenbogen KA, Thames MD, DiMarco JP, et al. Electrophysiological effects of adenosine in the transplanted human heart. Evidence of supersensitivity. *Circulation* 1990;81(3):821–828.

45. Goodman DJ, Rossen RM, Cannom DS, et al. Effect of digoxin on atioventricular conduction. Studies in patients with and without cardiac autonomic innervation. *Circulation* 1975;51(2):251–256.

46. Kubo SH, Naftel DC, Mills RM, Jr., et al. Risk factors for late recurrent rejection after heart transplantation: A multi-institutional, multivariable analysis. Cardiac Transplant Research Database Group. *J Heart Lung Transplant* 1995;14(3):409–418.

47. Mill MR. Cardiac transplantation. In: Tintinalli JE, Ruiz E, Krome RL (eds.), *Emergency Medicine*. 4th ed. New York: McGraw-Hill, 1996, pp. 399–403.

48. Dengler TJ, Zimmermann R, Braun K, et al. Elevated serum concentrations of cardiac troponin T in acute allograft rejection after human heart transplantation. *J Am Coll Cardiol* 1998;32(2):405–412.

49. Blankenberg FG, Strauss HW. Non-invasive diagnosis of acute heart- or lung-transplant rejection using radiolabeled annexin V. *Pediatr Radiol* 1999;29(5):299–305.

50. Auphan N, DiDonato JA, Rosette C, et al. Immunosuppression by glucocorticoids: Inhibition of NF-kappa B activity through induction of I kappa B synthesis. *Science* 1995; 270(5234):286–290.

51. Miller LW, Naftel DC, Bourge RC, et al. Infection after heart transplantation: A multiinstitutional study. Cardiac Transplant Research Database Group. *J Heart Lung Transplant* 1994; 13(3):381–392; discussion 93.

52. Montoya JG, Giraldo LF, Efron B, et al. Infectious complications among 620 consecutive heart transplant patients at Stanford University Medical Center. *Clin Infect Dis* 2001;33(5):629–640.

53. Onorato IM, Morens DM, Martone WJ, et al. Epidemiology of cytomegaloviral infections: Recommendations for prevention and control. *Rev Infect Dis* 1985;7(4):479–497.

54. Starling RC, McCarthy PM, Yamani MH. Surgical treatment of chronic congestive heart failure. In: Mann DL (ed), *Heart Failure*. Philadelphia, PA: W.B. Saunders, 2004, pp. 717–736.

55. Dor V, Sabatier M, Montiglio F, et al. Endoventricular patch reconstruction in large ischemic wall-motion abnormalities. *J Card Surg* 1999;14(1):46–52.

56. Batista RJ, Santos JL, Takeshita N, et al. Partial left ventriculectomy to improve left ventricular function in end-stage heart disease. *J Card Surg* 1996;11(2):96–97; discussion 8.

57. Batista RJ, Verde J, Nery P, et al. Partial left ventriculectomy to treat end-stage heart disease. *Ann Thorac Surg* 1997; 64(3):634–638.

58. Starling RC, McCarthy PM. Partial left ventriculectomy: Sunrise or sunset? *Eur J Heart Fail* 1999;1(4):313–317.

59. Bocchi EA, Bellotti G, Vilella de Moraes A, et al. Clinical outcome after left ventricular surgical remodeling in patients with idiopathic dilated cardiomyopathy referred for heart transplantation: Short-term results. *Circulation* 1997;96(9 Suppl):II-165–171; discussion II-171–172.

60. Starling RC, Young JB. Surgical therapy for dilated cardiomyopathy. *Cardiol Clin* 1998;16(4):727–737.

61. Moreira LF, Stolf NA, Braile DM, et al. Dynamic cardiomyoplasty in South America. *Ann Thorac Surg* 1996;61(1): 408–412.

62. Furnary AP, Jessup FM, Moreira LP. Multicenter trial of dynamic cardiomyoplasty for chronic heart failure. The American Cardiomyoplasty Group. *J Am Coll Cardiol* 1996;28(5):1175–1180.

63. Raman JS, Power JM, Buxton BF, et al. Ventricular containment as an adjunctive procedure in ischemic caridomyopathy: Early results. *Ann Thorac Surg* 2000;70(3): 1124–1126.

64. McCarthy PM, Fukamachi K, Takagi M. Left ventricular shape change reduced left ventricular wall stress in patients with dilated cardiomyopathy. *Circulation* 2000;102(Suppl II): 683.

65. Chachques JC, Shafy A, Duarte F, et al. From dynamic to cellular cardiomyoplasty. *J Card Surg* 2002;17(3): 194–200.

32

Future Diagnostics
Impedance Cardiography in the Assessment and Management of Acute Heart Failure

Richard L. Summers

HIGH YIELD FACTS

- Acute heart failure is physiologic state in which the circulation is unable to meet the needs of the body tissues due to a decompensation in the complex interactions between the heart and the peripheral vasculature.

- Adequate assessment of the central circulation in acute decompensated heart failure requires knowledge of hemodynamic data in addition to the traditional vital signs.

- Impedance cardiography (ICG) offers a potential means for noninvasive assessment and continuous monitoring of cardiac output and contractility in patients with acute heart failure in the emergency department setting.

- Goal-directed management of acute heart failure by optimizing physiologic parameters such as cardiac output is a preferred method of treatment that should improve outcomes.

INTRODUCTION

Determination of the hemodynamic status is one of the most important roles of the emergency physician in the assessment of the patient with acute decompensated heart failure. However, an accurate and complete analysis of circulatory function often cannot be made based on the traditional vital signs of blood pressure and heart rate alone.[1] While systemic pressures and rates of cardiac contractions are indicators of cardiovascular integrity, what we really want to know is flow. It is this flow (in the form of cardiac output) that is the measure of how well the circulation is delivering oxygen and nutrients to the vital organs and is the focus of all resuscitation efforts. In the past, the determination of cardiac output required the insertion of a catheter directly into the heart. As it becomes increasingly evident that these traditional invasive cardiac output monitoring methods may result in a greater patient morbidity and mortality, noninvasive techniques are commonly being considered as an acceptable alternative.[2] One of the most popular of the new noninvasive technologies is based on information generated as measured waveforms from the thoracic electrical bioimpedance (TEB). The study of the waveforms derived from TEB is collectively known as the field of ICG.

In addition to assessing cardiac output, the impedance waveform can also provide information concerning the cardiac contractility and thoracic fluid content. This constellation of measurements function, in combination with the technical aspects of ease of use and continuous monitoring capabilities, suggests that ICG could potentially be a tool for the emergent evaluation and management of patients with suspected or confirmed acute heart failure.

SCIENCE AND BACKGROUND

The technology of TEB was first developed by the National Aeronautics and Space Administration in the 1960s, and is similar to the pulse contour method for measuring stroke volume (SV).[3] Since its introduction aboard the space shuttle flight STS-8, TEB has been used clinically in many critical care areas as an alternative to invasive cardiac output determination.[3] The method is based on the idea that the human thorax is electrically a nonhomogeneous, bulk conductor.[4] In TEB, the patient interfaces with the transducer through a series of disposable surface electrodes providing the connection for measurements of current flowing in a direction parallel with the spine. In order to eliminate skin-to-electrode impedance, all modern TEB equipment uses a tetrapolar system of electrodes, separating the measurement current pathway from the TEB sensing pathway (Fig. 32-1). One set of the external surface pregelled electrodes, placed on the upper abdomen and upper neck, is the source and sink of a constant magnitude, high-frequency measurement current that provides homogeneous coverage of the thorax with an electrical field.

Voltage changes are then sensed by two pairs of electrodes placed at the beginning of the thorax (the line of the root of the neck) and the end of the thorax (the level of diaphragm—the xiphoid process level). These sensing

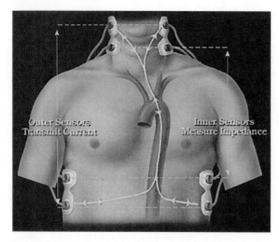

Fig. 32-1. Tetrapolar system of electrodes separating the current pathway from the sensing pathway. After injection of electricity by way of the outer electrodes, the impedance to flow of the current through the thorax along the path of least resistance (i.e., the great vessels) is sensed by way of the inner electrodes.

electrodes also detect the electrocardiogram (ECG) signal. "Z" is defined as the thoracic electrical resistance (impedance) to this high-frequency, very low magnitude measurement current and is indirectly proportional to the content of fluid in the thoracic cavity. TEB technology converts the measurement of the electrical resistance Z of the thorax into a variety of parameters related to different physiologic functions and phenomena.

The TEB changes (delta Z) are produced by fluid changes within the thorax consisting of:

a. Slow baseline changes of fluid levels in the intravascular, intraalveolar, and interstitial thoracic compartments (a result of volume increases, postural changes, or edema)
b. Tidal changes of intravascular blood volume caused by respiration
c. Volumetric and velocity changes of aortic blood produced by the heart's pumping

The predominate electrical conductor in humans is liquid. Since the lungs are mainly air filled, and of lower conductance for electrical current, the majority of fluid resides in the heart and great vessels. As the aorta and vena cava traverse the thoracic cavity, they act as a natural conduit of least resistance to flow for electrical current. Plasma is the most electrically conductive material in the thorax (plasma: $R = 65$ Ω/cm^3; whole blood: 130 Ω/cm^3; fat and lungs: $R = 300–500$ Ω/cm^3), the great vessels conduct more than 50% of the measurement current. Therefore, the rate of cardiovascular-induced TEB changes (dZ/dt) (i.e., the first derivative of impedance) is proportional to the aortic blood flow. Its maximum value, $[(dZ/dt)_{max}]$, is proportional to the aortic blood peak flow. The maximum rate of the second derivative of impedance, $[(d^2Z/dt^2)_{max}]$, is an reflection of aortic blood at maximum acceleration, and therefore a measure of the true inotropic state, much as the rate of maximum pressure change (dp/dt) has been used previously.

While the ECG depicts the electrical events of the heart, the TEB waveform (Fig. 32-2) is a fingerprint of

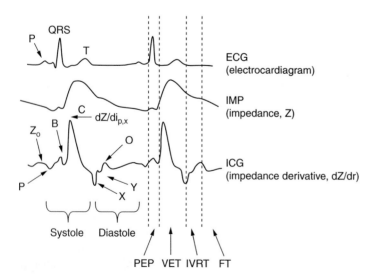

Fig. 32-2. Waveforms Z_0: baseline impedance; A: atrial wave; B: aortic valve opening; C: maximum aortic flow (dZ/dt_{max}); X: aortic valve closing; Y: pulmonic valve closing; O: mitral valve opening; PEP: preejection period; VET: ventricular ejection time; IVRT: isovolumic relaxation time; FT: ventricular filling time.

the mechanical events of cardiac contraction. When used in conjunction with the timing landmarks on the ECG, the dZ/dt signals enable measurement of the systolic time intervals. These include the ventricular ejection time (VET) and the preejection period (PEP), and can provide an analysis of other electromechanical activities. In addition to being noninvasive, safe and easily obtained, TEB-derived parameters have an obvious practical advantage in that they are acquired continuously, beat-by-beat, for continuous real-time monitoring.

PARAMETERS MEASURED

Stroke Volume and Cardiac Output

Stroke volume is determined from the magnitude of the changes in the electrical conductance of current as it traverses the thorax by way of the aorta.[4] The maximum deflection rate of the first waveform of the impedance cardiogram (dZ/dt_{max}) is related to the SV by the equation $SV = rho \times L^2/Z_0^2 \times ET \times dZ/dt_{max}$, where ET is the ejection time, rho is the resistance measure of blood, and L is the length of the thorax. The reliability of this very important parameter has been improved by using information concerning the patient's height and weight, and a direct measurement of the length between the thoracic electrodes. When combined with heart rate, this measure provides a continuous estimate of cardiac output, and parameters such as total peripheral resistance, aortic compliance, and other hemodynamic constants can be estimated. Some TEB instruments use waveform ensemble averaging, collecting data over a burst of 20–30 s, to improve the accuracy of the signal and to eliminate noise.

Central Fluid Volume Estimation

Central fluid volume status can sometimes be difficult to assess in patients with acute heart failure. Most methods for measuring blood and extracellular volume are either highly invasive, logistically cumbersome, or difficult to interpret. Baseline impedance of the thoracic cavity (Z_0) and its inverse (thoracic fluid volume content) have been strongly correlated with thoracic intravascular fluid volumes.[3–5] Therefore, Z_0 provides a noninvasive and continuous measure of the central fluid status in heart failure. It can also be used to monitor the effects of treatments or as a diagnostic adjunct when the underlying pathophysiologic state is uncertain.

Measurement of Cardiac Time Intervals

Different intervals and deflections within the bioimpedance waveform have now been correlated with many of the events of the cardiac cycle by phonocardiography, echocardiography, and ballistocardiograms.[6,7] It is simple to ascertain both the systolic and diastolic time intervals by ICG, and use these measures to make clinical determinations concerning physiologic parameters and pathophysiologic mechanisms.[6] Systolic and diastolic time intervals are available from the TEB tracings by the methodology of Lababidi et al.[7] In this method, the primary deflection of the bioimpedance waveform is correlated with the systolic time intervals and SV while diastolic time intervals such as the isovolumic relaxation time (IVRT: the period from aortic valve closure until mitral valve opening) are found by phonocardiogram to coincide with the second deflection of the TEB waveform (Fig. 32-2). The PEP is the time of isovolumic contraction, beginning with the initiation of the QRS complex at point Q and ending with the opening of the aortic valves. The left ventricular ejection time (LVET) begins at the end of the PEP and ends at the closure of the aortic valve when ejection ends as determined by the dZ/dt waveform. The X to O period represents the IVRT (Fig. 32-2). The beginning of the QRS complex on the ECG (Q) and the start of the primary TEB waveform indicates the end of diastole.

Contractility Indices

The calculated cardiac time intervals and the systolic waveform can be used to estimate the cardiac contractility. Several techniques can assess myocardial contractility from the systolic time intervals. The PEP/LVET ratio was first used by Weissler 30 years ago to noninvasively calculate the cardiac ejection fraction.[8] Capan has validated a similar method using ICG measurements.[9] However, this measurement method has not been well validated and is viewed with some skepticism. Other contractility estimates include the Heather Index (HI = $dZ/dt_{max}/QZ1$, where dZ/dt_{max} is the maximum deflection of the initial waveform and QZ1 is the time from the beginning of the Q wave to peak dZ/dt), the Minnesota Index, and acceleration contractility index (ACI) which are all based on the maximal slope of the systolic waveform, dZ/dt_{max}. These acceleration measures have been reported to demonstrate better accuracy in estimating contractility and are conceptually similar to the standard dp/dt measures.

POTENTIAL ROLE IN THE EMERGENCY SETTING

Diagnosis of Acute Heart Failure

The real impact of ICG measurements on the diagnosis of acute heart failure is uncertain. However, the sensitivity of the current ED tools of chest x-rays and physical examination is also questionable, though they are currently considered as the standard for early diagnosis. Even ED echocardiography findings of a suppressed ejection fraction might not necessarily indicate acute decompensation. Most experts in the field of heart failure think that advanced hemodynamic monitoring can play an important role in early diagnosis and management. Furthermore, noninvasive measures may be preferred due to the risks associated with right heart catheterization.[10–14] As long as the ICG values for SV and thoracic fluid volume appear to be relatively accurate, they can be considered an excellent addition to present diagnostic methods.

One area where ICG measurements may have the greatest impact is in the clinical categorization of the acute heart failure patient within the popular schemes of hemodynamic subsets.[13] Warm versus cold and wet versus dry are descriptive profiles indicating the degree of perfusion and pulmonary congestion and have implications in diagnosis and management. While the terminology of these profiles is somewhat subjective, the more objective measures of flow and thoracic fluid content offered by ICG could work to improve the determination of the clinical condition.

Assessment of Central Fluid Volume

The clinical assessment of the amount of fluid in the central vascular compartment is often based on information from chest x-rays, weight measurements, and findings on physical examination. While these methods may accurately estimate extracellular fluid volume changes and edema formation, they do not always reflect the intravascular volume status and may also vary with the patient's baseline pathology. In general, a cutoff baseline Z_0 value of 24.0 Ω has been found to predict an increased thoracic fluid volume with a sensitivity of 92% and a specificity of 79%. Impedance measurements can add information to assist in diagnosis in a significant number of patients.[5]

Peacock et al. found significant differences between patients with cardiomegaly ($Z_0 = 17.5 \pm 5.5$) and abnormal pulmonary fluid on chest x-ray ($Z_0 = 17.2 \pm 4.2$) when compared to normals ($Z_0 = 23.4 \pm 5.4$) but no differences between patients with cardiomegaly and abnormal pulmonary fluid.[15] They concluded that impedance measurement may detect pulmonary fluid not apparent on chest radiographs.

The O/C ratio (see Fig. 32-2) is calculated as the amplitude of the impedance cardiogram during diastole (point O) divided by the maximum height during systole (point C) and has been shown to strongly correlate to the invasively measured ventricular wedge pressures (PCWP) over a range of 3–30 mmHg ($r = 0.92$, standard error of the estimate, 3.2 mmHg).[16] The combined measurement of cardiac output and PCWP or Z_0 by ICG, is reflective of the state of the Starling curve, and might be a useful tool in detecting systolic heart failure.

Measurement of Diastolic Function

Differentiating systolic from diastolic congestive heart failure (CHF) is often difficult. ICG allows for the determination of relative cardiac contractility (HI or ejection fraction) and accurately measures diastolic time intervals such as IVRT (X to O period represents IVRT, a standard measure of diastolic function).[6,7] A previous study demonstrated that clinicians can distinguish systolic from diastolic mechanisms in the patient with acute heart failure in the emergency department using ICG-derived information.[6]

Diagnostic Adjunct

Generic complaints such as shortness of breath or weakness due to hypotension are common clinical scenarios often seen in the emergency department. Early differentiation of heart failure from other common serious conditions, such as emphysema or shock due to dehydration or sepsis, can significantly alter management plans and impact outcomes. Though ICG has previously been used primarily for continuous monitoring in the intensive care setting, recently it has been used in the emergency department to evaluate potentially unstable patients. This technology can be used in the acute setting as a diagnostic adjunct when the primary hemodynamic state is uncertain and information obtained from the application of a TEB device can be crucial to the determination of the patient's underlying pathophysiologic condition.[17] Distinguishing high from low flow states is important in the differentiation of conditions such as sepsis, dehydration, and cardiogenic shock. ICG often provides the missing piece of the hemodynamic puzzle and has been found to aid in the differentiation of conditions that mimic acute heart failure. In fact, changes in total intravascular volume as small 590 mL over 10 min can be detected by ICG.[18]

In patients presenting with a primary complaint of shortness of breath, the ED-IMPACT trial demonstrated that information acquired through ICG monitoring changed diagnosis and treatments 5.3 and 23.6% of the time, respectively.[19] This is a greater impact than was seen with the addition of pulse oximetry technology in vital sign determinations.

Monitoring Heart and Circulatory Function

Close clinical monitoring and assessment of the circulatory function of a patient in acute heart failure is critical to the determination of long-term outcome for these patients. This approach has become increasingly important with the advent of newer aggressive vasoactive therapies and our understanding of the role of neurohumoral factors in circulatory control. Traditional vital sign endpoints and subjective indicators of symptomatic improvement are inadequate measurements of response to treatment and do not portend eventual outcomes or recidivism potential. Thermodilution measures cardiac output at only one point in time and assumes a steady state. Furthermore, it tells us little about cardiac contractility and is usually impractical in the emergency department setting. Echocardiography is effective in determining contractility, but is not amenable to continuous monitoring and does not typically measure cardiac output without significant expertise. ICG monitoring overcomes these limitations, and has been used successfully to detect early changes in cardiac function and thoracic fluid content.[3,17]

In clinical trials using ICG, real-time monitoring of changes in thoracic fluid status was potentially useful in guiding and monitoring the results of therapeutic interventions or changes in clinical condition.[20] However, it may be most helpful in those patients whose thoracic fluid status is changing or unstable. It has also been used for monitoring circulatory responses to vasoactive therapy, as well as the impact of diuresis and noninvasive positive pressure ventilation on cardiac output.[21,22]

Goal-Directed Therapy

Therapy directed to optimize important physiologic parameters has been found to improve outcomes in a number of cardiovascular disease states.[23] Dramatic improvements in controlling resistant hypertension have been demonstrated using ICG measures as a tool in a goal-directed treatment approach.[24] There is also some evidence that the same may be true in the emergency management of acute heart failure.[25,26] Milzman et al. found improvement in symptoms and vital signs in acute heart failure patients when treatment was guided by ICG cardiac output measurements.[26] However, more studies are needed to determine which of the impedance-derived parameters, alone or in combination with other physiologic variables, would guide the greatest impact on outcomes.

UNRESOLVED ISSUES

Is ICG technology accurate? In the past, there has been some controversy with regard to the accuracy the cardiac output measurements of ICG when compared to the "gold standard" invasive measures such as thermodilution. As computer processing becomes more powerful and signal analysis more detailed, the ICG measurements have also become more reliable. A recent metaanalysis of over 200 studies found a correlation of 0.81 for ICG determined SV and cardiac output when compared to traditional measurements.[3] The patient group diagnosed as CHF was found to have a slightly better average correlation of 0.83 (0.63–0.99). Furthermore, ICG assessments are less variable and more reproducible then many standard techniques; certainly within the range of accuracy for practical use in clinical decision-making. Some of the ancillary ICG measurements of contractility and thoracic fluid content are considered less dependable but still can be used to monitor trends or changes with treatment.

Should I be monitoring my heart failure patients with ICG? While ICG has been shown to be very useful clinically and can impact diagnostic and treatment decisions, there are no studies documenting that overall outcomes in patients with heart failure are changed with the addition of this information. ICG researchers have spent the past 20 years just trying to create an accurate and practical methodology. We are only now reaching a point in the evolution of the technology where clinical trials that look at outcomes are being performed. However, some of the same invasively measured physiologic parameters that do make a difference in patient management are those that are also offered by ICG. It has long been expected that some noninvasive measure of cardiac output will emerge as a vital sign in much the same way that pulse oximetry measurements of oxygen saturation did within the past decade.

There are several limitations to the ICG technology that have been noted. Anything that creates noise within the system will affect the SV and other parameter measurements. Waveform ensemble averaging limits the effects of noise to distort the values obtained. Severe obesity and poor electrode skin contact may also lead to spurious measurements. Anthropomorphic information can be used to temper the influence of these factors. Aortic regurgitation can cause abnormally high estimations of SV. The extremes of heart rate (>140 or <40 bpm) or cardiac output (>8 or <1 L/min) may lead to inaccurate results. Pacemakers or natural rhythms in which it is difficult to identify the QRS morphology can cause faulty calculations of the PEP. Algorithms have been developed to correct for many of these problems but it is important to recognize situations that may limit the usefulness of the TEB. Though a certain level of skill is required to correctly interpret the results of the ICG measures, this technology is easier to master than either echocardiography or thermodilution.

What ICG parameters are most important to follow in heart failure management? While ICG was primarily intended for cardiac output determination, it is sometimes apparent that patients in heart failure may have a completely normal cardiac output. Likewise, a reduced cardiac output can be seen in conditions other than heart failure (i.e., dehydration, hemorrhage, advanced age). Hence, it is often useful to view the cardiac output in the context of the thoracic fluid content, Z_0. An elevated Z_0 in the face of an even slightly diminished cardiac output is a reflection of a depressed Starling curve. Regardless, the monitoring of cardiac output and Z_0 can be important as trending measurements and indicators of the response to therapy. Contractility measurements such as the acceleration indices and calculated ejection fractions have been more controversial and often harder to interpret. The acceleration index appears to be consistently lower in acute heart failure but the ejection fraction is frequently misleading. In general, it will take a period of collective experience in which emergency physicians become familiar with the ICG parameters and the clinical context of their meaning.

REFERENCES

1. Wo CCJ, Shoemaker WC, Appel PL, et al. Unreliability of blood pressure and heart rate to evaluate cardiac output in emergency resuscitation and critical illness. *Crit Care Med* 1993;21(2):218–223.
2. Sandham JD, Hull RD, Brant RF, et al. Canadian Critical Care Clinical Trials Group. A randomized, controlled trial of the use of pulmonary-artery catheters in high-risk surgical patients. *N Engl J Med* 2003;348:5–14.
3. Summers RL, Shoemaker W, Peacock WF, et al. Bench to bedside: Electrophysiologic and clinical principles of non-invasive hemodynamic monitoring using impedance cardiography. *Acad Emerg Med* 2003;10:(6):669–680.
4. Sramek BB. Thoracic electrical bioimpedance: Basic principles and physiologic relationship. *Noninvas Cardiol* 1994;3:83–88.
5. Saunders CE. The use of transthoracic electrical bioimpedance in assessing thoracic fluid status in emergency department patients. *Am J Emerg Med* 1988;6:337–340.
6. Summers RL, Kolb JC, Woodward LH, et al. Differentiating systolic from diastolic heart failure using impedance cardiography. *Acad Emerg Med* 1999;6:693–699.
7. Lababidi Z, Ehmke DA, Durnin RE, et al. The first derivative thoracic impedance cardiogram. *Circulation* 1970;41:651–658.
8. Garrard CL Jr., Weissler AM, Dodge HT. The relationship of alterations in systolic time intervals to ejection fraction in patients with cardiac disease. *Circulation* 1970;42:455–462.
9. Capan LV, Bernstein DP, Patel KP, et al. Measurement of ejection fraction by bioimpedance method. *Crit Care Med* 1987;5:402.
10. Strobeck JE, Silver MA, Ventura H. Impedance cardiography: Noninvasive measurement of cardiac stroke volume and thoracic fluid content. *Congest Heart Fail* 2000;6:56–59.
11. Rosenberg P, Yancy CW. Noninvasive assessment of hemodynamics: An emphasis on bioimpedance cardiography. *Curr Opin Cardiol* 2000;15:151–155.
12. Noble TJ, Morice AH, Channer KS, et al. Monitoring patients with left ventricular failure by electrical impedance tomography. *Eur J Heart Fail* 1999;1:379–384.
13. Yancy C, Abraham WT. Noninvasive hemodynamic monitoring in heart failure: Utilization of impedance cardiography. *Congest Heart Fail* 2003;9:241–250.
14. Peacock WF, Allegra J, Ander D, et al. Management of acute decompensated heart failure in the emergency department. *Congest Heart Fail* 2003;9(Suppl 1):3–18.
15. Peacock WF IV, Albert NM, Kies P, et al. Bioimpedance monitoring: Better than chest x-ray for predicting abnormal pulmonary fluid? *Congest Heart Fail* 2000;6:86–89.
16. Woltjer HH, Bogaard HJ, Bronzwaer JG, et al. Prediction of pulmonary capillary wedge pressure and assessment of stroke volume by noninvasive impedance cardiography. *Am Heart J* 1997;134:450–455.
17. Summers RL, Kolb JC, Woodward LH, et al. Diagnostic uses for thoracic electrical bioimpedance in the emergency department: Clinical case series. *Eur J Emerg Med* 1999;6:193–199.
18. Kosowsky JM, Collins SP, Han J, et al. Changes in stroke index measured by impedance cardiography in a human model of moderate acute blood loss. *Acad Emerg Med* 2000;7:1167–1168.
19. Peacock WF, Summers RL, Emerman CE. Bioimpedance monitoring changes therapy in dyspneic emergency department patients: The IMPACT Trial. *Ann Emerg Med* 2003;42:S82.
20. Noble TJ, Harris ND, Morice AH, et al. Diuretic induced change in lung water assessed by electrical impedance tomography. *Physiol Meas* 2000;21:155–163.
21. Domingo E, Gilabert MR, Alio J, et al. Effect of drugs on a noninvasive index of arterial compliance in healthy and heart failure patients. *Cathet Cardiovasc Diagn* 1991;24:93–98.
22. Summers RL, Patch J, Kolb JC. Effect of the initiation of noninvasive bi-level positive airway pressure on haemodynamic stability. *Eur J Emerg Med* 2002;9:37–41.
23. Rivers E, Nguyen B, Havstad S, et al. Early Goal-Directed Therapy Collaborative Group. Early goal-directed therapy

in the treatment of severe sepsis and septic shock. *N Engl J Med* 2001;345(19):1368–1377.

24. Taler SJ, Textor SC, Augustine JE. Resistant hypertension: Comparing hemodynamic management to specialist care. *Hypertension* 2002;39:982–988.

25. Drazner MH, Thompson B, Rosenberg PB, et al. Comparison of impedance cardiography with invasive hemodynamic measurements in patients with heart failure secondary to ischemic or nonischemic cardiomyopathy. *Am J Cardiol* 2002;89:993–995.

26. Milzman DP, Samaddar R, Moscowitz L, et al. Thoracic impedance monitoring of cardiac output in the emergency department improves heart failure resuscitation. *Ann Emerg Med* 1998;32:S61.

33

Clinical Utility of Heart Sounds in Heart Failure and Acute Coronary Syndromes

Sean P. Collins

HIGH YIELD FACTS

- Heart sounds have valuable prognostic information in the clinical management of patients.
- Auscultation is a difficult and dying art; consequently, the sensitivity of physician's detection of pathologic heart sounds is poor.
- While the S_3 may present when under 40 years old, with symptoms of heart failure, its presence is highly specific for left ventricular dysfunction.
- The S_4 is rarely present under 40, and if there are acute coronary syndrome (ACS) symptoms, it suggests a high likelihood of coronary artery disease.

ORIGIN OF S_3 AND S_4

The third heart sound (S_3) occurs 0.12–0.16 s after the second heart sound in early diastole[1] (Fig. 33-1). Of the many proposed theories, the most likely explanation is that excessive rapid filling of a stiff ventricle is suddenly halted, causing vibrations that are audible as the third heart sound.[2] Pathologic states where an S_3 is encountered include anemia, thyrotoxicosis, mitral regurgitation, hypertrophic cardiomyopathy, aortic and tricuspid regurgitation, and left ventricular dysfunction.[3] The fourth heart sound (S_4) occurs just before the first heart sound in the cardiac cycle. It is produced in late diastole as a result of atrial contraction causing vibrations of the LV muscle, mitral valve apparatus, and LV blood mass.[4] Disease processes that produce an S_4 include hypertension, aortic stenosis and regurgitation, severe mitral regurgitation, cardiomyopathy, and ischemic heart disease.[3]

AUSCULTATION OF THE S_3 AND S_4

Both S_3 and S_4 are auscultated in similar fashion. Harvey has suggested the "inching" technique as a way to distinguish the often times pathologic S_3 and S_4 from the physiologic S_1 and S_2.[5] In both situations, it is best to examine the patient in the left lateral position using the bell of the stethoscope. Starting at the aortic area (where the S_2 is the loudest) the examiner "inches" down to the cardiac apex, using the S_2 as a reference point. If one encounters an extra sound in diastole, just after the S_2, this is an S_3 or diastolic gallop. The S_3 is generally absent at the base, so that as the examiner moves toward the apex the S_3 is encountered.

The opposite maneuver results in detection of an S_4. In this instance, the examiner inches from the apex upward to the base. The first heart sound (loudest at the apex) is used as a reference because the S_4 occurs in late diastole, just before S1. If the stethoscope is moved away from the apex the S_4 disappears. A further method to distinguish a split S1 from an S_3/S_4 (both lower frequency sounds than an S1) is to place pressure on the bell of the stethoscope—an S_3/S_4 will disappear, while a fixed S_1 will remain.

THE ROLE OF HEART SOUNDS IN ACUTE CORONARY SYNDROMES

Significance of S_3 and S_4 in detection of ACS

The most common auscultatory finding in acute ischemia is the S_4 (Table 33-1). The incidence of an S_4 in acute ischemia and acute infarction approaches 100%.[6] A number of studies used phonocardiography in the 1970s to demonstrate the presence of an S_4 during episodes of angina, as well as in those patients with known coronary artery disease and subjects with ischemic exercise tests.[7,8] However, while highly sensitive for angina and coronary artery disease, the presence of an S_4 in hypertensive heart disease and cardiomyopathy reduce its specificity.[9] There is also some suggestion that it is a "normal" finding in subjects of all ages. Fourth heart sounds have been detected in patients with no clinical evidence of cardiovascular disease.[8,10,11]

Coronary heart disease without LV dysfunction does not produce an S_3. However, if coronary atherosclerosis results in LV dysfunction (either acute or chronic), an S_3 may develop even in asymptomatic patients. An S_3 during acute myocardial infarction suggests a large infarction and does not necessarily mean LV dysfunction that requires treatment. The intensity of an S_3 tends to decrease as the myocardium recovers from acute infarction.[12]

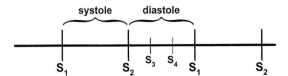

Fig. 33-1. Location of heart sounds in the cardiac cycle.

THE ROLE OF HEART SOUNDS IN HEART FAILURE

Significance of S_3 and S_4 detection in Congestive Heart Failure (CHF)

While detection of an S_3 can be normal in adolescents and young adults, its detection after the age of 40 is considered abnormal.[13–15] Traditionally not very sensitive for LV dysfunction, when detected, an S_3 can be very predictive of elevated left ventricular pressure. In a study of outpatients referred for cardiac catheterization, the detection of an S_3 was the most specific finding of left ventricular end-diastolic pressure (LVEDP) (95%).[16] A more recent study has also found that the detection of an S_3 has a high specificity and positive predictive value in detection of patients with low ejection fractions.[17] Unfortunately, while having a high specificity for elevated filling pressures, an S_3 has been reported to have a sensitivity of only 25%.[18] Even more importantly, it has been suggested patients with a detectable S_3 have an increased risk of hospitalization and death compared to those patients without a detectable S_3.[19–21]

Similarly, the presence of an audible S_4 appears to be suggestive of elevated LV pressures, although there have been conflicting data in previous studies. Spodick and Quarry found the presence of an S_4 to be no more common in patients with heart disease than those without.[11] However, the temporal relationship of the S_4 to the P wave may be more important than the mere presence of an S_4.[22] Those patients with increasing LVEDP have a decrease in the time interval between the onset of atrial contraction

(P wave) and the development of an S_4 (the P-S_4 interval [PS$_4$]). Furthermore, in patients with decreased ventricular compliance (i.e., heart failure) a greater proportion of filling occurs in late diastole. As a result the atrial component of ventricular filling is increased, resulting in a large amount of blood being forced into a stiff, non-compliant ventricle. The net result is an S_4.[23]

Unfortunately, identification of an S_3 or S_4 is difficult. The aforementioned studies, suggest a low incidence of S_3 detection in heart failure; perhaps abnormal heart sounds may have been present but physicians were unable to detect them.

Recent studies indicate that physicians are becoming less proficient at performing the physical examination, and physicians in residency programs have been shown to have poor cardiac auscultatory skills.[24–27] Furthermore, interobserver agreement of S_3 detection is poor, with board-certified cardiologists having no better agreement than house staff.[28–30] Compounding the difficulty of S_3 or S_4 detection is the loud ED environment, confounding illnesses such as chronic obstructive pulmonary disease and obesity that make detection difficult, and the inability of the patient to tolerate being placed in the ideal examining position (recumbent) because of their dyspnea.

PHONOCARDIOGRAPHY

While detection of an S_3 or S_4 may be useful as a diagnostic and prognostic tool in ED patients with dyspnea, the traditional method of auscultation is less than ideal. However, technology has been developed to aid the clinician at bedside diagnosis of an S_3/S_4. A phonocardiogram is under investigation that uses a dual sensor in conjunction with standard ECG electrodes. The dual sensor simultaneously acquires electrical and acoustical data from the V_3 and V_4 position on the standard 12-lead ECG. This allows simultaneous recording of both the 12-lead ECG and the acoustical information. The phonocardiogram attaches to the standard ECG machine. The sensors on leads V_3 and V_4 are only slightly larger than standard ECG leads. Diagnostic algorithms then analyze

Table 33-1. Clinical Relevance of Heart Sounds

Physical Examination Finding	Healthy Subjects Less than 40	With Symptoms of ACS	With Symptoms of Heart Failure
S_3	May be present	Indicative of CAD, but not as sensitive as S_4	Highly specific for LV dysfunction, likely poor sensitivity
S_4	Usually not present	High likelihood of CAD	Indicative of high LV pressure

both types of data and report on the presence of an S_3, S_4, and left ventricular hypertrophy (LVH). While limited, the initial data on the use of this technology appear promising. Using a gold standard of expert overread of printed acoustical heart sounds, this technology had a sensitivity of 71% and a specificity of 94% for detection of an S_3 in a study of 314 patients.[31] This technology has not been validated in a cohort of dyspneic ED patients. However, if this technology proves to be useful in the ED it may help in heart failure and ACS diagnosis and risk stratification. Future clinical applications of this technology may include following response to therapy by quantifying the change in amplitude of the heart sounds, as well as quantifying "normal" versus "abnormal" characteristics of S_3 and S_4 to better delineate pathologic from physiologic heart sounds.

REFERENCES

1. Sokolow M. Physical examination. *Clin Cardiol* 1990.
2. Joshi N. The third heart sound. *South Med J* 1999; 92(8):756–761.
3. Reddy PS, Salerni R, Shaver JA. Normal and abnormal heart sounds in cardiac diagnosis: Part II. Diastolic sounds. *Curr Probl Cardiol* 1985;10(4):1–55.
4. Abrams J. Current concepts of the genesis of heart sounds. II. Third and fourth sounds. *JAMA* 1978;239(26):2790–2791.
5. Harvey WP. Cardiac pearls. *Dis Mon* 1994;40(2):41–113.
6. Tavel M. The fourth heart sound: Current concepts. *Prac Cardiol* 1985;11(8).
7. Perez GL, Luisada AA. When does a fourth sound become an atrial gallop? *Angiology* 1976;27(5):300–310.
8. Aronow WS, Uyeyama RR, Cassidy J, et al. Resting and postexercise phonocardiogram and electrocardiogram in patients with angina pectoris and in normal subjects. *Circulation* 1971;43(2):273–277.
9. Thompson PL. Physical examination in ischaemic heart disease. *Med J Aust* 1976;1(14):492–495.
10. Rectra EH, Khan AH, Pigott VM, et al. Audibility of the fourth heart sound. A prospective, "blind" auscultatory and polygraphic investigation. *JAMA* 1972;221(1): 36–41.
11. Spodick D, Quarry V. Prevalence of the fourth heart sound by phonocardiography in the absence of cardiac disease. *Am Heart J* 1974;87(1):11–14.
12. Hill JC, O'Rourke RA, Lewis RP, et al. The diagnostic value of the atrial gallop in acute myocardial infarction. *Am Heart J* 1969;78(2):194–201.
13. Reddy PS. The third heart sound. *Int J Cardiol* 1985; 7(3):213–221.
14. Sloan A. Cardiac gallop rhythm. *Medicine* 1958;37:197–215.
15. Evans W. The use of phonocardiography in clinical medicine. *Lancet* 1951;1:1083–1085.
16. Harlan WR, Oberman A, Grimm R, et al. Chronic congestive heart failure in coronary artery disease: Clinical criteria. *Ann Intern Med* 1977;86(2):133–138.
17. Patel R, Bushnell DL, Sobotka PA. Implications of an audible third heart sound in evaluating cardiac function. *West J Med* 1993;158(6):606–609.
18. Davie AP, Francis CM, Caruana L, et al. Assessing diagnosis in heart failure: Which features are any use? *QJM* 1997;90(5):335–339.
19. Drazner MH, Rame JE, Stevenson LW, et al. Prognostic importance of elevated jugular venous pressure and a third heart sound in patients with heart failure. *N Engl J Med* 2001;345(8):574–581.
20. Rame JE, Dries DL, Drazner MH. The prognostic value of the physical examination in patients with chronic heart failure. *Congest Heart Fail* 2003;9(3):170–175, 178.
21. Glover DR, Littler WA. Factors influencing survival and mode of death in severe chronic ischaemic cardiac failure. *Br Heart J* 1987;57(2):125–132.
22. Schapira JN, Fowles RE, Bowden RE, et al. Relation of P-S4 interval to left ventricular end-diastolic pressure. *Br Heart J* 1982;47(3):270–276.
23. Shah PM, Gramiak R, Kramer DH, et al. Determinants of atrial (S4) and ventricular (S3) gallop sounds in primary myocardial disease. *N Engl J Med* 1968;278(14):753–758.
24. Fletcher RH, Fletcher SW. Has medicine outgrown physical diagnosis? *Ann Intern Med* 1992;117(9):786–787.
25. Adolph RJ. In defense of the stethoscope. *Chest* 1998; 114(5):1235–1237.
26. Weitz HH, Mangione S. In defense of the stethoscope and the bedside. *Am J Med* 2000;108(8):669–671.
27. Craige E. Should auscultation be rehabilitated? *N Engl J Med* 1988;318(24):1611–1613.
28. Lok CE, Morgan CD, Ranganathan N. The accuracy and interobserver agreement in detecting the 'gallop sounds' by cardiac auscultation. *Chest* 1998;114(5):1283–1288.
29. Held P, Lindberg B, Swedberg K. Audibility of an artificial third heart sound in relation to its frequency, amplitude, delay from the second heart sound and the experience of the observer. *Am J Cardiol* 1984;53(8):1169–1172.
30. Ishmail AA, Wing S, Ferguson J, et al. Interobserver agreement by auscultation in the presence of a third heart sound in patients with congestive heart failure. *Chest* 1987;91(6):870–873.
31. Inovise Medical I. Performance for Audicor 1.0. Data on file with Inovise Medical, Inc.

34

Valvular Heart Disease

Robert D. Welch
Phillip D. Levy

HIGH YIELD FACTS

- Diastolic murmurs are invariably pathologic and should be evaluated with an echocardiogram.

- Acute mitral regurgitation in the setting of acute coronary ischemia often has a very soft murmur even in severe cases, making diagnosis difficult.

- Mitral valve prolapse (MVP) is strongly associated with the development of infective endocarditis (IE), requiring consideration of antibiotic prophylaxis for high-risk procedures.

- Symptoms of syncope, angina, or heart failure in a patient with aortic stenosis (AS) are ominous and mandate hospitalization.

- Major shifts are taking place in the epidemiology of IE, with as many as 45% of cases now occurring in patients without previous heart disease, and staphylococcal species now surpassing viridans streptococci as the most common infective agent.

INTRODUCTION

Most heart valve diseases are slowly progressive and are followed long-term on an outpatient basis. There are a few scenarios that are of importance for emergency physicians. Patients with known valvular disease who present with symptoms such as weakness, shortness of breath, syncope, angina, congestive heart failure, cardiac arrhythmias, or thromboembolic disease have potential emergent conditions that may or may not be related to the valve abnormality. For patients without known valvular disease, these symptoms should prompt a careful examination for signs of valvular dysfunction. Anticoagulation for prosthetic valves (either under or overtreatment) and the diagnosis and management of endocarditis are potential emergent cardiac conditions.

The past quarter century has seen significant advances in the diagnosis and treatment interventions of patients with valvular heart disease. This has resulted in the need for an evidence-based approach to managing affected patients. In this context the American College of Cardiology/American Heart Association (ACC/AHA) guidelines for managing patients with valvular heart disease were developed and published in 1998.[1] The chapter will describe certain aspects of the ACC/AHA and European guidelines that are directed at the adult patients unless otherwise specified. The reader should continue to search for new information applicable to the evolving diagnostic studies and therapies.

Background

The etiology of valvular heart disease has changed over the past 50 years. Rheumatic fever has seen a marked decline in the United States and there has been an increase in age-related degenerative valve disease. In developing countries, rheumatic fever remains a serious and common cause of valvular heart disease.[1–3] A syndrome of anorexic drug-induced valvular heart disease has recently been described and this has resulted in removal of these pharmaceutical agents from the market.[4] A large multicenter study found that aortic regurgitation (AR) but not mitral regurgitation (MR) was associated with anorectic drug use.[5] Most cases have been mild or moderate and rarely required surgery. Discontinuation of the drugs has generally halted progression and resulted in improvements of the valve disorder.[6] The mechanism by which these agents produced valve diseases has not been fully elucidated but one proposed mechanism is a direct toxic effect similar to the pathogenesis of pulmonary hypertension from these same agents. A more likely explanation is the serotonin effect. Anorectic drugs have serotonin-like properties and histologically the valves are similar to those affected by the carcinoid syndrome or valves affected by ergot drugs.[7] Since these agents are no longer marketed they will receive little further attention here but the reader should be aware that future pharmaceutical agents could result in valvular heart disease.

Incidence and Natural History

The literature on valvular hear disease is often clouded by geographic differences in patients characteristics, etiologies of the valvular hear disease, and treatments. In a study comparing European and North American patients who underwent heart valve procedures in the Artificial Valve Endocarditis Reduction Trial (AVERT) between 1998 and 2000 it was found that the North American cohort was younger but required more extensive surgery.[8] Even among European centers differences exist among patients requiring surgery. North European patients were older, had more associated coronary artery disease, and had primarily aortic degenerative valve disease (72.7% aortic valve replacement [AVR]). South European patients had a higher fraction of primarily mitral valve procedures (46.1%) and had a worse baseline cardiac status.[9] Additionally, there are very little data available that describe the modern natural history and medical treatment of advanced valvular heart disease among the developed nations because many patients in those countries undergo surgical intervention before the disease becomes very advanced. The reader must consider these factors when reviewing the information provided.

Evaluation of a Heart Murmur

One of the challenges for physicians is to determine which murmurs require further testing even among asymptomatic patients. Among patients with symptoms of cardiac disease a murmur can be the clue needed to determine the etiology and treatment of those symptoms. The presence of a heart murmur is generally secondary to regurgitant flow through an incompetent valve or forward flow through a narrowed or stenotic valve. When anemia is present or in high-flow states (pregnancy, hyperthyroidism, atrial or ventricular septal defects) a murmur may be audible, despite the existence of normal valves (flow murmur). Murmurs are classified by when they occur in the cardiac cycle and are graded on a scale of increasing intensity (I-VI). Systolic murmurs may be present throughout (holo- or pansystolic murmur), in the early portion (systolic ejection murmur) or in the mid to late phase. Most systolic murmurs occur in the absence of significant underlying cardiac disease and are related to changes in flow rates. Diastolic murmurs however, are uniformly pathologic in origin. They may occur early in the cycle, with a low- or high-pitched quality, in the mid portion or toward the end (presystolic). Occasionally, a murmur may be continuous, noted during both systole and diastole. Attempts at differentiation of the underlying etiology of a murmur can be made through the use of dynamic auscultation, with associated changes induced by the performance of provocative maneuvers. In general, right-sided murmurs increase with inspiration and left-sided increase with expiration. A more complete description of valvular abnormalities, their associated murmurs, and selected interventions to alter the intensity can be found in Table 34-1.

The extent of initial evaluation of a murmur can be confusing. Electrocardiography and chest radiography may suggest more severe underlying etiologies through identification of ventricular hypertrophy, cardiomegaly, pulmonary vascular congestion or ischemia, but are relatively nonspecific. Echocardiography is the definitive test, enabling assessment of cardiac performance, determination of valvular pathology, and delineation of hemodynamic function. Deciding which patient will require an emergent echocardiographic evaluation can be difficult. A murmur with fever and/or signs of thromboembolic phenomenon in a patient at risk for IE is an absolute indication for at least a transthoracic, if not a transesophageal echocardiogram. All diastolic murmurs should be assessed by echocardiography. For a systolic murmur however, the decision should depend primarily on the qualities of the murmur and the associated clinical scenario. In an asymptomatic patient, an isolated systolic murmur is usually benign, and an echocardiogram can be delayed, provided the murmur has the following characteristics: ejection pattern, grade 1–2 intensity, location at the left sternal border, no accentuation with the Valsalva maneuver, no associated evidence of ventricular hypertrophy or dilatation, and a normal associated splitting of the second heart sound. Absence of these signs or presentation with syncope, angina, or heart failure requires a more aggressive approach. Continuous murmurs are likely to be associated with cardiac pathology, and should be evaluated by echocardiography as well. These murmurs are rarely resultant from valvular heart disease however and, of themselves, should not be taken as an indication of valve pathology.

MITRAL VALVE DISORDERS

Anatomic Overview

The mitral apparatus is composed of the annulus, two leaflets, the papillary muscles, and chordae tendineae

Table 34-1. Cardiac Murmurs with Corresponding Conditions and Response of Common Valvular Disorders to Selected Provocative Maneuvers

Murmur	Valvular or Cardiac Conditions	Valsalva	Standing Position*	Exercise	Amyl nitrate
Midsystolic	Flow murmur (aortic or pulmonic)	↓	↓	↑	↓
	Aortic stenosis (valvular)	↓	↓	↑	↑
	Subvalvular stenosis of HOCM	↑	↑	↓	↑
	Coarctation of the aorta				
	Aortic root dilatation				
	Pulmonic valve stenosis	↓	↓	↑	↑
	Pulmonic artery stenosis				
	Pulmonic leaflet reverberation (Still's)				
Late systolic	Papillary muscle dysfunction				
	Mitral valve prolapse	↑	↑	↓	↓ then ↑
Holosystolic	Mitral regurgitation	↓	↓	↑	↓
	Tricuspid regurgitation	↓	↓	↑	↑
	Ventricular septal defect	↓	↓	↑	↓
Early diastolic	Aortic regurgitation†	↓	↓	↑	↓
	Pulmonic regurgitation (Graham-Steele)	↓	↓	↑	↑
Middiastolic	Mitral stenosis	↓	↓	↑	↑
	Tricuspid stenosis	↓	↓	↑	↑
	Flow murmur (mitral or tricuspid)	↓	↓	↑	↑
	Acute rheumatic fever (Carey-Coombs)				
	Atrial myxoma				
Continuous	Patent ductus arteriosus				
	Coronary AV fistula				
	Ruptured sinus of Valsalva				
	Aortic septal defect				
	Cervical venous hum				
	Anomalous left coronary artery				
	Proximal coronary artery stenosis				
	Mammary soufflé				
	Pulmonary artery branch stenosis				
	Bronchial collateral circulation				
	Small AS with MS				
	Intercostal AV fistula				

*Opposite findings noted with squatting position.
†May have associated low pitch, mid to late diastolic murmur (Austin-Flint murmur) due to interference from backwash at mitral valve.

(Fig. 34-1). Papillary muscles connect to the valve leaflets by the chordae tendineae. The valve opens when left atrial pressure exceeds left ventricular pressure and closes when left ventricular pressure rises. Contraction of the papillary muscles and tightening of the chordae tendineae occurs during systole. This interaction helps keep the valve properly closed and prevents backflow of blood to the left atrium during systole.[10]

Mitral Stenosis

Epidemiology

The prevalence of mitral stenosis (MS) in Europe and the United States has markedly decreased over the past 40–50 years. Before the 1960s, rheumatic mitral disease was the most common finding among surgically excised mitral valves for all causes (89%) and this number

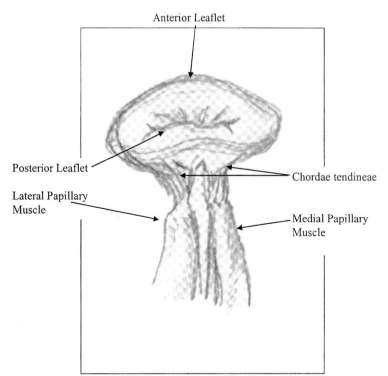

Anterior Leaflet

Posterior Leaflet

Lateral Papillary
Muscle

Chordae tendineae

Medial Papillary
Muscle

Fig. 34-1. Mitral valve. (Source: Schematic drawing compliments of Dana Welch.)

decreased to about 50% by the 1980s. By the early to mid-1990s, this number further decreased to 35%.[11] Improved living conditions and aggressive treatment of streptococcal infections has resulted in a decrease in rheumatic fever in developed countries. There was an outbreak of rheumatic fever in the United States in the 1980s and this was thought to be due to a virulent streptococcal strain and an increase in the immigrant population. However, an outbreak among nonimmigrant middle class families underscored the fact that there is incomplete understanding of the cycle of rheumatic fever.[11,12]

MS once comprised 43% of all valve disease but by 1985 MS accounted for only 9% of all valve disease at a European center.[13] More recent data from Europe (The Euro Heart Survey on Valvular Heart Disease) were published in a study that took place from April to July 2001. Five thousand patients were enrolled. Isolated MS accounted for 9.5% of all valve disease but was the cause of 12.1% of single native left side valve disease. Rheumatic fever was the etiology in 85.4% of cases of MS.[14]

In New England from 1990 to 1997 the percent of patients with MS of all causes who underwent mitral valve

repair or replacement ranged from 19.8 to 31.3%. This decreased to 11.0% (1998) and 12.4% (1999). During the same period however, the number of mitral valve procedures per 100,000/year increased 2.4 times mainly due to expanded indications for surgery. The population-based rate of MS showed an insignificant increase during the same time period.[15] This suggests that the prevalence of MS has remained stable in that area of the country in the most recent years. Despite the overall decreased incidence, rheumatic fever remains the most common cause of MS. Mixed MS and regurgitation are common. Females outnumber males by a 2:1 margin.[1] The immigrant population and sporadic outbreaks of rheumatic fever in the United States will result in a source of rheumatic MS at least for the near future.

With the exception of the Middle East, little decrease in the incidence of rheumatic fever and rheumatic heart disease has been seen in the developing world.[12] Among 319 patients undergoing mitral valve repair in Turkey for rheumatic disease between 1991 and 1998, 87.5% had MS.[16] However, a recent study does suggest there has been a decreased prevalence of rheumatic heart disease among rural Indian children.[17]

Etiology

Rheumatic fever is the leading cause of MS. About 50–60% of affected individuals report a history consistent with RF.[1,11] Pathology studies have shown that postinflammatory disease was found in 99% of valves excised for stenosis.[18] Multivalve involvement has been reported in nearly 40% of cases (most commonly aortic valve involvement). Other less common causes of MS include severe annular calcification, carcinoid disease, Fabry disease, mucopolysaccharidosis, Whipple disease, gout, rheumatoid arthritis, vegetations, and congenital MS.[1,2] Mitral annual calcification was found in less than 3% of cases in one series. Patients tended to be older and had associated aortic valve calcifications.[19] The etiology of MS at one center in Europe was rheumatic in 76.9% of all cases.[13] As noted above, the European survey found 85.4% of cases of isolated MS were rheumatic in origin, 12.5% were degenerative, and the remaining cases were of other etiologies.[14]

Pathophysiology

A mitral valve affected by rheumatic fever has leaflets that are thickened and calcified. The valve commissures progressively fuse and the subvalvular apparatus (wall of the left ventricle, chordea tendineae, and papillary muscles) can become matted. This leads to a narrowed funnel-shaped mitral apparatus. These findings are similar to those of other chronic inflammatory valve conditions and are often referred to as *postinflammatory* changes. In the absence of another etiology it is assumed that postinflammatory changes are due to rheumatic fever. It is debatable if the progressive pathologic lesions of MS result from a continued low-grade rheumatic process or by turbulent blood flow and repeated trauma to the damaged valve.[3,20,21] Patients with prior RF and valve disease have an elevate C-reactive protein level compared to patients with prosthetic valves or healthy controls. This suggests inflammation persists in chronic rheumatic fever.[22]

The normal valve orifice measures 4.0–5.0 cm^2 (or 6.0 cm^2) and mild symptoms of obstruction generally do not appear until there is about a 50% reduction in area. Moderate symptoms do not occur until the opening is less than 1.5 cm^2 and less than 1.0 cm^2 represents critical stenosis.[1,3,23]

The physiologic abnormalities seen among patients with MS are the result of obstruction of blood flow to the left ventricle at the mitral valve level. An increased transmitral pressure gradient occurs during diastole. In pure MS left ventricular contractility is normal. Function of the left ventricle may be normal or reduced due to decreased left ventricular filling. Scarring of the myocardium may result in regional hypokinesis. Rises in left atrial and pulmonary venous pressures can result in pulmonary congestion and edema.

Later in the course pulmonary hypertension will occur (or it may be due to other associated conditions). Pulmonary hypertension is often reactive and explained by the increased left atrial pressure. A reactive pulmonary hypertension that is out of proportion to the left atrial pressure occurs in some patients. Development of associated pulmonary hypertension can "protect" the patient from pulmonary edema but causes additional reductions in left ventricular volume. Long-standing pulmonary hypertension will eventually result in right heart failure. When right ventricular dilation occurs, the tricuspid valve can become incompetent and this worsens the patient's condition.

Increased left atrial pressure and dilation leads to atrial arrhythmias (particularly atrial fibrillation [AF] and flutter). Patients with MS are prone to the formation of thrombus and systemic embolization.[1,3,21,24]

Clinical Features

Early symptoms of MS are relatively nonspecific and include fatigue, decreased exercise tolerance, and those of left heart failure (dyspnea on exertion, orthopnea, and paroxysmal nocturnal dyspnea). Hemoptysis is a less common but often quoted finding. The natural history is that of a slow progressive disorder and in North America the course is even milder. In other areas, some patients will manifest a more rapid course. Acute decompensation may occur due to associated illness or other complications. Dyspnea often first appears after an emotional or physical stress such as exercise or infection. With long-standing disease the left atrium may become massively enlarged resulting in elevation of the left main stem bronchus and hoarseness from left recurrent laryngeal nerve palsy. Some patients present with symptoms of AF or systemic embolism.[1,3,21,24]

The right ventricle must pump blood against an increased pressure load that is reflected back from the left atrium. This results in signs of pulmonary hypertension and right-side heart failure (loud P$_2$, jugular venous distention, right ventricular heave, peripheral edema, and so on). Pulmonary pressures may exceed that predicted by the left heart pressures indicating there are other mechanisms involved in the production of pulmonary hypertension. As noted above, pulmonary hypertension may "protect" the patient from pulmonary edema but this is at the expense of decreased left heart filling.[1,3,21,24]

Heart failure or pulmonary edema occurs when pulmonary capillary pressure exceeds oncotic tissue pressure. This can be rather insidious with long-standing MS. Acute heart failure or pulmonary edema can occur in patients with noncritical stenosis if other conditions that elevated left atrial pressure and transmitral flow exist. Precipitators include but are not limited to AF or other tachycardias, thyrotoxicosis, infections, or pregnancy and the physician should carefully look for these conditions. Patients will have the same pulmonary findings as heart failure of other causes. A left ventricular S_3 is usually absent unless there is another condition that results in left ventricular dysfunction such as mitral or AR because in pure MS ventricular filling is slow and the left ventricle is normal size.

Atrial arrhythmias frequently occur in otherwise asymptomatic patients. Overall, 40% of patients with MS develop AF. AF it is less frequent in younger individuals and increases with age and left atrial size or pressure increases.[1,21]

Thromboembolic events are a feared complication of MS. The exact incidence is hard to determine because they may go unreported but 10–20% is a reasonable estimate. Cerebral emboli account for 60–70% of systemic emboli. Systemic embolic events are associated with age, duration of valvular disease, and AF but not necessarily with the size of the left atrium.[1,21,24]

Physical Examination

The classic auscultatory findings of MS include a diastolic rumble murmur and a loud opening snap. Other findings are dependent on coexisting disorders and include a systolic murmur, a loud P_2, and signs of left or right heart failure. The diastolic murmur is best heard at the apex with the patient in the left lateral position. It increases during expiration and decreases with Valsalva maneuver. The intensity of the murmur does not correlate with the degree of stenosis but a longer duration murmur is associated with more severe stenosis. The Carey-Coombs murmur of acute active valvulitis differs from the established MS murmur being a softer, higher pitched sound. A pansystolic murmur indicates associated mitral or tricuspid regurgitation (TR). In rheumatic heart disease, aortic valve disease often coexists with MS and murmurs of AS or regurgitation will be noted.

The opening snap occurs just after S_2 and is best heard at the apex. The S_2-OS interval ranges from 0.03 to 0.1 s. An interval less than 0.08 s indicates tight MS due to the increased left atrial pressure and resultant earlier opening of the mitral valve. The opening snap is a result of the chordae tendineae tightening. It can be difficult to differ-

entiate from S_2. When stenotic, the mitral valve stays open longer due to the increased pressure gradient. If the valve is relatively mobile its closure is signaled by a loud S_1 but if the leaflets are thickened and severely calcified S_1 is decreased. The findings of MS are often overlooked in otherwise asymptomatic patients. In a loud busy emergency department these heart sounds may be very difficult to characterize or hear even among more advanced cases.

Diagnosis

Electrocardiography

An electrocardiogram should be done for all patients with suspected MS or with exacerbations of known disease. Almost all patients with advanced MS who are in sinus rhythm show signs of left atrial enlargement on the electrocardiogram. "P mitrale" is noted by a widened and notched P wave in lead II. AF develops in 30–40% of patients with MS.[1,21] Signs of right heart pressure overload (right ventricular hypertrophy–QRS axis >90, RS ratio > 1:1) may be noted.[1,3,21,24] Proposed criterion to diagnose left atrium enlargement is by P-wave area measured in lead II for patients with MS. A P-wave area ≥24 milliseconds × millivolts had an 85.8% sensitivity and 93.7% specificity for left atrial enlargement.[25]

Chest Radiography

One of the earliest chest radiograph finding is left atrial enlargement. This can be subtle or reveal an extremely large left atrium with elevation of the left main stem bronchus. Other findings include those of left or right heart failure and calcification of the mitral valve or left atrium.[1,13,21,24]

Echocardiography

Echocardiography is the mainstay for the evaluation of patients with MS (Fig. 34-2). There are various criteria for the diagnosis and evaluation of MS by echocardiography but a detailed discussion is beyond the scope of this text. M-mode echocardiography findings include a decreased rate of valve closure and valve calcifications. Under normal conditions, the posterior leaflet normally moves away from the anterior leaflet in early diastole. A specific finding of MS is the posterior leaflet moving anterior during early diastole. M-mode echocardiography is unreliable for determining severity of disease. Two-dimensional (2D) echocardiography will also demonstrate valve calcifications but its main advantage is the ability to

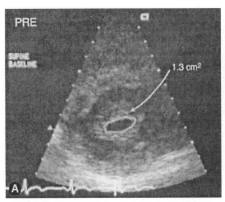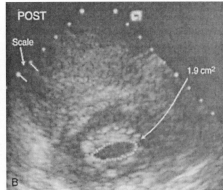

Fig. 34-2. Mitral stenosis. Echocardiogram—short-axis view of mitral stenosis. (Source: Reprinted from Otto CM. *Valvular Heart Disease*. The Netherlands: Elsevier, 1999, p. 255.)

determine valve mobility, thickening, orifice size, and the presence of subvalvular disease. Echocardiography provides important additional information including chamber size and function, the presence of coexisting MR, involvement of other valves, and an estimated pulmonary artery pressure.

Doppler echocardiography is used to measure flow rates across the valve and other indices that are used to estimate orifice size. Transesophageal echocardiography (TEE) is useful when the transthoracic window is inadequate and it is superior to transthoracic echocardiography (TTE) for detecting chamber thrombus. Because balloon valvuloplasty is contraindicated when left atrial thrombus is present, TEE is indicated prior to that procedure.[1,3,21,24] Three-dimensional TEE may offer additional information to assist in selecting patients for percutaneous balloon valvotomy but this is still early in development.[26]

Cardiac Catheterization

Cardiac catheterization has been replaced by echocardiography for the diagnosis and follow-up management of many patients with MS. Cardiac catheterization is indicated if an accurate measure of pulmonary artery pressures is needed for clinical management, when echocardiographic studies conflict with other clinical data or the results are nondiagnostic, or coronary artery disease is suspected. It is a also requirement to perform balloon valvulotomy.[1,21,24]

Treatment

It has been thought that MS has a relatively good prognosis with surgery indicated only when symptoms appeared. This thinking is being reconsidered based on the risk of systemic embolization and the development of low-risk percutaneous mitral commissurotomy.

Medical Management

Medical management has generally been the mainstay of management for asymptomatic cases of MS. The goals of medical treatment are to: (1) follow the progression of disease and determine the optimal timing and type of surgical intervention, (2) prevent and treat the complications of disease progression, (3) prevent recurrent rheumatic fever, and, less ideally, (4) treat symptoms of congestive heart failure until definitive therapy is accomplished.[1,3,21,24] The 1998 ACC/AHA guidelines recommend low-level physical conditioning[1] and there are guidelines for determining if a patient can complete in more strenuous events.[27] Although the emergency department is not involved in following disease progression or determining the timing of surgical therapy, recognition of the occurrence of symptoms does warrant consultation with a cardiologist or cardiovascular surgeon. There is no proven therapy that will halt or reverse the progression of the disease process.

The goal of modern therapy is not to allow the disease to progress to that of symptoms. There are situations where this is unavoidable such as among patients who have elected not to undergo surgical therapy for advancing disease or those with hemodynamic stressors (significant exertion, infections, pregnancy, and so on). Early symptoms typically result from a physical stress. The fixed obstruction of MS results in an increase in left atrial pressure when either flow increases or the heart rate increases, the latter resulting in a decrease in diastolic filling time. Beta-blocking agents or other negative chronotropic agents may reduce symptoms that are due to high heart rates. If there is evidence of pulmonary congestion diuretics may be prescribed. Digoxin is not of benefit unless there is coexisting left ventricular failure and the patient requires heart rate control for AF.[1,3,21,24]

The evaluation and treatment of AF is discussed in Chap. 21 and is similar to the treatment of AF due to other cardiac causes. In patients with MS AF commonly reoccurs or persists despite surgical therapy and is associated with a worse outcome. The European guidelines for managing asymptomatic valvular disease recommend not performing cardioversion before intervention if the obstruction is severe but suggest that cardioversion may be attempted prior to surgical treatment if the obstruction is mild or moderate.[28] The AHA/ACC guidelines state that surgical treatment prior to cardioversion is controversial.[1] In any case, if acute hemodynamic compromise occurs emergent cardioversion may be urgently needed. Heparin should be administered prior to attempted cardioversion and continued after the procedure.[1,28]

Prevention of systemic emboli is particularly important in patients with MS and AF or those with a prior embolic event. Anticoagulation is indicated in patients with AF (chronic or paroxysmal) and those with a history of an embolic event (class I recommendation). Anticoagulation should also be considered when the left atrium is enlarged (≥50 or 55 mm; class IIb).[1] It is controversial if severe cases of MS in patients with normal sinus rhythm require anticoagulation therapy and this should be individualized.[1,28,29] Patients with MS presenting to the emergency department with any potential serious complaint should undergo an assessment of their anticoagulation state.

Patients undergoing procedures in the emergency department present a special challenge. Unfortunately, there is a paucity of evidence as to prophylaxis and in particular, prophylaxis in the emergency department. In an emergency situation the patient may not be able to provide a history of valvular heart disease. Fortunately, most procedures commonly performed in the emergency department do not fall in the category of recommended endocarditis prophylaxis for acquired valvular heart disease. Acquired valve disease is considered to be a moderate risk for subsequent bacterial endocarditis. Procedures where prophylaxis is not recommended include oral-endotracheal intubation, urethral catheterization (if uninfected), and endoscopy without gastric biopsy.[1] There are no good studies or recommendations as to prophylaxis of a multiple-trauma patient but the authors recommend treatment for patients with serious genitourinary, gastrointestinal, or respiratory tract injuries (even though the prophylaxis is *late*). Good clinical judgment should guide the need to deviate from the recommendations. A more detailed discussion is found under the endocarditis section.

Rheumatic fever prophylaxis is critical. Primary prevention is accomplished by treating all cases of group A streptococci infections. Patients with a previous episode of rheumatic fever should receive long-term prophylaxis. This most easily accomplished with 1.2 million units of benzathine penicillin G every month (or every 3 weeks for high-risk patients with residual carditis or those who are economically disadvantaged). Other treatments require daily therapy. Options for oral therapy include penicillin V, 250 mg twice daily or sulfadiazine, 0.5 g daily (≤27 kg) or 1.0 g daily (>27 kg). For penicillin or sulfadiazine allergic patients erythromycin, 250 mg, twice daily is recommended.[1,28,30]

Surgical Management

Percutaneous mitral balloon valvotomy (PMBV) has become the procedure of choice in selected patients. It was first introduced in 1984[31] and over 30,000 patients had undergone the procedure by 1996.[21] The cost of a disposable balloon catheter makes this procedure expensive for underdeveloped nations. A reusable metallic device (percutaneous metallic commissurotomy) has been developed that is effective and costs are about 25% that of PMBV.[32,33]

There has been a worldwide trend toward performing percutaneous mitral commissurotomy at an earlier stage of disease. Patients with little or no symptoms, favorable valve morphology, and significant stenosis (valve area ≤1.5 cm^2 or ≤1.0 cm^2/m^2 body surface area) are now being treated. Asymptomatic patients with pulmonary hypertension and those with increased risk of a thromboembolism should strongly be considered for PMBV (the latter group requires 4 weeks of anticoagulant therapy and a transesophageal echocardiogram to exclude left atrial thrombus prior to the procedure).[28] Factors that favor PMBV include a pliable valve with minimal calcification or subvalvular disease, minimal MR, pregnancy, advanced age, and coexisting pulmonary disease. It is relatively contraindicated in patients with left atrial thrombus or significant MR. This should be the procedure of choice in capable centers for patients with moderate to severe disease and no contraindications.[1,28] Generally, only patients with moderate to severe stenosis (≤1.5 cm^2) are considered for surgical intervention. Patients with mild MS do not require PMBV (class III recommendation).[1] Table 34-2 summarizes the 1998 ACC/AHA guidelines for PMBV.

PMBV is successful in 80–95% of patients and the success rate is higher in more experienced centers.

Table 34-2. ACC/AHA Guidelines Percutaneous Mitral Balloon Valvotomy for Mitral Stenosis

Indication	Class
Symptomatic patients* with moderate to severe† MS and favorable valve morphology.‡ Patients must not have either left atrial thrombus or moderate to severe associated mitral regurgitation (MR).	I
Asymptomatic patients with moderate to severe MS, favorable valve morphology, and pulmonary hypertension.§	IIa
Severe symptoms** in patients with moderate to severe MS, unfavorable valve morphology§ and are high-risk surgical candidates. There must not be left atrial thrombus or moderate to severe MR.	IIa
Asymptomatic patients with moderate to severe MS, favorable valve morphology, but having new onset atrial fibrillation. There must not be associated left atrial thrombus or moderate to severe MR.	IIb
Severe symptoms in patients with moderate to severe MS, favorable valve morphology, and low-risk surgical candidates	IIb

*Symptomatic patient, New York Heart Association (NYHA) functional class II, III, or IV
**Severe symptoms (NYHA) functional class III or IV
†Mitral valve area ≤1.5 cm².
‡Favorable valves are noncalcified and pliable. Unfavorable characteristics include calcifications, thickened leaflets, decreased mobility, and subvalvular apparatus fusion.
§Pulmonary artery pressures >50 mmHg at rest or >60 mmHg with exercise.
Source: Adapted from ACC/AHA guidelines (reference 1).

Complications of the procedure include severeMR, a large atrial septal defect, perforation of the left ventricle, embolic events, and myocardial infarction. In properly chosen patients the mortality rate associated with the procedure should be <1%.[1]

A recent study showed that patients <55 years have a better hemodynamic response than older patients. The older group had worse baseline symptoms and a higher degree of stenosis making comparisons difficult.[34] There are instances where emergency PMBV has been done successfully on critically ill patients.[35] It is hoped the disease will not progress this far among patients in developed nations but it may be noted among the immigrant population.

Closed mitral commissurotomy is often done in developing countries (where the disposable balloon catheter cost can be prohibitive) but in the United States the open technique is preferred. Any type of valvulotomy must be considered a palliative procedure as restenosis invariably occurs.

Mitral valve repair is not indicated if the valve area is >1.5 cm² despite symptoms. Class I recommendations for mitral valve repair include moderate or severe stenosis (≤1.5 cm²) with valve morphology that is favorable for repair and the patient has New York Heart Association (NYHA) class III or IV symptoms under the following conditions:

1. PBMV is not available.

2. Left atrial thrombus exist despite anticoagulation therapy.

3. The valve is calcified or nonpliable and a decision to repair or replace the valve is made at the time of surgery.

For patients with moderate or severe stenosis and NYHA class I symptoms who have recurrent embolic events despite anticoagulation the evidence for surgical repair is class IIb.[1] The European guidelines recommend considering surgery in NYHA class II symptoms with tight stenosis and high embolic risk when there are contraindications to PBMV.[28]

Mitral valve replacement is indicated in symptomatic (NYHA III-IV) patients with moderate or severe stenosis who are not candidates for PMBV or repair (class I). For patients with no or mild symptoms, significant stenosis, and severe pulmonary hypertension valve replacement is indicated if PBMV or repair cannot be done (class IIa). The need for anticoagulation and the operative mortality rate (average 6.4%) must be considered when recommending valve replacement surgery. The emergency complications of valve replacement are valve thrombosis, embolism, valve dehiscence, or infection.[1] This is discussed in more detail in the mechanical valve section.

In the developing world monitoring anticoagulation can be difficult. A stentless bovine pericardial quadrileaflet mitral valve (Quattro valve) is a potential answer for those needing replacement and has shown satisfactory intermediate results. Long-term results are unknown.[36,37] Emergent valve replacement surgery has been successfully performed on patients considered to be terminal within 24 hours from rheumatic valve disease.[38]

Prognosis

MS in European and North American patients is a slowly progressive disease. The average time from the episode of rheumatic fever to symptoms was 16.3 ± 5.2 years[13] and can be even longer (20–40 years).[1] The age at which the typical North American of European patient undergoes a procedure for MS is 45–55 years of age and more than a third are over 65. This contrasts with the shorter interval and lower age range (27–37 years) among patients undergoing valvuloplasty in developing nations.[1,24]

Without surgery the overall 10-year mortality rate for all patients ranges from 33 to 70%. Most of this information is from studies prior to widely available surgical therapy and included a large number of asymptomatic cases.[24] For asymptomatic patients the 10-year survival rate is much better (>80%) and in only about 40% will symptoms become evident. The wide range of mortality is reflected by the heterogeneous age and frequency of symptoms in the various studies.[1,13,21,24] Among symptomatic patients who refused surgery 5-year survival was only 44% in the modern era.[13] A recent study from England examined 405 patients with MS who required a procedure. Older patients were found to have more symptomatic limitations, more degenerative valve disease, and a higher frequency of a severe degree of MS. The incidence of AF, mitral reflux, left ventricular impairment, coronary artery disease, and aortic valve disease increased progressively with age.[34] This confirms the poor outcome of symptomatic nonsurgically treated cases.

Mitral Regurgitation

Epidemiology

Like other valve disorders, the prevalence of MR in the United States is difficult to estimate. There are about 500,000 discharge diagnoses of MR but only about 18,000 mitral valve procedures performed each year in the United States. Many adults have benign flow murmurs and up to 80% of adults have nonpathologic regurgitation detected by echocardiography.[39] In Europe, 24.8% of all valve disease and 31.5% of single left side native valve diseases was MR. It is the second most common heart valve disease trailing only AS.[14] The prevalence of MR appears

to be increasing. This may be due to shifts in the etiology of MR and longevity as the prevalence increases with age.[40] Finally, the number of mitral valve procedures done in New England increased 2.4 times in the decade spanning 1990–1999.[15]

Etiology

The main causes of MR include MVP, ischemic heart disease, rheumatic heart disease, dilated cardiomyopathy, connective tissue and collagen vascular diseases, endocarditis, and anorexic drugs.[1,41] Acute MR is classified into ischemic and nonischemic. A detailed list of causes can be found in Table 34-3. Table 34-4 outlines the general causes of MR and their associated frequencies. Emergency physicians must be keenly aware of acute MR resulting from ischemic heart disease, acute heart failure, and endocarditis. MVP will be discussed separately.

Pathophysiology

Mitral regurgitation can result from a number of different pathologic processes. The valve leaflets can shorten and stiffen or become deformed and unable to close properly. Endocarditis can cause valve perforations or vegetations. Dilation of the mitral annulus results in regurgitation. Calcification of the mitral annulus is a very common finding at autopsy and is usually of no significance. When severe it can, however, interfere with valve closure. Lengthening or rupture of the chordae tendineae and papillary muscle dysfunction or rupture results in MR. Ischemia can cause a transient papillary muscle dysfunction. Left ventricular dilation alters the normal anatomy of the papillary muscles and size of the orifice.[3,41] In the case of ischemic MR, the valve morphology is normal but ischemia-induced changes in the geometry of the ventricle and the subvalvular apparatus result in regurgitation. In this instance, the left ventricular abnormalities are the primary cause of the MR as opposed to the result of valvular abnormalities.[42]

The volume of regurgitation is related to the orifice area and the blood flow velocity where velocity is a function of the left ventricular-left atrial pressure gradient. MR occurs mainly during systole.[43] MR impacts three heart chambers (left ventricle, left atrium, and right ventricle) as opposed to AS which mainly affects one ventricle.[40] Regurgitation of blood results in increased volume in the left atrium during systole and in the left ventricle during diastole. In chronic MR the continued overload of the left ventricle results in both left ventricular hypertrophy and an increase in left ventricular end-diastolic volume (dilation). This

Table 34-3. Causes of Mitral Valve Regurgitation

Etiology	Pathophysiology
Acute	
Acute ischemia	Altered left ventricular geometry and/or papillary muscle dysfunction or rupture
Chordal rupture	Myxomatous degeneration
Endocarditis	Destruction and perforations of the valve
Trauma	Rupture of the chords
Chronic	
Postinflammatory	Valve thickening, retraction, and decreased mobility
Rheumatic heart disease	
Systemic lupus erythematosus	
Postradiation changes	
Other collagen-vascular diseases	
Tumors	Decreased mobility, unable to close
Degeneration	Prolapsed valve, ruptured chords
MVP	
Marfan syndrome	
Ehlers-Danlos syndrome	
Chordae tendineae lesions	Infection, trauma, muscle strain,
Papillary muscle pathology	Ischemia, left ventricular dilation
Ischemic heart disease	
Left ventricular dysfunction	
Trauma	
Dilated mitral annulus (cardiomyopathy)	Left ventricular dilation
Congenital disorders	
Failure of prosthetic valve	
Drugs	Thickening and decreased mobility
Diet drugs (controversial)	
Ergots	
Carcinoid syndrome	
Hypereosinophilic syndrome	

Table 34-4. Etiologies of Chronic Aortic and Mitral Regurgitation

Etiology	Chronic Mitral Regurgitation	Chronic Aortic Regurgitation
Degenerative	61.3	50.3%
Rheumatic	14.2	15.2%
Congenital	4.8	15.2%
Other	8.1	7.7%
Endocarditis	3.5	7.5%
Ischemic	7.3	0
Inflammatory	0.8	4.1%

Source: Adapted from The Euro Heart Survey (reference 14).

increased volume can cause annular dilation and a cycle of worsening MR, further dilation, and worsening regurgitation.[3,41]

The left atrium size is determined by compliance. If the compliance is normal or slightly reduced, then left atrium will not enlarge and pressures increase dramatically resulting in pulmonary congestion. This is more characteristic of acute MR. In another subgroup of patients in which MR is longstanding, left atrial compliance is increased and the left atrium will massively dilate. The pressures in the left atrium and pulmonary vasculature remain normal or minimally elevated. AF is common in that situation due to increased left atrial size. Most patients fall somewhere in between these two extremes.[3]

The most common manifestation of MR is the situation where there is some increased compliance but there is also a significant increase in left atrial pressure. As the condition progresses the increased pulmonary venous pressures cause increased pulmonary pressure. Some patients will develop a reactive pulmonary hypertension. If this is allowed to progress the pulmonary artery walls develop the changes of chronic pulmonary hypertension and right heart failure will ensue.[3,43] During the chronic phase forward flow may be normal or reduced but the total left ventricular output (forward and regurgitation) is elevated. Despite these changes, patients can remain asymptomatic for long periods.

Acute Ischemic Mitral Regurgitation

Myocardial infarction can lead to rupture of the papillary muscles. This rare event typically occurs days after the infarction. The emergency physician is more likely to be confronted with acute papillary muscle dysfunction that is seen during acute ischemia or infarction. Acute myocardial infarction (AMI) resulting in MR is most commonly (80%) a complication of right coronary or circumflex occlusions. It carries a worse prognosis than MR of other causes.[1,43] Mortality rates in patients with an ejection fraction (EF) <0.4 were 29% among AMI patients with mild MR versus 12% at 3.5 years if MR was not present.[44] Patients with MR due to previous myocardial infarction (defined as more than 16 days old) have higher long-term cardiac mortality rates compared to those without MR.[45] When ischemic MR is more severe, the 1-year mortality rates postmyocardial infarction were over 50%.[46] A study from the SHould we emergently revascularize Occluded Coronaries in cardiogenic shocK (SHOCK) registry compared patients with postacute myocardial cardiogenic shock due to severe MR with that caused by left ventricular failure. In-hospital unadjusted mortality was 55% and 61% for the severe MR and left ventricular failure groups, respectively. Adjusting for patient differences did not alter that conclusion (odds ratio [OR] = 0.97, 95% confidence interval [CI] 0.60–1.56).[47]

In addition to ischemia, acute MR can occur as a result of trauma, valvular degeneration, chordal rupture, endocarditis, and hypovolemia in patients with mitralvalve prolapse. Acute MR results in a sudden volume overload of the left heart. There is an increased left ventricular end-diastolic volume and sarcomeres stretch. Contractility is normal or increased due to Frank-Starling forces. The ability of blood to regurgitate to the atrium reduces left ventricular afterload and the end-systolic volume decreases. These conditions result in an increased stroke volume. As discussed above, however, the left atrium is usually of normal size and compliance so a marked increase in pressure results in pulmonary edema and elevated pulmonary artery pressures. Overall, the heart size remains normal in the acute phase.[3,46]

Clinical Features

Mild to severe MR can be associated with little or no symptoms. In slowly progressing cases, some patients will modify their activity and other medical therapy will mask changing symptoms. Progressive disease symptoms are fatigue and those of congestive heart failure. Physiologic stressors such as infections or pregnancy can result in acute symptoms. AF may be a presenting feature but sudden death is rare. If the etiology is ischemia patients may present with symptoms of ischemic heart disease and those with dilated cardiomyopathy often present with those signs. Patients with serious acute MR are almost always symptomatic including pulmonary edema.[3,41,43]

Physical Examination

Peripheral pulses feel normal in mild cases. The carotid upstroke is brisk in patients with severe MR and this is different from the delayed upstroke of AS. Blood pressure and pulse pressure are normal. In more advanced cases AF and signs of heart failure are evident.

A third heart sound is often present but does not always indicate heart failure. The classic murmur of MR is the systolic murmur that is loudest at the apex and radiates to the axilla. The murmur is often holosytolic but can occur during any part of the cycle. S_1 is soft or normal in intensity and the murmur can obscure A_2. The intensity of the murmur does not correlate with the degree of regurgitation.

Acute MR presents a significant challenge to the emergency physician because the murmur can be very soft even in severe cases and there may be no audible murmur in 50% of cases of acute MR.[3,41,43]

Diagnosis

Electrocardiography

The ECG findings are nonspecific and are dependent on the associated pathology. Findings include signs of left atrial enlargement, left ventricular hypertrophy, AF, and right ventricular hypertrophy. ECG findings do not correlate well with severity of MR.[1,3,41]

Chest Radiography

The chest radiograph can be anywhere from normal to signs of left atrial and ventricular enlargement and decompensation. Right heart enlargement is a late finding. Calcification of the annulus may be noted in the elderly patient with MR.[1,3,41]

Echocardiography and Doppler Studies

Echocardiography is invaluable for the initial evaluation in the outpatient setting. It provides baseline left atrial and ventricle volumes and function. It also provides information on valve and subvalvular anatomy. Estimates of severity are based on Doppler studies. In cases of acute MR echocardiography is extremely useful. In myocardial infarction it will show wall motion abnormalities but papillary muscle rupture may be difficult to demonstrate. In cases of endocarditis echocardiography may demonstrate the typical findings (see endocarditis). TEE is superior to TTE but is often not available to the emergency department. It is indicated when transthoracic studies are inadequate.[1,3,41] Mitral annular calcification noted on echocardiography in patients ≤65 years of age has been associated with severe coronary artery disease.[48]

Cardiac Catheterization

The main indication for cardiac catheterization is to perform coronary angiography for cases of ischemic MR or when coronary artery disease is suspected or coexists in patients where valve surgery is contemplated. Patients with AMI and acute MR may undergo cardiac catheterization and revascularization if appropriate as dictated by clinical conditions and the indications based on the myocardial infarction.[1,3,41] In cases of acute MR bedside right heart catheterization is often performed to assess hemodynamics.[46]

Magnetic Resonance Imaging

Magnetic resonance is an accurate method for evaluating the mitral valve (and other valves) but at this time has no use in the emergency setting.[3,49] This diagnostic modality will not be discussed in detail.

Treatment

Medical Management

The main goals of medical management are to determine the need for surgery, prevent recurrent rheumatic fever, or endocarditis, and treat heart failure if the condition has progressed. Prophylaxis for procedures and rheumatic fever is similar to that of other acquired valve disorders. Patients who are in AF should have their heart rate controlled. The risk for systemic embolization may be less than that of patients with MS and AF. There are no firm guidelines as to anticoagulation therapy but it is suggested that the international normalized ratio (INR) be maintained in the 1–3 range.[1]

Afterload reduction for asymptomatic patients is controversial. There is no convincing evidence as to the efficacy of prophylactic afterload reduction therapy to prevent disease progression and to delay the need for surgery among asymptomatic patients.[1,28] Afterload reduction is of use for symptomatic patients with left ventricular dysfunction in whom surgery cannot be performed. Vasodilator therapy has been shown to be of use in patients with MR that is associated with a dilated poorly functioning left ventricle. Acutely vasodilators reduce the regurgitation fraction but there are no trials that demonstrate clinical benefit for chronic MR. Beta-blocker therapy should be considered when there is left ventricular systolic dysfunction. These agents reduce the regurgitation volume and have favorable effects on left ventricular remodeling.[28,42,43] Standard treatment for heart failure is used in this situation. Long-term prognosis for patients with heart failure treated only medically is poor.[43] In cases of acute MR, emergent afterload reduction with nitroprusside or a balloon pump may stabilize the patient long enough to arrange for surgical intervention.[1,3]

Surgical Management

Mitral valve repair (which consists of annuloplasty with a prosthetic ring and/or valve reconstruction) is more often possible in patients with degenerative valve disease than rheumatic disease or endocarditis. It generally has better operative and long-term prognoses than valve replacement. Left ventricular function is maintained, the incidence of thromboembolism is lower, and there is a reduced risk of endocarditis.[41] A possible exception to this is in severe MR due to ischemia or myocardial infarction. In these cases, it has been suggested that revascularization alone may suffice but that is becoming more debatable. Regardless, operative and long-term mortality rates are high in patients with AMI and MR.[1,44,46]

The timing of mitral valve surgery for nonischemic MR will be outlined below. Some expert centers are repairing mitral valves among asymptomatic patients with normal left ventricular function in order to prevent the complications of chronic MR.[1,41] Class I recommendations for mitral valve surgery for nonischemic MR are as follows: (1) acute symptomatic MR when repair is likely, (2) any patient who is symptomatic (NYHA functional class II or greater) despite normal left ventricular function should undergo valve surgery, and (3) any patient (symptomatic or asymptomatic) where echocardiography indicates signs of mild (EF 0.5–0.6 and left ventricular end-systolic dimension 45–50 mm) or moderate (EF >0.3.0–0.5 and/or left ventricular end-systolic dimension 50–55 mm) left ventricular dysfunction (even when valve repair is unlikely).[1] The European guidelines recommend surgery in selected asymptomatic patients with severe MR and any of the following conditions: (1) either an EF <0.6 or left ventricular end-systolic diameter >45 mm when repair is likely, (2) AF or, (3) pulmonary hypertension but normal left ventricular function when repair is likely.[28]

Class IIa evidence for surgery are as follows: (1) patients with pulmonary hypertension and normal left ventricular function, (2) AF when left ventricular function is normal, (3) asymptomatic patients with either an EF 0.5–0.6 with normal ventricular end-diastolic dimension or an EF >0.6 but dimension 45–55 mm, and finally in patients with severe left ventricular dysfunction (EF <0.3 and/or dimensions >55 mm) in whom chordal preservation is likely. Class IIb evidence was noted for asymptomatic patients with normal left ventricular function when repair is highly likely or in patients with MVP who have ventricular arrhythmias despite medical therapy.[1]

The recommendations for earlier surgery resulted from improved techniques, decreased surgical mortality, and the recognition that long-term outcomes are poor when surgery is delayed until left ventricular dysfunction or AF have appeared. Minimally invasive mitral valve surgery is another factor that makes early surgery more attractive.[29,50] A recent study showed that the incidence of postoperative left ventricular dysfunction was higher in patients with a preoperative EF <55% or left ventricular end-systolic diameter ≥40 mm. It was concluded that in patients with MR, when either a decrease in function or increase in diameter is detected mitral valve repair should be considered to preserve postoperative left ventricular function. This lends further evidence to the concept of earlier valve repair and a left ventricular end-systolic diameter of ≥40 mm may become the new standard.[51] Percutaenous mitral repair is in current development.[52]

Surgical therapy for MR that is secondary to severe left ventricular dilated cardiomyopathy and left ventricular

dysfunction (EF <30%) is more controversial. In that case, there may be a worsening of cardiac function due to an increased afterload and altered mitral annular and papillary muscle anatomy. When valve repair is possible these patients may be considered for surgery.[1,3,53] Recent data, however, suggest that mitral valve repair for patients with advanced heart failure can be done with a relatively low operative mortality rate and with good functional outcome.[54,55]

The surgical approach to ischemic pathology is still controversial. It is not always predictable if coronary artery bypass alone will suffice and if or when mitral valve repair or replacement is optimal or feasible.[1,46,56] A study from the Society of Thoracic Surgeons National Cardiac Database looked at patients undergoing mitral valve surgery. Of the 5401 patents with who underwent coronary artery bypass graft (CABG) and an isolated mitral valve procedure from 1999 to 2000 valve repair was done in 46.3% and the remainder underwent replacement.[57]

Mitral surgery is generally indicated for acute severe ischemic MR.[1,40] Surgery should be considered for patients in myocardial infarction-related shock and with severe MR despite the high mortality rates.[58] Some recommend that many patients undergoing CABG who have moderate ischemic MR should undergo concomitant mitral annuloplasty.[59,60] Papillary muscle repair is another method that has been used to repair MR in selected cases.[61] Bitran et al. described good short-term results for patients with ischemic MR and poor left ventricular function.[62] Long-term survival among patients undergoing both CABG and mitral valve surgery was related to the degree of coronary artery disease and left ventricular dysfunction rather than the etiology of the MR.[63] Prospective trials comparing CABG alone or CABG with mitral valve surgery are needed to determine optimal therapy for patients with moderate ischemic MR.[60]

It has been suggested that percutaneous coronary intervention is relatively contraindicated for non-AMI patients who require revascularization. Although not designed to answer the question, the study suggests that valve surgery and another revascularization method (such as CABG) could improve survival.[64]

Prognosis

Chronic MR is often a slow progressing disorder and in mild cases prognosis is excellent. Average time of diagnosis to symptom onset was 16 years in one study. Once patients become symptomatic surgical therapy improves survival. Without intervention the 5- and 8-year survival was 45 and 33%, respectively. More severe cases progress faster and have higher mortality. The variation in progression is partially due to the condition of the myocardium and the etiology of the regurgitation. Mortality is usually related to congestive heart failure but arrhythmias and sudden death can occur.[3,41,43]

Mitral Valve Prolapse

Epidemiology

Mitral valve prolapse is a disorder characterized by retrograde movement of the mitral valve into the left atrium during systole. The estimated prevalence of MVP is close to 2.5%, making it one of the most common forms of valvular heart disease.[65] While classically thought of as a disease of younger patients, recent data suggest the mean age at first diagnosis may be closer to 50.[65,66] Data from the same series show a gender predilection, with females outnumbering males by a ratio of 1.5:1.[65,66]

Etiology

Although MVP can result from anatomic variation in any component of the mitral valve apparatus, the primary form develops through myxomatous proliferation of the spongiosa layer of the leaflets of the valve itself, with resultant thickening and redundancy.[1] Most cases of primary MVP are idiopathic and sporadic, but the occurrence may be familial with autosomal-dominant inheritance or associated with generalized connective tissue disorders such as Marfan syndrome.[1] Secondary MVP may occur in the absence of primary valve leaflet pathology, developing as a complication from cardiac ischemia, rheumatic heart disease, an untreated atrial septal defect, or long-standing hypertrophic cardiomyopathy.[1]

Clinical Features

Most patients with MVP remain asymptomatic. Clinical manifestations, when present, are heterogeneous and correlate most directly with the presence and degree of MR. Presenting symptoms are often nonspecific (chest pain, dyspnea, and syncope) and occur with a frequency no greater than that of the general population.[1,65] MVP is not an independent risk factor for cardiac ischemia, and recurrent presentations with anginal symptoms despite appropriate coronary evaluation may be related to underlying neuropsychiatric syndromes such as panic disorder. Rarely, dyspnea or syncope may be related to a variant of MVP characterized by intermittent, exercise-induced MR.[1] For the vast majority of patients with MVP (>85%), MR is either absent or trivial,[65,66] diminishing the

likelihood of a causational relationship between symptoms of dyspnea and disease. Progressive development of heart failure may complicate MVP over the course a lifetime however, occurring insidiously with gradually worsening LV dysfunction from MR or more acutely from chordae rupture.[1,66,67]

Palpitations are a common complaint of patients with MVP. Susceptibility to the development of supraventricular arrhythmias has been noted, and may be due to an increased incidence of left-sided atrioventricular (AV) bypass tracts.[1] Additionally, MVP is associated with the development of AF in 10–15% of patients within 10 years of diagnosis, with a greater risk in older individuals with moderate to severe MR and left atrial enlargement of ≥40 mm.[68] Initial electrocardiographic evaluation is most often normal. Holter monitoring is not routinely indicated and when performed, generally shows non-life-threatening arrhythmias.[1] Overall, the long-term incidence of sudden death from presumed ventricular tachyarrhythmias is low, although familial forms of MVP may carry a slightly greater risk because of an association with QT prolongation.[1]

An increased incidence of ischemic neurologic events (transient ischemic attacks and strokes) is commonly attributed to the existence of MVP, but the exact relationship is unclear. While early analyses, based largely on case series, suggested a correlation, more recent reports refute an association.[69,70] Combined information from several studies which applied more specific echocardiographic criteria, demonstrates a significant lifetime excess rate of occurrence (relative risk 2.2; 95% CI 1.5–3.2),[68] but the effect appears to be age dependent.[68–70] While age >50 years has been demonstrated to be an independent predictor, patients <45 years with MVP seem to be at no greater risk.[68] Other identified risk factors, including the development of AF after an initial diagnosis of MVP and the need for cardiac surgery during follow-up, appear to be time dependent, complicating the interaction.[68,70] Mitral valve leaflet thickening may also be an important prognostic indicator, but it is difficult to determine if the effect is independent or related to the natural progression of MVP.[68,70]

Physical Examination

The presence of MVP may be suspected by cardiac examination with auscultation of a midsystolic click and a late systolic murmur. Dynamic provocation with the Valsalva maneuver or a positional change from supine to standing may intensify these findings through a decrease in LV end-diastolic volume.[1]

Diagnosis

A clinical diagnosis of MVP lacks sensitivity and mandates further evaluation. Electrocardiography and chest radiography have limited utility in this regard. Confirmation of a suspected diagnosis requires 2D echocardiography.[1,65] The recent development of echocardiographic diagnostic criteria has resulted in a lower rate of false positive diagnoses and a redefinition of the incidence of MVP.[65–70] The diagnosis of MVP is established through visualization, during systole (in the parasternal long-axis view), of mitral leaflet displacement >2 mm superior to the plane of the mitral annulus.[65–67] Associated leaflet thickness, defined as ≥5 mm, is a frequent finding, noted in about 55% of cases.[65,66] Flail movement of the leaflet may be seen and reflects involvement of the papillary muscles or chordae tendineae.[1,66] MR appears to accompany nearly 60% of patients with MVP, with up to 25% of these graded semi-quantitatively as moderate or severe.[65–67] Higher grades of MR may be more frequent with posterior rather than anteriorleaflet prolapse, but are unrelated to valve thickening.[66] Secondary effects of MR may include left atrial enlargement, left ventricular hypertrophy, and left ventricular dysfunction.

Treatment

Treatment of MVP is symptom based and reassurance may be the most important intervention for the majority of patients. Patients with recurrent palpitations, chest pain, or dyspnea in the absence of significant underlying cardiac morbidity should be counseled to avoid stimulants such as caffeine, alcohol, and cigarettes. Pharmacotherapy with beta-blockers may be particularly effective.[1] Referral for electrophysiologic (EPS) testing may be required for those with recurrent tachyarrhythmias, recurrent unexplained syncope, sustained ventricular tachycardia, or aborted sudden death.[1] Aspirin therapy (81–325 mg/day) should be initiated in patients who develop ischemic neurologic events. Long-term anticoagulation with warfarin may be indicated as well, particularly for those with AF, especially if ≥65 years of age with moderate to severe MR and a history of heart failure.[1] For patients with moderate to severe MR with development of LV dysfunction (defined as an EF = 0.60 or an LV end-systolic dimension ≥45 mm), valve replacement or repair is generally indicated.[1,67]

MVP is the leading cardiovascular cause of IE and the diagnosis mandates consideration of antibiotic prophylaxis for those undergoing risky procedures (see Tables 34-10 and 34-11). Although the association between MVP and IE is strong (OR 8.2; 95% CI 2.4–28.4), the overall incidence is rare, developing in only 4 of 833 (0.48%) patients in one series with 10 years of observation.[66] Class I indications for antibiotic prophylaxis include diagnosed MVP with an audible systolic click-murmur complex or an isolated systolic click with echocardiographic evidence of MR.[1] Patients with valve thickening (generally due to primary MVP) and men older than 45 years also exhibit greater susceptibility to IE and should receive prophylaxis prior to high-risk procedures.[30,71] A more complete discussion of IE and antibiotic prophylaxis can be found in a subsequent section.

Prognosis

In general, prognosis for patients with MVP is good. Although 10% will require eventual surgical treatment for progressive cardiac morbidity, the overall mortality rate is similar to the general population.[65–67] Certain patients may be at an elevated risk for either however, and stratification can be performed, based on evaluation of several primary (EF <50% or MR ≥ moderate) and secondary factors (slight MR, flail leaflet, left atrial diameter >40 mm, AF or age ≥50 years).[66] Using this scheme, 1 in 5 patients can be categorized as high-risk (≥1 primary risk factor) with significant excess morbidity and mortality, 1 in 3 will be moderate-risk (no primary, ≥2 secondary risk factors) with excess morbidity, but equivalent mortality, and 1 in 2 will be low-risk (no primary, 1 secondary risk factor) with neither excess morbidity nor mortality.[66] It is important to remember that MVP can be an evolving process, and that patients may develop clinical deterioration with progression of risk over the lifetime of the disorder.

AORTIC VALVE DISORDERS

Anatomical Overview

The anatomy of the aortic and pulmonary valves is very similar. The aortic valve is attached to the myocardium, the anterior mitral valve, and the aorta. It has three fibrous cusps and the right and left coronary ostia arise next to two of the cusps (see Fig. 34-3). The valve opens during systole and closes when aortic pressure is greater than left ventricular pressure.[10]

Aortic Stenosis

Epidemiology

The prevalence of AS is difficult to determine but calcific AS is the third most common heart disease in developed

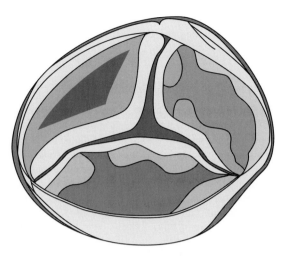

Fig. 34-3. Aortic valve. (Source: Schematic by Dana Welch.)

countries. In many countries in Europe, it is estimated that over 5% of people over 75 years of age have moderate AS.[28] The most recent data available are from Europe where isolated AS was the most frequent finding (43.1%) among patients with single left side native valve disease and accounted for 33.9% of all valve disease.[14]

Etiology

In adults, AS is most commonly caused by degenerative changes, rheumatic fever, or calcification of congenital abnormalities (unicuspid, bicuspid, or tricuspid valves). Calcification is a common finding in older adults regardless of the cause. AS is more common in males. The developed countries have seen a shift in the etiology of AS. In the United States about 50% of surgically treated cases of AS in 1990 were due to degenerative valve disease, 36% were bicuspid valves, and only 9% form postinflammatory disease (mostly rheumatic fever). This is in stark contrast to earlier years (pre-1980) where postinflammatory valves disease was noted in over 30% of cases.[72] Recent data from Europe show that 81.9% of cases of single native valve AS were degenerative in etiology and 11.2% were rheumatic in origin.[14]

Aortic sclerosis without stenosis is found in up to 37% of patients who are aged 75 or greater.[73] Risk factors for atherosclerotic disease correlate with both sclerosis and stenosis.[3,74] In particular, chronic *Chlamydia pneumoniae* infection and high lipoprotein levels have been implicated by some.[75–77] Others have found no relation between calcific AS and *C. pneumoniae* infections.[78] Further work needs to be done in this area to determine if there is an actual cause and effect relationship.

Aortic outflow obstruction may be caused by pathology in the supravalvular or subvalvular areas or by hypertrophic cardiomyopathy. The other causes of aortic outflow obstruction must be differentiated from valvular AS.

Pathophysiology

Aortic stenosis usually is a gradual process. Obstruction results in an increase in blood velocity across the valve and an associated increased pressure gradient. The left ventricle is exposed to increased pressure and it adapts by increasing wall thickness (left ventricular hypertrophy) while maintaining chamber size. During this period, the patient usually remains asymptomatic but there can be signs of diastolic dysfunction. The hypertrophied heart is subject to ischemia because of increased demand (reduced blood flow per amount of tissue), decreased coronary reserve, and maldistribution of blood flow. Hypertrophy is more common in women in whom it is frequently excessive. Not all develop adequate hypertrophy and these patients will have depressed contractility and low EFs.[1,74,79]

Clinical Features

The physician must be keenly aware of the symptoms of AS. Initially, patients may complain of decreased exercise tolerance. Angina pectoris symptoms are more frequent with AS than any other valve disease and angina can occur with isolated AS or in those with coexisting coronary artery disease. Dizziness and syncope can occur. Less commonly acute heart failure or pulmonary edema may be the presenting symptom and sudden death can occur. Systemic emboli occur and can be clinically silent.[1,74,79] Gastrointestinal bleeding, either from angiodysplasia or other sources, has been associated with AS. Some authorities have suggested a direct link and that severe recurrent or massive bleeding often stops after AVR.[74] Others argue there is no association between angiodysplasia and AS.[80]

Physical Examination

The key findings of AS are a decreased and delayed carotid upstroke and a systolic murmur best heard at the base in the right second intercostal space. The murmur is typically crescendo/decrescendo in character. The second heart sound may be singular if the aortic valve is severely immobile or may have reversed splitting due to prolonged left ventricular ejection time. An S_4 can be heard in many patients. Left ventricular hypertrophy can result in a heaving or thrusting apical impulse but the apical impulse will be in the normal position unless there is increased left ventricular chamber size. Signs of heart failure are found in advanced cases and this can be a result of AS or coexisting diseases. Right heart failure is rarely seen but when present may be due to the Bernheim effect (hypertrophy of the ventricular septum causing impaired right ventricular filling).[3,79]

Diagnosis

Electrocardiography

Left ventricular hypertrophy is classic for AS but many patients will not exhibit this finding. Other findings are non-specific and include left atrial abnormalities, left bundle branch block or conduction delays, and arrhythmias. AF should suggest concomitant cardiac disease. Exercise-induced electrocardiogram changes are common in adults but do not correlate with the presence of coronary artery abnormalities and the prognostic significance of ST depression is not clear. However, hemodynamic instability during exercise testing is reason to explore the possibility of valve replacement.[1] Positive stress test results in patients with AS are listed in Table 34-5. Positive results predict a 2-year survival of 19% compared to 85% if negative.[28]

Chest Radiography

The radiographic findings are often normal or non-specific. Occasionally calcified valve cusps are seen and

Table 34-5. Positive Exercise Stress Testing in Aortic Stenosis

Symptoms occur during study (dyspnea, angina, syncope, or near-syncope)

Systolic blood pressure rise less than 20 mmHg or a fall in blood pressure

Patient not reaching 80% of adjusted normal level of exercise tolerance

Greater than 2 mm of ST-segment depression not attributable to other causes

Ventricular tachycardia or more than four consecutive PVCs

Source: Adapted from "Recommendations on the management of the asymptomatic patient with valvular heart disease," 2002 (reference 28).

with ventricular dilatation and decompensation, cardiomegaly and the pulmonary signs of heart failure will be observed.

Echocardiography and Doppler Studies

The echocardiogram is highly effective in the diagnosis of AS and in delineating the left ventricular size and function. Doppler studies assist in determining the degree of stenosis by measuring the pressure gradient and valve area. Patients with moderate or severe calcifications and a rapid increase in the peak aortic jet velocity (≥ 0.3 m/s/year) are at higher risk for rapid progression. TEE is rarely needed.[1,28]

Cardiac Catheterization

Cardiac catheterization is indicated when the possibility of coronary artery disease exists or when noninvasive tests are inconclusive or conflict with clinical findings. Some still prefer to perform the study before planned valve replacement even when noninvasive studies are adequate.[1]

Treatment

Medical Management

Like other valve disorders, the goal of medical therapy is to prevent the complications and to determine when surgical therapy is needed. The disease is usually slow in progression. There is marked individual variation in the rate of progression with some showing little or no progression and others with a more rapid course. The incidence of first occurrence of symptoms ranges from 5 to 23% per year. Interpretation of these figures is complicated by the heterogeneous severity of disease and by classification of patients who underwent valve replacement while asymptomatic as an "event." Physical activity should be restricted for asymptomatic patients with moderate or severe AS. Echocardiography and Doppler studies are the studies of choice to follow patients and determine the need for surgery.[1,28]

Any patient with mild symptoms of AS (weakness or fatigue) should be referred to a cardiologist. Those with more emergent symptoms (syncope, angina, or heart failure) should be hospitalized for observation and further diagnostic studies.

There is no specific medical therapy for AS. Endocarditis prophylaxis is similar to other valve diseases (Tables 34-10 and 34-11). Rheumatic fever prophylaxis is required if AS was rheumatic in origin. Isolated calcified valves or bicuspid valves do not require rheumatic fever prophylaxis. For symptomatic patients who cannot undergo surgery, standard treatment of heart failure and arrhythmias are used to control symptoms. Excessive preload reduction should be avoided as cardiac output will be reduced.[1] Nitroprusside has been recommended as a bridge to surgery for patients with severe AS and severe left ventricular systolic dysfunction.[81] Statin therapy has been used in an attempt to prevent progression but clinical trials examining this therapy need to be done.[82]

Surgical Management

The degree of AS is determined by diagnostic studies and is classified as mild (valve area >1.5 cm^2), moderate (area > 1.0–1.5 cm^2), and severe (≤1.0 cm^2). The ACC/AHA guidelines recommend valve replacement for symptomatic patients with severe stenosis (class I). Other class I indications include patients with severe AS who are undergoing coronary artery bypass or other valve or aortic surgery. For patients with moderate AS, valve surgery should be considered for patients undergoing the other aforementioned surgeries (class IIa). While surgery should be considered for asymptomatic patients who have severe AS accompanied by left ventricular systolic dysfunction or an abnormal response to exercise (class IIa), the evidence for asymptomatic patients with either ventricular tachycardia, left ventricular hypertrophy, or valve area <0.6 cm^2 is limited (class IIb).[1]

For asymptomatic patients the decision to proceed with AVR should be balanced against the surgical morbidity and mortality and the long-term consequences of an artificial valve.[1] The European guidelines for the treatment of asymptomatic patients recommend surgery for those with severe AS (valve area <1.0 cm^2, or defined as <0.6 cm/m^2 body surface area) and any of the following conditions: left ventricular dysfunction (EF < 50%), parameters predictive of a more rapid progression (moderate to severe calcifications with high peak jet velocities and an accelerated progression of peak velocities), or an abnormal response to exercise test (Table 34-5). It was also recommended that surgery be considered for those with severe AS and either excessive left ventricular hypertrophy not due to hypertension, or severe ventricular arrhythmias.[28] Patients with no or only minimal valve calcifications may represent a low-risk group in whom surgery can be delayed.[83]

Among 1400 patients surgically treated between 1996 and 2001 the operative mortality rate within 30 days was 3.8%. Simultaneous CABG was performed in 572 patients. Independent predictors of mortality were previous bypass surgery, emergency operations, simultaneous MVR, renal dysfunction, age greater than 80 years. Although others

have reported concomitant bypass to be a risk for increased mortality, this study found only females with a high body mass index undergoing coronary bypass to be at increased risk. Finally small patients over 71 years were at increased risk.[84] Valve replacement surgery had been considered relatively risky for patients with severe left ventricular dysfunction but it now carries an acceptable risk.[85,86] Minimally invasive AVR surgery appears to be gaining acceptance and in skilled hands can be performed on elderly patients with good results.[87]

Percutaneous aortic valvuloplasty is generally not indicated in asymptomatic older adult patients but may be used as a bridge to surgery in unstable patients or as palliation for patients with other serious comorbid conditions. It has also been used for patients who require urgent noncardiac or aortic surgery. Aortic balloon valvuloplasty is successful and indicated in children and young adults.[1,28] Because of the histology of calcific AS it is unlikely that valve sparing surgery will have good long-term results. Endovascular valve replacement is early in development.[88]

For young patients the Ross procedure (a pulmonary autograft to replace the aortic valve and a cadaver pulmonary valve replacement) is often done. The patient's own pulmonary valve is better able to withstand the high pressure in the aortic side and the more fragile cadaver graft is implanted in the lower pressure pulmonary side.[79]

Prognosis

Like other valve diseases much of the data on progression are based on older retrospective data and more modern studies are often interrupted by valve surgery. The normal valve area is about 3.0–4.0 cm^2 but significant circulatory changes are not evident until the area is reduced to one-fourth normal size.[1] AS in adults is generally defined by a long latent period. Cardiac catheterization studies have shown some patients to have a 0.1–0.3 cm^2/year decrease in valve area and a transaortic pressure gradient increase of 10–15 mmHg increase per year. Limited data based on noninvasive studies have shown an average decrease in aortic valve area of 0.1 cm^2/year and an average increase in transaortic pressure gradient of 6–7 mm/year. The rate of progression however, is highly variable among individuals with some patients undergoing little or no change.[1,79,89]

The development of signs or symptoms marks a critical point of disease progression for patients with AS. Once signs and symptoms appear the average survival depends on the symptom. Average times of death for patients with syncope, angina, or dyspnea are 5, 3, and 2 years, respectively. The average time to death for symptomatic patients is less than 3 years. Symptoms mark a critical period in the disease progression.[1,89]

Aortic Regurgitation

Epidemiology

Isolated AR accounted for 10.4% of all cases and 13.3% of single left side native valve disease in Europe.[14] Doppler studies have revealed AR in almost 30% of people older than 75 years. Most of these cases are of no hemodynamic significance.[90]

Etiology

The causes of AR are many (some being uncommon) and include idiopathic dilatation, congenital valve abnormalities, calcific or other degenerative (myxomatous), rheumatic heart disease, endocarditis, aortic dissection, and Marfan syndrome. Less common causes include ankylosing spondylitis, syphilitic aortitis, trauma, rheumatoid arthritis, giant cell arteritis, Ehlers-Danlos syndrome, anorectic drugs, and others. A dilated aortic root can result from a variety of disorders and causes AR. Acute severe AR is most often a result of aortic dissection, trauma, or endocarditis.[1,91] Table 34-4 outlines the general causes of chronic AR and their associated frequencies.

Pathophysiology

In chronic AR the left ventricle responds by increasing end-diastolic volume and compliance resulting in concentric hypertrophy. New sarcomeres are produced and this results in eccentric hypertrophy. Early in the course there is a normal left ventricular preload and the left ventricle is able to maintain normal function by increasing stroke volume. Left ventricular afterload is increased and as the disease progresses both volume and pressure overload occur. Many patients remain asymptomatic for decades during this phase. Eventually, the compensatory balance cannot be maintained and patients become symptomatic. In some cases, symptoms do not appear until advanced left ventricular dysfunction has occurred. Left ventricular dysfunction can be reversed after valve replacement.[1,90,91]

AR affects coronary blood flow due to a decrease in aortic diastolic pressure. Coronary vessels increase in size to compensate for the degree of ventricular hypertrophy. Eventually the increase in size may not keep up with the demand particularly when the demand is increased by fever, exercise, or other conditions.[90]

Acute Aortic Regurgitation

In serious acute AR, the abrupt volume overload causes a rise in left ventricular and left atrial pressures. Cardiac output falls and it cannot be compensated by an increased heart rate. There is reduced blood flow to peripheral, major organ, and coronary vessels. Pulmonary edema and cardiogenic shock are common presentations.[1,91]

Clinical Features

Acute severe AR results in symptoms of pulmonary congestion and heart failure and shock. In acute cases pulse pressure may not be increased and heart size can be normal. Other symptoms are related to causative pathology such as aortic dissection, trauma, or endocarditis. In chronic cases patients may remain asymptomatic for decades. Some notice dizziness or vigorous cardiac contractions. Angina can occur in the presence or absence of significant coronary artery disease. Heart failure is the most common symptom to develop. Atrial or ventricular dysrhythmias occur late in the course. Syncope and sudden death can rarely occur even in the absence of symptoms[1,91,92]

Physical Examination

The classic findings of chronic AR include a low diastolic pressure with a widened pulse pressure, a bounding carotid pulse, signs of left ventricular dilation, and a diastolic murmur. The diastolic murmur is classically described as soft, high-pitched, holodiastolic, and decrescendo in character. It is heard best at the left sternal border but can be heard almost anywhere. Sitting the patient forward will increase the perceived volume of the murmur. The Austin-Flint murmur, another potential finding, is a lower-pitched mid to late diastolic murmur that may be confused with the murmur of MS. A systolic murmur may be present because of the increased forward flow and in the absence of other valvular abnormalities. The increased pulse pressure is the result of increases in forward and backward flow in the ascending aorta. The carotid pulse may be biphasic (bisferiens pulse) and when AR is severe a systolic thrill may be noted.

The peripheral signs of chronic AR are classic and have been described in detail. A "water-hammer" or Corrigan's pulse is the rapid hard pulse that quickly disappears. Quincke's pulse is the alternate reddening and blanching of the fingernails at each systole and diastole (augmented by gentle pressure on the nail bed). Head bobbing is another characteristic finding in severe chronic AR. Duroziez's sign is the presence of a systolic and diastolic bruit heard over the femoral arteries by gently compressing with the stethoscope.[3,90,91]

In acute AR the signs of heart failure occur more suddenly, the pulse pressure may not be wide, and systolic blood pressure can be normal or low. The diastolic murmur is soft and short. Findings consistent with the etiology of acute AR will be found such as fever and petechiae (suggestive of endocarditis), unequal pulses or a Marfan's appearance (aortic dissection), or trauma may be evident.[90,92]

Diagnosis

Electrocardiography

The electrocardiogram frequently shows signs of left ventricular hypertrophy and left axis deviation for chronic cases of AR. Conduction disturbances can be seen. Exercise testing is useful to assess the functional capacity of patients with equivocal symptoms (class I). Other potential indications for exercise testing are to evaluate symptoms and function before athletic activities and to assess prognosis before valve replacement among patients with left ventricular dysfunction (class IIa).[1] In patients with AR, exercise may not induce an appropriate rise in left ventricular EF. Stress nucleotide studies or echocardiographies have been used to determine the effect of AR on left ventricular function. The evidence that the latter studies have prognostic implications however is less well established.[90,91]

Chest Radiography

The chest radiograph may show an enlarged cardiac silhouette and a dilated aortic root is frequently dilated when the disease is long standing. In cases of acute AR, the radiograph may show signs of heart failure but unless there was preexisting cardiomegally, the heart size will be normal. A widened mediastinum or other radiographic signs of aortic dissection may be seen in acute AR due to aortic dissection.[90,91]

Echocardiography

Echocardiography and Doppler studies are indicated to confirm the diagnosis and severity of disease, to diagnose equivocal cases, define the etiology of AR, assess left ventricular function, and estimate severity of disease (Fig. 34-4). It is also used to reevaluate patients with moderate to severe disease and who have new or changing symptoms and to reevaluate those patients with enlarged aortic roots. Finally, among patients with severe disease it is used to reevaluate left ventricular size and function. These studies are essential for cases of acute AR and can provide clues to the etiology of that condition.[1,90]

Radionuclide Angiography

This study is indicated when echocardiography is suboptimal, equivocal, or when the echocardiography results are discordant with clinical findings. Cardiac magnetic resonance imaging may be used in place of radionuclide angiography when available.[1]

Cardiac Catheterization

This study is generally not needed for isolated chronic AR. It is indicated prior to valve replacement in patients with known or suspected coronary artery disease or to assess left ventricular function or the severity of AR when the noninvasive studies are inconclusive or at odds with clinical findings (class I).[1] For acute AR due to suspected aortic dissection aortic angiography will be needed if other studies are not diagnostic or not available.

Treatment

Medical Management

The goals of medical therapy for patients with AR are to improve stroke volume (forward flow), reduce regurgitated blood volume, and prevent endocarditis. Class I indications for the long-term use of vasodilator agents in chronic AR are as follows: (1) patients with severe AR who are symptomatic and/or left ventricular dysfunction who cannot undergo surgery, (2) patients with severe AR and left ventricular dilatation but normal systolic function, (3) asymptomatic patients with hypertension and any degree of AR, (4) angiotension converting enzyme inhibitors for patients with persistent left ventricular systolic dysfunction after valve replacement. Short-term therapy is indicated (class I) for patients with severe symptoms and left ventricular dysfunction prior to valve replacement. Therapy is not indicated for asymptomatic patients with mild to moderate AR and normal systolic function as they have a good prognosis with no therapy. Vasodilator therapy is not an alternative to valve replacement when replacement is indicated and possible.[1,91]

Endocarditis is a potential complication of AR. Bicuspid aortic valves and degenerative valvular diseases are commonly associated with endocarditis. Prophylactic therapy should be administered as per Tables 34-10 and 34-11. Patients with trivial AR detected by echocardiography have not been studied well and the decision to

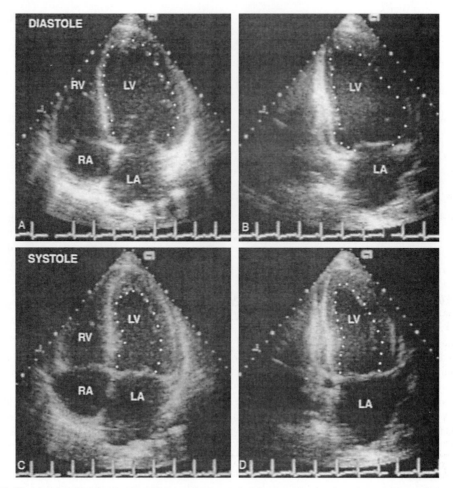

Fig. 34-4. Cardiac chamber dilatation due to aortic regurgitation. Apical four-chamber (A, C) and two-chamber (B, D) views of left ventricular dilation in a patient with aortic regurgitation. The cardiac cycles are end-diastole (A, B) and end-systole (C, D). (Source: Reprinted from Otto CM. *Valvular Heart Disease*. The Netherlands: Elsevier, 1999, p. 267.)

administer prophylaxis in this group should be individualized.[90] However, in the emergency situation time may not allow for intensive record searching and consultation. In situations where time is critical, patients should receive prophylactic therapy for procedures as indicated.

In cases of acute AR supportive care is needed until surgery can be performed. Heart failure and pulmonary edema should be treated as indicated. Nitroprusside therapy and inotropic agents may be required during this bridging period. Aortic balloon counterpulsation is relatively contraindicated. If the AR is from an ascending aortic dissection some recommend that beta-blocker therapy should be used cautiously or not at all because the compensatory tachycardia is needed to maintain cardiac output.[1,90] Others recommend the use of beta-

blockers similar to that of any aortic dissection to control the heart rate.[92] It is reasonable to use beta-blockers in this setting if the pressure is extremely high, the patient is tachycardic, and no other contraindications exist. Patients with aortic dissection and AR should undergo emergency surgery.

Surgical Management

For chronic AR, valve replacement is not required for the asymptomatic patient with normal left ventricular systolic function (rest EF >0.50) and only mild left ventricular dilatation (end-diastolic <70 mm and end-systolic <50 mm dimensions). Other indications for AVR per the 1998 ACC/AHA guidelines are given in Table 34-6.[1]

Table 34-6. Indications for Aortic Valve Replacement for Patients with Chronic Severe Aortic Regurgitation

Indication	Class
NYHA class III or IV symptoms and normal ejection fraction (EF, defined as ≥0.50) at rest	1
NYHA class II symptoms and normal EF but either a declining EF or progressive left ventricular (LV) dilatation on serial testing or decreased exercise tolerance	1
Canadian Heart Association class II or greater angina	1
Any patient with an EF 0.25 to 0.49 at rest	1
Patients undergoing coronary artery bypass surgery, aortic surgery, or other valve surgery	1
Patients with NYHA class II symptoms, EF ≥0.50, and stable LV size and function	IIa
Asymptomatic patients with normal LV function but severe LV dilation (LV end-systolic dimension >55 mm or end-diastolic dimension >75 mm)	IIa
Patients with severe LV dysfunction (<0.25)	IIb
Asymptomatic patients with normal LV function but progressive moderately severe LV dilatation	IIb
Asymptomatic patients with normal LV function at rest but a decline in EF noted on exercise radionuclide angiography	IIb

Source: Adapted from the ACC/AHA guidelines for the management of patients with valvular heart disease (reference 1).

The European guidelines for asymptomatic patients recommend valve replacement or possibly valve sparing operations under the following conditions: (1) evidence of progressive left ventricular dysfunction (end-diastolic diameter >70 mm or end-systolic diameter >50 mm) (consider using body surface area for measurements) or an EF ≤0.05 or (2) aortic root dilatation >55 or >50 mm in patients with bicuspid valves or Marfan syndrome when valve sparing is likely. It is suggested that surgery should be considered when an observed to predicted aortic root diameter >1.3 is evident.[28]

Symptomatic patients with impaired cardiac function represent a group at higher surgical and long-term risk whereas those with a normal left ventricular function have an excellent prognosis. For patients with impaired left ventricular function, those with less severe symptoms, less severe left ventricular dysfunction, and shorter duration of symptoms are more likely to significantly improvement after surgery. For those with less dramatic improvement, valve surgery will facilitate the medical management of heart failure.[1,91] A recent retrospective study suggests that AVR can be done in patients with severe left ventricular dysfunction (EF <30%) with good results (90% NYHA functional class III/IV presurgery to 45% NYHA class III/IV postsurgery and 5-year survival 74%).[86] Another study of patients with AR who underwent valve replacement compared those with an EF <35% to those with an EF>35%. Patients with low EFs did have higher operative and postoperative mortality rates. However, postoperative EFs improved markedly and most patients had

good long-term survival without heart failure after undergoing valve replacement surgery.[93] The acute volume reduction noted after aortic valve surgery has a favorable effect on left ventricular mechanics and hemodynamics.[94] It is clearly preferable to perform valve replacement surgery prior to severe symptoms or markedly depressed left ventricular function but patients with advanced disease should not be denied therapy.

There has been renewed interest in valve repair as opposed to replacement in recent years due to the complications of long-term anticoagulant therapy. Short-term results are similar to other standard procedures but the long-term results are unclear. Rheumatic aortic valvular disease appears to be less amenable to repair.[95] For younger patients the Ross procedure may be indicated. In cases of acute AR due to proximal aortic dissection, surgery is indicated and valve sparing operations are promising.[96,97]

Prognosis

There are no large studies that examine patients with AR and normal left ventricular function. A summary of seven studies that included 490 patients (different selection criteria) and a mean 6.4-year follow-up period showed a rate of progression to symptoms and/or left ventricular dysfunction of 4.3% per year. The average mortality rate (sudden death) was <0.2% per year but some developed left ventricular dysfunction without symptoms. About one-fourth who die or develop systolic dysfunction did so before symptoms developed. Among symptomatic patients the mortality rate is >10% per year for those with angina and >20% per year for those with heart failure.[1]

RIGHT-SIDED VALVE DISORDERS

The right ventricle is affected by right-sided valve disorders. Tricuspid or pulmonary regurgitation (PR) results in right ventricular volume overload where pulmonary stenosis (PS) or pulmonary hypertension results in a pressure overload. The right ventricle response to a volume overload is similar to that of the left ventricle but the pressure overload response differs. When the volume overload process is slow there is some wall thickening but the ventricle dilates sooner. This can cause tricuspid annular dilation, TR, and worsening of right heart function.[98]

The tricuspid valve is similar in morphology and function to the mitral valve but is anatomically more variable. It is comprised of three leaflets (anterior, posterior, and septal). The pulmonary valve is similar to the aortic valve but is a bit thinner as it is not exposed to the high pressures of the left heart. Right side valve disorders should be classified as primary valve disorders or secondary to pulmonary hypertension. PS is almost always congenital in origin.[2,11]

Tricuspid Valve Disease

Epidemiology and Eiology

The European survey found that only 1.2% of all valve disease was due to isolated tricuspid or pulmonary valve disorders.[14] The clinical diagnosis of tricuspid valve disease can be difficult and the clinical significance is often unclear. The most common cause of tricuspid valve disease is secondary valve regurgitation due to annular dilatation. Right side annular dilatation can result from left heart disease and the resulting pulmonary hypertension, primary pulmonary hypertension or lung disease and cor pulmonale, or right ventricular infarction and failure.

Other causes of TR include endocarditis, rheumatic heart disease, penetrating or nonpenetrating trauma, tricuspid valve prolapse, carcinoid heart disease, connective tissue diseases, myxomas, endomyocardial fibrosis, systemic lupus erythematosus, iatrogenic causes (attempted right ventricular biopsy, catheter- and pacemaker-induced pathology, radiation therapy, or migrated Greenfield filter), and other extremely rare causes. Tricuspid valves excised for endocarditis results in significant regurgitation. Congenital abnormalities can directly affect tricuspid function. Ebstein's anomaly can result in severe TR (see congenital heart disease).

Tricuspid stenosis (TS) is a rare disorder and is mainly a result of rheumatic heart disease but can be caused by myxomas or carcinoid heart disease.[3,98,99]

Clinical Features

Isolated TR is usually well tolerated. Symptoms can include fatigue, peripheral edema, and decreased appetite. Patients with TS invariably have other valve involvement and symptoms are difficult to differentiate.

The physical findings noted in patients with TR are those of right heart disease. In severe long-standing cases jugular venous distention and a prominent CV (also termed S or systolic) wave are evident. The CV wave consists of a slow rising impulse that differs from the rapid rise of Cannon A waves. The C wave occurs in early systole when the tricuspid valve bulges into the right atrium. The V wave is a continuation of atrial filling through the incompetent valve during systole. The right ventricular impulse is hyperdynamic and heaving in character, the liver is enlarged and tender, and ascites and peripheral edema will be present. Auscultation usually reveals a right ventricular S_3. P_2 will be accentuated when pulmonary hypertension exits. Patients are often in AF. The systolic murmur of TR is best heard at the left or right sternal border and increases with inspiration (Carvallo's sign) or with the application of abdominal (hepatic) pressure. It can be very soft and is heard in less than 20% of patients with documented valve dysfunction. The murmur can be minimal or absent in cases of severe regurgitation. AF can confound these classic signs.

TS will result in an increased height of the jugular venous A wave but this finding is more commonly noted when there is decreased right ventricular compliance. The right side opening snap and diastolic murmur is best heard at the lower left sternal area. It is higher pitched that of MS and it has a crescendo-decrescendo character. Since the findings of MS are more obvious, TS is often missed or attributed to MS.[1,3,98,99]

Diagnosis

The chest radiograph and electrocardiogram are not sensitive for the diagnosis of TR or TS. Features that suggest either on the chest radiograph include cardiomegaly with right heart border displacement and right atrial prominence. Among patients with advanced TS the cardiomegaly is marked and dilation of the superior vena cava and azygous vein will be present but without accompanying dilation of the pulmonary artery.

The electrocardiogram in patients with TS can reveal signs of right atrial or biatrial enlargement (in the absence of AF and if MS coexists). AF is common. In cases of TR the electrocardiogram may show right atrial enlargement, Q waves in V_1, an incomplete right bundle branch block, and the AF.

Echocardiography is the mainstay of diagnosis. In cases of TR it is used to evaluate severity, pulmonary artery pressure, and right ventricular function. Echocardiography may identify the actual cause. The echocardiographic findings of TS parallel those of MS. The use of echocardiography and Doppler studies has virtually replaced the need for cardiac catheterization.[3,98,99]

Treatment

There is no proven medical therapy for either TS or TR. If pulmonary artery pressures are elevated treatment should be directed at lowering the pressure. Peripheral edema associated with TR can be managed with diuretics.

The ACC/AHA guidelines do not provide recommendations for isolated TS because of its unique rarity. It is noted that valvulotomy has been recommended but experience is limited and TR is a frequent result. This seems to limit the utility of the procedure. Tricuspid commissurotomy with annuloplasty for the associated regurgitation is performed most commonly in association with mitral valve surgery.

For acquired TR, annuloplasty has become the procedure of choice when feasible. Valve replacement is performed when repair is not possible. A bioprosthetic valve is preferred in tricuspid valve replacement due to the increased thrombogenic potential of a mechanical tricuspid valve and durability of a bioprosthesis relative to other valves. Others suggest a mechanical valve may be preferred in young patients or those who require anticoagulation for other reasons.[3,98]

The ACC/AHA guidelines make the following recommendations for surgery for TR: (1) annuloplasty for severe TR and pulmonary hypertension for patients undergoing mitral valve surgery (class I), (2) valve replacement for severe TR due to diseased or abnormal valves not amenable to annuloplasty or repair or in cases of symptomatic TR with pulmonary artery pressures ≤60 mmHg (class IIa), or (3) annuloplasty for mild TR in patients with pulmonary hypertension resulting from mitral valve disease and undergoing mitral surgery (class IIb). Surgery is not recommended for asymptomatic patients, in those with pulmonary artery pressures <60 mmHg with normal mitral valves, or in symptomatic patients who have not been treated with diuretics.[1]

Prognosis

Little is known about the natural history of tricuspid valve disease. It is rarely an isolated finding but it is a slow progressing disease. Severe TR was actually well tolerated for years among patients who underwent valve resection for endocarditis.[98]

Pulmonary Valve Disorders

Epidemiology and Eiology

Pulmonary stenosis is most commonly congenital in origin. Acquired stenosis is rare but can be seen in cases of rheumatic fever or carcinoid syndrome. When congenital in origin it is most often associated with other structural heart abnormalities. Most (80%) are "isolated" valve abnormalities that include other types of structural heart abnormalities. The rheumatic form is usually associated with other valve involvement.

PR is rare in adults. The most common cause is dilation of the valve ring or artery secondary to pulmonary hypertension. Other disorders that cause pulmonary artery dilation are Marfan syndrome or idiopathic. Endocarditis can result in PR. Less common causes of PR are carcinoid syndrome, blunt or penetrating trauma, rheumatic fever, and syphilis. Iatrogenic causes such as pulmonary artery catheter-induced injury, valve procedures (valvulotomy or surgery), or other cardiac surgeries are becoming more frequent.[3,98,100]

Clinical Features

Pulmonary stenosis is frequently asymptomatic when moderate but also in some severe cases. When symptomatic, dyspnea and fatigue are common. Other signs of right ventricular dysfunction such as venous congestion are evident in advanced cases. Light-headedness, syncope, and angina-like chest pain are less common symptoms. On auscultation, a systolic murmur that is crescendo-decrescendo in character best heard at the upper left sternal border radiating to the suprasternal notch or neck will be heard. P_2 will be widely split in more severe cases due to the prolonged right ventricular ejection time. Pulmonary valve stenosis must be differentiated from other causes of right ventricular outflow obstruction.

PR is often asymptomatic as well and often results from right ventricular volume overload and failure. The primary pathologic disorder (endocarditis, pulmonary hypertension, and so on) frequently overshadows the clinical findings of PR. Auscultation of the heart reveals an absent P_2 in cases of congenital absence of the pulmonary valve otherwise the second heart sound is widely split due to increased right ventricular ejection time. A systolic ejection click and midsystolic ejection murmur may be heard when the pulmonary artery is significantly dilated. The classic diastolic decrescendo murmur is low pitched (in contrast to then higher pitch of AR) and best heard at the upper and mid-left sternal border. When there is associated pulmonary hypertension the murmur is an early diastolic higher pitched blowing murmur similar to the murmur of AR and is classically described by the eponym "Graham-Steele murmur." A right ventricular S_3 or S_4 are often heard.[3,98,100]

Diagnosis

The chest radiograph of patients with PS will show a normal size heart and poststenotic dilatation of the pulmonary artery unless the stenosis is severe and long standing. In the latter case, right atrial and ventricular enlargement will be observed. The peripheral pulmonary vasculature is usually normal. The electrocardiogram is often normal but as disease progresses it can show signs of right ventricular hypertrophy and a right atrial abnormality (combination of frontal plane right axis deviation, R waves in the right precordial leads, or tall P waves in the inferior leads). Certain congenital abnormalities can have other electrocardiographic findings that may not include the right axis deviation.

The chest radiograph in patients with PR commonly shows only a prominent pulmonary artery but more advanced cases will reveal right ventricular dilatation. The electrocardiogram will be normal or show signs of right ventricular overload (rSR′ or similar pattern in the right precordial leads) and if it is accompanied by pulmonary hypertension, right ventricular hypertrophy will be evident.

Echocardiography and Doppler studies are the studies of choice. Echocardiographic findings of patients with PS are thickened and immobile leaflets that become dome shaped during systole. Pulmonary artery dilatation is seen. Doppler studies are used to measure the degree of obstruction and pressure gradient and to evaluate for associated regurgitation. For patients with moderate or severe PR, right ventricular dilatation is seen and the intraventricular septal motion is flat or paradoxical. Regurgitation will be detected by Doppler studies. Diagnostic cardiac catheterization is rarely needed.

Treatment

The vast majority or pulmonary valve abnormalities are congenital and it is the least likely valve to be affected by acquired disorders. Treatment of congenital anomalies will not be described here.

Medical therapy for patients with pulmonary valve disease is mainly directed at preventing endocarditis (which rarely affects pulmonary valves). There are no exercise limits for asymptomatic patients. If right heart failure does appear medical therapy directed at treating congestion should be started but surgical therapy is indicated. In cases of PR right heart failure is unusual. When it does occur it is often due to severe PR that resulted from surgically corrected tetralogy of Fallot. PS when minimal or mild (pressure gradients <25 and <50 mmHg, respectively) does not require intervention. Patients should undergo routine follow-up examinations to detect progression of stenosis and increased pressure gradients that warrant intervention.[1]

The ACC/AHA guidelines for intervention for PS in adolescents or adults are as follows. Symptomatic patients with dyspnea, angina, presyncope, or syncope and asymptomatic patients with normal cardiac outputs and a pressure gradient >50 mmHg should undergo surgical therapy (class I). Surgical therapy should be considered for asymptomatic patients with a transvalvular pressure gradient 40–49 mmHg (class IIa) but is generally not needed if the pressure is 30–39 mmHg (class IIb). Surgical intervention is not indicated when the pressure gradient is <30 mmHg (class III).[1]

Balloon valvulotomy is the procedure of choice if valve morphology is favorable for the procedure. The balloon is oversized (relative to the pulmonary annulus) and at times a double balloon technique is used.[100] After balloon valvulotomy there may be some residual subvalvular stenosis resulting from the pressure overload-induced hypertrophy of the right ventricle myocardium. This often subsides over time but some have recommended the use of beta-blocking medications until resolution has occurred. Surgical valvulotomy may be required if balloon valvulotomy results are inadequate or valve morphology is unfavorable. If valve replacement is required a homograft pulmonary valve is the optimal choice.[1,98]

PR generally does not require surgical therapy. In severe cases or when the right ventricle is extremely dilated and systolic function is poor valve replacement has been done. A homograft is preferred but little data regarding long-term outcomes are available.[1,3,98,100]

Prognosis

Patients with mild PS (valve gradient <50 mmHg) are often asymptomatic and many do well even without surgical intervention. Those with gradients ≥80 mmHg often are symptomatic with right heart failure and generally benefit from relief of the obstruction. Studies of patients with gradients 50–79 mmHg are less clear with some doing well and others progressing.

Isolated PR rarely progresses or requires specific therapy. In contrast, the history of patients with PR that accompanies other disorders is dependent on that associated disorder. Those with pulmonary hypertension, COPD, or thromboembolic disease tend to have a significant right heart burden and develop right ventricular failure. The prognosis of patients with idiopathic pulmonary artery dilatation or PR from valvuloplasty is good.[98,100]

MULTIPLE VALVE DISORDERS

Single Valve Stenosis and Regurgitation

Patients with single valve disease often have both stenosis and regurgitation but one is usually the predominant lesion. Combined AS and AR is very common among patients with calcific AS but is also noted in rheumatic and congenital bicuspid aortic valve disease. Most mixed mitral lesions are rheumatic in origin but may be noted in calcified mitral disease, left atrial tumors, or endocarditis.[101] In these cases echocardiography and Doppler studies are useful for diagnosis but cardiac catheterization is often necessary for full hemodynamics assessment. Exercise hemodynamics may reveal abnormalities that indicate the need for mechanical correction that are not apparent on normal noninvasive testing. There are no hard and fast guidelines for management but surgical correction of the dominant lesions producing more than mild symptoms (or in the case of AS even mild symptoms) should be considered. For cases of MS where there is severe MR, PMBV may worsen the regurgitation and therefore is contraindicated.[1]

Multiple Valve Involvement

The Euro heart survey found that 20.2% of all patients in the study had multiple valve disorders (more than one valve).[14] Rheumatic heart disease is the most common cause of multiple valve disorders and the mitral valve is almost always involved. Most other conditions such as Marfan syndrome, other connective tissue disorders, degenerative and calcific valve diseases, cardiac camber, or aortic and pulmonary root dilatation can affect multiple valves. Two different pathologies may affect different valves (e.g., calcified AS and ischemic MR). Each valve disorder will produce its own effects on the heart and circulation. The most severe lesion frequently results in the predominant clinical finings. If the valves are near equally affected the more upstream or proximal valve frequently produces the symptoms. Some valve lesions will "protect" a cardiac chamber from the full effects of the other valve lesion.[3,101] The Society of Thoracic Surgeons National Database has shown an increased mortality rate for multiple valve replacements (9.6%) compared to single valve replacement procedures (4.3 and 6.4% for aortic valve and mitral valve replacement, respectively).[102]

Mitral Stenosis and Aortic Regurgitation

The combination of severe MS and severe AR is uncommon. In most cases of severe MS the AR is of little importance. When AR is severe the typical signs may be absent (an example of the proximal valve causing the symptoms and "protecting" the other heart chamber). Echocardiography and cardiac catheterization may be required to determine the significance of the valve lesions. When MS is severe it is often treated by PBMV first followed by AVR due to the high short- and long-term risks incurred from double valve replacement.[1,3,101]

Mitral Stenosis and Aortic Stenosis

This is most always due to rheumatic heart disease and regurgitation of at least one valve is the norm. The symptoms are predominantly those of MS but the physical findings of AS can overshadow those of MS. Associated findings such as systemic emboli and AF are more common than in pure AS alone. Noninvasive evaluation should determine if PBMV is acceptable and if AS is mild. If valve morphology is acceptable PBMV should be attempted and the aortic valve is then reevaluated. If both are severe PBMV may result in a sudden load to the left ventricle and result in early serious symptoms of AS.[1,3,101]

Aortic Stenosis and Mitral Regurgitation

This is relatively uncommon and is most frequently of rheumatic in origin. Other causes are congenital AS and MVP (young patients), or degenerative AS and MR (elderly). The AS and resultant increased pressure will cause an increase in MR and the regurgitation decreases the left ventricular end-systolic volume. These abnormalities cause a reduction in cardiac output and pulmonary venous hypertension. AF will further reduce forward flow. When both valves are severely affected AVR and mitral valve repair or replacement is warranted. If AS is the predominant lesion AVR alone may improve the MR component.[1,101]

Aortic Regurgitation and Mitral Regurgitation

This is a relatively frequent combination and results from rheumatic heart disease, prolapsed valves due to degenerative valve disease, or dilation of both annuli. The left ventricular dilatation that results from long-standing AR can result in MR due to annular dilation. When both are severe it is poorly tolerated due to the high pressures that are reflected back to the left atrium and pulmonary veins and an increased AR volume. At this time it is recommended that the dominant lesion should be treated accordingly. If MR is a result of AR and left ventricular dilatation the MR may be reduced by AVR alone but annuloplasty of the mitral valve may be needed.[1,3,101]

Tricuspid Regurgitation and Other Valve Disorders

Tricuspid regurgitation is often a functional disorder due to pulmonary hypertension and annular dilatation or a direct result of organic pathologies such as rheumatic fever (see the section on TR for a complete list). When TR and MS coexist there is usually some element of pulmonary hypertension. If mitral valve morphology is suitable PBMV should be done when indicated and a reduction of pulmonary hypertension and TR can be expected. If mitral valve surgery is required tricuspid annuloplasty should be considered. For other cases of multiple valve diseases, if the tricuspid valve is seriously damaged by organic causes it often must be replaced.[1,101]

INFECTIVE ENDOCARDITIS

Epidemiology

Infective endocarditis results from microbial proliferation on the endocardial surface of the heart, typically involving the valves. Because intact endothelium is generally resistant to infection or thrombus formation, there is a propensity for IE to develop primarily in patients with surgical or structural cardiac conditions that have the potential to induce endothelial injury or aberrant flow (Table 34-7). Valvular conditions, such as MVP, have a substantially higher risk for development of IE. Prosthetic valves are responsible for up to 25% of cases of IE, with an equivalent lifetime risk for mechanical and biologic prostheses.[71]

Recent reports have noted a decade-long epidemiologic shift, with an increasing percentage (approximately 35–45%) of IE in patients without previous heart disease.[103–105] Many of these cases appear to be nosocomial or iatrogenic in origin, which has been attributed to changes in general medical practice, with more frequent use of

Table 34-7. Risk Stratification for Conditions Associated with Infective Endocarditis[30,149]

High risk
Prosthetic valves (mechanical or bioprosthetic)
Previous episode of infective endocarditis
Complex congenital cyanotic heart disease
    Transposition of the great vessels
    Tetralogy of Fallot
    Single ventricle states
Surgically constructed systemic-pulmonary shunts

Moderate risk
Congenital cardiac malformations
    Primum atrial septal defect
    Ventricular septal defect
    Patent ductus arteriosus
    Coarctation of the aorta
    Bicuspid aortic valve
Acquired valvular dysfunction (stenosis or regurgitation)
    Rheumatic heart disease
    Collagen vascular diseases
Hypertrophic cardiomyopathy
Mitral valve prolapse with regurgitation and/or leaflet
  thickening

Minimal risk[*]
Physiologic or innocent heart murmurs
Mitral valve prolapse without regurgitation
Secundum atrial septal defect
Surgically repaired atrial or ventricular septal defect

[*]Risk no greater than the general population and prophylaxis is generally not indicated.

invasive procedures (central venous catheter placement, percutaneous pacemaker or defibrillator implantation, and hemodialysis), and greater employment of immunosuppressive therapy.[103,104,106,107] An aging population with concomittant, but undiagnosed degenerative valvular disease may be a contributing factor as well.[71,103] Intravenous drug abuse (IVDA), which is highly associated with the development of IE, especially in younger patients with normal valves, does not seem to be causational in this trend, accounting for a similar proportion of cases (5–7%) over time.[103,108] Overall rates of IE within this subgroup however have been decreasing and now average 1–2 cases per 1000 IV drug users.[109] Interestingly, this trend has been noted despite a substantial rise in the prevalence of coinfection (44–90%) with human immunodeficiency virus (HIV).[109] Reasons for this are uncertain, but may be related to increased awareness of the infectious associations with IVDA and the availability of clean needles. Although the profile of IE appears to be changing, the crude incidence remains steady at 1.7–6.2 cases per 100,000 person years.[71] Older individuals are disproportionately affected, as evidenced a mean age at diagnosis of 47–69 years and an incident rate nearly five times greater (15–30 cases per 100,000) for those between 70 and 80 years of age.[103,108]

Etiology

The microbial etiology of IE is reflective of the transforming epidemiology, with increasing prominence of organisms capable of infecting native valves such as *Staphylococcus aureus*.[106,107,110,111] In recent series, staphylococci species have emerged as the most common cause of IE, surpassing viridans streptococci (*Streptococcus mitis, S. mutans, S. oralis, S. sanguis*, and the like).[71,112] *S. aureus* IE is generally associated with cutaneous inoculation from IVDA (often methicillin-resistant) or nosocomial exposure (usually methicillin-susceptible).[103,112] Coagulase-negative staphylococci (*S. epidermidis*) are the most frequent cause of prosthetic valve IE within the first 12 months of surgery, with methicillin-resistance noted in >85% of cases.[112] Coagulase-negative staphylococci may occasionally cause native valve IE, with extensive tissue destruction from species such as *S. lugdunensis*.[113]

Viridans species remain the most common streptococci, but the incidence of group D infection (*S. bovis, S. gallolyticus, S. infantarius*, and the like) appears to be rising.[103] IE caused by *S. bovis* is particularly prevalent in the elderly and is strongly associated with underlying colonic pathology including polyps and villous adenoma. Enterococcal IE represents 5–15% of cases, often arising as a secondary complication of nosocomial bacteremia.[71] The bacteremia frequently seeds from the urinary tract, possibly related to procedural manipulation, and associated resistance to medical therapy is common. Enterococcus is associated with left-sided IE in patients with a history IVDA, but may not be the sole cause; as such vegetations are frequently polymicrobial. *Pseudomonas aeruginosa* is a common isolate from left-sided lesions in IVDAs as well, and represents the second most frequent infectious agent found in such cases (*S. aureus* is the most common). This organism is associated with a high mortality rate and usually causes a fulminant clinical picture. Overall however, gram-negative bacilli such as *P. aeruginosa* and members of the Enterobacteriaceae family (*Salmonella* spp., *Escherichia coli, Serratia marcescens, Klebsiella* spp.) cause 1.3–4.8% of IE cases. They are particularly refractory to nonsurgical treatment.[114] On rare occasions, diptheroids (*Cornybacteium* spp.) may be isolated as the causative agent of IE, more often with damaged or prosthetic valves. Anaerobic bacteria, typically

Bacteroides fragilis formerly caused ~1% of all IE, but recent reports have placed the incidence between 5 and 10%. Particularly high morbidity is associated with these infections, in part due to the production of heparinase and resultant embolization.

In 5–10% of cases, no organism is isolated.[115,116] Culture-negative IE may result from inadequate microbiological techniques, infection with fastidious bacteria or fungi, or more commonly, administration of antimicrobial agents prior to specimen collection. When the latter occurs, bacterial recovery rates are reduced by 35–40%.[114] In instances unrelated to the timing of antibiotic therapy, prolonged incubation, subculture on enriched mediums, use of serology or DNA hybridization and immunofluoresence techniques may improve the diagnostic yield.[71,115] Commonly implicated organisms include the gram-negative coccobacilli of the HACEK group (*Haemophilus* spp., *Actinobacillus actinomycetemcomitans, Cardiobacterium hominis, Eikenella corrodens*, and *Kingella kingae*) and *Abiotrophia* spp. (formerly classified as nutritionally variant streptococci), which requires pyridoxine (vitamin B_6) or L-cysteine in subculture medium.[71,115] Q fever (*Coxiella burnetti*) is thought to be the cause of IE in 3–5% of cases, with a higher occurrence in immunocompromised patients and those with previous valve damage.[117] Up to 3% of cases, particularly those involving homeless, alcoholic patients, are caused by *Bartonella* species (*B. quintana* and *B. henslae*).[118–120] Although an uncommon etiology overall, IE may develop in 20–55% of patients with Whipple disease (*Tropheryma whipplei*) often developing in those with previously normal valves.[119–121] Other less common bacteria include *Brucella* spp. (highest prevalence in rural Spain) and *Legionella* spp.[115] Fungal IE is relatively rare (1.2–2.6% of all cases), resulting primarily from infection with *Candida* spp., or *Aspergillus* spp., but may involve a number of other organisms, including *Histoplasma, Crytpococcus*, and *Coccidiodies*. Cases usually develop in association with a history of IVDA, immunosuppressive therapy, or prolonged intravenous antibiotic or nutritional therapy.[122]

Pathophysiology

The defining lesion of IE, termed as "vegetation," begins with progressive accumulation of fibrin, and platelets, generally in response to endothelial damage. The vegetation may remain sterile, termed nonbacterial thrombolytic endocarditis (NBTE), or may be infiltrated by microorganisms during an episode of bacteremia or fungemia. In the absence of valve injury, primary infection of the endocardial surface can occur, but requires a more virulent organism. Secondary infection of nondamaged valves is also possible with systemic conditions that cause development of NBTE. A high rate of occurrence of NBTE has been noted in patients with systemic lupus erythematosus (termed Libman-Sacks endocarditis),[123] particularly those with antiphospholipid antibodies.[124]

Clinical Features and Physical Examination

The clinical presentation of IE is variable, often depending on the organ system involved and reflects the acuity of the underlying process (acute vs. subacute). While fever is the most common symptom and sign, noted in 78–95%, its absence should not be used to exclude the diagnosis.[71,103,107] Other nonspecific but relatively common symptoms include dyspnea, malaise, anorexia, weight-loss, arthralgias, and night sweats.[71,125] Pulmonary symptoms predominate with right-sided IE, which is found almost exclusively in patients with a history of IVDA. These patients often complain of a nonproductive cough and pleuritic chest pain is noted in 30%.[126]

Classic immunologic vascular manifestations such as splinter hemorrhages, subconjunctival hemorrhages, Janeway lesions (nontender, hemorrhagic, or pustular macules on the palms or soles), Roth's spots (retinal lesions with central clearing and surrounding hemorrhage), and Osler's nodes (painful, subcutaneous nodules usually found on the distal, volar surface of the digits) are more indolent findings, seen in less than 15% of cases.[103,107,114] As such, these peripheral signs have minimal sensitivity, particularly for those with isolated right-sided IE in whom they do not develop. In contrast, immune complex glomerulonephritis (focal or diffuse) is a frequent sequelae, noted in up to 88% of cases.

Cardiac abnormalities are the most common clinical feature of IE. While the majority (~85%) of patients have a murmur at baseline,[71] a new heart murmur or a change in the quality of a preexisting murmur can be detected in 30–40% and is indicative of worsening valvular regurgitation.[107,125] The development of congestive heart failure, which may be closely related, occurs in 20–40% and is a particularly important prognostic indicator.[103,107,114,125] When heart failure is noted, aortic valve lesions are more frequently involved than mitral valve infections (29% vs. 20%).[71,114] Rapid deterioration may occur with leaflet perforation, rupture of infected mitral chordae, or valve obstruction from bulky vegetations.[114] Rare instances of myocardial infarction with heart failure have resulted from coronary artery occlusion from vegetative emboli.[71] Heart failure is common with periannular extension, which complicates 10–40% of native valve IE cases.[114]

Aortic valve lesions have a greater susceptibility to this complication. The incidence is particularly high with prosthetic valves (56–100%) because the annulus, rather than the leaflet tends to be the primary site of infection.[114,127] Subsequent perivalvular abscess formation is common. Extension into the membranous septum may occur, leading to involvement of the AV node with potential for the development of conduction delays.[128] New ECG abnormalities including AV, fascicular, and/or bundle branch blocks can be seen by in 20–30% of patients with IE, and are moderately predictive (PPV = 88%) of more invasive infection.[127,128] Alternatively, fistulae may form, producing intracardiac shunts, which can cause refractory hemodynamic compromise.[71,114]

Embolization represents a significant source of added morbidity. Systemic lesions occur in 22–50% of cases with left-sided IE and septic pulmonary emboli are found in 87% of those with right-sided involvement.[114,126] Systemic emboli are associated with larger (>10 mm in length), mobile vegetations and more frequently arise from mitral valve.[129] Significant risk also exists for IE due to *S. aureus*, particularly with left-sided vegetations in those on chronic anticoagulant therapy.[111] Overall, 65% of embolic events involve the central nervous system, making it the most common location. Neurologic manifestations such as focal deficits or mental status changes may be the presenting sign in 47% of patients.[130] The incidence of actual complications ranges from 20 to 40%, with the majority caused by ischemia in the distribution of the middle cerebral artery.[130,131] Hemorrhagic transformation may be a fatal consequence and occurs with increased frequency in patients on chronic anticoagulation for mechanical valves.[131] The development of an intracranial mycotic aneurysm (bacterial seeding of the vascular intima) may be particularly problematic, with an associated overall mortality rate of 60%.[114] The reported occurrence is 1.2–5%, with lesions tending to form at bifurcation points along the middle cerebral artery.[114] Variable presentation is common, ranging from slow leaks with mild meningeal irritation to sudden, massive intracranial hemorrhage.[71] Although routine screening is not warranted, preliminary evaluation with contrast-enhanced computed tomography (CT) or magnetic resonance (MR) angiography for suspected cases (severe headache, focal neurologic signs, "sterile" meningitis) is appropriate, with conventional four-vessel cerebral angiography reserved for diagnostic confirmation and follow-up.[114]

Mycotic aneurysms may form elsewhere as well, and can be recognized by the appearance of a tender, pulsatile mass. In a patient with IE, the presence of hematemesis, hematobilia, or jaundice suggests hepatic artery involvement; hematochezia, mesenteric artery involvement; and hematuria, renal artery involvement.[114] Bacterial embolization to the splenic artery is relatively common with IE, occurring in nearly 40% of cases, often resulting in an isolated splenic infarction. Patients may complain of back, flank, or abdominal pain, but are frequently asymptomatic. Splenomegaly may be noted in 30–60% of patients with IE and is not a specific finding. In 5% of cases, a splenic abscess develops, either from hematogenous seeding of the infracted zone, or direct embolic infection.[114] A splenic abscess is suggested by the recurrent bacteremia, persistent fever, or poor response to antibiotic therapy. CT or MR imaging is 90–95% sensitive and specific for the diagnosis, and splenectomy is the definitive treatment.[114]

Diagnosis

Suspicion of IE is the cornerstone of diagnosis. Definitive determination requires an integrative approach, combining clinical, laboratory, and radiographic information. Unfortunately, much of this information will be unavailable in the ED setting necessitating admission for patients in whom the diagnosis is strongly considered. General recommendations in this regard include admission for all febrile IVDA patients and all patients with valve prostheses plus fever, malaise, or signs of vasculitis. Admission should also be considered for those patients with underlying cardiac illness and persistent (>2 weeks), unexplained fever and those patients with a new or changed murmur in association with fever or signs of embolization/immune complex deposition.

General Diagnostic Approach

An ECG should be performed to assess for the presence of new conduction abnormalities and a chest x-ray should be obtained to evaluate for cardiomegaly and signs of heart failure. Routine lab tests may show leukocytosis, anemia, thrombocytopenia, creatinine elevations, hypoalbuminemia, and abnormal urinalysis results, but these findings are not uniform.[132] Nonspecific markers of inflammation such as C-reactive protein and erythrocyte sedimentation rate are frequently elevated as are measures of immune system activity like rheumatoid factor.[71,132] Blood cultures should be obtained prior to initiation of antibiotic therapy, with three sets (aerobic and anaerobic bottles) taken from individual sites. Although IE is associated with a continuous bacteremia, the intensity may be low (<50 colony-forming units per mL of blood) and yields may be increased if samples are spaced over

the course of 1–2 hours.[114] Use of a polymerase chain reaction (PCR) assay primed for a universal, highly conserved region of the bacterial-specific 16S rRNA gene may allow rapid detection of bacterial presence in whole blood samples.[133] Preliminary analysis comparing this technique with blood cultures showed promising results with a sensitivity and specificity of 86.7 and 86.9%, respectively.[133]

Clinical Criteria

Although definitive diagnosis of IE requires vegetation sampling with microbiologic and histologic confirmation, reliable clinical criteria have been developed to help clinicians predict the likelihood of a true diagnosis of IE in suspected cases. Named after the institution where it was formulated, the Duke Criteria enables the stratification of patients into 1 of 3 categories: definite IE, possible IE, or rejection of the diagnosis.[134] The criteria are divided into major and minor categories (Table 34-8). The presence of 2 major, 1 major and 3 minor, or 5 minor criteria enables a definite clinical diagnosis of IE. Absence of these criterion, establishment of an alternative diagnosis, symptom resolution without recurrence if given antibiotic therapy or absence of pathologic evidence of IE at surgery or autopsy when given less than 4 days of antibiotic therapy. A diagnosis of possible IE can be assigned to those cases, which are neither definite nor rejected. The original schema was shown to have a specificity of 99%, a negative predictive value close to 92%, and a good diagnostic correlation (72–90%) when retrospectively compared to blinded expert clinical opinion.[135-137] Several modifications have been recently proposed (Table 34-8), which add clinical information to the minor criteria and adapt the major criteria to reflect current bacteriologic trends (i.e., the shift in organism prominence from streptococcal to staphylococcal and recognition of the etiologies of what may have been previously termed culture-negative IE).[128,138,139] Additionally, the inherent ambiguity of the original Duke Criteria in assignment of the diagnosis of "possible IE," has led to the suggestion that such cases now be defined by the presence of at least 1 major and 1 minor, or 3 minor criteria.[138]

Echocardiography

The role of echocardiography is emphasized in the Duke Criteria and is considered central to the diagnostic evaluation of suspected IE. TTE is a technique with high specificity (98%) but poor sensitivity (60–70%) for the detection of a vegetative lesion.[71,140] Additionally, the study may be inadequate in 20% due to large body

Table 34-8. The Duke Criteria[34] (with Proposed Modifications) for the Clinical Diagnosis of Infective Endocarditis

Major criteria
Positive blood culture for IE
  Typical microorganisms from 2 separate specimens
    Viridans streptococci, *Streptococcus bovis*, HACEK group, or *Staphylococcus aureus*[*]
                           Or
  Community acquired enterococci, without a primary focus
  Persistently positive in
    At least 2 samples, drawn > 12 h apart
                           Or
    All of 3 or a majority of 4 separate cultures, with the first and last drawn > 1 h apart
    Single positive sample for *Coxiella buretti* or antiphase IgG antibody titer > 1:800[†]
Evidence of endocardial involvement
  Positive echocardiogram
    Oscillating intracardiac mass on valve or supporting structures, in the path of regurgitant jets or on implanted material
      in the absence of an alternative anatomic explanation
                           Or
    Visualization of an abscess
                           Or
    New partial dehiscence of a prosthetic valve
  New valvular regurgitation (excludes change in character of preexisting murmur)

Minor criteria
Predisposition or history of injection drug use
Temperature = 38.0°C
Vascular phenomena: major arterial emboli, septic pulmonary infarcts, mycotic aneurysm, intracranial hemorrhage,
  conjunctival hemorrhage or Janeway's lesions
Immunologic phenomena: glomerulonephritis, Osler's nodes, Roth's spots, or rheumatoid factor
Microbiological evidence: positive blood culture, not meeting major criteria or serologic evidence of active infection
  with an organism consistent with IE (excludes single positive culture for coagulase-negative staphylococci or
  organisms not known to cause IE)
Echocardiogram consistent with IE, but not meeting major criteria[*]
The presence of newly diagnosed clubbing, Splenomegaly, splinter hemorrhages or petechiae[†]
An elevated ESR or C-reactive protein[†]
The presence of central non-feeding lines, peripheral lines or microscopic hematuria[†]
New-onset heart failure[‡]
New conduction disturbances[‡]

---

[*]Modifications proposed by Li, et al.; includes recognition of increasing prominence of *Staphylococcus aureus* and removal of echocardiogram findings from minor criteria.[138]
[†]Modifications proposed by Lamas and Eykyn.[139]
[‡]Modifications proposed by Perez-Vazquez, et al.[128]

habitus or a history of emphysema.[115] TEE is more invasive, but offers significant improvement in sensitivity (75–95%) at no detriment to specificity (85–98%).[71] TEE has been shown to improve the diagnostic sensitivity of the Duke Criteria to such a degree, that its use could potentially result in a reclassification from probable to definite in one out of four patients.[141] TEE is particularly useful in patients with prosthetic valves and those with suspected periannular extension or perivalvular abscesses (sensitivity > 85%) and is the test of choice.[138,140,141] Although TEE has a negative predictive value of 92%[71] there is inadequate diagnostic accuracy to completely rule out a diagnosis of IE if clinical suspicion is high enough and a repeat TEE at 7–10 days may be needed.[114] In the absence of valve prosthesis or suspicion of complicated infections, an evaluation of pretest probability can assist with determination of the appropriate initial test.[140] For patients with a low pretest probability (<4%), a TTE is sufficient, with a negative result capable of ruling out the diagnosis.[142] For patients with an intermediate (4–60%) or greater pretest probability, which includes those with fever and a history of IVDA, gram-positive coccus bacteremia without a source or catheter-associated *S. aureus* bacteremia, a TEE is more cost-effective and diagnostically efficient.[71,142]

Treatment

Medical Management

The mainstay of treatment for IE is antibiotic therapy. Though some early reports suggested a potential benefit from the addition of acetylsalyicylic acid (ASA),[143] this has recently been refuted.[144] In the emergency department setting, information regarding the etiology of suspected IE is likely to be incomplete, forcing the clinician to weigh the risk of providing an intervention (potential detriment to bacterial yield) against the benefit (inhibition of disease progression). In most circumstances, after proper collection of blood culture specimens, initiation of empiric treatment is justified. Early antibiotic therapy results in a 10-fold reduction in the rate of embolic events and can serve as a temporizing measure in unstable patients.[130,145] Many hospital pharmacies, in concert with infectious disease specialists, offer therapeutic regimens based on regional susceptibility patterns, and consultation in this regard may be helpful. In the absence of this resource, antibiotic coverage should be selected with the anticipation of resistant strains of common organisms. Because streptococci or staphylococci cause 80–90% of all cases of IE, the combination of vancomycin (15 mg/kg IV q 12h) and gentamicin (1–2 mg/kg IV q 8h) is recommended. This regimen provides a synergistic effect through the interaction of a cell-wall inhibitor and a bactericidal agent. It is broad enough to cover both native and prosthetic valve infections and is safe for patients with penicillin allergy.[112,145] Teicoplanin (unavailable in the United States) can be used in the absence of vancomycin, but may not be as effective.[112,145] Tobramycin (2–3 mg/kg) substitution offers improved pseudomonal coverage, and should be considered in any patient with a history of IVDA. This change in empiric aminoglycoside coverage, however, must be avoided if enterococcus is suspected due to the resistance of enterococci to agents of this class except gentamicin.[112] Enterococci are also resistant to nafcillin, oxacillin, and most cepaholsporins, limiting the empirical utility of these agents. Ampicillin and penicillin G are effective for enterococci and many strains of streptococci, but these agents should not be administered as

first-line therapy, because of the high prevalence (95%) of beta-lactamase production in staphylococcal isolates.

In patients with prosthetic valves, rifampin is an essential component of antibiotic therapy because of its ability to eradicate bacteria adherent to the foreign material. Current recommendations however, suggest a delay in initiation by 48–72 hours to enable assessment of the effectiveness of concurrent medications, and minimize development of early resistance.[71]

Once culture and susceptibility results return, treatment can be tailored and the empirical regimen adapted (for selected organisms, see Table 34-9). With methicillin-susceptible staphylococcal infections, a change from vancomycin to appropriate beta-lactam therapy is more effective, resulting in an earlier sterilization of blood cultures (3–5 days vs. 7–9 days).[112] Continuation of gentamicin has been shown to enhance staphylococcal clearance rates, but its use has no effect on survival or overall cure and increases the potential for nephrotoxicity.[112,145] Because of this, in cases of native-valve IE caused staphylococci, it is recommended that gentamicin be discontinued after 3–5 days, and avoided in those with baseline renal dysfunction. With purely right-sided involvement or in the presence of prosthetic valves however, gentamicin should be continued for at least 2 weeks. In cases of IE due to any isolate of enterococcus or resistant strains of streptococcus, it is recommended that gentamicin therapy (in combination with a cell-wall inhibiting agent) be maintained for 4–6 weeks.[112,145]

For culture-negative IE, maintenance of vancomycin and gentamicin is appropriate until an organism can be identified. When such a case involves a prosthetic valve >12 months postsurgery, ceftriaxone (2 g/day) or cefotaxime (2 g/day) should be added to treat for potential HACEK infection.[71] Q fever is highly fatal and when the causative organism is isolated (*C. burnetti*), early initiation of appropriate treatment is important. *C. burnetti* responds well to combination of doxycycline and one of the following: hydroxychloroquine, trimethoprim-sulfamethoxazole, or rifampin. For fungal infections, teatment with amphotericin B and 5-fluorocytosine should be initiated on identification, but a high rate of failure is usual with medical therapy alone.

In general, patients with native valve disease will require 4–6 weeks of therapy. Some patients with uncomplicated IE caused by viridans streptococci or *S. bovis* may be eligible for shorter courses (2 weeks), but this practice is not routine.[145] Those with prosthetic valves will require at least a full 6-week regimen, with recommendation for an 8 weeks course in some instances. Blood cultures should be obtained daily until bacteria are no longer isolated, and repeated 1–2 months after completion

Table 34-9. Antimicrobial Therapy for Infective Endocarditis[*,71,112,145]

Infecting Organism	Antimicrobial	Penicillin Allergy	Comments
Streptococci			
Penicillin-susceptible viridans or S. *bovis*	Penicillin G 2–4 million units IV q4h × 4 weeks or Penicillin G 2–4 million units IV q4h *plus* gentamicin 1–2 mg/kg IV q8h × 2 weeks or Ceftriaxone 2 g IV qd × 4 weeks	Vancomycin 15 mg/kg IV q12 × 4 weeks	Treat all streptococci for 6 weeks with prosthetic valve. Include gentamicin × 2 weeks if prosthetic valve
Relatively penicillin-resistant	Penicillin G 3–4 million units IV q4th × 4–6 weeks *plus* gentamicin 1–2 mg/kg IV q8h × 2 weeks	Substitute vancomycin 15 mg/kg IV q12h × 4–6 weeks for penicillin	Continue gentamicin × 4 weeks with prosthetic valve
Penicillin-resistant and Abiotrophia spp.	Penicillin G 3–4 million units IV q4h *plus* gentamicin 1–2 mg/kg IV q8h × 4–6 weeks		Treat for 6 weeks if symptoms present for 3 months or longer or complications (abscess, and so on). Treat for 6 weeks with all prosthetic valves
Enterococci			
	Penicillin G 3–4 million units IV q4h *plus* gentamicin 1–2 mg/kg IV q8h × 4–6 weeks or Ampicillin 2 g IV q4h *plus* gentamicin 1–2 mg/kg IV q8h × 4–6 weeks	Vancomycin 15 mg/kg IV q12h *plus* gentamicin 1–2 mg/kg IV q8h × 4–6 weeks	
Staphylococci Native-valve			
Methicillin-susceptible	Nafcillin or oxacillin 2 g IV q4h × 4–6 weeks *plus* gentamicin (optional) 1–2 mg/kg IV q8h × 3–5 days	Substitute cefazolin 2 g IV q8h for nafcillin or oxacillin or Vancomycin 15 mg/kg IV q12h *plus* gentamicin 1–2 mg/kg IV q8h × 4–6 weeks	Cefazolin if minor allergy. Vancomycin if major allergy
Methicillin-resistant	Vancomycin 15 mg/kg IV q12h × 4–6 weeks		

(Continued)

Table 34-9. Antimicrobial Therapy for Infective Endocarditis[*,71,112,145] (*Continued*)

Infecting Organism	Antimicrobial	Penicillin Allergy	Comments
Prosthetic valve			
Methicillin-susceptible	Nafcillin or oxacillin 2 g IV q4h *plus* rifampin 300 mg PO q8h × 6–8 weeks *plus* gentamicin 1–2 mg/kg IV q8h for 2 weeks	Substitute cefazolin 2 g IV q8h for nafcillin or oxacillin or Use same regimen as for methicillin-resistant	Withhold addition of rifampin for 72 h to enable determination of antibiotic susceptibility
Methicillin-resistant	Vancomycin 15 mg/kg IV q12h *plus* rifampin 300 mgpo q8h × 6–8 weeks *plus* gentamicin 1–2 mg/kg IV q8h for 2 weeks		
***HACEK* organisms**	Ceftriaxone or cefotaxime 2 g IV qd × 4 weeks or Ampicillin 2 g IV q4h plus gentamicin 1–2 mg/kg IV q8h × 4 weeks	Vancomycin 15 mg/kg IV q12h plus gentamicin 1–2 mg/kg IV q8h × 4	Treat for 6 weeks with prosthetic valve Avoid with B-lactamase producing isolates
P. aeruginosa	Ticaricillin or piperacillin 3 g IV q4h *plus* tobramycin 2–3 mg/kg IV q8h × 6 weeks	Aztreonam 1–2 g IV q8h *plus* tobramycin 2–3 mg/kg Iv q8h × 6 weeks	Antibiotics curative in 75% with right-sided IE
***Candida, Aspergillus* spp.**	Amphotericin B 1–5 mg/kg IV qd plus fluorocytosine 150 mg/kg day × 6–8 weeks	Primary regimen is safe	Surgery usually required for left-sided IE Surgery usually required

[*]Dosages are based on a CrCl > 50 mL/min; adjustments may be required for patients with renal failure.

of treatment to ensure eradication. Complete bacterial elimination may be difficult in some cases, due in large part to inadequate antibiotic penetration of the vegetation and the presence of resilient organisms. Although data are limited, newer antibiotics such as quinupristin-dalfopristin (Synercid), linezolid, daptomycin, and evernimicin may be useful for vancomycin-resistant gram-positive infections.[112]

Surgical Management

Surgical treatment for IE has been steadily increasing for the past decade, with 25–50% of patients now undergoing operative repair, and a tendency toward higher rates in those with aortic valve involvement.[103,112,146] Long-term outcome is improved by early surgical intervention when compared to medical treatment alone,[103,125] with a reported decrease in 5-year mortality from 75 to 54%.[147] The most robust indication for surgery is the development of heart failure. Severity of heart failure is the principal predictor of surgical outcome and the optimal time for operative management is early, prior to the onset of severe ventricular decompensation. The importance of this has been demonstrated by data that show a mortality rate 17–33% in those with heart failure at the time of operation compared to 6–11% for those without heart failure.[114]

Echocardiographic evidence of valvular dysfunction that may result in heart failure, such as acute aortic or mitral insufficiency, dehiscence or rupture, or an unstable appearing prosthetic valve should also be taken as an indication for surgical intervention, as they are unlikely to improve with medical therapy alone. TEE evidence of perivalvular extension or an abscess, especially in the presence of cardiac conduction abnormalities, should prompt surgical treatment as well.[112,114]

Vegetation characteristics which predispose to development of emboli, including size >10 mm (especially if on the anterior leaflet of the mitral valve), significant mobility or persistence after an episode of systemic embolization may influence the decision to perform surgery.[114] Vegetations that increase in size during antibiotic treatment are associated with higher rates of complication and may also warrant surgical intervention.[71] In some instances, usually involving tricuspid IE in an IVDA, removal of the vegetation (*vegetectomy*) without valve replacement may be performed.

Recurrence of embolic events (1) during the first 2 weeks of antibiotic treatment or (2) during subsequent treatment or after completion can be regarded as a secondary indication for surgery.[114] Early operative intervention for those with central nervous system involvement may worsen outcome though, with neurologic deterioration in up to 44% if performed within 1 week. If delayed until the second week however, the risk decreases to 16.7% and only 2.3% when postponed until the fourth week.[71] For this reason, when there is a documented cerebral embolic event, valve surgery is usually delayed 2–3 weeks; when there is evidence of a cerebral hemorrhage, the delay to 4 weeks is recommended.[112]

Refractory response to medical therapy, as indicated by a persistence of fever 1 week after initiation of antimicrobial therapy or continuous positive blood cultures may merit surgical evaluation as well, for both treatment and tissue diagnosis.[112] Particularly poor response to medical therapy mandating surgical debridement or valve replacement is common with vancomycin-resistant enterococci, gram-negative bacilli (especially *P. aeruginosa*), fungal infections, *Brucella* spp., and *C. burnetti*.[114] *S. aureus* infection with aortic or mitral prosthetic valve involvement has a particularly high complication rate with medical treatment alone and of itself may also be an indication for surgical management.[107] In situations of relapse despite optimal antibiotic therapy, especially with involvement of prosthetic valves, surgery may be the only curative option. Recurrence rates are variable, ranging from <2% for native valve IE with penicillin-susceptible-streptococci, to 10–15% for cases involving prosthetic

valves.[71] When a relapse does occur, consideration must be given to the possibility of perivalvular extension or existence of ectopic foci such as a splenic abscess.

Prognosis

The prognosis for patients with IE is variable. Six-month mortality for both native valve and prosthetic IE ranges from 16 to 26%,[103,125,148] with a significantly lower rate (<10%) seen in IVDAs with right-sided lesions.[126] Survival rates are clearly better for those who undergo surgical treatment, particularly in the subgroup with prosthetic valve IE.[103,125,147] The causative organism is an important factor with a higher mortality for gram-negative bacilli (>50%), fungal infections (>50%), *S. aureus* (25–46%), and Q fever (5–37%), equivalent mortality with enterococci (15–25%), and a lower rate with streptococci, both viridans and group D (4–16%).[71,107,117,122,125] Baseline characteristics including HIV with a low CD4 count, age >60, and the presence of excessive comorbidity (coronary artery disease, history of CVA, diabetes mellitus) are associated with an increased risk of mortality.[109,125,148] Clinical parameters indicative of complications such as heart failure, neurologic manifestations, renal failure, and the development of periannular extension or perivalvular abscess also strongly correlate with worse outcomes.[107,125,130] The presence of these risk factors should prompt consideration of close observation, with cardiac monitoring in an intensive care unit setting.

Prevention

Prevention may be one way to avoid the excessive morbidity and mortality resulting from IE. Patients with moderate to high-risk cardiac conditions may develop IE from bacteremia induced by certain invasive procedures (Table 34-10) and should be advised to take prophylactic antibiotics (Table 34-11). The rationale behind this stems from numerous reports and case series demonstrating a causal relationship, but the benefit has not been substantiated by randomized trials.[30,112] Recommendations for antibiotic prophylaxis are based on the most commonly isolated organisms; viridans streptococci for dental and oral procedures, enterococci for those involving the genitourinary or nonesophageal gastrointestinal tract, and staphylococci for dermal procedures. The incidence of IE attributable to such procedures has been estimated to be between 4 and 19%, but has not been precisely quantified.[149] The majority of cases of IE are unrelated to procedural seeding however,[30] and the actual risk may be closer to 0.5–2% per year.[149] It also has been shown that recent exposure to predisposing procedures is

Table 34-10. Procedures Requiring Antimicrobial Prophylaxis[30,112,149]

Dental or oropharyngeal

Tooth extractions

Periodontal procedures including cleaning, scaling, and probing

Implant placement and reimplantation of avulsed teeth

Endodontic instrumentation (root canal) or surgery only beyond apex

Subgingival placement of antibiotic fibers or strips

Initial placement of orthodontic bands but not brackets

Intraligamentary local anesthetic injections

Prophylactic cleaning of teeth or implants where bleeding may occur

Tonsillectomy or adenoidectomy

Respiratory

Nasotracheal intubation

Rigid bronchoscopy

Surgery involving upper respiratory mucosa

Gastrointestinal*

Esophageal stricture dilation

Variceal sclerotherapy

Endoscopic retrograde cholangiography

Biliary tract surgery

Operative manipulation of intestinal mucosa

Genitourinary

Cystoscopy or urethral dilation

Prostatic surgery

Foley catheter placement, if urinary tract infection is present

Cutaneous

Incision through infected tissue (abscess drainage)

---

*Consider prophylaxis for colonoscopy and sigmoidoscopy as well, but not endoscopy.

no more frequent in those who develop IE than in matched, unaffected controls.[150] In analyses of the effectiveness of antibiotic prophylaxis, risk reduction has varied widely, from 20 to 90%.[112] Poor compliance or knowledge on the part of both patients and providers may be a contributing factor to lower rates.[151] It has been suggested though that overall, the use of prophylaxis may result in prevention of only 6% of cases of IE per year.[149]

Nevertheless, recognition of the potential for some procedures to precipitate bacteremia is important. When bacteremia does occur, it is transient, usually lasting <10 min and the peak effect occurs within 30 s.[149] Dental or oropha-

ryngeal manipulation carry the highest risk, with an incidence of bacteremia ranging from 40% for simple tooth brushing or irrigation to 88% for periodontal surgery.[149] Maintenance of good oral and dental hygiene may prevent significant colonization and is of particular benefit in high-risk patients.[114,150] The use of chlorhexidine hydrochloride mouth rinse (15 cc) 30 s prior to dental treatment may also be useful, through a reduction in magnitude of subsequent bacteremia.[114] Intermediate risk is generally associated with genitourinary procedures, although catheterization in the presence of a urinary tract infection may increase this. The lowest risk occurs with gastrointestinal procedures.[112,149] The time to onset of procedural-related IE is generally 2 weeks or less, and a longer incubation period diminishes the likelihood of a true correlation.[114]

PROSTHETIC VALVES

Overview

As evident by the preceding discussion, surgical management of valvular disorders is a relatively common occurrence. In fact, heart valve replacement surgery has been steadily increasing since its inception in 1960. In the United States, between 60,000 and 75,000 valve replacement procedures are performed each year.[152] Prosthetic valves may be mechanical or biologic in nature. In the United States and other developed countries, the majority of implanted prosthetic valves are biologic (55%), while in the remainder of the world the opposite is true.[152] Since the advent of this form of treatment for valvular disorders, more than 80 different models have been developed and employed. Mechanical valves are generally composed of metal alloys or titanium with pyrolytic carbon-coated graphite components. All have similar fundamental structures consisting of the housing, an occluder (a poppet, disc, or hinged leaflet) and a synthetic fabric-sewing cuff. Three basic mechanical valve designs are currently approved by the Food and Drug Administration (FDA): caged-balls, single-tilting discs, and bileaflet-tilting discs (Fig. 34-5). Mechanical valves that are commonly encountered in the practice of emergency medicine are listed in Table 34-12. Biologic valves on the other hand, are almost entirely of tissue-based, with harvest from one of several sources. Autograft valves arise from the same individual (i.e., the Ross procedure, where the aortic valve is replaced by the pulmonic valve) as do autologous valves (formed from the patient's own pericardial tissue). Homograft (allograft) valves come from human donors. Heterograft valves originate from another

Table 34-11. Prophylactic Antibiotic Regimens[30,112,114]

Dental, oropharyngeal, respiratory, or esophageal procedures	
Standard procedure	Amoxicillin 2 g (50 mg/kg in children) PO 1 h prior to procedure
	Or
	Ampicillin 2 g (50 mg/kg in children) IV 30 min prior to procedure if unable to take oral medications
Penicillin allergy	
Mild	Cephalexin 2 g (50 mg/kg in children) PO 1 h prior to procedure
	Or
	Cefazolin 1 g (25 mg/kg in children) IV 30 min prior to procedure if unable to take oral medications
Severe procedure	Clindamycin 600 mg (20 mg/kg in children) PO 1 h prior to procedure
	Or
	Azithromycin or clarithromycin 500 mg (15 mg/kg in children) PO 1 h prior to procedure
	Or
	Clindamycin 600 mg (20 mg/kg in children) IV 30 min prior to procedure if unable to take oral medications
Genitourinary or gastrointestinal procedures	
High-risk patients	Ampicillin 2 g (50 mg/kg in children) IM or IV
	plus
	Gentamicin 1.5 mg/kg (max 120 mg) IM or IV 30 min prior to procedure
	followed in 6 h by
	Ampicillin 1 g (25 mg/kg in children) IM or IV or
	Amoxicillin 1 g (25 mg/kg in children) PO
High-risk, penicillin allergy	Vancomycin 1 g (20 mg/kg in children) over 1–2 h
	plus
	Gentamicin 1.5 mg/kg (max 120 mg) IM or IV, with both completed 30 min prior to procedure
Moderate-risk patients	Amoxicillin 2 g (50 mg/kg in children) PO 1 h prior to procedure
	Or
	Ampicillin 2 g (50 mg/kg in children) IV 30 min prior to procedure if unable to take oral medications
Moderate-risk, penicillin allergy	Vancomycin 1 g (20 mg/kg in children) over 1–2 h, completed 30 min prior to procedure
Cutaneous	
Standard	Cephalexin 2 g (50 mg./kg in children) po 1 hr prior to procedure
	Or
	Cefazolin 1 g (25 mg/kg in children) IV 30 min prior to procedure if unable to take oral medications
Penicillin allergy	Clindamycin 600 mg (20 mg/kg in children) po 1 hr prior to procedure
	Or
	Clindamycin 600 mg (20 mg/kg in children) IV 30 min prior to procedure if unable to take oral medications
Known MRSA	Vancomycin 1 g (20 mg/kg in children) over 1-2 hrs, completed 30 min prior to the procedure

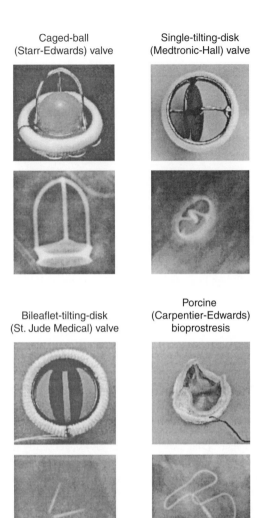

Caged-ball
(Starr-Edwards) valve

Single-tilting-disk
(Medtronic-Hall) valve

Bileaflet-tilting-disk
(St. Jude Medical) valve

Porcine
(Carpentier-Edwards)
bioprostresis

Fig. 34-5. Prosthetic valves with corresponding radiographic appearance. (Source: Reproduced with permission from Vongpatanasin W, Hillis LD, Lange RA. Prosthetic heart valves. *N Engl J Med* 1996;335(6):407–416.)

species and may be transplanted whole (porcine), or configured on a stented frame from pericardial tissue (bovine).

Long-term (10–15 years) comparison trials have demonstrated improved postoperative survival with mechanical valves (aortic position only), lower reoperative rates, and better maintenance of structural integrity.[153] Mechanical valves are associated with an overall increase in thrombogenicity, necessitating life-long warfarin therapy. Biologic valves generally carry less potential for

thromboembolism but do have a greater frequency of primary valve failure, particularly for those <65 years of age with mitral valve replacement.[153] Current guidelines for choosing which prosthetic valve to insert reflect these findings. Bioprostheses are recommended for patients = 65 years without risk factors for thromboembolism (AF, hypercoaguable state, and so on), in those who have an increased potential for bleeding or will not take anticoagulants and those with a life expectancy = 10–12 years. Mechanical valves are indicated for younger patients (<60 years for aortic, <65 years for mitral) and those already on life-long anticoagulation.[153]

Valve Function

An understanding of normal prosthetic valve function is essential to enable appropriate evaluation of patients with valve replacement. Auscultatory findings vary depending on valve type and location, with dysfunction suggested by a change in preexisting characteristics or a new murmur. In general, biologic valves sound similar to native valves, but often have an audible opening snap and an early midsystolic ejection murmur. Mechanical prosthetics are more distinctive, producing readily perceptible opening and closing clicks. A degree of incompetence is inherent to most mechanical valves. Most valves are designed to allow backwash and inhibit thrombosis. This can be detected as an early systolic ejection murmur with aortic valves or a soft diastolic murmur with mitral valves.[154]

Complications

Complications are not uncommon in those with prosthetic valves. Although the higher overall rates are associated with mechanical valves in the first 5 postoperative years, the cumulative risk equilibrates over time with convergence by the tenth year.[1] Primary concern is given to the potential for development of valve thrombosis. The incidence of this complication ranges from 0.1 to 5.7%, with greater risk associated with the mitral valve replacement and inadequate anticoagulation.[154] Patients with acute valve thrombosis often present with hemodynamic compromise mandating immediate medical attention. Clinical manifestations may include pulmonary edema, diminished peripheral perfusion, or systemic embolization. Artificial valve leaflets may become obstructed, causing significant and life-threatening regurgitation with cardiogenic shock. When the diagnosis is suspected, intravenous heparin should be started and consultation with a cardiothoracic surgeon should be obtained. Rapid thrombolytic infusion with streptokinase (1.5 million units over 3 hours) or tissue plasminogen

Table 34-12. Commonly Encountered Mechanical Prosthetic Valves[152]

Caged-ball
Starr-Edwards

Single-tilting disc
Björk-Shiley monostrut[*]
Omnicarbon and omniscience
Medtronic-Hall

Bileaflet-tilting disc
St. Jude Medical (SJM)[†]
CarboMedics
Edwards Mira[‡]
Advancing the Standard (ATS) open pivot
On-X and Conform-X Medical Carbon Research Institute (MCRI)
Sorin Biomedica Cardio Bicarbon and Bicarbon Slimline

[*]The single leaflet model was removed from the North American market in 1986 due to as series of strut fractures with disc dislodgement.
[†]The most frequently implanted valve worldwide; second generation model with Silzone coating withdrawn from the market in 2000 due to high rates of paravalvular leakage.
[‡]Replaced the Edwards-Duromedics and Edwards Tekna models; available for use in Europe and Canada, but awaiting FDA approval in the United States.

activator (tPA 10 mg bolus, then 90 mg over 3–5 hours), may result in thrombus resolution in 70–80%, but carries the risks of embolism (18%), major bleeding (5%), and recurrence (11%).[1,155] Continuous infusion of streptokinase (60,000–100,000 U/hour for 15–24 hours) may be useful as well, with guidance of duration by repeat echocardiographic evaluation. Because of the inherent risks of thrombolytic therapy, emergent valve replacement is generally preferred for those with hemodynamic stability. With either treatment, the immediate mortality may be substantial, ranging from 6 to 15%.[1,154]

Even in the absence of acute valve thrombosis, systemic thromboembolism remains a major complication. The risk is increases for those with mechanical values, with an annual incidence of approximately 4% without anticoagulant therapy vs. 1–2% with its use.[156] The latter is roughly equivalent to the overall risk for non-anticoagulated patients with biologic prosthesis (0.7%). Other risk factors include mitral valve prostheses, the presence of >1 mechanical valve, the use of caged-ball valves, age >70 years, AF, and decreased LV function.[157]

The development of IE is relatively frequent (compared to those without prosthetic valves) and particularly concerning, due to an association with excessive morbidity and mortality. The presence of IE is a high-risk condition, requiring life-long antibiotic prophylaxis for certain procedures (Table 34-10 and 34-11). The clinical manifestations, diagnosis, and treatment of IE have been discussed, but some aspects pertaining to prosthetic valves

deserve further mention. The lifetime risk of IE with artificial valves is 3–6%,[154] with the majority of infections occurring 2–3 months subsequent to replacement. After 12 months, the rate declines significantly to 0.4% per year. The onset is divided into "early" (<60 days after surgery) and "late" (>60 days postoperatively) stages. Early IE is primarily due to skin- or wound-related bacterial seeding or contaminated devices, with a predominance of cases caused by staphylococci (*S. epidermidis* > *S. aureus*). Less common isolates may include gram-negative bacilli, diptheroids, and fungi. Staphylococci also cause the majority of late IE, followed by streptococci, enterococci, and the so-called culture-negative organisms. Because staphylococci may be particularly adherent to the prosthetic valve surface, treatment requires the addition of rifampin (Table 34-9). A complication somewhat specific to prosthetic valve IE is paravalvular regurgitation, which results from infection at the suture lines with subsequent leakage. When significant this may contribute to the development of heart failure and hemolytic anemia.

Other complications noted with prosthetic valves are seldom seen in the ED setting. With several older mechanical valve models (Björk-Shiley single tilting-disc or Starr-Edwards caged-ball) cardiovascular collapse has resulted from housing or strut fracture with embolization of the disc or poppet. This is a rapidly fatal event if occurring at the aortic position, but may be survivable when the mitral valve is involved.[1,154] Structural failure of biologic prostheses may also occur, noted in 10% of homografts and up to 30% of heterografts within 10–15 years of placement. The course is usually indolent, marked by progressive rather than acute symptoms of heart failure. Lastly, although hemolysis is a near uniform occurrence, it is usually subclinical, noted by laboratory findings (elevated serum lactate dehydrogenase, decreased serum haptoglobin, and reticulocytosis) alone without symptomatology.[1,154]

Evaluation of Suspected Complications

Prosthetic valves are readily visible on plain chest radiography (Fig. 34-5). Although this modality may enable visualization of associated pulmonary edema, it offers limited information in the setting of a potential malfunction. Assessment of suspected abnormalities can be performed using TTE or TEE, but may be limited with mechanical valves due to reverberation artifact. Comparison with baseline studies is likely to provide the most useful information. Cinefluoroscopy is rarely used in the modern era, but remains a rapid, inexpensive, and potentially valuable technique, particularly for mechanical valves with questionable compromise of structural composition. MRI can be safely performed with all currently marketed prosthetics valves (mechanical and biologic) and may enable delineation of regurgitation or paravalvular leakage when visualization is inadequate with echocardiography. Cardiac catheterization can be used for the same purpose, but allows the additional capability of measuring transvalvular pressure gradients. Because it is invasive and has the potential for catheter entrapment with induction of acute regurgitation in those with mechanical valves, it should be reserved for situations where noninvasive methods are inconclusive.[154]

Anticoagulation Considerations

All patients with mechanical valves (and some with bioprosthetic valves) should receive chronic anticoagulation therapy. Recommendations are based on the thrombogenic potential of the different valve subtypes (Table 34-13). The risk of thromboembolism increases

Table 34-13. Recommended Antithrombotic Therapy for Patients with Valve Prostheses[1,157,159]

Valve Type	Thrombogenic Potential	Target INR	Comments
Bioprosthetic			
First 3 months	++	2.5 (2.0–3.0)	Disproportionate risk exists during first 3 months postsurgery
>3 months	+	No anticoagulation, but long-term aspirin, 81 mg/day should be given	Add warfarin with atrial fibrillation or left atrial thrombus
Mechanical (aortic)			
Single-tilting disc	++/+++	2.5 (2.0–3.0)	For all mechanical valves, patients with atrial fibrillation, previous systemic embolization, left atrial thrombus or severe
Bileaflet-tilting disc	++	2.5 (2.0–3.0)	LV dysfunction are at higher risk INR should be kept ≥3 (2.5–3.5) with aspirin, 81 mg/day added
Caged-ball	++++	3.0 (2.5–3.5) plus aspirin 81 mg/day	
Mechanical (mitral)			
Single-tilting disc	+++	3.0 (2.5–3.5)	
Bileaflet-tilting disc	++/+++	3.0 (2.5–3.5)	
Caged-ball	++++	3.0 (2.5–3.5) plus aspirin 81 mg/day	

when the INR < 2.0.[157] When a patient presents with a subtherapeutic INR, consideration must be given to temporary anticoagulation with heparin. Whether to select outpatient bridging therapy with subcutaneous low-molecular weight heparin (LMWH) or inpatient admission for intravenous unfractionated heparin (UFH) may be difficult and the decision should be made in concert with the patient's cardiothoracic surgeon or cardiologist. Caution should be exercised in those considered high risk or in whom there is inadequate follow-up with strong consideration of admission for parenteral anticoagulation administration.

In cetain instances, a patient may have had an adjustment in his/her normal anticoagulation regimen. This practice is common and may be required for specific circumstances such as a planned surgical intervention or pregnancy (Table 34-14).

The degree of anticoagulation must be carefully balanced against the risk of hemorrhagic complications. The latter increase significantly when the INR >4.8.[158] Overall, the incidence of major bleeding episodes is 2.7% per year, with CNS hemorrhage in nearly 0.5% per year, and extracranial hemorrhage in approximately 2%.[158]

Table 34-14. Guidelines for Antithrombotic Therapy in Special Circumstances[1,159,160]

Circumstance	Recommendation	Comments
Procedures no bleeding risk	Continue normal therapy	
Minor surgery (dental procedures, minor noncardiac procedures, with minimal bleeding risk)	Stop warfarin 72 h prior; restart day of procedure. Stop aspirin 1 week prior; restart day after procedure. Tranexamic acid (4.8%) mouth wash can be used to control bleeding from dental procedures	For high-risk patients (atrial fibrillation, LV dysfunction, previous embolic event, or hypercoaguable state) or mechanical prosthesis in mitral position, heparin, or low-molecular weight heparin should be strongly considered
Major noncardiac surgery	Stop warfarin 72 h prior and stop aspirin 1 week prior initiate UFH when INR <2, then hold 4–6 h before procedure. Restart heparin and warfarin within 24 h of procedure; continue heparin until INR = 2	
Cardiac procedures, including catheterization	Stop warfarin 72 h prior and initiate UFH when INR <1.5–2 then hold UFH 4–6 h before procedure, and restart 12 h after. If transseptal puncture is planned, INR should be <1.2 and no heparin should be given	Warfarin therapy is not a contraindication in emergent or semiemergent situations
Pregnancy	Subcutaneous UFH throughout pregnancy, adjusted to maintain PTT to 2 × control Or Weight-adjust LMWH throughout pregnancy, adjusted to maintain factor Xa level = 0.5 U/mL Or UFH or LMWH as above, until gestational week 13, then start warfarin, with target INR = 3 (2.5–3.5) Discontinue at 32–34 weeks and restart UFH or LMWH, with continuation until delivery	

Table 34-15. Management of Excessive Anticoagulation in Patients with Prosthetic Valves[161]

INR	Recommendations
Below 5.0	Halve or omit next dose of warfarin
Between 5.0 and 9.0	No active hemorrhage and no concurrent aspirin therapy: omit next several doses of warfarin
	Active hemorrhage or high risk of hemorrhage: omit next warfarin dose and give oral vitamin K_1 (1–2.5 mg)
Between 9.0 and 20.0	Hold warfarin and give oral vitamin K_1 (3–5 mg)
Greater than 20.0 (or active hemorrhage with need for rapid reversal)	Hold warfarin indefinitely and give vitamin K_1 (10 mg) IM or IV* (q12 as needed) with fresh frozen plasma or prothrombin complex concentrate

*IV route provides negligible additional benefit and may result in severe anaphylactoid reaction.

Management of patients with a mechanical valve and major hemorrhage may require withholding warfarin or complete reversal of anticoagulation with vitamin K or fresh frozen plasma (FFP). If required, such treatment, at least during the initial 2 weeks, appears to be associated with a low risk of thromboembolism and can be safely recommended.[158] Guidelines for the management of excessive anticoagulation, with or without active bleeding, are outlined in Table 34-15.

CONCLUSIONS

The approach to the diagnosis and management of valvular heart disease will continue to evolve and hopefully improve. Emergency physicians will encounter many patients with valvular heart disease. Most cases can be managed in the outpatient setting after careful evaluation. Some patients will have potential serious or life-threatening disorders that require emergency therapy, specially consultation, and hospital admission. More in-depth knowledge, as previously outlined will aid the physician in providing emergency care for patients with these valvular pathologies.

REFERENCE

1. ACC/AHA guidelines for the management of patients with valvular heart disease. A report of the American College of Cardiology/American Heart Association. Task Force on Practice Guidelines (Committee on Management of Patients with Valvular Heart Disease). *J Am Coll Cardiol* 1998;32(5):1486–1588.

2. Otto CM. Etiology and prevalence of valvular heart disease. In: Otto CM (ed.), *Valvular Heart Disease*. 2nd ed. Philadelphia, PA: W.B. Saunders, 2004, pp. 1–17.

3. Braunwald E. Valvular heart disease. In: Braunwald E, Zipes DP, Libby P (eds.), *Heart Disease*, 6th ed. Philadelphia, PA: W.B. Saunders, Vol. 2, 2001, pp. 1643–1714.

4. Connolly HM, Crary JL, McGoon MD, et al. Valvular heart disease associated with fenfluramine-phentermine. *N Engl J Med* 1997;337(9):581–588.

5. Gardin JM, Schumacher D, Constantine G, et al. Valvular abnormalities and cardiovascular status following exposure to dexfenfluramine or phentermine/fenfluramine. *JAMA* 2000;283(13):1703–1709.

6. Weissman NJ, Panza JA, Tighe JF, et al. Natural history of valvular regurgitation 1 year after discontinuation of dexfenfluramine therapy. A randomized, double-blind, placebo-controlled trial. *Ann Intern Med* 2001;134(4):267–273.

7. Seghatol FF, Rigolin VH. Appetite suppressants and valvular heart disease. *Curr Opin Cardiol* 2002;17(5):486–492.

8. Englberger L, Carrel T, Schaff HV, et al. Differences in heart valve procedures between North American and European centers: A report from the Artificial Valve Endocarditis Reduction Trial (AVERT). *J Heart Valve Dis* 2001;10(5):562–571.

9. Roques F, Nashef SA, Michel P. Regional differences in surgical heart valve disease in Europe: Comparison between northern and southern subsets of the EuroSCORE database. *J Heart Valve Dis* 2003;12(1):1–6.

10. Flinger CL, Reichenbach DD, Otto CM. Pathology and etiology of heart disease. *Valvular Heart Disease*. 2nd ed. Philadelphia, PA: W.B. Saunders, 2004, pp. 18–50.

11. Farb A, Virmani R, Burke AP. Pathogenesis and pathology of valvular heart disease. In: Alpert JS, Dalen JE, Rahimtoola SH (eds.), *Valvular Heart Disease*. Philadelphia, PA: Lippincott Williams & Wilkins, 2000, pp. 1–39.

12. Chandrashekhar Y, Narula J. Rheumatic Fever. In: Alpert JS, Dalen JE, Rahimtoola SH (eds.), *Valvular Heart Disease*. Philadelphia, PA: Lippincott Williams & Wilkins, 2000, pp. 41–73.

13. Horstkotte D, Niehues R, Strauer BE. Pathomorphological aspects, aetiology and natural history of acquired mitral valve stenosis. *Eur Heart J* 1991;12(Suppl B):55–60.

14. Iung B, Baron G, Butchart EG, et al. A prospective survey of patients with valvular heart disease in Europe: The Euro Heart Survey on Valvular Heart Disease. *Eur Heart J* 2003;24(13):1231–1243.

15. Nowicki ER, Weintraub RW, Birkmeyer NJ, et al. Mitral valve repair and replacement in northern New England. *Am Heart J* 2003;145(6):1058–1062.

16. Mavioglu I, Dogan OV, Ozeren M, et al. Valve repair for rheumatic mitral disease. *J Heart Valve Dis* 2001; 10(5):596–602.

17. Jose VJ, Gomathi M. Declining prevalence of rheumatic heart disease in rural schoolchildren in India: 2001–2002. *Indian Heart J* 2003;55(2):158–160.

18. Olson LJ, Subramanian R, Ackermann DM, et al. Surgical pathology of the mitral valve: A study of 712 cases spanning 21 years. *Mayo Clin Proc* 1987;62(1):22–34.

19. Hammer WJ, Roberts WC, deLeon AC. "Mitral stenosis" secondary to combined "massive" mitral anular calcific deposits and small, hypertrophied left ventricles. Hemodynamic documentation in four patients. *Am J Med* 1978;64(3):371–376.

20. Turgeman Y, Atar S, Rosenfeld T. The subvalvular apparatus in rheumatic mitral stenosis: Methods of assessment and therapeutic implications. *Chest* 2003;124(5):1929–1936.

21. Dalen JE, Fenster PE. Mitral stenosis. In: Alpert JP, Dalen JE, Rahimtoola SH (eds.), *Valvular Heart Disease*, 3rd ed. Philadelphia, PA: Lippincott Williams & Wilkins, 2000, pp. 75–112.

22. Golbasi Z, Ucar O, Keles T, et al. Increased levels of high sensitive C-reactive protein in patients with chronic rheumatic valve disease: Evidence of ongoing inflammation. *Eur J Heart Fail* 2002;4(5):593–595.

23. Rahimtoola SH, Durairaj A, Mehra A, et al. Current evaluation and management of patients with mitral stenosis. *Circulation* 2002;106(10):1183–1188.

24. Otto CM. Mitral stenosis. In: Otto CM (ed.), *Valvular Heart Disease*. 2nd ed. Philadelphia, PA: W.B. Saunders, 2004, pp. 247–271.

25. Zeng C, Wei T, Zhao R, et al. Electrocardiographic diagnosis of left atrial enlargement in patients with mitral stenosis: The value of the P-wave area. *Acta Cardiol* 2003;58(2):139–141.

26. Langerveld J, Valocik G, Plokker HW, et al. Additional value of three-dimensional transesophageal echocardiography for patients with mitral valve stenosis undergoing balloon valvuloplasty. *J Am Soc Echocardiogr* 2003;16(8):841–849.

27. Cheitlin MD, Douglas PS, Parmley WW. 26th Bethesda Conference: Recommendations for determining eligibility for competition in athletes with cardiovascular abnormalities. Task Force 2: Acquired valvular heart disease. *J Am Coll Cardiol* 1994;24(4):874–880.

28. Iung B, Gohlke-Barwolf C, Tornos P, et al. Recommendations on the management of the asymptomatic patient with valvular heart disease. *Eur Heart J* 2002;23(16):1252–1266.

29. Casselman FP, Van Slycke S, Wellens F, et al. Mitral valve surgery can now routinely be performed endoscopically. *Circulation* 2003;108(Suppl 1):II48–II54.

30. Dajani AS, Taubert KA, Wilson W, et al. Prevention of bacterial endocarditis. Recommendations by the American Heart Association. *Circulation* 1997;96(1):358–366.

31. Inoue K, Owaki T, Nakamura T, et al. Clinical application of transvenous mitral commissurotomy by a new balloon catheter. *J Thorac Cardiovasc Surg* 1984;87(3):394–402.

32. Bhat A, Harikrishnan S, Tharakan JM, et al. Comparison of percutaneous transmitral commissurotomy with Inoue balloon technique and metallic commissurotomy: Immediate and short-term follow-up results of a randomized study. *Am Heart J* 2002;144(6):1074–1080.

33. Zaki AM, Kasem HH, Bakhoum S, et al. Comparison of early results of percutaneous metallic mitral commissurotome with Inoue balloon technique in patients with high mitral echocardiographic scores. *Catheter Cardiovasc Interv* 2002;57(3):312–317.

34. Shaw TR, Sutaria N, Prendergast B. Clinical and haemodynamic profiles of young, middle aged, and elderly patients with mitral stenosis undergoing mitral balloon valvotomy. *Heart* 2003;89(12):1430–1436.

35. Lokhandwala YY, Banker D, Vora AM, et al. Emergent balloon mitral valvotomy in patients presenting with cardiac arrest, cardiogenic shock or refractory pulmonary edema. *J Am Coll Cardiol* 1998;32(1):154–158.

36. Middlemost SJ, Manga P. The Quattro valve in rheumatic mitral valve disease: Four-year follow up. *J Heart Valve Dis* 2003;12(6):758–763.

37. Walther T, Lehmann S, Falk V, et al. Midterm results after stentless mitral valve replacement. *Circulation* 2003; 108(Suppl 1):II85–II89.

38. Doshi H, Shukla V, Korula RJ. Emergency valve replacement in rheumatic heart disease. *J Heart Valve Dis* 2003; 12(4):516–519.

39. Otto CM. Clinical practice. Evaluation and management of chronic mitral regurgitation. *N Engl J Med* 2001; 345(10):740–746.

40. Borer JS, Bonow RO. Contemporary approach to aortic and mitral regurgitation. *Circulation* 2003;108(20):2432–2438.

41. Enriquez-Sarano M, Schaff HV, Tajik AJ, et al. Chronic mitral regurgitation. In: Alpert JP, Dalen JE, Rahimtoola SH (eds.), *Valvular Heart Disease*, 3rd ed. Philadelphia, PA: Lippincott Williams & Wilkins, 2000, pp. 113–142.

42. Iung B. Management of ischaemic mitral regurgitation. *Heart* 2003;89(4):459–464.

43. Otto CM. Mitral regurgitation. In: Otto CM (ed.), *Valvular Heart Disease*. 2nd ed. Philadelphia, PA: W.B. Saunders, 2004, pp. 336–367.

44. Lamas GA, Mitchell GF, Flaker GC, et al. Clinical significance of mitral regurgitation after acute myocardial infarction. Survival and Ventricular Enlargement Investigators. *Circulation* 1997;96(3):827–833.

45. Grigioni F, Enriquez-Sarano M, Zehr KJ, et al. Ischemic mitral regurgitation: Long-term outcome and prognostic implications with quantitative Doppler assessment. *Circulation* 2001;103(13):1759–1764.

46. Carabello BA. Acute mitral regurgitation. In: Alpert JP, Dalen JE, Rahimtoola SH (eds.), *Valvular Heart Disease*, 3rd ed. Philadelphia, PA: Lippincott Williams & Wilkins, 2000, pp. 143–155.

47. Thompson CR, Buller CE, Sleeper LA, et al. Cardiogenic shock due to acute severe mitral regurgitation complicating acute myocardial infarction: A report from the SHOCK Trial Registry. SHould we use emergently revascularize Occluded Coronaries in cardiogenic shocK? *J Am Coll Cardiol* 2000;36(3 Suppl A): 1104–1109.

48. Atar S, Jeon DS, Luo H, et al. Mitral annular calcification: A marker of severe coronary artery disease in patients under 65 years old. *Heart* 2003;89(2):161–164.

49. Didier D. Assessment of valve disease: Qualitative and quantitative. *Magn Reson Imaging Clin N Am* 2003; 11(1):115–134, vii.

50. Greelish JP, Cohn LH, Leacche M, et al. Minimally invasive mitral valve repair suggests earlier operations for mitral valve disease. *J Thorac Cardiovasc Surg* 2003;126(2):365–371; discussion 371–363.

51. Matsumura T, Ohtaki E, Tanaka K, et al. Echocardiographic prediction of left ventricular dysfunction after mitral valve repair for mitral regurgitation as an indicator to decide the optimal timing of repair. *J Am Coll Cardiol* 2003; 42(3):458–463.

52. Block PC. Percutaneous mitral valve repair for mitral regurgitation. *J Interv Cardiol* 2003;16(1):93–96.

53. Christenson JT, Simonet F, Bloch A, et al. Should a mild to moderate ischemic mitral valve regurgitation in patients with poor left ventricular function be repaired or not? *J Heart Valve Dis* 1995;4(5):484–488; discussion 488–489.

54. Badhwar V, Bolling SF. Mitral valve surgery in the patient with left ventricular dysfunction. *Semin Thorac Cardiovasc Surg* 2002;14(2):133–136.

55. Gummert JF, Rahmel A, Bucerius J, et al. Mitral valve repair in patients with end stage cardiomyopathy: Who benefits? *Eur J Cardiothorac Surg* 2003;23(6):1017–1022; discussion 1022.

56. Hamner CE, Sundt TM, 3rd. Trends in the surgical management of ischemic mitral regurgitation. *Curr Cardiol Rep* 2003;5(2):116–124.

57. Savage EB, Ferguson TB, Jr., DiSesa VJ. Use of mitral valve repair: Analysis of contemporary United States experience reported to the Society of Thoracic Surgeons National Cardiac Database. *Ann Thorac Surg* 2003;75(3): 820–825.

58. Webb JG, Lowe AM, Sanborn TA, et al. Percutaneous coronary intervention for cardiogenic shock in the SHOCK trial. *J Am Coll Cardiol* 2003;42(8):1380–1386.

59. Aklog L, Filsoufi F, Flores KQ, et al. Does coronary artery bypass grafting alone correct moderate ischemic mitral regurgitation? *Circulation* 2001;104(12 Suppl 1): 168–175.

60. Adams DH, Filsoufi F, Aklog L. Surgical treatment of the ischemic mitral valve. *J Heart Valve Dis* 2002;11(Suppl 1): S21–S25.

61. Fasol R, Lakew F, Pfannmuller B, et al. Papillary muscle repair surgery in ischemic mitral valve patients. *Ann Thorac Surg* 2000;70(3):771–776; discussion 776–777.

62. Bitran D, Merin O, Klutstein MW, et al. Mitral valve repair in severe ischemic cardiomyopathy. *J Card Surg* 2001; 16(1):79–82.

63. Dahlberg PS, Orszulak TA, Mullany CJ, et al. Late outcome of mitral valve surgery for patients with coronary artery disease. *Ann Thorac Surg* 2003;76(5):1539–1487; discussion 1547–1538.

64. Ellis SG, Whitlow PL, Raymond RE, et al. Impact of mitral regurgitation on long-term survival after percutaneous coronary intervention. *Am J Cardiol* 2002;89(3):315–318.

65. Freed LA, Levy D, Levine RA, et al. Prevalence and clinical outcome of mitral-valve prolapse. *N Engl J Med* 1999;341(1):1–7.

66. Avierinos JF, Gersh BJ, Melton LJ 3rd, et al. Natural history of asymptomatic mitral valve prolapse in the community. *Circulation* 2002;106(11):1355–1361.

67. St John Sutton M, Weyman AE. Mitral valve prolapse prevalence and complications: An ongoing dialogue. *Circulation* 2002;106(11):1305–1307.

68. Avierinos JF, Brown RD, Foley DA, et al. Cerebral ischemic events after diagnosis of mitral valve prolapse: A community-based study of incidence and predictive factors. *Stroke* 2003;34(6):1339–1344.

69. Gilon D, Buonanno FS, Joffe MM, et al. Lack of evidence of an association between mitral-valve prolapse and stroke in young patients. *N Engl J Med* 1999;341(1):8–13.

70. Oppenheimer S. Editorial comment: Is MVP an MVP in ischemic cerebral events? *Stroke* 2003;34(6):1345.

71. Mylonakis E, Calderwood SB. Infective endocarditis in adults. *N Engl J Med* 2001;345(18):1318–1330.

72. Dare AJ, Veinot JP, Edwards WD, et al. New observations on the etiology of aortic valve disease: A surgical pathologic study of 236 cases from 1990. *Hum Pathol* 1993; 24(12):1330–1338.

73. Stewart BF, Siscovick D, Lind BK, et al. Clinical factors associated with calcific aortic valve disease. Cardiovascular Health Study. *J Am Coll Cardiol* 1997;29(3):630–634.

74. Levison GE, Alpert JP. Aortic stenosis. In: Alpert JS, Dalen JE, Rahimtoola SH (eds.), *Valvular Heart Disease*. Philadelphia, PA: Lippincott Williams & Wilkins, 2000, pp. 183–243.

75. Wilmshurst PT, Stevenson RN, Griffiths H, et al. A case-control investigation of the relation between hyperlipidaemia and calcific aortic valve stenosis. *Heart* 1997;78(5):475–479.

76. Juvonen J, Juvonen T, Laurila A, et al. Can degenerative aortic valve stenosis be related to persistent Chlamydia pneumoniae infection? *Ann Intern Med* 1998;128(9):741–744.

77. Glader CA, Birgander LS, Soderberg S, et al. Lipoprotein(a), Chlamydia pneumoniae, leptin and tissue plasminogen activator as risk markers for valvular aortic stenosis. *Eur Heart J* 2003;24(2):198–208.

78. Kaden JJ, Bickelhaupt S, Grobholz R, et al. Pathogenetic role of Chlamydia pneumoniae in calcific aortic stenosis: Immunohistochemistry study and review of the literature. *J Heart Valve Dis* 2003;12(4):447–453.

79. Otto CM. Aortic stenosis. In: Otto CM (ed.), *Valvular Heart Disease*. 2nd ed. Philadelphia, PA: W.B. Saunders, 2004, pp. 197–246.

80. Bhutani MS, Gupta SC, Markert RJ, et al. A prospective controlled evaluation of endoscopic detection of angiodysplasia and its association with aortic valve disease. *Gastrointest Endosc* 1995;42(5):398–402.

81. Khot UN, Novaro GM, Popovic ZB, et al. Nitroprusside in critically ill patients with left ventricular dysfunction and aortic stenosis. *N Engl J Med* 1 2003;348(18):1756–1763.

82. Bellamy MF, Pellikka PA, Klarich KW, et al. Association of cholesterol levels, hydroxymethylglutaryl coenzyme-A reductase inhibitor treatment, and progression of aortic stenosis in the community. *J Am Coll Cardiol* 2002; 40(10):1723–1730.

83. Rosenhek R, Binder T, Porenta G, et al. Predictors of outcome in severe, asymptomatic aortic stenosis. *N Engl J Med* 2000;343(9):611–617.

84. Florath I, Rosendahl UP, Mortasawi A, et al. Current determinants of operative mortality in 1400 patients requiring aortic valve replacement. *Ann Thorac Surg* 2003; 76(1):75–83.

85. Sharony R, Grossi EA, Saunders PC, et al. Aortic valve replacement in patients with impaired ventricular function. *Ann Thorac Surg* 2003;75(6):1808–1814.

86. Rothenburger M, Drebber K, Tjan TD, et al. Aortic valve replacement for aortic regurgitation and stenosis, in patients with severe left ventricular dysfunction. *Eur J Cardiothorac Surg* 2003;23(5):703–709; discussion 709.

87. Sharony R, Grossi EA, Saunders PC, et al. Minimally invasive aortic valve surgery in the elderly: A case-control study. *Circulation* 2003;108(Suppl 1):II43–II47.

88. Cribier A, Eltchaninoff H, Bash A, et al. Percutaneous transcatheter implantation of an aortic valve prosthesis for calcific aortic stenosis: First human case description. *Circulation* 2002;106(24):3006–3008.

89. Lester SJ, Heilbron B, Gin K, et al. The natural history and rate of progression of aortic stenosis. *Chest* 1998; 113(4):1109–1114.

90. Otto CM. Aortic regurgitation. In: Otto CM (ed.), *Valvular Heart Disease*. 2nd ed. Philadelphia, PA: W.B. Saunders, 2004, pp. 302–335.

91. Bonow RO. Chronic aortic regurgitation. In: Alpert JS, Dalen JE, Rahimtoola SH (eds.), *Valvular Heart Disease*. Philadelphia, PA: Lippincott Williams & Wilkins, 2000, pp. 245–268.

92. Alpert JP. Acute aortic insufficiency. In: Alpert JS, Dalen JE, Rahimtoola SH (eds.), *Valvular Heart Disease*. Philadelphia, PA: Lippincott Williams & Wilkins, 2000, pp. 245–268.

93. Chaliki HP, Mohty D, Avierinos JF, et al. Outcomes after aortic valve replacement in patients with severe aortic regurgitation and markedly reduced left ventricular function. *Circulation* 2002;106(21):2687–2693.

94. Morita S, Ochiai Y, Tanoue Y, et al. Acute volume reduction with aortic valve replacement immediately improves ventricular mechanics in patients with aortic regurgitation. *J Thorac Cardiovasc Surg* 2003;125(2):283–289.

95. Carr JA, Savage EB. Aortic valve repair for aortic insufficiency in adults: A contemporary review and comparison with replacement techniques. *Eur J Cardiothorac Surg* 2004;25(1):6–15.

96. Kuroczynski W, Dohmen G, Hake U, et al. Aortic valve preservation in acute type A dissection: Mid-term results. *J Heart Valve Dis* 2001;10(6):779–783.

97. Graeter TP, Langer F, Nikoloudakis N, et al. Valve-preserving operation in acute aortic dissection type A. *Ann Thorac Surg* 2000;70(5):1460–1465.

98. Otto CM. Right-sided valve disease. *Valvular Heart Disease*. Philadelphia, PA: W.B. Saunders, 1999, pp. 362–379.

99. Ewy GA. Tricuspid valve disease. In: Alpert JS, Dalen JE, Rahimtoola SH (eds.), *Valvular Heart Disease*. Philadelphia, PA: Lippincott Williams & Wilkins, 2000, pp. 377–392.

100. Rao PS. Pulmonic valve disease. In: Alpert JS, Dalen JE, Rahimtoola SH (eds.), *Valvular Heart Disease*. Philadelphia, PA: Lippincott Williams & Wilkins, 2000, pp. 339–376.

101. Paraskos JA. Combined valvular disease. In: Alpert JS, Dalen JE, Rahimtoola SH (eds.), *Valvular Heart Disease*. Philadelphia, PA: Lippincott Williams & Wilkins, 2000, pp. 291–337.

102. Jamieson WR, Edwards FH, Schwartz M, et al. Risk stratification for cardiac valve replacement. National Cardiac Surgery Database. Database Committee of the Society of Thoracic Surgeons. *Ann Thorac Surg* 1999;67(4): 943–951.

103. Hoen B, Alla F, Selton-Suty C, et al. Changing profile of infective endocarditis: Results of a 1-year survey in France. *JAMA* 2002;288(1):75–81.

104. Castillo JC, Anguita MP, Torres F, et al. Comparison of features of active infective endocarditis involving native cardiac valves in nonintravenous drug users with and without predisposing cardiac disease. *Am J Cardiol* 2002;90(11):1266–1269.

105. Mouly S, Ruimy R, Launay O, et al. The changing clinical aspects of infective endocarditis: Descriptive review of 90 episodes in a French teaching hospital and risk factors for death. *J Infect* 2002;45(4):246–256.

106. Cabell CH, Jollis JG, Peterson GE, et al. Changing patient characteristics and the effect on mortality in endocarditis. *Arch Intern Med* 2002;162(1):90–94.

107. Roder BL, Wandall DA, Frimodt-Moller N, et al. Clinical features of Staphylococcus aureus endocarditis: A 10-year experience in Denmark. *Arch Intern Med* 1999;159(5): 462–469.

108. Hogevik H, Olaison L, Andersson R, et al. Epidemiologic aspects of infective endocarditis in an urban population. A 5-year prospective study. *Medicine (Baltimore)* 1995; 74(6):324–339.

109. Ribera E, Miro JM, Cortes E, et al. Influence of human immunodeficiency virus 1 infection and degree of immunosuppression in the clinical characteristics and outcome of infective endocarditis in intravenous drug users. *Arch Intern Med* 1998;158(18):2043–2050.

110. Hoen B, Selton-Suty C, Danchin N, et al. Evaluation of the Duke criteria versus the Beth Israel criteria for the diagnosis of infective endocarditis. *Clin Infect Dis* 1995; 21(4):905–909.

111. Tornos P, Almirante B, Mirabet S, et al. Infective endocarditis due to Staphylococcus aureus: Deleterious effect of anticoagulant therapy. *Arch Intern Med* 1999;159(5): 473–475.

112. Delahaye F, Hoen B, McFadden E, et al. Treatment and prevention of infective endocarditis. *Expert Opin Pharmacother* 2002;3(2):131–145.

113. Patel R, Piper KE, Rouse MS, et al. Frequency of isolation of Staphylococcus lugdunensis among staphylococcal isolates causing endocarditis: A 20-year experience. *J Clin Microbiol* 2000;38(11):4262–4263.

114. Bayer AS, Bolger AF, Taubert KA, et al. Diagnosis and management of infective endocarditis and its complications. *Circulation* 1998;98(25):2936–2948.

115. Prendergast BD. Diagnosis of infective endocarditis. *Br Med j* 2002;325(7369):845–846.

116. Lamas CC, Eykyn SJ. Blood culture negative endocarditis: Analysis of 63 cases presenting over 25 years. *Heart* 2003;89(3):258–262.

117. Fenollar F, Fournier PE, Carrieri MP, et al. Risks factors and prevention of Q fever endocarditis. *Clin Infect Dis* 2001;33(3):312–316.

118. Spach DH, Kanter AS, Dougherty MJ, et al. Bartonella (Rochalimaea) quintana bacteremia in inner-city patients with chronic alcoholism. *N Engl J Med* 1995;332(7): 424–428.

119. Raoult D, Fournier PE, Drancourt M, et al. Diagnosis of 22 new cases of Bartonella endocarditis. *Ann Intern Med* 1996;125(8):646–652.

120. Raoult D, Fournier PE, Vandenesch F, et al. Outcome and treatment of Bartonella endocarditis. *Arch Intern Med* 2003;163(2):226–230.

121. Fenollar F, Lepidi H, Raoult D. Whipple's endocarditis: Review of the literature and comparisons with Q fever, Bartonella infection, and blood culture-positive endocarditis. *Clin Infect Dis* 2001;33(8):1309–1316.

122. Ellis ME, Al-Abdely H, Sandridge A, et al. Fungal endocarditis: Evidence in the world literature, 1965–1995. *Clin Infect Dis* 2001;32(1):50–62.

123. Roldan CA, Shively BK, Crawford MH. An echocardiographic study of valvular heart disease associated with systemic lupus erythematosus. *N Engl J Med* 1996; 335(19):1424–1430.

124. Hojnik M, George J, Ziporen L, et al. Heart valve involvement (Libman-Sacks endocarditis) in the antiphospholipid syndrome. *Circulation* 1996;93(8):1579–1587.

125. Hasbun R, Vikram HR, Barakat LA, et al. Complicated left-sided native valve endocarditis in adults: Risk classification for mortality. *JAMA* 2003;289(15):1933–1940.

126. Hecht SR, Berger M. Right-sided endocarditis in intravenous drug users. Prognostic features in 102 episodes. *Ann Intern Med* 1992;117(7):560–566.

127. Meine TJ, Nettles RE, Anderson DJ, et al. Cardiac conduction abnormalities in endocarditis defined by the Duke criteria. *Am Heart J* 2001;142(2):280–285.

128. Perez-Vazquez A, Farinas MC, Garcia-Palomo JD, et al. Evaluation of the Duke criteria in 93 episodes of prosthetic valve endocarditis: Could sensitivity be improved? *Arch Intern Med* 2000;160(8):1185–1191.

129. Di Salvo G, Habib G, Pergola V, et al. Echocardiography predicts embolic events in infective endocarditis. *J Am Coll Cardiol* 2001;37(4):1069–1076.

130. Heiro M, Nikoskelainen J, Engblom E, et al. Neurologic manifestations of infective endocarditis: A 17-year experience in a teaching hospital in Finland. *Arch Intern Med* 2000;160(18):2781–2787.

131. Roder BL, Wandall DA, Espersen F, et al. Neurologic manifestations in Staphylococcus aureus endocarditis: A review of 260 bacteremic cases in nondrug addicts. *Am J Med* 1997;102(4):379–386.

132. Wallace SM, Walton BI, Kharbanda RK, et al. Mortality from infective endocarditis: Clinical predictors of outcome. *Heart* 2002;88(1):53–60.

133. Rothman RE, Majmudar MD, Kelen GD, et al. Detection of bacteremia in emergency department patients at risk for infective endocarditis using universal 16S rRNA primers in a decontaminated polymerase chain reaction assay. *J Infect Dis* 2002;186(11):1677–1681.

134. Durack DT, Lukes AS, Bright DK. New criteria for diagnosis of infective endocarditis: Utilization of specific echocardiographic findings. Duke Endocarditis Service. *Am J Med* 1994;96(3):200–209.

135. Hoen B, Beguinot I, Rabaud C, et al. The Duke criteria for diagnosing infective endocarditis are specific: Analysis of 100 patients with acute fever or fever of unknown origin. *Clin Infect Dis* 1996;23(2):298–302.

136. Dodds GA, Sexton DJ, Durack DT, et al. Negative predictive value of the Duke criteria for infective endocarditis. *Am J Cardiol* 1996;77(5):403–407.

137. Sekeres MA, Abrutyn E, Berlin JA, et al. An assessment of the usefulness of the Duke criteria for diagnosing active infective endocarditis. *Clin Infect Dis* 1997;24(6): 1185–1190.

138. Li JS, Sexton DJ, Mick N, et al. Proposed modifications to the Duke criteria for the diagnosis of infective endocarditis. *Clin Infect Dis* 2000;30(4):633–638.

139. Lamas CC, Eykyn SJ. Suggested modifications to the Duke criteria for the clinical diagnosis of native valve and prosthetic valve endocarditis: Analysis of 118 pathologically proven cases. *Clin Infect Dis* 1997;25(3):713–719.

140. Lindner JR, Case RA, Dent JM, et al. Diagnostic value of echocardiography in suspected endocarditis. An evaluation

based on the pretest probability of disease. *Circulation* 1996;93(4):730–736.

141. Roe MT, Abramson MA, Li J, et al. Clinical information determines the impact of transesophageal echocardiography on the diagnosis of infective endocarditis by the duke criteria. *Am Heart J* 2000;139(6):945–951.

142. Heidenreich PA, Masoudi FA, Maini B, et al. Echocardiography in patients with suspected endocarditis: A cost-effectiveness analysis. *Am J Med* 1999;107(3):198–208.

143. Kupferwasser LI, Yeaman MR, Shapiro SM, et al. Acetylsalicylic acid reduces vegetation bacterial density, hematogenous bacterial dissemination, and frequency of embolic events in experimental Staphylococcus aureus endocarditis through antiplatelet and antibacterial effects. *Circulation* 1999;99(21):2791–2797.

144. Chan KL, Dumesnil JG, Cujec B, et al. A randomized trial of aspirin on the risk of embolic events in patients with infective endocarditis. *J Am Coll Cardiol* 2003;42(5):775–780.

145. Chemotherapy. WPotBSfA. Antibiotic treatment of streptococcal, enterococcal, and staphylococcal endocarditis. *Heart* 1998;79(2):207–210.

146. Vlessis AA, Khaki A, Grunkemeier GL, et al. Risk, diagnosis and management of prosthetic valve endocarditis: A review. *J Heart Valve Dis* 1997;6(5):443–465.

147. Vlessis AA, Hovaguimian H, Jaggers J, et al. Infective endocarditis: Ten-year review of medical and surgical therapy. *Ann Thorac Surg* 1996;61(4):1217–1222.

148. Watanakunakorn C, Burkert T. Infective endocarditis at a large community teaching hospital, 1980–1990. A review of 210 episodes. *Medicine (Baltimore)* 1993;72(2):90–102.

149. Durack DT. Prevention of infective endocarditis. *N Engl J Med* 1995;332(1):38–44.

150. Strom BL, Abrutyn E, Berlin JA, et al. Risk factors for infective endocarditis: Oral hygiene and nondental exposures. *Circulation* 2000;102(23):2842–2848.

151. Knirsch W, Hassberg D, Beyer A, et al. Knowledge, compliance and practice of antibiotic endocarditis prophylaxis of patients with congenital heart disease. *Pediatr Cardiol* 2003;24(4):344–349.

152. Butany J, Ahluwalia MS, Munroe C, et al. Mechanical heart valve prostheses: Identification and evaluation. *Cardiovasc Pathol* 2003;12(6):322–344.

153. Rahimtoola SH. Choice of prosthetic heart valve for adult patients. *J Am Coll Cardiol* 2003;41(6):893–904.

154. Vongpatanasin W, Hillis LD, Lange RA. Prosthetic heart valves. *N Engl J Med* 1996;335(6):407–416.

155. Ozkan M, Kaymaz C, Kirma C, et al. Intravenous thrombolytic treatment of mechanical prosthetic valve thrombosis: A study using serial transesophageal echocardiography. *J Am Coll Cardiol* 2000;35(7):1881–1889.

156. Cannegieter SC, Rosendaal FR, Briet E. Thromboembolic and bleeding complications in patients with mechanical heart valve prostheses. *Circulation* 1994;89(2):635–641.

157. Stein PD, Alpert JS, Bussey HI, et al. Antithrombotic therapy in patients with mechanical and biological prosthetic heart valves. *Chest* 2001;119(1 Suppl):220S–227S.

158. Ananthasubramaniam K, Beattie JN, Rosman HS, et al. How safely and for how long can warfarin therapy be withheld in prosthetic heart valve patients hospitalized with a major hemorrhage? *Chest* 2001;119(2):478–484.

159. Goldsmith I, Turpie AG, Lip GY. Valvar heart disease and prosthetic heart valves. *Br Med J* 2002;325(7374):1228–1231.

160. Ginsberg JS, Chan WS, Bates SM, et al. Anticoagulation of pregnant women with mechanical heart valves. *Arch Intern Med* 2003;163(6):694–698.

161. Ansell J, Hirsh J, Dalen J, et al. Managing oral anticoagulant therapy. *Chest* 2001;119(1 Suppl):22S–38S.

35

Pericarditis

Ronny M. Otero
Abhinav Chandra

HIGH YIELD FACTS

- Patients with cardiac tamponade may present in extremis or decompensate slowly depending on the etiology and magnitude of ventricular compromise.
- Pericarditis recurs in 15–30% of patients.
- Hemodynamic compromise from pericardial tamponade is manifested by Bechs Triad:
  · elevated central venous pressure (jvd)
  · arterial hypotension
  · decreased heart sounds
- Pulsus paradoxus is the exaggerated decrease of systolic BP, >10 mmHg, between inspiration and expiration.
- Cancer is the most common cause of tamponade in medical patients; most frequently a lung or breast malignancy.

INTRODUCTION

Pericarditis is one of the causes of acute chest pain assessed by emergency physicians (EP). It is an inflammatory process, usually confined to the pericardial lining surrounding the heart, and often involves the epicardial surface of the heart. Pericarditis may present acutely or in an indolent form. In the emergency department (ED) setting, the spectrum of symptomatology ranges from acute distress with chest pain and dyspnea to nonspecific complaints of malaise, general weakness, and fever. The EP must recognize and differentiate pericarditis, acute coronary syndrome, causes of noncardiac chest pain, and dyspnea. Once the EP identifies a patient with pericarditis, it is important to appreciate the potential complications occurring with either an acute or chronic manifestation.

ANATOMY

The pericardial space is defined as a potential space between the visceral and parietal layers of pericardium.

The visceral layer is composed of mesothelial cells closely adherent to the epicardial surface of the heart. The outer most fibrous parietal layer has reflections around the heart creating the potential spaces of the oblique and transverse sinuses. Normally there is between 15 and 50 cc of serous fluid contained within this space.[1] The pericardial space accommodates relatively slow changes in pericardial fluid volume over time.

DEFINITIONS

Pericarditis is classified by its duration and complications, and may be described as either acute or chronic in presentation. Acute pericarditis is clinically identified by characteristic chest pain, the presence of a pericardial friction rub, and may demonstrate classic electrocardiographic changes.[2] The duration of symptoms in acute pericarditis may last up to 6 weeks. Patients may have recurrent bouts of pericarditis or persistent symptoms lasting greater than 6 months termed chronic pericarditis.[3] Pericarditis may be "dry" or noneffusive, and confined to the pericardial space, or alternatively present with an inflammatory exudate (effusive pericarditis).[4]

Cardiac tamponade is a cardiac emergency resulting from a cascade of increased intrapericardial pressure, diminished preload, and impaired cardiac output.[5] Patients may present in extremis or decompensate slowly depending on the etiology and magnitude of ventricular compromise. Restrictive pericarditis refers to the condition in which patients develop a thickened and unyielding pericardium from chronic inflammation and scarring.[6,7] The diagnosis is difficult to make because symptoms are similar to congestive heart failure.[5]

HISTORY

Patients with acute pericarditis usually present with complaints of chest pain, shortness of breath, and fever. Obtaining a preceding history of illness may suggest a particular etiology for pericarditis. A prodrome of fever, cough, and myalgia often precede acute idiopathic primary pericarditis or viral pericarditis.[4] The characteristics of precordial pain are described as sharp with recumbent provocation. The pain usually develops over days to weeks. The clinician may also elicit a history of trapezial ridge pain. This pain is often mistakenly described as shoulder pain.[8] Pain in the trapezial ridge is fairly specific for acute pericarditis and can be the main area of discomfort on presentation.[9] Pericarditis can be recurrent in up to 15–30% of patients with acute pericarditis occurring with or without effusions.[6] It is helpful to define previous treatment measures and whether they were effective.

The following characteristics for each symptom should be elicited and explored:

Onset: sudden or gradual

Current condition: improving, fluctuating, or worsening

Location: left lower sternal border, trapezial ridge pain

Radiation

Quality: sharp, dull, burning

Timing: frequency, duration

Severity: mild, moderate, severe

Precipitating and aggravating factors: recumbency

Relieving factors: seated position

Associated symptoms: nausea, vomiting, fever, weakness, dyspnea

Previous diagnosis of similar episodes

Previous treatments: non-steroidal anti-inflammatory drugs (NSAIDs), steroids, pericardiocentesis

Efficacy of previous treatments

PAST HISTORY

A patient's past history may reveal predisposing factors for pericarditis, cardiac tamponade, or restrictive pericarditis. A history of malignancy can suggest effusive pericarditis. In patients with worsening renal disease, uremic pericarditis can develop. Patients with recent myocardial infarction (MI) or preexisting coronary disease may have had recent interventions and develop Dressler syndrome or postpericardiotomy syndrome, respectively. Specific medical history may point to an etiology such as hypothyroidism, autoimmune disease, metastatic malignancy, chemotherapy, or radiation therapy-induced pericarditis.[6] Multiple historical factors overlap with risks for acute coronary syndromes, and often pericarditis and myocardial ischemia must be concurrently investigated. Elements of a patient's past history which should be surveyed include:

Hypertension

Hypercholesterolemia

Coronary artery disease/MI

Heart murmurs, rheumatic heart disease

Diabetes mellitus, thyroid disease

Gout, rheumatoid arthritis

Chronic renal disease: severity

Chronic obstructive pulmonary disease (COPD)

Systemic lupus erythematosus or other autoimmune disease

Recent viral illness

Recent cardiac surgery or bypass

Organ transplantation

History of malignancy: type, therapies instituted

Additional history: recent or remote travel to nonindustrialized region

Exposure to person with confirmed or suspected tuberculosis

PHYSICAL EXAMINATION

Pericarditis

Physical examination in patients with pericarditis may reveal fever, tachycardia, and a pericardial friction rub. The friction rub is specific for pericarditis, and is best auscultatated by applying the diaphragm of the stethoscope against the left sternal border and leaning the patient forward. During auscultation one can hear the "scratchy," "leathery," or "velcro-like" rub heard in atrial systole, ventricular systole, and early diastole.[8,9] The ventricular component tends to be the loudest. Rubs tend to be loudest during inspiration owing to increased venous return and closer approximation of visceral and parietal pericardium of the anteriorly located right ventricle.[8,9] Pericardial rubs are evanescent and can disappear and later reappear. Pericardial friction rubs will often be preserved in the presence of a pericardial effusion.[5] An infrequent finding is friction between the parietal pericardium and thoracic pleura referred to as an exopericardial rub.[8]

A maneuver used to augment the volume of the rub is to ask the patient to lift all four extremities simultaneously, thereby enlarging the right ventricle by increasing venous return. Patients with acute pericarditis may present tachycardic due to pain, fever, or as a compensatory response to an enlarging pericardial effusion.[10]

Cardiac Tamponade

Cardiac tamponade occurs in the setting of a large pericardial effusion or increased intrapericardial pressure. Claude Beck first described the triad of symptoms representing the clinical manifestations of hemodynamic compromise from acute pericarditis. These consist of an elevated central venous pressure, low systemic arterial pressure, and decreased heart sounds.[11] An elevated venous pressure correlates with jugular venous distention. Hypotension occurs when cardiac output cannot compensate for a decrease in venous return and reduced stroke volume.[5] In some patients early increased sympathetic output can initially provide a hypertensive response in tamponade.[5,9]

Heart sounds can appear distant in patients with a large pericardial effusion. Large effusions increase the risk of developing cardiac tamponade.[12] However, there have been reports of patients with echocardiographic evidence of large pericardial effusions without significant hemodynamic decompensation.[12] Other causes of distant heart sounds include obesity and lung hyperinflation.

Pulsus paradoxus is the exaggerated decrease in systolic pressure of >10 mmHg between inspiration and expiration seen during cardiac tamponade. Pulsus paradoxus may also be seen in other clinical conditions, including COPD and pulmonary embolism.[5,6] Pulsus paradoxus may be detectable only by sphygmomanometry. It is measured with the patient breathing quietly and the blood pressure cuff inflated to a pressure higher than the systolic blood pressure. The cuff pressure is then lowered slowly until the first heart sounds are heard. This is noted, and the cuff pressure lowered until sounds can be heard throughout the respiratory cycle. Pulsus paradoxus is present if the two readings are greater than 10 mmHg apart.

Constrictive Pericarditis

Constrictive pericarditis may develop from any of the etiologies causing acute or chronic pericarditis, but most commonly is associated with uremia, radiation, and infectious pericarditis. Patients present with symptoms of systemic congestion including peripheral edema, hepatic enlargement, or orthopnea. The diagnosis is difficult to make based on clinical grounds alone and often must be supported by cardiac catheterization, echocardiography, or MRI.[7,13–15] Jugular venous pressure wave monitoring demonstrates a steep y-descent, representing elevated diastolic pressure, followed by right ventricular systole. Kussmaul's sign, the presence of persistent or augmented jugular venous pressure during inspiration is not specific for constrictive pericarditis.[14] In constrictive pericarditis, a rare pericardial knock describes the high-pitched sound of left ventricular filling being halted by the pericardium.[6]

INCIDENCE

The reported incidence of pericarditis discovered on postmortem examinations is between 2 and 6%, and 1/1000 patients have clinical symptoms when admitted to the hospital.[3] The exact incidence of specific etiologies of pericarditis, see Tables 35-1 and 35-2, is difficult to determine.[16] In one study, definitive diagnosis was established in only 25% of cases of pericarditis.[17] Even in patients in whom a thorough evaluation was carried out, idiopathic primary pericarditis comprises a large portion of the etiologies.[17] Infectious etiologies vary in their demographics and presentation. Overall, viral pericarditis is one of the most frequent causes in developed countries. Tuberculous and bacterial pericarditis are seen more frequently in developing countries. Procedurally related pericarditis, such as postpericardiotomy pericarditis, has been reported to be as high as 25% in one series.[18] The incidence of this etiology may be expected to increase as more interventions are performed.[19]

Cardiac tamponade is associated with many of the causes of pericarditis especially those presenting with

Table 35-1. Etiologies of Pericarditis

Idiopathic
Infectious
Viral (coxsackie B, enteroviruses, CMV, HIV)
Bacterial (*Staphylococcus, Pneumococcus, Hemophilus, Tuberculous*)
Fungal (toxoplasmosis)
Parasitic (amebiasis)
Malignancy
Lung
Breast
Leukemic
Lymphoma
Metabolic
Hyperuricemia
Uremic
Myxedematous
Therapy related
Postradiation therapy
Postcardiotomy/thoracotomy
Cardiac catheterization
Medications (hydralazine, procainamide, minoxidil, anticoagulants, chemotherapy)
Connective tissue disease
Mixed connective tissue disease, SLE, scleroderma, rheumatoid arthritis
Cardiac injury
Postmyocardial infarction (Dressler syndrome), blunt trauma
Miscellaneous
Pulmonary embolism, pleuritis, pneumonia

Table 35-2. Etiologies of Pericarditis Identifiable in the ED

Infectious (viral)
Malignancy
Cardiac injury (postmyocardial infarction, blunt trauma)
Uremic or dialysis pericarditis
Hypothyroid

large effusions such as malignancy, uremia, idiopathic pericarditis, infections and autoimmune connective tissue disorders, Dressler syndrome, and postpericardiotomy syndrome.

PATHOPHYSIOLOGY

The pathophysiology of pericarditis is a result of pericardial inflammation that irritates the subjacent epicardial myocytes, leading to the characteristic electrocardiographic findings. The magnitude of inflammation varies from clinical symptoms of chest pain and associated electrocardiographic changes, to biochemical evidence of myocardial injury.[8,20] One example of the extent of inflammation is the friction rub. The presence of a friction rub on examination is believed to be due to depletion of phospholipids which lubricate the visceral and parietal pericardium.[9]

Patients with effusive pericarditis have variable accumulations of fluid in the pericardial space. The absolute volume of effusion does not correlate directly to an increase in intrapericardial pressure. A small but rapid increase in the amount of effusion can markedly elevate intrapericardial pressure. A large effusion is often a reflection of a more protracted course of disease.[5,12]

Normally there is a bimodal increase in venous return during a regular cardiac cycle. Venous return increases during ventricular systole and in early diastole. When intrapericardial pressure rises, as occurs with an enlarging pericardial effusion, there is progressive diminution of venous return (preload). As intrapericardial pressure exceeds right heart pressures, the pressure gradient for venous return also decreases. Decreasing cardiac output results in reflexive tachycardia, which allows for even less venous return during diastole. The bimodal influx of venous return is diminished until a single pressure wave results. Normally the jugular venous pressure consists of an x- and y-descent.[4] The y-descent represents tricuspid closure and right ventricular filling. In cardiac tamponade the diminished filling during diastole leads to a loss of the y-descent. This nonlinear relationship between intrapericardial volume, pressure, and cardiac output and the intersection of these values at a threshold value has been previously described.[5]

Constrictive pericarditis develops from long-standing inflammation or scarring. As the pericardium becomes more thickened and limits diastolic filling, several clinical features are seen. Due to venous congestion hepatomegaly, peripheral edema and even ascites may be observed. The elevated venous pressure can be recognized by examination of the jugular venous wave. A prominent x-descent and y-descent are seen in contrast to cardiac tamponade. Venous return is not impeded as much during systole as is observed during cardiac tamponade. Early diastolic filling is more rapid during constrictive pericarditis. At the end of rapid filling, the left ventricle is filled and diastolic pressure remains elevated. This leads to the "dip and plateau" pattern or "square root sign" described with constrictive pericarditis.[13,14]

ASSOCIATED CONDITIONS

Infections

Viral infections are the most common infectious etiology of acute pericarditis. Viral etiologies are often difficult to prove because of difficulty in isolating the virus or the need for acute and convalescent titers. Viral causes of pericarditis include coxsackie virus B, echovirus, adenovirus, and influenza. Putative coxsackie-like receptors have been described as a possible explanation for the greater propensity of this virus to invade myocardial tissue.[19]

Infectious pericarditis due to bacteria is often life threatening. Patients with bacterial pericarditis present severely ill, and mortality from bacterial pericarditis with effusion has been reported as high as 80%.[20] Bacterial sources may be from contiguous sources, such as pneumonia or other bacterial infections. Specific agents causing infectious pericarditis include *Streptococcus*, *Hemophilus*, and *Staphylococcus*. *Hemophilus* vaccination is believed to be linked to a decrease in reported cases resulting from this specie. The arrival of pneumococcal vaccination is also expected to have a similar impact. Tuberculous pericarditis is found in underdeveloped countries and immunocompromised patients, e.g., HIV.

End-Stage Renal Disease

Patients with end-stage renal disease (ESRD) may present with various degrees of pericardial involvement. Uremic pericarditis may affect patients before, or within 8 weeks after starting renal replacement therapy (hemodialysis, chronic ambulatory peritoneal dialysis). These patients will generally have other signs or symptoms of the uremic syndrome: confusion, pruritus, anorexia, vomiting, and multiple electrolyte abnormalities.

Dialysis pericarditis is defined as pericarditis developing after establishment of renal replacement therapy (>8 weeks).[21] The development of uremic and dialysis pericarditis is thought to be due to accumulations of toxic metabolites in pericardial space or a nonspecific immunologic reaction to the pericardium.[21]

The overall incidence of uremic pericarditis is estimated to be less than 20% of ESRD patients. Similarly, dialysis pericarditis is present in approximately 2–21% of patients.[22] Both forms of pericarditis tend to occur in younger patients. Constrictive pericarditis may result from chronic recurrent fibrinous pericarditis in 12% of ESRD patients. Uremic pericarditis appears to respond well to an intensification of hemodialysis sessions to a greater extent than dialysis pericarditis.[21,22] Both conditions can lead to cardiac tamponade. Clinical presentation of uremic or dialysis pericarditis is similar to that of patients without ESRD except that diffuse ST-segment elevations seen on electrocardiogram are less commonly found with uremic and dialysis pericarditis, presumably due to decreased inflammatory cell penetration into subjacent epicardium.[22]

Malignancy-Related Pericarditis

The clinical presentation of patients with malignant pericarditis is highly variable. The history of malignancy, stage, or state of remission may not be known. Patients complain of weakness, fatigue, and difficulty breathing. A history of fever or recumbent chest pain is sometimes lacking with malignant pericarditis. Patients with pericardial effusions may present with hemodynamic compromise as a result of cardiac tamponade.

Malignant pericardial effusions can coexist with other complications of malignancy. In a review at the Roswell Institute, 26% of patients with malignancy-related pericarditis were found to have decreased breath sounds on physical examination signifying a high incidence of concurrent pleural effusions.[23]

Cancer is the most common cause of tamponade in medical patients.[24] An estimated 2–31% of autopsies in cancer patients revealed pericardial involvement.[24] In general, autopsies revealed a 3–4% incidence of pericardial involvement. A study by Wilkes implies malignant pericardial effusion contributed to death in 86% of patients with symptomatic pericarditis.[24] The most common malignancies known to invade into the pericardial space include breast and lung carcinoma.[25]

Neoplastic masses and thrombi can also occupy the pericardial space. Characteristic malignant effusions vary, and can be hemorrhagic, serosanguinous, fibrinous, or thrombotic, thus rendering the appearance and analysis of an effusion nondiagnostic.

Medications, Chemotherapy, and Radiation Therapy

Multiple therapeutic agents, ranging from antibiotics to chemotherapeutic agents, have been implicated in causing pericarditis and pericardial effusions. Medications associated with pericarditis include azathioprine, and either hydralazine or procainamide, both of which have been implicated in a systemic lupus-like autoimmune syndrome. Cephalosporins, cromolyn, and dantrolene can create an eosinophilic serositis.[25] Minoxidil and 5-aminosalicylic acid have also been associated with pericarditis by an unknown mechanism.

Among chemotherapeutic agents known to cause effusive pericarditis, cyclophosphamide used in high doses is associated with myopericarditis. All-trans retinoic acid (ATRA), used in the treatment of acute promyelocytic leukemia, can cause pleural or pericardial effusions.[24] Patients receiving treatment for non-Hodgkin's lymphoma or Hodgkin's lymphoma may be treated with radiation therapy and later develop subacute myopericarditis.

Therapeutic radiation may also result in pericarditis. Its development corresponds to the dose and field of irradiation. Chronic pericardial inflammation can result many years after treatment and cause weakness, chest pain, or shortness of breath as a result of constrictive pericarditis.[24] A clue to previous irradiation is the observation of small ink skin tattoos denoting the field of radiotherapy.

Dressler Syndrome, Postcardiotomy Syndrome

Dressler syndrome (post-MI syndrome) and postcardiotomy syndrome are two pericardial conditions which develop after a MI or cardiac surgery that involved opening of the pericardial lining, respectively. Clinically the syndromes are similar to other causes of pericarditis, except in their association with direct cardiac injury or contact. These syndromes are suspected to be due to an autoimmune process. It is postulated that after an MI, myocardial antigens are released into pericardial fluid which triggers an autoimmune process.[26]

Dressler syndrome is described in 5% of post-MI patients, whereas postcardiotomy syndrome is seen in 10–40% after cardiac surgery.[26] Dressler syndrome occurs at least 2 weeks after an MI, with symptoms suggestive of pericarditis, whereas postcardiotomy syndrome occurs from 4 weeks to up 6 months after surgery. Patients with postcardiotomy syndrome present with fever, leukocytosis (predominantly eosinophils), and characteristic chest pain, with a positional component. Studies reviewing the use of thrombolytics for the treatment of MI have shown a decrease in the incidence of pericarditis with the institution of thrombolytic therapy.[27]

Autoimmune Pericarditis

Multiple autoimmune diseases have been associated with the development of pericarditis, including systemic lupus erythematosus (SLE), mixed connective tissue disease (MCTD), scleroderma, rheumatoid arthritis, and polymyositis. SLE is a relatively common systemic autoimmune disease. It can involve various organ systems, including the skin, kidney, brain, arteries, and the heart in 25% of cases, as pericarditis.[28] MCTD, an "overlap" syndrome consisting of characteristics similar to SLE, rheumatoid arthritis, polymyositis, and scleroderma, had a 30% reported incidence of acute pericarditis in one study.[29] Pericarditis is discovered at autopsy in 50% of cases of patients with scleroderma.[30,31] There is a low incidence of cardiac tamponade with autoimmune disease-related pericarditis, presumably due to its favorable response to treatment.

DIAGNOSTICS

Electrocardiogram

Characteristic ECG Findings and Stages of Pericarditis

Knowledge of the various electrocardiographic findings in pericarditis must be coupled with historic features of a patient's presentation. The electrocardiographic findings of pericarditis are divided into stages.

Stage 1
  Lasts from a few days to a week with concave ST-segment elevations and concurrent upright T waves. In leads aVR and V_1, ST segments may be depressed. PR depression can occur in any lead but are best described in leads II, V_5, and V_6.

Stage 2
  Lasts from 1 to 3 weeks, ST segments have returned to baseline without concurrent T-wave abnormalities.

Stage 3
  Begins after 3 weeks with the appearance of T-wave inversions.

Stage 4
  The ECG returns to normal after several weeks as pericarditis resolves.[32]

There are multiple causes for ST-segment elevation on electrocardiogram and a thorough familiarity with key features of these conditions is necessary.[33] Misinterpretation of ST elevation can have serious ramifications. Brady found emergency physician's misinterpret the etiology of ST-segment elevation in up to 6% of patients with ST-segment elevation on their ECG.[34] The conditions which cause confusion include left ventricular aneurysm and acute pericarditis.[35]

T-wave inversions, seen in stage 3 of pericarditis, must be differentiated from a number of other conditions including normal variants, early repolarization, cerebrovascular events, strain pattern, digitalis effect, and myocardial ischemia.[33,36] Upwardly concave ST changes may have an atypical appearance in up to 43% of cases.[37] ST-segment changes are more commonly seen in acute or viral pericarditis than in post-MI-associated pericarditis, and less than half of patients with pericarditis progress through all electrocardiographic changes[37,38] (see Fig. 35-1).

Emergency physician's will likely evaluate patients in any of the above stages, but typically in the early stage. Dysrhythmias are infrequently seen in pericarditis, but may be due to preexisting cardiac disease.[39,40] Electrical alternans is described in effusive pericarditis. This is an alternation of the QRS amplitude, varying from one complex to the next, due to changes in the ECG axis. This occurs because the heart, normally static in position, is now "floating" within a large effusion, and may change position with each systolic cyclic.[5,32]

Differentiating Acute Pericarditis from Myocardial Ischemia

Pericarditis and myocardial ischemia may be difficult to differentiate by electrocardiogram; however, some distinct features exist (see Table 35-3). In pericarditis, ST segments are elevated with a concave up shape (see Fig. 35-1). ST segments in myocardial ischemia tend to have a convex appearance. The PR segment is often depressed in the early stages of pericarditis; a feature seldom seen with myocardial ischemia. In pericarditis, the T wave inverts before the ST-segment abnormality has resolved. In myocardial ischemia, the ST segment resolves and then T wave inverts. The ratio of the ST segment to the T wave in pericarditis is greater than 0.25. This feature is also not present in myocardial ischemia.[6,41]

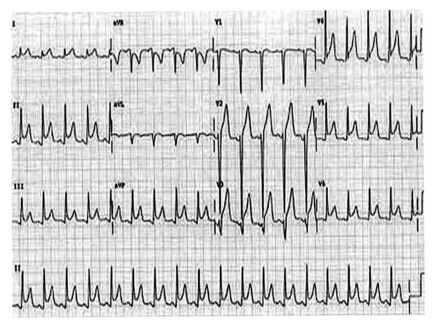

Fig. 35-1. EKG demonstrating diffuse ST segment elevation with a "concave up" deflection of the ST segment. Also note PR depression, seen most prominently in the inferior leads.

Radiographic

The chest x-ray can be of value in patients with suspected pericarditis. The chest radiograph of a patient with a large effusion or tamponade may demonstrate a cardiac shadow described as a "water bottle" shape due to its large and rounded appearance (see Fig. 35-2). A "double density" sign can be seen on lateral chest x-ray, and may represent thickening or calcification of the pericardium, as seen with effusion or constrictive pericarditis.[42] The radiograph can also demonstrate the presence of a coexistent pleural effusion. Although not suggestive of hemodynamic significance, comparison chest radiographs may help determine significant interval changes. The finding of an enlarged cardiac silhouette can also signify the end product of existing hypertensive heart disease or congestive heart failure. Chest radiographs also assist by pointing to an underlying cause of pericarditis such as pneumonia or tuberculosis.

Echocardiogram

The echocardiogram has become the preferred modality to diagnose and quantify pericardial effusion associated with pericarditis. Echocardiograms can be performed by either a transthoracic or transesophageal approach. With either modality, an effusion appears as an echo-free area anterior to the right ventricle. Quantification of fluid is classified by dimension: an echo-free area of <10 mm denotes a small effusion, 10–20 mm of echo-free space is moderate effusion, and a large effusion is >20 mm anteriorly and posteriorly during diastole.[43]

Although not studied in an ED setting, recent guidelines recommend specific indications for echocardiography in patients with pericarditis.[44] Echocardiogram has become the main modality to define the presence and extent of

Table 35-3. Differentiation between Pericarditis and Ischemia

Pericarditis	Ischemia
ST-segments concave	ST-segments convex
PR depression	No PR depression
T-wave inversion occurs before ST-segment resolution	T wave changes after ST segment
Low amplitude T waves	Less common
ST/T-wave ration	>0.25 in V_4–V_6

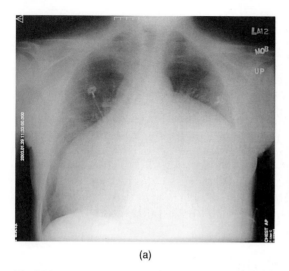

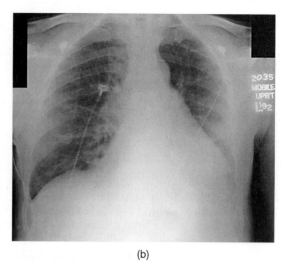

(a)   (b)

Fig. 35-2. (a) X-rays of patient with massive pericardial effusion prior to drainage performed in cardiac catheterization laboratory. (b) Patient's x-ray after pericardiocentesis, notice significant clearing of right hemithorax. Approximately 1500 cc of clear exudate was drained in this patient who had previously been treated with minoxidil.

pericardial involvement.[9] The presence of an isolated pericardial effusion without symptoms does not mandate immediate therapy.

The two-dimensional echocardiogram has assisted clinicians in detecting the presence of fibrinous exudates, pericardial effusions, thickened pericardium, and the characteristic findings of tamponade.[9] Echocardiography is less sensitive and specific for detection of constrictive pericarditis.[9] A recent study evaluating the ability of EP to use bedside echocardiography found a sensitivity of 96% and specificity of 98% for the detection of a pericardial effusion.[45] Sierzenski found that emergency physicians performed echocardiography decreased the length of time for diagnosis and overall length of stay for patients with pericardial disease.[46] It is expected that as emergency physicians become more proficient with cardiac echocardiography, earlier detection will lead to earlier referral to the appropriate consultant.

Echocardiographic findings which suggest pericardial tamponade include a large pericardial effusion with evidence of right atrial or right ventricular diastolic collapse. It is uncommon to see left ventricular collapse (see Fig. 35-3).

Computed Tomography

Computed tomography (CT) is an option for patients with a suboptimal sonographic window due to habitus when using transthoracic echocardiography or when transesophageal echocardiography is not available. The CT scan may reveal a thickened pericardium, as may be seen in fibrinous or constrictive pericarditis.[42] An additional value of CT of the chest is to help distinguish restrictive pericarditis from restrictive cardiomyopathy by the finding of a calcified pericardium.[42] These syndromes are often difficult to differentiate clinically.

Laboratory Studies

Laboratory studies have limited utility in diagnosing patients with pericarditis. Their use may be relegated to ruling out other possible causes of chest pain, or as preceding other investigations. Prothrombin time, international normalized ratio (INR), and a complete blood count may be indicated in patients with effusive pericarditis on oral anticoagulants. In patients with presumed bacterial pericarditis, blood and sputum cultures should be obtained. A new assay, adenosine deaminase, is specific for tuberculosis and may be measured in pleural or pericardial fluid.[6,47]

TREATMENT

Emergency Department Management

Pericarditis should be considered when suggested by the differential diagnosis, based on history, physical, and

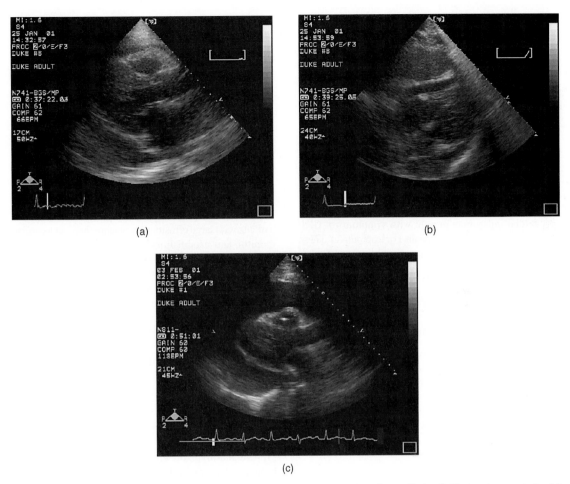

Fig. 35-3. (a) Pericardial fluid anterior to right ventricle demonstrating diastolic collapse. Notice fluid extends posteriorly. (b) Echocardiogram demonstrating RV collapse. (c) A large pericardial effusion is seen surrounding the heart completely. (Source: Echocardiogram courtesy of James G. Jollis, MD.)

clinical presentation. Initial management is focused on determination of hemodynamic stability and may drive the acute interventions described below. If the patient is hemodynamically unstable, demonstrating hypotension and tachycardia, despite evidence of elevated filling pressures, in the presence of a significant pericardial effusion, cardiac tamponade must be considered. Initial stabilization measures are appropriate as for all with cardiogenic shock, and include airway control, assessment of intravascular filling, fluid administration, and hemodynamic support, all concurrent with a rapid evaluation directed at determining the underlying etiology.

If the patient appears hemodynamically stable, the ED work up should focus on determining the potential for compromise. Admission should be considered for all with a moderate-to-large pericardial effusion, when the etiology is associated with conditions of known adverse outcome or is not benign, or when patient conditions suggest a difficult outpatient environment (e.g., homeless). The presence of pulsus paradoxicus may provide some index of the systemic reserve.

When the clinical presentation is of lower acuity, and the differential diagnosis is limited to low-risk conditions, initiating outpatient treatment and arranging for a complete evaluation may be appropriate. Others require admission and work up within the hospital environment. Whether inpatient or outpatient, appropriate consultation should be considered in the ED.

Expectant management is important in cases of effusive pericarditis with abnormal vital signs. The clinician must be aware of the potential for hemodynamic compromise in these patients. When a patient's pain is refractory or there is a suspicion of a large effusion an echocardiogram may help characterize or quantify the effusion.

If bacterial etiologies (including tuberculosis) are suspected, a thorough evaluation including echocardiography is warranted. Patients should be treated empirically, pending the results of cultures. Bacterial pericardial effusions should be drained completely.

In patients with myopericarditis, defined as having evidence of concurrent myocardial injury, efforts should be made to avoid overexerting patients. Patients with myocardial injury may present with symptoms of CHF with positive biomarkers (troponin-I or troponin-T). These patients should be admitted for observation and further cardiac assessment.

THERAPY

Non-Steroidal Antiinflammatory Drugs

These medications have proven effective in idiopathic, viral, postpericardiotomy, and uremic pericarditis. Aspirin may be prescribed if not contraindicated, at doses up to 650 mg orally four times a day.[6] Additional medications which may be used include indomethacin, ketorolac, and ibuprofen.[10,48,49] Caution should be used in patients with a history of gastrointestinal bleeding, renal insufficiency, or on concurrent anticoagulants.

Corticosteroids

Corticosteroids should be reserved for patients in whom the diagnosis of idiopathic, autoimmune, or Dressler syndrome is suspected but have not responded to NSAIDs.[50] A recommended regimen is prednisone 60–80 mg orally once a day. Steroids are generally avoided in suspected infectious etiologies. Before beginning this type of therapy it would be prudent to discuss this with the appropriate consultant, e.g., infectious disease, cardiology. Recurrent pericarditis can occur in patients being weaned from steroids

Colchicine

Colchicine was first described as an effective treatment of Familial Mediterranean fever with serositis. Recent literature supports its use for the treatment of acute and recurrent pericarditis including patients who have failed corticosteroids.[50] Care should be taken in patients with known intolerance to colchicine, impaired renal or hepatic functions.

Antibiotics

Empiric antibiotics should be started in patients who are suspected to have bacterial pericarditis. Arrangements should be made to have infected pericardial effusion drained surgically. Tuberculous pericarditis mandates triple therapy with isoniazid, rifampin, and pyrazinamide.[51] Early consultation with cardiothoracic surgery and infectious disease is recommended.

PROCEDURE

Pericardiocentesis

The emergency physician should prepare symptomatic patients with large effusions by placing them on a cardiac monitor and establishing two large bore intravenous catheters. Boluses of crystalloid fluids should be infused in hemodynamically compromised volume depleted patients. Central venous access may be necessary for administration of vasoactive medications as well as central venous pressure monitoring. Inotropic support should be considered after preload has been addressed with crystalloids. Patients with large effusions may have elevated vagal tone and administering atropine (0.5 mg IV) has been suggested before pericardiocentesis to prevent hemodynamic collapse.[4,53] Consider dobutamine to augment inotropy in patients with a SBP >100 mmHg.

Procedure

Prepare and drape the chest in a sterile fashion using a bacteriocidal agent. If the patient is conscious, explain to them the need for intervention and obtain informed consent. Sedation and pain medications may be titrated carefully if time permits. After identifying the site where needle will be inserted, an initial small incision may facilitate passing of pericardial needle. Using a subxiphoid approach, and holding the pericardial needle at approximately 30–45° from neutral position, direct the needle in the direction of the left shoulder (aspirating while advancing the needle). When fluid begins to drain into syringe, continue to advance the catheter. Commercially available kits allow for the placement of a pig-tail catheter over a wire, which can be left in pericardial space for further drainage.

Although not possible in the hemodynamically unstable patient, in preparation for pericardiocentesis it is ideal to have checked coagulation studies if time permits. Ultrasound or echocardiographic guidance is recommended to minimize complications.[52] Ultrasound is helpful in localizing whether the effusion is anterior, posterior, or loculated. It is often difficult to see an advancing needle in the pericardial space. Pericardial drainage kits are commercially available which normally include pericardial drainage needle, catheter, scalpel, and other supplies. The clinician should be familiar with the contents of the kit before embarking on drainage of effusion. Ultimately, these patients will require the placement of a surgical pericardial window, or fluoro-scopically guided pericardiocentesis, if a catheter was not left in place when pericardial fluid was initially drained. Choice of sedation should be based on patient's clinical status.

POTENTIAL COMPLICATIONS

Performance of blind pericardiocentesis is associated with a number of possible complications that include: acute right or left ventricular dysfunction, hypotension, pulmonary edema, myocardial injury by lacerating the right ventricle, coronary vein or artery.[6,54,55] In addition, depending on the angle and depth of placement of the needle, pulmonary lac-eration may result. As mentioned previously, reflex hypotension can occur and irritation of the myocardium can cause cardiac arrhythmias.

CONCLUSION

Recognition of the pattern and symptomatology of peri-cardial disease is integral to early identification. The importance of history and physical examination cannot be overemphasized in making the diagnosis of peri-carditis. An electrocardiogram supports the clinical suspicion and must be meticulously reviewed. The emergency physician must have the knowledge of pre-disposing conditions, and a heightened clinical suspicion for appropriate patient management. In the future, echocardiography may have applications for cardiac diagnostics and therapeutics. The emergency physician must understand the indications and how to perform emergent pericardiocentesis. Pericardiocentesis can be a life-saving technique, but should be undertaken with the utmost respect for potential complications.

REFERENCES

1. Ling LH, Oh JK, Tajik AJ. *Diagnostic Evaluation in Constrictive Pericarditis and Differentiation from Restrictive Cardiomyopathy. In Imaging in Cardiovascular Disease.* Baltimore, MD: Lippincott Williams & Wilkins, 2000, pp. 759–766.
2. Permanyer-Miralda G, Sagrista-Sauleda J, Shebatai R, et al. Acute pericardial disease: An approach to etiologic diagnosis and treatment. In: Soler-Soler-Soler J, et al. (eds.), *Pericardial Disease: New Insights and Old Dilemmas.* Dordrecht: Kluwer Academic Publishers, 1990.
3. Lorell BH, Pericarditis. In: Braunwald E (ed.), *Heart Disease*, 5th ed. Philadelphia, PA: W.B. Saunders, 1997, pp. 1478–1534.
4. Hoit BD. *Disease of the Pericardium in Hurst's: The Heart*, 10th ed. New York: McGraw-Hill, Vol. 2, 2001, pp. 2061–2062.
5. Spodick DH. Acute cardiac tamponade. *N Engl J Med* 2003;349:684–690.
6. Aikat S, Ghaffari S. A review of pericardial diseases: Clinical, ECG and hemodynamic features and management. *Cleve Clin J Med* 2000;67(12):903–914.
7. Mehta A, Mehta M, Jain A. Constrictive pericarditis. *Clin Cardiol* 1999;22:334–344.
8. Spodick DH. Acute pericarditis: Current concepts and practice. *JAMA* 2003;289(9):1150–1153.
9. Spodick DH, Roldan CA. *The Patient with Pericardial Disease. In Evaluation of the Patient with Heart Disease: Integrating the Physical Exam & Echocardiography.* Baltimore, MD: Lippincott Williams & Wilkins, 2002, pp. 339–364.
10. Goyle KK, Walling AD. Diagnosing pericarditis. *Am Fam Phys* 2002;66(9):1695–1702.
11. Beck CS. Two cardiac compression triads. *JAMA* 1935;104:714–716.
12. Fowler NO. Cardiac tamponade: A clinical or an echocar-diographic diagnosis? *Circulation* 1993;87(5):1738–1741.
13. Myers RBH, Spodick DH. Constrictive pericarditis: Clinical and pathophysiologic characteristics. *Am Heart J* 1999;138 (2 Pt 1):219–232.
14. Hancock EW. Cardiomyopathy: Differential diagnosis of restrictive cardiomyopathy and constrictive pericarditis. *Heart* 2001;86:343–349.
15. Osterberg L, Vagelos R, Atwood JE. Case presentation and review: Constrictive pericarditis. *West J Med* 1998;169(4): 232–239.
16. Sagrista-Sauleda J, Angel J, Permanyer-Miralda G, et al. Long-term follow-up of idiopathic chronic pericardial effusion. *N Engl J Med* 1999;341:2054–2059.
17. Zayas R, Anguita M, Torres F, et al. Incidence of specific etiology and role of methods for specific etiologic diagnosis of primary acute pericarditis. *Am J Cardiol* 1995;75(5):378–382.
18. Tsang TSM, Enriquez-Sarano M, Freeman WK, et al. Consecutive 1127 therapeutic echocardiographically guided pericardiocenteses: Clinical profile, practice patterns, and outcomes spanning 21 years. *Mayo Clin Proc* 2002;775(5): 429–436.
19. Oakley CM. Myocarditis, pericarditis and other pericardial diseases. *Heart* 2000;84:449–454.
20. Tierney LM, McPhee SJ, Papadakis MA. Disease of the peri-cardium. In: Tierney LM (ed.), *Current Medical Diagnosis and Treatment*, 39th ed. Lange Medical Books, 2000, pp. 433–436.
21. Alpert MA, Ravenscraft MD. Pericardial involvement in end-stage renal disease. *J Med Sci* 2003;325(4):228–236.
22. Gununkula SR, Spodick DH. Pericardial disease in renal patients. *Semin Nephrol* 2001;21(1):52–56.

23. Wilkes JD, Fidias P, Vaickus L, et al. Malignancy-related pericardial effusion. *Cancer* 1995;76:1377–1387.

24. Keefe DL. Cardiovascular emergencies in the cancer patient. *Semin Oncol* 2000;27(3):244–255.

25. Davey P, Lalloo DG. Drug induced chest pain-rare but important. *Postgrad Med J* 2000;76:420–422.

26. Prince SE, Cunha BA. Postpericardiotomy syndrome. *Heart Lung* 1997;26(2):165–168.

27. Correale E, Maggioni AP, Romano S, et al. Peicardial involvement in acute myocardial infarction in the post-thrombolytic era: Clinical meaning and value. *Clin Cardiol* 1997;20:327–331.

28. Moder KG, Miller TD, Tazelaar HD. Cardiac involvement in systemic lupus erythematosus. *Mayo Clin Proc* 1999; 74:275–284.

29. Alpert MA, Goldberg SH, Singsen BH, et al. Cardiovascular manifestations of mixed connective tissue disease in adults. *Circulation* 1983;68:1082–1193.

30. Sackner MA, Akgun N, Kimbel P, et al. The pathophysiology of scleroderma involving the heart and respiratory system. *Ann Intern Med* 1964;60:611–630.

31. D'Angelo WA, Fries JF, Masi AT, et al. Pathologic observation in systemic sclerosis (scleroderma): A study of 58 autopsy cases and 58 matched controls. *Am J Med* 1969;46:428–440.

32. Chan TC, Brady WJ, Pollack M. Electrocardiographic manifestations : Acute myopericarditis. *J Emerg Med* 1999;17(5): 865–872.

33. Hayden GE, Brady WJ, Perron AD, et al. Electrocardiographic T-wave inversion: Differential diagnosis in the chest pain patient. *Am J Emerg Med* 2002;20(3):252–262.

34. Brady WJ, Perron AD, Ullman EU. Errors in emergency physicians interpretation of ST-segment elevation in emergency department chest pain patients. *Acad Emerg Med* 2000;7:1256–1260.

35. Brady WJ, Perron AD, Chan T. Electrocardiographic ST-segment elevation: Correct identification of acute myocardial infarction (AMI) and non-AMI syndromes by emergency physicians. *Acad Emerg Med* 2001;8(4):349–360.

36. Bruce MA, Spodick DH. Atypical electrocardiogram in acute myopericarditis: Characteristics and prevalence. *J Electrocardiol* 1980;13:61–66.

37. Krainin H, Cole JS, Surawicz B. Negative U wave: A highly specific but poorly understood sign of heart disease. *Am J Cardiol* 1976;38:157.

38. Marinella MA. Electrocardiographic manifestations and differential diagnosis of acute myopericarditis. *Am Fam Phys* 1990;57:699–704.

39. Spodick DH. Arrhythmias during acute myopericarditis: A prospective study of 100 consecutive cases. *JAMA* 1976; 235:39–41.

40. Spodick DH. Significant arrhythmias during myoperi-carditis are due to concomitant heart disease. *J Am Coll Cardiol* 1998;32:551–352.

41. Ginzton LE, Laks MM. The differential diagnosis of acute pericarditis from normal variant: New electrocardiographic criteria. *Circulation* 1982;65:1004.

42. Shabetai R. *Acute and Chronic Pericardial Disease in Imaging in Cardiovascular Disease.* Baltimore, MD: Lippincott Williams & Wilkins, 2000, pp. 741–758.

43. Sagrista-Sauleda J, Merci J, Permanyer-Miralda G, et al. Clinical clues to the cause of large pericardial effusion. *Am J Med* 2000;109:95–101.

44. Committee on Clinical Application of Echocardiography ACC/AHA: Guidelines for the Clinical Application of Echocardiography. *Circulation* 1997;5:1686–1744.

45. Mandavia DP, Hoffner RJ, Mahaney K, et al. Bedside echocardiography by emergency physicians. *Ann Emerg Med* 2001;38(4):377–382.

46. Sierzenski PR, Leech SJ, Gukhool J, et al. Emergency physician echocardiography decreases time to diagnosis of pericardial effusions. *Acad Emerg Med* 2003;10(5):561.

47. Cairns JA, Camm AJ, Fallen EL, et al. Pericardial disease: An evidence-based approach to diagnosis and treatment in evidence based cardiology. *Br Med J* 2003;735–748.

48. Arunsalam S, Siegel RJ. Rapid resolution of symptomatic acute pericarditis with ketorolac tromethamine: A parenteral nonsteroidal anti-inflammatory agent. *Am Heart J* 1993; 125:1455–1458.

49. Fowler RS, Mc Cully RB, Oh JK, et al. Mycoplasma associated pericarditis. *Mayo Clin Proc* 1997;72:33–36.

50. Adler Y, Finkelstein Y, Guindo J, et al. Colchicine treatment for recurrent pericarditis. A decade of experience. *Circulation* 1998;97:2183–2185.

51. Cohn DL, Catlin BJ, Peterson KL, et al. A 62 dose month 6 month therapy for pneumonia and extrapulmonary tuberculous. A twice-weekly directly observed cost-effective regimen. *Ann Intern Med* 1990;112:407–415.

52. Lindenberger M, Kjellberg M, Karlsson E, et al. Pericardiocentesis guided by 2-D echocardiography: The method of choice for treatment of pericardial effusion. *J Intern Med* 2003;253:411–417.

53. Soler-Soler J, Sagrista-Sauleda J, Permanyer-Miralda G. Management of Pericardial effusion. *Heart* 2001;86: 235–240.

54. Hoit BD. Management of effusive and constrictive peri-cardial heart disease. *Circulation* 2002;105:2939–2942.

55. Pawsat DE, Lee JY. Inflammatory disorders of the heart. *Emerg Med Clin North Am* 1998;16(3):665–681.

36

Myocarditis

Eric A. Gross
Steve D. Slauson

HIGH YIELD FACTS

- Congestive heart failure (CHF) is the most common presenting symptom of acute myocarditis in the emergency department.
- Other than endomyocardial biopsy, no diagnostic modality offers clinically useful specificity in the diagnosis of myocarditis.
- Supportive care remains the mainstay of therapy.
- Antiviral agents and immunomodulation may be useful in some types of myocarditis.
- Anti-inflammatory drugs may worsen outcomes and should not be used the in acute phase of the disease.

EPIDEMIOLOGY AND ETIOLOGY

The true incidence of myocarditis is difficult to ascertain because many cases go undetected. Postmortem studies over the years suggest that myocarditis may be the cause of sudden death in 20% of young adults and in 16% of infants who die of sudden infant death syndrome (SIDS).[1] Another confounding factor has been a lack of precise definition for myocarditis.

The classification of diseases affecting the myocardium was changed by the 1995 World Health Organization/ International Society and Federation of Cardiology Task Force.[2] A cardiomyopathy is considered a myocardial disease associated with myocardial dysfunction. Many categories exist, including dilated cardiomyopathy, hypertrophic cardiomyopathy, restrictive cardiomyopathy, and arrhythmogenic right ventricular cardiomyopathy. Inflammatory cardiomyopathy is a subset of dilated cardiomyopathy and is defined as myocarditis associated with myocardial dysfunction.

Cardiac inflammation may be caused by a variety of agents: viral, immune-mediated, toxin or idiopathic. In North America, viral agents are the most common, especially adenovirus and coxsackievirus B.[3,4] A large number of infectious causes have been identified (Table 36-1). Human immunodeficiency virus (HIV) is also becoming a more prevalent cause of myocarditis, either alone or in association with other viruses.[5] Worldwide, Chagas disease is the leading cause of myocarditis. Many other infectious agents have been implicated as well and are discussed below. Drugs may also cause inflammation of the myocardium either through direct toxic effect or autoimmune-mediated mechanisms.[6] Although not discussed in depth here, these include cocaine and doxorubicin. Readers are referred to the review by Feenstra et al.[6]

SYMPTOMS, SIGNS, AND NATURAL HISTORY

There is no pathognomonic presentation of myocarditis. The clinical presentation ranges from an asymptomatic state with ECG changes to fulminant cardiac failure or sudden death. Vague, nonspecific complaints, such as fatigue, cough or myalgias, are common, especially among children. This may be associated with a viral prodrome. In other patients, arrhythmias may be the only presenting finding.

Symptoms of CHF are common in symptomatic myocarditis; these include respiratory distress, diaphoresis, and possibly chest pain. Younger children and infants may show poor feeding or irritability. Signs of CHF, such as an S_3 gallop, poor peripheral perfusion, peripheral edema, or hepatomegaly may also be present.

The outcome following acute viral myocarditis is variable (Fig. 36-1). Subclinical cases may recover fully, without ever being detected, or may be the precursor to the development of dilated cardiomyopathy later in life. Acute myocarditis may spontaneously resolve, progress to dilated cardiomyopathy (DCM), or require transplantation to avoid death.[1] Past difficulties in the detection and classification of myocarditis, as described above, have made defining the incidence of these complications problematic.

DIAGNOSTIC TESTING

Laboratory Findings

The laboratory findings in myocarditis are generally nonspecific. Sixty percent of patients have an elevated erythrocyte sedimentation rate and 25% have an elevated white blood cell count. Additional findings may include a white cell differential with lymphocyte predominance and an elevated C-reactive protein.[7] Elevated cardiac

Table 36-1. Infectious Causes of Myocarditis

Viral	**Protozoal/Metazoal**
Adenovirus	Cysticercosis
Arbovirus A and B	Echinococcus
Coxsackie A and B	Heterophyiasis
Cytomegalovirus	Schistosomiasis
Echovirus	Toxoplasmosis
Epstein-Barr virus	Trichinosis
Hepatitis viruses	Trypanosomiasis
Herpes simplex	Visceral larva
Human	migrans
Immunodeficiency	
Virus	**Rickettsial and**
Influenza	**spirochetal**
Mumps	Q fever
Poliomyelitis	Rocky mountain
Rabies	spotted fever
Rubella	Scrub typhus
Rubeola	Leptospirosis
Vaccinia	Relapsing fever
Varicella	
Variola	**Fungal**
Viral Encephalitides	Aspergillosis
Yellow fever	Actinomycosis
	Blastomycosis
Bacterial	Cryptococcus
Brucellosis	Candidiasis
Clostridia	Coccidiodomycosis
Diptheria	Histoplasmosis
Meningiococcus	
Mycoplasma	
Psittacosis	
Salmonella	
Streptococcus	
Tuberculosis	

enzymes are also seen in some but not all patients with myocarditis. Increases in CK-MB are observed in 2–6% of patients while elevated cardiac troponin levels have been identified in 34–53% of the patients with biopsy-proven myocarditis.[8]

Elevated titers to cardiotropic viruses may also be suggestive of myocarditis. A fourfold increase in a specific titer from the acute to convalescent phase identifies response to a recent acute viral infection; however, it does not confirm the presence of viral myocarditis.[9]

Rheumatologic screening may be helpful in patients who present with unexplained heart failure and signs and symptoms of connective tissue disease.[10]

ECG

ECG changes in myocarditis are common, however generally nonspecific. Sinus tachycardia is the most frequent finding. Diffuse ST- and T-wave changes, prolongation of the QTc interval, low voltage, and even myocardial infarct pattern have been observed.[11] Conduction delay is common, with left bundle branch block identified in 20% of patients. Complete heart block may be seen but is typically transient. Supraventricular and less frequent ventricular arrhythmias may also occur.[12]

CXR

The chest radiograph is highly variable in patients with myocarditis. The heart size and lung fields range from normal size and clear to marked biventricular enlargement with pulmonary congestion or edema.

Echocardiography

Echocardiography may provide additional information about ventricular function but often is not diagnostic. Global hypokinesis is the most common finding; however, segmental wall motion abnormalities that mimic regional ischemia may be observed.[13] Left ventricular systolic dysfunction with normal-sized left ventricular cavities may be seen. Wall thickness may also be increased, particularly early in the course of the disease. Ventricular thrombi are detected in 15% of those studied.[14] Newer echocardiographic techniques using digital image processing in which ventricular wall texture is analyzed may prove to be more diagnostic; however, these techniques are still considered experimental.[15]

Other Noninvasive Modalities

In addition to echocardiography, several noninvasive strategies have been used to identify myocarditis. Radionucleotide scanning after administration of indium-111 antimyosin antibody can identify myocardial necrosis with a sensitivity of 71–83% and specificity of 53–66%.[16] Radionucleotide scanning combined with resting thallium imaging may assist in distinguishing myocarditis and myocardial infarction.[17] At the present time however, the utility of scintigraphy is limited by radiation exposure, availability, and expense.

Contrast-enhanced MRI may also be useful for the noninvasive localization and assessment of the extent of inflammation in patients with presumed myocarditis. Gadolinium-DTPA accumulation in inflammatory lesions, visualized by MRI, correlates with both clinical status and left ventricular function and may prove to be a

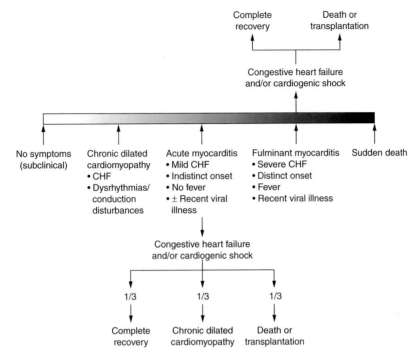

Fig. 36-1. Clinical presentation of acute viral **myocarditis**. Most children with viral **myocarditis** are asymptomatic and probably escape detection. There is a wide spectrum of clinical presentation ranging from a mild, indistinct illness to sudden death. Classically, it is thought that one third of patients with acute viral **myocarditis** recover normal cardiac function, one third show signs of chronic heart failure, and one-third either die or require heart transplantation. (Reprinted with permission from wheeler and Kooy, A formidable challenge: the diagnosis and treatment of viral myocarditis in children. *Critical Care Clinics*, 2003;19:365–369, with permission from Elsevier.)

valuable technique in the diagnosis and monitoring of disease activity.[18] Its clinical utility however is still under investigation.

Endomyocardial Biopsy

Despite the increased availability of an array of specialized diagnostic tests, many investigators still consider endomyocardial biopsy to be the gold standard for the diagnosis of myocarditis. The preferred approach is transvenous endomyocardial biopsy of the right ventricular septum. Studies evaluating the accuracy of biopsy for diagnosing myocarditis are variable. Reports of sensitivity and ranges from 35 to 63%; specificity approximates 80%.[19] Because of the high false negative rate and the low likelihood that biopsy will yield a specific diagnosis for which there is effective therapy, the utility of endomyocardial biopsy has been challenged.[20]

The yield of the endomyocardial biopsy may be improved with the application of newer molecular biology

techniques for the detection of viral nucleic acid in myocardial cells. These techniques are rapid, sensitive, and may become the test of choice for the diagnosis of viral myocarditis.[21]

MANAGEMENT

Supportive

Supportive care is the first line of therapy for patients with myocarditis. Bed rest is recommended in the acute phase of disease. This is based on the negative effects of activity in animal models and the recognition that myocarditis has been lethal in young athletes.[22] During the initial phase of acute myocarditis, hospitalization and monitoring are recommended to permit early detection of asymptomatic yet potentially life-threatening arrhythmias or conduction defects. In the subacute phase of the disease, physical activity should be restricted for 6 months and until the heart size and function have normalized.[10]

Arrhythmias are common in patients with acute myocarditis and should be managed with usual antiarrhythmic agents. Patients with complete AV block may require temporary transvenous pacing; however, this abnormality is typically transient. Unnecessary medications should be discontinued to reduce the chance of allergic myocarditis, particularly in the presence of eosinophilia.[10]

Congestive Heart Failure

The treatment of heart failure in patients with active myocarditis remains primarily supportive and responds to routine management including angiotensin-converting enzyme (ACE) inhibitors and diuretics. Severe failure may require high-dose inotropic support, vasodilators, and possibly the use of mechanical circulatory support.

Captopril in particular has been shown to be beneficial in several experimental models as it decreases cellular inflammation and necrosis.[23] Beta-blocking agents are recommended once the patient is clinically stable; however, there have been few reports of their use in humans with myocarditis.[24] Digoxin is recommended by some authors; however, it increases the expression of proinflammatory cytokines and mortality in animal models and should be used with caution.[25]

Mechanical Cardiac Support

Fulminant myocarditis frequently causes rapidly progressive cardiac decompensation resulting in death or need for cardiac transplantation. A substantial number of reports have shown success using temporary ventricular assist devices or extracorporal membrane oxygenation systems as a bridge to recovery or to transplantation for heart failure that is refractory to maximal medical therapy.[26] Patients presenting with signs and symptoms consistent with acute myocarditis should be rapidly transferred to a site capable of ventricular support.[10]

Transplantation

Cardiac transplantation may be necessary for myocarditis presenting with persistent heart failure. The surgical risk, allograft rejection rates, and 1-year survival are poorer for this group as compared to those transplanted for other reasons.[27]

Antivirals

Given the presence of replicating enterovirus RNA in some patients with myocarditis, the use of antiviral therapy in the acute phase of disease has been studied. Antiviral therapy with ribavirin or alpha interferon reduces the severity of myocardial lesions and mortality in experimental animal models of myocardial enteroviral infection when started prior to or soon after infection.[28]

Several case reports in humans have documented successful treatment of myocarditis with antiviral therapy.[29] In a small preliminary study of patients with persistence of myocardial viral genomes, beta-interferon eliminated viral nucleic acid and improved left ventricular function.[30] The clinical value of antiviral therapy is being assessed in the European Study of Epidemiology and treatment of cardiac inflammatory disease.[31]

Vaccinations

Attenuated vaccines have prevented the development of myocarditis following viral challenge in several animal models; however, further studies are needed to confirm these initial reports.[32]

Immunomodulating Therapy

Since the latter phases of myocarditis appear to be related to activation of cellular and humoral autoimmunity, immunosuppressive therapy has been evaluated. A large number of small uncontrolled studies have supported the use of a variety of immunosuppressive drugs. More recent randomized-controlled trials of anti-inflammatory-immunosuppressive agents including corticosteroids, azathioprine, and cyclosporine fail to demonstrate benefit in acute or chronic myocarditis.[33] Although immunosuppression is not routinely recommended, these agents may have role in myocarditis caused by systemic autoimmune diseases such as idiopathic giant cell myocarditis (GCM) or systemic lupus erythematosus (SLE).[34] A recent retrospective study suggests that certain subsets of patients, those with high circulating levels of cardiac autoantibodies and low levels of viral genome in the myocardium, may show improvement with immunosuppressive therapy[35]; however, more work needs to be done in this area.

High-dose IV gamma-globulin has been shown to be beneficial in a number of case reports.[36] However, a subsequent randomized-controlled trial failed to show an effect of high-dose IVIG in adult patients.[37]

Nonsteroidal Anti-inflammatories

Nonsteroidal anti-inflammatory drugs including indomethacin, aspirin, and ibuprofen are contraindicated in the acute phase of viral myocarditis as they have been shown to increase myocardial damage in animal models.[9]

SPECIFIC ENTITIES

Giant Cell Myocarditis

Giant cell myocarditis is a rare and frequently fatal form of myocardial inflammation. Histologically, GCM is defined by myocyte necrosis associated with multinucleated giant cells and a mixed inflammatory infiltrate. Although its etiology remains unknown, GCM has been associated with autoimmune and inflammatory conditions in up to 20% of cases, including inflammatory bowel disease, Hashimoto's thyroiditis, myasthenia gravis, and different forms of inflammatory arthritis.[34] Myocarditis resembling human GCM can be induced in rats by immunization with cardiac myosin, further supporting an autoimmune mechanism.[38]

GCM typically affects young to middle aged adults. Patients typically present with heart failure, although conduction disturbance, ventricular arrhythmia, sudden death or, rarely, a syndrome mimicking acute myocardial infarction have also been described. The clinical course typically follows a rapid deterioration of left ventricular function despite conventional heart failure treatment. In one study of 63 patients, the rate of death or cardiac transplantation was 89% and the median survival was less than 6 months from onset of symptoms.[34]

Diagnosis is made by endomyocardial biopsy, which has a sensitivity of approximately 85% compared with the gold standards of open heart biopsy, cardiectomy, or autopsy.[39] No controlled clinical trial has compared different treatment regimens. Retrospective analysis suggests that multidrug immunosuppression may prolong survival, although outcomes with medical treatment are highly variable and remain poor.[40] A prospective treatment trial is currently underway to determine the optimal therapeutic approach.[41] At this time, transplantation remains the therapy of choice for severe disease, although GCM recurs in the transplanted heart in about a quarter of the cases.

Lyme Disease

Lyme disease is caused by the spirochete *Borrelia burgdorferi* and transmitted by the Ixodes tick. The disease usually begins during the summer months with flu-like illness and characteristic rash (erythema migrans). This is followed weeks to months later by joint, neurologic, or cardiac involvement. Although cases are concentrated in certain endemic areas, foci of Lyme disease are widely spread throughout the United States, Europe, and Asia.[42]

Four to ten percent of patients with Lyme disease develop evidence of cardiac involvement, the most common manifestation being self-limited atrioventricular blocks. Myocardial involvement leading to cardiomegaly, echocardiographic left ventricular dysfunction, or clinical CHF occurs in 10–15% of patients.[43,44] Pericarditis, pericardial effusion, tachyarrhythmias occur infrequently. The clinical course of disease is typically benign and complete recovery is expected. However, rare instances of death have been reported.[45]

Diagnosis is based on clinical and historical features of Lyme disease in the setting of ECG abnormalities and symptoms of chest pain, syncope, palpitations, or dyspnea. Diffuse ST- and T-wave changes, although nonspecific, may suggest myocardial involvement.[46] Serologic studies and identification of spirochete in endomyocardial biopsies can also support the diagnosis.[47,48] A screening ECG is recommended whenever the diagnosis of Lyme disease is suspected.

Although no treatment has been shown to attenuate or prevent the development of Lyme carditis, antibiotics are used routinely.[46] Intravenous penicillin G or ceftriaxone is the therapy of choice for more severe disease and oral therapy with doxycycline or amoxicillin may be used in milder cases. The efficacy of anti-inflammatory agents (corticosteroids or salicylates) for hastening recovery of conduction disease is unproven. Patients with second-degree or complete heart block should be hospitalized with continuous cardiac monitoring. Temporary pacing may be necessary in up to 30% of patients.[49]

Diphtheria

Although rare in the United States, diphtheria continues to be of importance in some developing countries.[50] Diphtheria is caused by the gram-positive bacillus *Corynebacterium diphtheriae*. Humans are the only known reservoir for infection, which is spread primarily via airborne respiratory droplets from the nose and throat or contact with exudate from infected skin lesions. Clinical manifestations vary from asymptomatic or mild cutaneous infection to severe inflammation of the upper respiratory tract. Toxin from the organism may affect the heart or nervous system, resulting in polyneuropathies or damage to the myocardium and conduction system.

Myocardial involvement is seen in about 25% of cases and is the most common cause of death.[50] The risk of cardiac involvement is proportional to the severity of local disease. Myocarditis typically develops 1 week after the onset of illness when local symptoms are often resolving. Clinically, patients may present with cardiomegaly and overt failure or with less severe signs and symptoms, including dyspnea, weakness, decreased heart sounds, or gallop rhythm.[51,52] ECG changes often include ST-T-wave changes and first-degree heart block. Progression to bundle branch block or complete heart block is an ominous sign and usually associated with extremely poor prognosis.[53]

Hospitalization and monitoring is necessary for suspected cases because patients without clinical evidence of disease may have significant conduction abnormalities. In addition to supportive treatment, therapy includes antitoxin and high-dose penicillin. Overall, cardiac-related mortality is about 30%. Prognosis for patients that survive the acute phase of illness is good, although cardiomyopathy and conduction disturbances may persist in some cases.[53]

Chagas Disease

Chagas disease is caused by the parasite *Trypanosoma cruzi*. The vast majority of cases (85%) are due to certain species of triatomine bugs that inhabit human dwellings and act as the vector.[54] Approximately 10% of cases are transfusion related.[55] Maternal-fetal transmission and oral transmission from contaminated food or drink are responsible for a smaller number of cases.

Cardiac involvement occurs in both the acute and chronic phases of the disease. The acute phase is most commonly seen in children. Sinus tachycardia is common. The electrocardiogram frequently shows low QRS voltage, prolonged PR and/or QT intervals, and primary T-wave changes. Ventricular extrasystoles, atrial fibrillation, or advanced grade right bundle branch block are rare and indicate a poor prognosis. Five to ten percent of symptomatic, untreated patients will die from cardiac failure or encephalomyelitis during the acute phase.

The chronic disease manifestations in Chagas follow a latent period also known as the indeterminate form. Cardiac involvement may be mild or severe. Mild disease is characterized by mild or no symptoms of CHF. ECG changes are typically primary ST-T changes, right bundle branch block of nonadvanced degree, first-degree AV block, premature ventricular beats, and low voltage QRS. Severe disease shows more advanced ECG changes, including atrioventricular blocks, intraventricular blocks, sinus bradycardia (with premature ventricular contractions or primary and diffuse alterations of ventricular repolarization), and premature ventricular contractions (5 or more per minute).[55] Arrhythmias are common; episodes of nonsustained ventricular tachycardia are observed in 40% of patients with mild wall motion abnormalities and in 90% of patients with heart failure.[56] Ventricular aneurysms are seen in 19% of the endemic population and are directly related to severity of disease.[57] Sudden death occurs in 38% of patients with or without CHF. Thrombosis in the left atrium and ventricle is seen in 44% of autopsies and is associated with cardiomegaly. Lastly, intermittent precordial pain occurs in 15% of Chagas patients.[55]

Treatment in the acute phase is indicated with benznidazole, preferably, or nifurtimox to reduce parasitemia and affect cure. Disagreement exists about these treatments in the chronic phase; therefore, treatment should be aimed at CHF, thromboembolic complications, and arrhythmias. Beta-blockers should be avoided due to bradyarrhythmias and conduction disturbances. Pacemakers are the treatment of choice for severe bradyarrhythmias. Amiodarone is the treatment of choice for ventricular tachycardia.[58] Implantable defibrillators should be used in patients with recurrent ventricular tachycardia. Chagas is not a contraindication to cardiac transplantation.

Trichinosis

Trichinosis is a parasitic disease caused by tissue-dwelling roundworms of the species *Trichinella spiralis*. The organism is acquired by eating *Trichinella*-infected meat products, most often wild game meat or undercooked pork.[59] The acute illness typically consists of fever, myalgias, muscle tenderness, intestinal symptoms, and periorbital edema. Larvae may invade the myocardium resulting in an eosinophilic inflammatory response and muscle necrosis. Reported incidences of cardiac involvement in outbreaks range from 1 to 68%, with most studies reporting less than 15%.[60–63]

The most common ECG findings are pericardial effusion (75%), nonspecific ST-T-wave changes (75%), and ventricular repolarization abnormalities (66%). The majority of these ECG and echocardiographic changes resolve within 6 months.[62,64] Treatment with corticosteroids and a benzimidazole, begun in consultation with an infectious disease specialist, is indicated.

Kawasaki Disease

Kawasaki disease (KD) is an acute vasculitis of unknown cause that occurs predominantly in infancy and early childhood. The disorder occurs worldwide, with Asians at highest risk. KD is the most common cause of acquired pediatric heart disease in developed nations. Cardiac complications often appear early in the illness and may include myocarditis, pericarditis, pericardial effusion, aortic or mitral valve insufficiencies, or dysrhythmias. Coronary artery abnormalities including ectasia and aneurysm, with the potential for myocardial infarction, aneurysm rupture, and sudden death also occur in about 20% of untreated children.[65,66]

Myocarditis, manifested by tachycardia and decreased ventricular function, occurs during the initial phase of the disease in at least 50% of patients. This may progress to CHF in a small fraction of patients, most commonly in those younger than 6 months and older than 9 years of age. The diagnosis of KD is based on presence of fever, bilateral nonexudative conjunctivitis, erythema of the lips and oral mucosa, periungual desquamation, rash, and cervical lymphadenopathy. The ECG in acute KD may show mild abnormalities, most commonly a prolonged PR interval and nonspecific ST-T-wave changes.[65] Early evaluation with echocardiography or angiography is essential to evaluate for coronary dilation and LV function.[67]

In addition to conventional supportive therapy for myocarditis or CHF, treatment of the acute stage of KD includes intravenous gamma-globulin and high-dose aspirin. These agents reduce the prevalence of coronary artery abnormalities and rapidly improve myocardial function, often within days.[68] The use of corticosteroids in KD remains controversial. Long-term cardiac sequelae are uncommon in children treated during the acute phase of KD and the overall mortality rate is less than 1%.[65]

HIV-related

HIV-infected patients may manifest a variety of cardiovascular abnormalities, including pericarditis, myocarditis, cardiomyopathy, endocarditis, pulmonary hypertension, malignant neoplasms, and coronary artery disease.[69] Cardiac illness related to HIV infection tends to occur late in the disease course and is therefore becoming more prevalent as therapy and longevity improve. The prevalence of cardiac pathology in AIDS patients has been reported to range between 28 and 73% and is thought to be a cause of death in at least 6% of AIDS patients.[70]

Myocarditis is found in approximately 30–50% of all autopsies performed in AIDS patients although only about 6% of patients manifest clinically symptomatic disease.[71,72] Among HIV patients with myocarditis, bacterial, fungal, and protozoal pathogens can be identified in about 15% of cases. Cytomegalovirus, coxsackievirus, and herpes simplex infections are frequently reported causes.[69,70] The etiology of the remaining apparently idiopathic HIV-related heart muscle disease is uncertain, although it is most likely multifactorial. Direct or indirect effects of HIV on the myocardium, potential infection by other cardiotropic organisms, nutritional deficiencies, and toxic effects of drug treatment have all been implicated.[73]

Clinical manifestations and diagnosis of myocarditis in AIDS patients is similar to that of other causes of acute myocarditis. Heart failure typically occurs in the late stages

of AIDS and is associated with poor survival, ranging from 1 to 3 months. Isolation and identification of specific etiologic agents may provide additional helpful information although the necessity of performing myocardial biopsy in these patients remains controversial. Immunomodulatory therapy and nutritional supplementation may be helpful in HIV-infected patients with myocarditis; however, further study is necessary.[74]

REFERENCES

1. Wheeler DS, Kooy NW. A formidable challenge: The diagnosis and treatment of viral myocarditis in children. *Crit Care Clin* 2003;19(3):365–391.
2. Richardson P, McKenna W, Bristow M. Report of the 1995 World Health Organization/International Society and Federation of Cardiology Task Force on the Definition and Classification of Cardiomyopathies. *Circulation* 1996;93:841–842.
3. Bowles K, Gibson J, Wu J. Genomic organization and chromosomal localization of the human coxsackievirus B-adenovirus receptor gene. *Hum Genet* 1999;105:354–359.
4. Martin AB, Webber S, Fricker FJ. Acute myocarditis: Rapid diagnosis by PCR in children. *Circulation* 1994;90:330–339.
5. Barbaro G, Lorenzo GD, Grisorio B. Incidence of dilated cardiomyopathy and detection of HIV in myocardial cells of HIV-positive patients. *N Engl J Med* 1998;339:1093–1099.
6. Feenstra J, Grobbee DE, Remme WJ. Drug induced heart failure. *J Am Coll Cardiol* 1999;35(5):1152–1162.
7. Investigators MTT. Incidence and clinical characteristics of myocarditis. *Circulation* 1991;84:II-2.
8. Smith SC, Ladenson JH, Mason JW. Elevations of cardiac troponin I associated with myocarditis. *Circulation* 1997;95:163.
9. Mason JW. Myocarditis. *Adv Intern Med* 1999;44:293.
10. Feldman AM, McNamara D. Myocarditis. *N Engl J Med* 2000;349:1388–1398.
11. Dec G, Waldman H, Southern J. Viral myocarditis mimicking acute myocardial infarction. *J Am Coll Cardiol* 1992;20:85–89.
12. Karjalainen J, Viitasalo M, Kala R. 24-Hour electrocardiographic recordings in mild acute infectious myocarditis. *Ann Clin Res* 1984;16:34–39.
13. Nieminen MS, Heikkila J, Karjalainen J. Echocardiography in acute infectious myocarditis: Relation to clinical and electrocardiographic findings. *Am J Cardiol* 1984;53:1331–1337.
14. Pinamonti B, Alberti E, Cigalotto A. Echocardiographic findings in myocarditis. *Am J Cardiol* 1988;62:285–291.
15. Lieback E, Hardouin I, Meyer R. Clinical value of echocardiographic tissue characterization in the diagnosis of myocarditis. *Eur Heart J* 1996;17:135–142.
16. Dec GW, Palacios I, Yasuda T. Antimyosin antibody cardiac imaging: Its role in the diagnosis of acute myocarditis. *J Am Coll Cardiol* 1990;16:97–104.

17. Sarda L, Colin P, Boccara F. Myocarditis in patients with clinical presentation of myocardial infarction and normal coronary angiograms. *J Am Coll Cardiol* 2001;37:786–792.

18. Friedrich MG, Strohm O, Schulz-Menger J. Contrast media-enhanced magnetic resonance imaging visualizes myocardial changes in the course of viral myocarditis. *Circulation* 1998;97:1802.

19. Hauck AJ, Kearney DL, Edwards WD. Evaluation of post-mortem endomyocardial biopsy specimens from 38 patients with lymphocytic myocarditis: Implications for role of sampling error. *Mayo Clin Proc* 1989;64:1235.

20. Abelmann WH, Baim DS, Schnitt SJ. Endomyocardial biopsy: Is it of clinical value? *Postgrad Med J* 1992;68 (Suppl 1):S44.

21. Why HJ, Meany BT, Richardson PJ. Clinical and prognostic significance of detection of entero-viral RNA in the myocardium of patients with myocarditis or dilated cardiomyopathy. *Circulation* 1994;89:2582.

22. Pisani B, Taylor DO, Mason JW. Inflammatory myocardial diseases and cardiomyopathies. *Am J Med* 1997;102:459.

23. Rezkalla S, Kloner RA, Khatib G, et al. Effect of delayed captopril therapy on left ventricular mass and myonecrosis during acute coxsackievirusmurine myocarditis. *Am Heart J* 1990;120:1377.

24. Popovic Z, Miric M, Vasiljevic J, et al. Acute hemodynamic effects of metoprolol +/− nitroglycerin in patients with biopsy proven lymphocytic myocarditis. *Am J Cardiol* 1998;81:801–804.

25. Matsumori A, Igata H, Ono K, et al. High doses of digitalis increase the myocardial production of proinflammatory cytokines and worsen myocardial injury in viral myocarditis: A possible mechanism of digitalis toxicity. *Jpn Circ J* 1999;63:934–940.

26. Rockman HA, Adamson RM, Dembitsky WP, et al. Acute fulminant myocarditis: Long-term follow-up after circulatory support with left ventricular assist device. *Am Heart J* 1991;121:922.

27. O'Connel JB, Dec GW, Goldenberg IF, et al. Results of heart transplantation for acute lymphocytic myocarditis. *J Heart Transplant* 1990;9:351.

28. Kishimoto C, Abelmann WH. Ribavirin treatment of murine coxsackievirus B3 myocarditis with analyses of lymphocyte subsets. *J Am Coll Cardiol* 1988;12:1334.

29. Baykurt C, Calgar K, Cerviz N, et al. Successful treatment of Epstein-Barr virus infection associated with myocarditis. *Pediatr Int* 1999;41:389–391.

30. Kuhl U, Pauscchinger M, Schwimmbeck PL, et al. Interferon-beta treatment eliminates cardiotropic viruses and improves left ventricular function in patients myocardial persistence of viral genomes and left ventricular dysfunction. *Circulation* 2003;107:2793.

31. Maisch B, Hufnagel G, Schonian U, et al. The European study of epidemiology and treatment of cardiac inflammatory disease. *Eur Heart J* 1995;16:173–175.

32. Chapman NM, Ragland A, Leser JS, et al. A group B coxsackievirus/poliovirus 5′ nontranslated region chimera can act as attenuated vaccine strain in mice. *J Virol* 2000; 74:4047–4056.

33. Mason JW, O'Connell JB, Herskowitz A, et al. A clinical trial of immunosuppressive therapy in inflammatory myocarditis. *N Engl J Med* 1995;333:269.

34. Cooper Jr LT, Berry GJ, Shabetai R. Idiopathic giant-cell myocarditis-natural history and treatment. *N Engl J Med* 1997;336:1860–1866.

35. Frustaci A, Chimenti C, Calabrese F, et al. Immunosuppressive therapy for active lymphocytic myocarditis: Virological and immunologic profile of responders versus nonresponders. *Circulation* 2003;107(6):857–863.

36. Tedeschi A, Airaghi L, Giannini S, et al. High-dose intravenous immunoglobulin in the treatment of acute myocarditis. A case report and review of the literature. *J Intern Med* 2002;251:169–173.

37. McNamara DM, Starling RC, Dec GW, et al. Intervention in myocarditis and acute cardiomyopathy with immune globulin: Results from the randomized placebo controlled IMAC trial [abstract]. *Circulation* 1999;100(Suppl 1):21.

38. Kodama M, Zhang S, Hanawa H, et al. Immunohistochemical characterization of infiltrating mononuclear cells in the rat heart with experimental autoimmune giant cell myocarditis. *Clin Exp Immunol* 1992;90(2):330–335.

39. Cooper LT Jr. Giant cell myocarditis: Diagnosis and treatment. *Herz* 2000;25(3):291–298.

40. Menghini VV, Savcenko V, Olson LJ, et al. Combined immunosuppression for the treatment of idiopathic giant cell myocarditis. *Mayo Clin Proc* 1999;74(12):1221–1226.

41. Cooper L. The giant cell treatment trial and registry. Design and methods (abstract). *J Heart Failure* 2000;6:133.

42. Steere AC. Lyme disease. *N Engl J Med* 2001;345(2): 115–125.

43. Pinto DS. Cardiac manifestations of Lyme disease. *Med Clin North Am* 2002;86:285–296.

44. van der Linde MR. Lyme carditis: Clinical characteristics of 105 cases. *Scand J Infect Dis* 1991;77(Suppl):81–84.

45. Cary NR, Fox B, Wright DJ, et al. Fatal Lyme carditis and endodermal heterotopia of the atrioventricular node. *Postgrad Med J* 1990;66(772):134–136.

46. Steere AC, Batsford WP, Weinberg M, et al. Lyme carditis: Cardiac abnormalities of Lyme disease. *Ann Intern Med* 1980;93(1):8–16.

47. Duray PH. Clinical pathologic correlations of Lyme disease. *Rev Infect Dis* 1989;11(Suppl 6):S1487–S1493.

48. de Koning J, Hoogkamp-Korstanje JA, van der Linde MR, et al. Demonstration of spirochetes in cardiac biopsies of patients with Lyme disease. *J Infect Dis* 1989;160:150–153.

49. Nagi KS, Thakur RK. Lyme carditis: Indications for cardiac pacing. *Can J Cardiol* 1995;11(4):335–338.

50. Kadirova R, Kartoglu HU, Strebel PM. Clinical characteristics and management of 676 hospitalized diphtheria cases, Kyrgyz Republic, 1995. *J Infect Dis* 2000;181(Suppl 1): S110–S115.

51. Boyer NH, Weinstein L. Diphtheritic myocarditis. *N Engl J Med* 1948;239:913.

52. Morgan BC. Cardiac complications of diphtheria. *Pediatrics* 1963;32:549–557.

53. Havaldar PV, Patil VD, Siddibhavi BM, et al. Fulminant diptheretic myocarditis. *Indian Heart J* 1989;41(4):265–269.

54. Schofield CJ, Dujardin JP. Chagas disease vector control in Central America. *Parasitol Today* 1997;13:141–144.

55. Prata A. Clinical and epidemiological aspects of Chagas disease. *Lancet Infect Dis* 2001;1(2):92–100.

56. Rassi Jr A, Rassi A, Little WC. Chagas heart disease. *Clin Cardiol* 2000;23:883–889.

57. Borges-Pereira J. Chagas disease in Virgem da Lapa, Minas Gerais, Brazil. IV. Clinical and epidemiological aspects of left ventricular aneurysm. *Rev Soc Bras Med Trop* 1998; 31(5):457–463.

58. Rassi Jr A, Rassi SG, Rassi AG. Sudden death in Chagas disease. *Arq Bras Cardiol* 2001;76:86–96.

59. Roy SL, Lopez AS, Schantz PM. Trichinellosis surveillance— United States, 1997–2001. *MMWR Surveill Summ* 2003; 52(6):1–8.

60. Knezevi K, Jovanovi J. Clinical characteristics of trichinosis. *Med Pregl* 1996;49:473–477.

61. Vujisic B, Najdanovic L, Simic N. Cardiac trichinosis— echocardiographic study. *Glas Srp Akad Nauka* 1991; 40:113–116.

62. Siwak E, Pancewicz S, Zajkowska J. Changes in ECG examination of patients with trichinosis. *Wiad Lek* 1994; 47:499–502.

63. Blondheim DS, Klein R, Ben-Dror G. Trichinosis in southern Lebanon. *Isr J Med Sci* 1984;20:141–144.

64. Lazarevi AM, Neskovi AN, Goronja M, et al. Low incidence of cardiac abnormalities in treated trichinosis: A prospective study of 62 patients from a single-source outbreak. *Am J Med* 1999;107(1):18–23.

65. Rowley AH, Shulman ST. Kawasaki syndrome. *Pediatr Clin North Am* 1999;46(2):313–329.

66. Barron KS, Shulman ST, Rowley A, et al. Report of the National Institutes of Health Workshop on Kawasaki Disease. *J Rheumatol* 1999;26(1):170–190.

67. Sundel R, Szer I. Vasculitis in childhood. *Rheum Dis Clin North Am* 2002;28(3):625–654.

68. Moran AM, Newburger JW, Sanders SP, et al. Abnormal myocardial mechanics in Kawasaki disease: Rapid response to gamma-globulin. *Am Heart J* 2000;139(2 Pt 1):217–223.

69. Rerkpattanapipat P, Wongpraparut N, Jacobs LE, et al. Cardiac manifestations of acquired immunodeficiency syndrome. *Arch Intern Med* 2000;160(5):602–608.

70. Kaul S, Fishbein MC, Siegel RJ. Cardiac manifestations of acquired immune deficiency syndrome: A 1991 update. *Am Heart J* 1991;122(2):535–544.

71. Barbarinia G, Barbaro G. Incidence of the involvement of the cardiovascular system in HIV infection. *Aids* 2003; 17(Suppl 1):S46–S50.

72. Yunis NA, Stone VE. Cardiac manifestations of HIV/AIDS: A review of disease spectrum and clinical management. *J Acquir Immune Defic Syndr Hum Retrovirol* 1998;18(2):145–154.

73. Currie PF, Boon NA. Immunopathogenesis of HIV-related heart muscle disease: Current perspectives. *Aids* 2003; 17(Suppl 1):S21–S28.

74. Barbaro G. HIV-associated cardiovascular complications: A new challenge for emergency physicians. *Am J Emerg Med* 2001;19:566–574.

37

Aortic Emergencies

Evan C. Leibner

HIGH YIELD FACTS

Aortic Aneurysm

- Aneurysms often remain asymptomatic while slowly enlarging, with eventual rupture in 25–50% of untreated cases. Overall mortality for rupture is 90%.
- Early diagnosis and surgical repair of asymptomatic lesions is key to reducing overall morbidity and mortality.
- Rupture risk exceeds surgical risk if the aneurysm exceeds 5.5 cm in diameter.
- Ultrasound is the diagnostic test of choice for aneurysm, but is not ideal for rupture. Surgical intervention can proceed based on strong suspicion alone. If time permits, the location and extent of the aneurysm can be identified by computed tomographic angiography (CTA), magnetic resonance angiography (MRA), or aortography.

Aortic Dissection

- Aortic dissection occurs by intimal violation, allowing blood to dissect between the aortic tissue planes. The variable location and involvement of other vessels allows for a plethora of clinical symptoms.
- Aortic imaging can be done by aortography, transesophageal echocardiography, CTA, or MRA.
- Treatment is by lowering dP/dt, by a combination of short-acting vasodilators that have negative chronotropicity. A short-acting β-blocker (e.g., esmolol) and vasodilation with nitroprusside is common, but labetalol (with both α- and β-blockade) is acceptable.
- While not all types are surgically repaired, early surgical consultation is needed.

INTRODUCTION

Aortic emergencies account for an increasing number of emergency department (ED) visits primarily due to the aging of the population. Aortic aneurysm, dissection, and occlusion are the primary lesions that can be seen and diagnosed in the ED. Pseudoaneurysms, ulcers, and atherosclerotic diseases are also encountered. Traumatic aortic injuries are beyond the scope of this chapter, but are a major cause of immediate death and morbidity, associated primarily with blunt deceleration injuries.

Identification of these lesions is often difficult in the ED setting. Symptoms can range from subtle to catastrophic, and are often nonspecific. By the time hemodynamic instability occurs, mortality rates markedly increase. It is therefore imperative to maintain a high index of suspicion for these lesions and to initiate appropriate diagnostic testing and therapeutic interventions early in the course of evaluation. Elective management of aortic aneurysm can improve outcome. Management of acute emergencies is best performed in conjunction with the vascular surgeon, as early surgical referral can improve morbidity and mortality.

ABDOMINAL AORTIC ANEURYSM

Abdominal aortic aneurysm (AAA) is defined as dilatation of the abdominal aorta to greater than 3 cm in the antero-posterior diameter.[1–6] Aneurysms can occur at any point along the thoracic and abdominal aorta, and can range in length. True aneurysms involve all three layers of the aorta: intima, media, and adventitia. Pseudoaneurysms are caused by local damage to a portion of the media, and are an expansion of only the adventitia. This damage can occur as a result of trauma, infection, or other insults (Fig. 37-1). The primary difference between true and false aneurysms is the integrity of the media.

AAA affects approximately 1–5% of adults over age 50. Ruptured AAA accounts for greater than 16,000 deaths per year in the United States, and is the tenth leading cause of death in men older than 55 years of age.[7,8] Important risk factors for AAA include increasing age, male sex, coronary artery disease, smoking, hypercholesterolemia, and family history of AAA.[1] Aneurysms often remain asymptomatic while slowly enlarging, with eventual rupture in 25–50% of untreated cases.[9] Rupture is associated with an overall mortality exceeding 90%.[10]

AAAs are described anatomically by the relationship of the aneurysm to the renal arteries: suprarenal, transrenal, and infrarenal, with the majority being infrarenal. Most are fusiform, but can be ectatic in form. Aneurysms can also

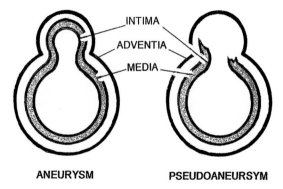

Fig. 37-1. True aneurysm vs. pseudoaneurysm in cross-section. In true aneurysm, all layers are involved. In false aneurysm, the intimae and media are disrupted, and the aneurysm is contained primarily by the adventitia (Original artwork by Georgiann Stevens).

extend above the diaphragm, or exist entirely above the diaphragm. These are described as thoracoabdominal aortic aneurysms (TAAAs) and thoracic aortic aneurysms (TAAs), respectively. TAAs are less common, occurring at a rate of 5 per 100,000 per year. They are often confused with thoracic dissections, but are different in etiology and epidemiology, although a complication of untreated thoracic aortic dissection can be the formation of an aneurysm (Table 37-1).[11,12]

Early diagnosis and repair of asymptomatic lesions is key to reducing overall morbidity and mortality. Elective operative mortality ranges from 2 to 4%, whereas emergent operative mortality for ruptured AAA is estimated at 50%.[2,13] Aneurysms that are less than 6 cm in diameter grow at an average rate of between 4[2] and 7.9 mm/year.[3] Laplace's law describes wall tension as a function of pressure and radius. As the radius increases, wall tension also increases. The aneurysm then has a greater tendency to dilate, leading to further growth. Risk of rupture is low for aneurysms less than 5 cm, but the rate of rupture increases to 76% once the aneurysm is greater than 7 cm in diameter.[3] The risk of rupture generally outweighs the risk of elective surgical repair when the aneurysm exceeds 5.5 cm in diameter, but a risk-benefit assessment needs to be made individually on each patient in whom surgery is considered.

Given the prevalence of AAA in the population older than 50, generalized mass screening has been evaluated extensively. Although some controversy remains, most large, recent studies show benefit in screening men, but not asymptomatic women. Screening with ultrasound between 65 and 74 years of age has shown a 42% risk reduction in an intention to treat analysis. This reduction is due to surgical intervention on asymptomatic individuals, with an aneurysm-related death rate dropping from 0.33% in the nonscreened control group to 0.19% in the group invited to be screened.[14] Conversely, the lower prevalence rate of aneurysm in women compared to men aged 65–80 (1.3% vs. 7.6%) results in no mortality improvement seen with screening women. In this study, the incidence of AAA rupture was the same in the screened and the control group of women.[15] ED bedside ultrasound screening has been shown to appropriately identify asymptomatic patients with AAA in men over 65 years of age.[4,16]

Most aortic aneurysms are the result of degeneration of the elastin and collagen in the media of the aorta,

Table 37-1. Abdominal Aortic Aneurysm and Thoracic Aortic Dissection

Characteristic	Abdominal Aortic Aneurysm	Thoracic Aortic Dissection
Primary location	Infrarenal	Proximal ascending aorta
Typical age	>65	50–70
Male:female ratio	5:1	2:1
Clinical presentation:		
Unruptured	Asymptomatic	Sudden, severe chest or back pain
Ruptured	Hemodynamic collapse	Hemodynamic collapse
Frequency	1–5% >50 years	5–30 per million per year
Primary diagnostic tool	Abdominal Ultrasound	TEE or CTA
ED treatment	BP support	Supportive; limit dP/dt
Definitive therapy	Endovascular stent or surgery	Open surgical repair and/or stenting

leading to decreased structural integrity. While atherosclerosis is often associated with AAA, no causative link has been identified. Many other factors, including genetics, age-related degeneration, hypertension, inflammatory changes, and infections may also be involved. Although a strong familial pattern has been shown, no specific genetic cause has been described.[17]

The role of inflammation in the pathogenesis of arterial disease, including AAA, has become an area of increasing research interest. Several potential infectious etiologies, including *Chlamydia pneumoniae* and cytomegalovirus, have shown suspicious links to AAA,[18,19] and studies have looked at the stabilization or slowing of growth of aneurysms with chronic use of doxycycline and roxithromycin.[20,21,22] The presence of elevated levels of matrix metaliproteinase-2, an inflammatory mediator involved in the destruction of aortic medial matrix, is another line of evidence linking inflammation to the formation of AAA.

Most patients with AAA are asymptomatic. It is often discovered when imaging is performed for other etiologies, such as for cholelithiasis or nephrolithiasis. Thoracic aneurysms are often discovered during routine chest radiography. Some patients will have nonspecific complaints, such as diffuse abdominal, back, or chest pain. The discomfort may radiate to the legs, mimicking sciatica or radiculopathy. A rapidly expanding aneurysm can cause more severe pain. Sudden onset of severe pain, in the setting of a known AAA, is associated with impending rupture.

Physical examination is poor for diagnosing AAA, particularly with small aneurysms.[23] Accuracy improves as the aneurysm enlarges, but unruptured aneurysms larger than 5 cm in diameter are found only 75% of the time on physical examination.[24] Large body habitus and abdominal tenderness complicate the physical examination. Bruits are rarely heard.

Many patients with acute rupture of AAA will die prior to arrival at the ED. For those who arrive alive, the classic findings of hypotension, abdominal and back pain, and a pulsatile abdominal mass, are rarely seen. Flank and periumbilical ecchymosis associated with retroperitoneal hemorrhage are also rare. Other rare presentations include lower extremity paralysis, massive gastrointestinal hemorrhage from aorto-enteric fistula, high output cardiac failure from aorto-caval fistula, and marked hematuria.

History and physical examination are not specific enough to rule out AAA. If suspected, imaging must be performed. No serum markers have been identified which adequately differentiate patients with and without aneurysm, or to distinguish between ruptured and unruptured aneurysms. The traditional gold standard for the diagnosis of AAA is aortography, but this has been largely supplanted by ultrasound in clinical practice, and was first described in 1972.[25] Computed tomography angiography (CTA) and magnetic resonance angiographic (MRA) are also used in the diagnosis and evaluation of AAA.[26] MRA and color Doppler ultrasonography are essentially equivalent in their ability to describe size, location, and involvement of the renal arteries.[26–28] Ultrasound has become the test of choice, as it is low cost, noninvasive, repeatable, and rapid. In critical or hemodynamically unstable patients, ultrasound can be performed at the bedside with a high degree of accuracy (Fig. 37-2).

Bedside emergency physician-performed ultrasound has become a frequently performed modality (Fig. 37-2).[4,5,16,29] While in some instances aortic rupture can be strongly suspected or identified on ultrasound, it is most often not visualized.[29,30] If suspected, surgical consultation is required immediately. An evaluation of the aorta is also advocated as part of a multiview ultrasound examination of the undifferentiated patient with hypotension in the ED.[31]

ED management of AAA depends on the clinical scenario. A small aneurysm discovered incidentally requires follow-up. Aneurysms between 3.0 and 4.4 cm in diameter have a rate of rupture of 2.1% per year, lower than reported operative mortality rates.[32] In another study, no long-term benefit was seen in survival of surgically treated patients with aneurysms between 4.0 and 5.5 cm in diameter who were randomized to immediate repair versus surveillance.[33]

Patients who present with signs or symptoms of impending or ruptured aortic aneurysm need to be treated

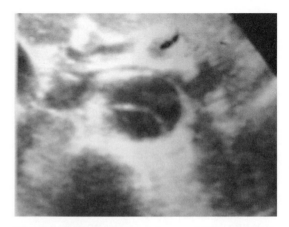

Fig. 37-2. Bedside ultrasound image of abdominal aortic aneurysm with dissection and a false lumen. (Source: Courtesy of Barry Simon, MD.)

aggressively in the ED. Surgical involvement at the earliest possible point is indicated. While ultrasound is the diagnostic test of choice for aneurysm, it is not ideal for diagnosing or localizing rupture.[29] Surgical intervention can proceed based on strong suspicion alone, but some surgeons prefer to know the extent and location of the aneurysm if time permits. This can be identified by CTA, MRA, or aortography. The key is early surgical consultation to determine the ideal diagnostic strategy in the hemodynamically stable patient, and to intervene as early as possible in the unstable patient. While operative mortality of a ruptured AAA remains high, a metaanalysis has shown improved survival in published trials between 1955 and 1998, with an estimated operative morality rate for the year 2000 of 41%.[34] Endovascular stenting procedures may further reduce operative mortality, but are currently primarily used for unruptured aneurysms.

Supportive care is the mainstay of the emergency physicians' intervention for ruptured AAA. The current practice is to maintain a perfusing blood pressure, through fluid resuscitation, blood transfusion, and use of pressor agents when necessary. Inadequate perfusion leads to increased risk of renal failure in the postoperative period, but overhydration carries the risk of worsening rupture and dilutional coagulopathy.[35] If vascular surgical intervention is not available, rapid stabilization and transport to a higher level of care is indicated.

While overall mortality has decreased for AAA, surgical complications remain high. Endovascular repair has become more common, with lower perioperative morbidity and more rapid recovery.[36] Endovascular intervention can be used for patients with high risk of complications, but have a high rate of need for reintervention. The durability of repair and the long-term outcome of patients treated endovascularly are still unknown. Endovascular repairs are currently used primarily for unruptured infrarenal aneurysms.[37] Most procedures for AAA are still traditional open surgical intervention. The specific plan is dependent on the surgeon, and the characteristics of the patient and the aneurysm.

Patients who have previously been treated for AAA are a challenge to the emergency physician. Recurrent aneurysm, leakage, stent migration, stenosis, and occlusion have been reported in postoperative patients.[38,39] Patients with endovascular procedures are often able to be discharged from the hospital rapidly, and therefore postoperative complications that had formerly been seen in hospitalized patients may present to the ED. The evaluation and management of these patients follows the same pattern described above for the evaluation of primary aneurysm, and should be performed in conjunction with the surgeon.

AAA is a disease frequently seen in elderly men. As the population ages, this illness will be diagnosed more frequently. Clinical findings may be subtle and early diagnosis reduces mortality. The emergency physician must consider this diagnosis and intervene early to prevent unnecessary deaths.

THORACIC AORTIC DISSECTION

Aortic dissection occurs when there is a violation of the intima, allowing blood to dissect between and along the tissue planes of the aorta. It is estimated to occur in 5–30 people per million per year. It affects men more than women, with an approximate two to one predominance, and typically affects those between 50 and 70 years of age. Dissection can originate anywhere along the thoracic aorta, but most commonly occurs proximally. Acute aortic dissection is defined as those that present within 2 weeks of symptom onset, and chronic dissection as those that are discovered later (Table 37-1).[40–43]

Aortic dissections are classified in several different ways. The DeBakey classification describes three types, with type I involving the ascending and descending aorta, type II involving only the ascending aorta, and type III involving only the descending aorta.[44] The Stanford classification describes two types. Type A includes the ascending aorta, regardless of the involvement of the arch and descending aorta. This is analogous to DeBakey types I and II. Type B involves the aorta only distal to the takeoff of the left subclavian artery, similar to DeBakey type III.[45] Neither classification system covers dissections which are isolated to the arch. It is probably best to describe the dissections by their actual anatomic extent for the planning of intervention, but the DeBakey and Stanford classifications remain useful for comparing literature and groups of patients (Fig. 37-3).

Intimal violation is theorized to be the initiating event in acute aortic dissection. Once pulsatile blood flow enters the media, it is able to dissect between tissue layers. In this three-dimensional environment, it will dissect both circumferentially and longitudinally along the aorta. While it tends to dissect in the direction of flow, retrograde dissection also occurs. The dissection originates at an area of weakness of the intimae, and/or at an area where wall stress is elevated. When blood flow is turbulent, such as at a bicuspid aortic valve, stenotic aortic outflow track, aortic coarctation, or other anatomic abnormality, dissection is more likely to occur. Blood in the false lumen may rupture back into the true lumen, may clot, or may catastrophically rupture outside of the aorta.[41] Intramural hematoma is considered a variant of aortic dissection.[46]

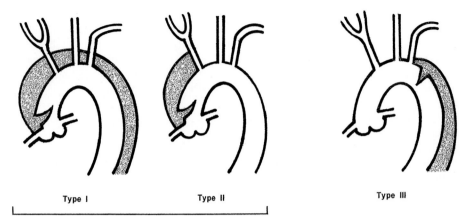

Fig. 37-3. DeBakey and Stanford classifications of thoracic aortic dissection. Stanford type A includes those classified as DeBakey type I and II. Stanford B and DeBakey III are analogous. Neither system describes an aneurysm that is isolated to the arch (Original artwork by Georgiann Stevens).

Age-related degenerative aortic change is the most common risk factor for aortic dissection. Hypertension is present acutely in 70% of patients with proximal dissection, and 35% of those with distal dissection.[40–42] Turner and Noonan syndromes are associated with significantly increased risk for aortic dissection. Patients who have dissection younger than age 40 tend to have a connective tissue disorder such as Marfan or Ehlers-Danlos syndrome.[41] Deceleration trauma can disrupt the intimae and allow for traumatic dissection, particularly at tethered points along the aorta, such as at the root or ligamentum arteriosa. Spontaneous hemorrhage has also been described as an inciting event for dissection.[46] Cocaine use, alone or in combination with other agents, has also been described as a causative factor in acute aortic dissection.[47–49] Mechanisms that increase the change in pressure over time (dP/dt) or weaken the intimae or media are implicated in the formation of aortic dissection.

Aortic dissection can present with a myriad of clinical findings. History and physical examination are non-specific and cannot be relied on to rule in or rule out dissection.[50] The International Registry of Acute Aortic Dissection (IRAD) notes that almost all patients have complaints of sudden onset of chest and or back pain as their primary complaint.[40] The location of pain may vary depending on the location of the dissection, and pain that migrates may indicate extension of the dissection. Classic tearing or ripping pain occurs in 51% of patients.[40] The absence of sudden onset of pain lowers the likelihood of dissection, but cannot rule it out.[50] In a pooled analysis,

approximately half the patients had hypertension on initial evaluation, and 31% had either pulse deficits or blood pressure differentials on examination.[50]

The variable location and involvement of other vessels allows for a plethora of clinical symptoms. Acute aortic regurgitation and congestive heart failure can occur from dissection back toward or initiating at the aortic root. At the same site, involvement of the ostia of the coronary arteries can lead to ischemia and mimic myocardial infarction. Involvement of the innominate or carotid arteries can lead to stroke symptoms, and the presence of new neurologic deficit in the face of chest pain, should lead the physician to strongly consider the possibility of acute aortic dissection. Involvement of penetrating arteries, which supply the spinal cord, can lead to lower extremity paralysis. Dissection into the renal or mesenteric vessels can complicate the clinical picture further.

Hypotension, shock, and syncope are also common presentations.[40–42,50] Many patients die within the first 24 hours of symptoms, with 38% missed on initial evaluation and 28% discovered at autopsy.[40,42,50]

The diagnosis of acute aortic dissection in the ED requires maintaining a high degree of suspicion. Imaging is required. A clinical probability model (Table 37-2) has been described, with the low probability group having a 7% risk of acute aortic dissection and high probability having more than 83% risk of dissection.[51] Absence of aortic or mediastinal widening on chest radiograph lowers the suspicion; however, chest radiography by itself is not adequate to diagnose or exclude dissection.[52]

Table 37-2. Risk Stratification for Thoracic Aortic Dissection

Predictor	Risk with Presence of Predictor
Chest pain with sudden onset and/or ripping or tearing sensation	Intermediate risk: 31%
Aortic or mediastinal widening on chest radiograph	Intermediate risk: 39%
Pulse deficit or blood pressure differentials	High risk: 83%
Presence of 2 or 3 above predictors	High risk: 83%
Absence of all 3 predictors	Low risk: 7%

Source: von Kodolitsch Y, Schwartz AG, Nienaber CA. Clinical prediction of aortic dissection. *Arch Int Med* 2000;160:2977–2982.

Electrocardiography is also nonspecific in the evaluation of aortic dissection, and may show evidence of ischemia or infarction, related to global hypoperfusion or involvement of the coronary arteries.[50] Elevated serum levels of smooth muscle heavy chain myosin has been proposed as a biochemical marker of aortic dissection, but is not yet proven or clinically available.[53]

Clinicians can image the aorta with aortography, transesophageal echocardiography (TEE), CTA, and MRA with a high degree of accuracy. CTA is usually the initial test of choice, and has an overall sensitivity of 93%, similar to aortography with an overall sensitivity of 87%. MRI has a 100% sensitivity, but its use is limited currently by the long duration of the procedure and the need to remove the patient from the care environment for a prolonged period of time. Aortography is invasive, and MRI, CTA, and aortography all require dye administration. Transthoracic echocardiography has limited use in identifying dissection, but can be used to evaluate cardiac function and the pericardium at the bedside.[31] TEE can be done at the bedside with minimal sedation, and is a good choice in patients with a contrast allergy, but is often not immediately available.[46,54,55] All imaging modalities have some ability to visualize other potential etiologies and complications of aortic dissection, but TEE is ideal for evaluation of valvular involvement and pericardial effusion/tamponade.

When dissection is strongly suspected on clinical grounds, involvement of the surgeon is indicated prior to extensive diagnostic testing. CTA is rapid, readily available, and sensitive, and is often the first choice for testing. Supportive care should be initiated immediately, and other causes of patient symptomatology need to be excluded. Lowering dP/dt is the traditional approach to limiting extension of the aneurysm. This is best accomplished with the combination of short-acting agents that

are vasodilatory and have negative chronotropicity. A combination of β-blockade with a short-acting agent such as esmolol, and vasodilation with nitroprusside is often used, but labetalol as a single medication with both α- and β-blockade, and other agents are acceptable alternatives.[41] Adequate blood pressure to perfuse end-organs needs to be maintained. Patients with uncomplicated, type B distal aortic dissections may be managed nonsurgically.

Traditionally, proximal dissections in patients who are good candidates have been treated with open surgical intervention.[56] There are a number of surgical approaches, and the particular approach depends on the surgeon, and the clinical scenario.[57] In addition to resection and replacement of the aorta, gelatin resorcin formalin tissue adhesive has been used to reapproximate and seal the dissected tissue layers.[58] More recently, endovascular stenting has been used, either as the only procedure or as an adjunct to operative intervention.[59,60] Aortic valve replacement and coronary artery bypass grafting may be required. With a lower mortality, higher risk patients and some with distal aortic dissections are being treated with endovascular procedures. Endovascular stent grafting has also been used successfully in the treatment of acute traumatic aortic dissection.[61]

Delayed complications of aortic dissection are common. Recurrent dissections, aneurysms at the location of dissection, and pseudoaneurysm at anastomosis or graft sites are among the complications that can be seen in the ED after intervention for dissection. Imaging with TEE, TTE, CTA, or MRI is often indicated if there is a concern for a complication related to the initial dissection. Supportive care and surgical consultation are indicated for hemodynamically unstable patients. Radiologic investigations in the stable patient should be performed in consultation with the vascular surgeon.[41]

ACUTE AORTIC OCCLUSIVE DISEASE

Acute aortic occlusion is rare, and is often severe and life threatening. It often occurs as a result of thromboembolus or plaque rupture in an aorta with underlying severe atherosclerosis. Severe atherosclerotic disease is seen more commonly in men, and is associated with coronary artery and peripheral vascular disease. Smoking, diabetes mellitus, high cholesterol, and hypertension are risk factors.[62,63] Takayasu's giant cell arteritis is an uncommon cause of occlusive aortic disease, seen mainly in women of Japanese descent. It is an autoimmune inflammatory disease, and can cause progressive distal aortic occlusion over time. Treatment can be medical or surgical.[64]

Chronic aortic occlusive disease is often manifest by claudication symptoms, primarily in the buttocks, thighs, and calves. Male sexual dysfunction, Leriche syndrome, occurs as a result of bilateral aortoiliac occlusion. Acute occlusion of the aorta as a result of embolization is often sudden in onset and associated with severe pain. The "5 Ps" of acute arterial occlusion—pallor, pulselessness, poikilothermia, paresthesias, and paralysis—may also be present.[62] Anesthesia and paralysis may represent irreversible ischemia.[65]

ED evaluation and management of acute aortic occlusion includes diagnostic evaluation, supportive care, and intervention in consultation with the vascular surgeon. The diagnosis can be strongly suspected on clinical grounds. Definitive diagnosis can be made with Doppler ultrasound, CTA, MRI, or aortography. Echocardiography, in particular TEE, can be used as an adjunct to diagnose residual cardiac thrombus. Ankle-brachial indices (ABI), the ratio of the calf to upper arm systolic blood pressures, are used to diagnose peripheral vascular disease. An ABI of less than 0.9 suggests disease, and less than 0.4 indicates severe, limb-threatening ischemia.[62,63]

Heparinization and supportive care is the initial treatment in the ED. Interventions may include thrombectomy, systemic- or catheter-directed thrombolysis, and bypass grafting.[63,65] In cases of irreversible ischemia, amputation is indicated to prevent reperfusion-related complications. For chronic obstruction, specific management in the ED should be decided in conjunction with the vascular surgeon.

SUMMARY AND CONCLUSIONS

Acute aortic disease is seen frequently in the ED. The diagnosis is often challenging, due to the subtle and non-specific nature of the clinical presentation. Aortic dissection, aneurysm, and occlusion should be considered in a wide variety of complaints and patient populations.

Supportive care is the mainstay of ED treatment. The emergency physician should be familiar with the appropriate diagnostic tests for each of these entities. A close working relationship with the vascular surgeon and radiologist is key to the rapid diagnosis and treatment of patients with acute aortic emergencies.

REFERENCES

1. Lederle FA, Johnson GR, Wilson SE, et al. Prevalence and associations of abdominal aortic aneurysm detected through screening. Aneurysm Detection and Management (ADAM) Veterans Affairs Cooperative Study Group. *Ann Intern Med* (United States) 1997;126(6):441–449.

2. LaRoy L, Cormier P, Matalon T, et al. Imaging of the abdominal aortic aneurysms. *Am J Radiogr* 1989;152: 785–792.

3. Littooy F, Steffan G, Greisler H, et al. Use of sequential B-mode ultrasonography to manage abdominal aortic aneurysms. *Arch Surg* 1989;124:419–421.

4. Kuhn M, Bonnin RL, Davey MJ, et al. Emergency department ultrasound scanning for abdominal aortic aneurysm: Accessible, accurate, and advantageous. *Ann Emerg Med* 2000;36(3):219–223.

5. Lanoix R, Leak LV, Gaeta T, et al. A preliminary evaluation of emergency ultrasound in the setting of an emergency medicine training program. *Am J Emerg Med* 2000;18(1):41–45.

6. Akkersdijk GJ, Puylaert JB, de Vries AC. Abdominal aortic aneurysm as an incidental finding in abdominal ultrasonography. *Br J Surg* 1991:78(10):1261–1263.

7. US Public Health Service: Vital statistics of The United States, Vol II Mortality, Part A. Department of Health and Human Service, Publication NO (PHS) 87–1101. Washington DC: US Government Printing Office, 1987.

8. National Center for Health Statistics. Vital Statistics of the United States 2000. Available at: http://www.cdc.gov/nchs. Accessed February 20, 2004.

9. Lederle F, Walker J, Reinke D. Selective screening for abdominal aortic aneurysms with physical examination and ultrasound. *Arch Intern Med* 1988;148:1753–1756.

10. Rohrer MJ, Cutler BS, Wheeler HB. Long-term survival and quality of life following ruptured abdominal aortic aneurysm. *Arch Surg* 1988;123:1213–1217.

11. Fann JI. Descending thoracic and thoracoabdominal aneurysms. *Coron Artery Dis* 2002;13:93–103.

12. Moon MR, Sundt TM. Aortic arch aneurysms. *Coron Artery Dis* 2002;13:85–92.

13. Collin J. Screening for abdominal aortic aneurysms. *Br J Surg* 1985;72:851–852.

14. Ashton HA, Buxton MJ, Day NE, et al. The Multicentre Aneurysm Screening Study (MASS) into the effect of abdominal aortic aneurysm screening on mortality in men: A randomised controlled trial. *Lancet* 2002;360(9345): 1531–1539.

15. Scott RA, Bridgewater SG, Ashton HA. Randomized clinical trial of screening for abdominal aortic aneurysm in women. *Br J Surg* 2002;89(3):283.

16. Salen P, Melanson S, Buro D. ED screening to identify abdominal aortic aneurysms in asymptomatic geriatric patients. *Am J Emerg Med* 2003;21:133–135.

17. Wassef M, Baxter BT, Chisholm RL, et al. Pathogenesis of abdominal aortic aneurysms: A multidisciplinary research program supported by the National Heart, Lung, and Blood Institute. *J Vasc Surg* 2001;34:730–738.

18. Epstein SE, Zhou TF, Zhu J. Infection and atherosclerosis: Emerging mechanistic paradigms. *Circulation* 1999;100: e20–e28.

19. Lindholt JS, Juul S, Vammen S, et al. Immunoglobulin A antibodies against *Chlamydia pneumoniae* are associated with expansion of abdominal aortic aneurysm. *Br J Surg* 1999;86:634–638.

20. Morrison M, Juvonen J, Biancari F, et al. Use of doxy-cycline to decrease the growth rate of abdominal aortic aneurysms: A randomized, double-blind pacebo-controlled pilot study. *J Vasc Surg* 2001;34:606–610.

21. Vammen S, Lindholt JS, Ostergaard L, et al. Randomized, double-blind controlled trial of roxithromycin for pre-vention of abdominal aortic aneurysm expansion. *Br J Surg* 2001;88:1066–1072.

22. Goodall S, Crowther M, Hemmingway DM. Ubiquitous elevation of matrix metalloproteinase-2 expression in the vas-culature of patients with abdominal aneurysms. *Circulation* 2001;104(3):304–309.

23. Fink HA, Lederle FA, Roth CS, et al. The accuracy of physical examination to detect abdominal aortic aneurysm. *Arch Intern Med* 2000;160:833–836.

24. Lederle FA, Simel DL. The rational clinical examination. Does this patient have abdominal aortic aneurysm? *JAMA* (United States) 1999;281(1):77–82.

25. Leopold GR, Goldberger LE, Bernstein EF. Ultrasonic detection and evaluation of abdominal aortic aneurysms. *Surgery* 1972;72:939–945.

26. Flak B, Li DK, Knickerbocker WJ, et al. Magnetic resonance imaging of aneurysms of the abdominal aorta. *Am J Roentgenol* 1985;144:991–996.

27. Carriero A, Iezzi A, Magarelli N, et al. Magnetic resonance angiography and colour-Doppler sonography in the evaluation of abdominal aortic aneurysm. *Eur Radiol* 1997;7(9):1495–1500.

28. Amparo EG, Hoddick WK, Hricak H, et al. Comparison of magnetic resonance imaging and ultrasonography in the evaluation of abdominal aortic aneurysms. *Radiology* 1985;154:451–456.

29. Shuman WP, Hastrup W, Kohler TR, et al. Suspected leaking abdominal aortic aneurysm: Use of sonography in the emergency room. *Radiology* 1988;168(1):117–119.

30. Miller J. Small ruptured abdominal aneurysm diagnosed by emergency physician ultrasound. *Am J Emerg Med* 1999;17(2):174–175.

31. Rose JS, Bair AE, Mandavia D, et al. The UHP ultrasound protocol: A novel ultrasound approach to the empiric evaluation of the undifferentiated hypotensive patient. *Am J Emerg Med* 2001;19(4):299–302.

32. Scott RA, Tisi PV, Ashton HA, et al. Abdominal aortic aneurysm rupture rates: A 7-year follow-up of the entire abdominal aortic aneurysm population detected by screening. *J Vasc Surg* 1998;28(1):124–128.

33. Lederle FA, Wilson SE, Johnson GR, et al. Immediate repair compared with surveillance of small abdominal aortic aneurysms. *N Engl J Med* 2002;346(19):1437–1444.

34. Brown MJ, Sutton AJ, Bell PR, et al. A meta-analysis of 50 years of ruptured aortic aneurysm repair. *Br J Surg* 2002;89(6):714–730.

35. Donaldson MC, Rosenberg JM, Buckman CA. Factors affecting survival after ruptured abdominal aortic aneurysm. *J Vasc Surg* 1985;2:564–570.

36. Brewster DC, Cronenwett JL, Hallett JW, et al. Guidelines for the treatment of abdominal aortic aneurysms. Report of a subcommittee of the Joint Council of the American Association for Vascular Surgery and Society for Vascular Surgery. *J Vasc Surg* 2003;37(5):1106–1117.

37. Bush RL, Lin PH, Lumsden AB. Endovascular management of abdominal aortic aneurysms. *J Cardiovasc Surg* 2003; 44(4):527–534.

38. Becquemin JP, Kelley L, Zubilewicz, et al. Outcomes of secondary interventions afterabdominal aortic aneurysm endovascular repair. *J Vasc Surg* 2004;39(2):298–305.

39. Parodi JC, Ferreira LM. Ten-year experience with endovascular therapy in aortic aneurysms. *J Am Coll Surg* 2002;194(1 Suppl):S58–S66.

40. Hagan PG, Nienaber CA, Isselbacher EM, et al. The International Registry of Acute Aortic Dissection (IRAD): New insights into an old disease. *JAMA* 2000;283:897–903.

41. Khan IA, Nair CK. Clinical, diagnostic, and management per-spectives of aortic dissection. *Chest* 2002;122(1):311–328.

42. Spittell PC, Spittell JA, Joyce JW, et al. Clinical features and differential diagnosis of aortic dissection: Experience with 236 cases (1980 though 1990). *Mayo Clin Proc* 1993;68:642–651.

43. Meszaros I, Morocz J, Szlavi J, et al. Epidemiology and clini-copathology of aortic dissection. *Chest* 2000;117:1271–1278.

44. DeBakey ME, Henly WS, Cooley DA, et al. Surgical man-agement of dissecting aneurysms of the aorta. *Thorac Cardiovasc Surg* 1965;49:130–148.

45. Dailey PO, Trueblood HW, Stinson EB, et al. Management of acute aortic dissections. *Ann Thorac Surg* 1970;10:237–246.

46. O'Gara PT, DeSanctis RW. Acute aortic dissection and its variants: Toward a common diagnostic and therapeutic approach. *Circulation* 1995;92:1376–1378.

47. Perron AD, Gibbs M. Thoracic aortic dissection secondary to crack cocaine ingestion. *Am J Emerg Med* 1997;15:507–509.

48. Hsue PY, Salinas CL, Bolger AF, et al. Acute aortic dis-section related to crack cocaine. *Circulation* 2002;105(13): 1592–1595.

49. Famularo G, Polchi D, DiBona G, et al. Acute aortic dissection after cocaine and sildenafil abuse. *J Emerg Med* 2001;21(1):78–79.

50. Klompas M. Does this patient have an acute thoracic aortic dissection? *JAMA* 2002;287(17):2262–2272.

51. von Kodolitsch Y, Schwartz AG, Nienaber CA. Clinical prediction of aortic dissection. *Arch Intern Med* 2000; 160:2977–2982.

52. von Kodolitsch Y. Chest radiography for the diagnosis of acute aortic syndrome. *Am J Med* 2004;116(2):73–77.

53. Suzuki T, Katoh H, Tsuchio Y, et al. Diagnostic implications of elevated levels of smooth-muscle myosin heavy-chain protein in acute aortic dissection: The smooth muscle myosin heavy chain study. *Ann Intern Med* 2000;133:537–541.

54. Moore AG, Eagle KA, Bruckman D. Choice of computed tomography, transesophageal echocardiography, magnetic resonance imaging, and aortography in acute aortic dissection: International Registry of Acute Aortic Dissection (IRAD). *Am J Cardiol* 2002;89:1235–1237.

55. Penco M, Paparoni S, Dagianti A, et al. Usefulness of transesophageal echocardiography in the assessment of aortic dissection. *Am J Cardiol* 2000;86(Suppl):53G–56G.

56. Borst HG, Laas J. Surgical treatment of thoracic aortic aneurysms. *Adv Card Surg* 1993;4:47–87.

57. Guilmet D, Bachet J, Goudot B, et al. Aortic dissection: Anatomic types and surgical approaches. *J Cardiovasc Surg (Torino)* 1993;34:23–32.

58. Hata M, Shiono M, Orime Y, et al. The efficacy and midterm results with use of gelatin resorcin formalin (GRF) glue for aortic surgery. *Ann Thorac Cardiovasc Surg* 1999;5:321–325.

59. Dake MD, Kato N, Mitchell RS, et al. Endovascular stent-graft placement for the treatment of acute aortic dissection. *N Engl J Med* 1999;340:1546–1552.

60. Fleck T, Hutschala D, Czerny M, et al. Combined surgical and endovascular treatment of acute aortic dissection type A: Preliminary results. *Ann Thorac Surg* 2002;74:761–766.

61. Thompson CS, Rodriguez JA, Ramaiah VG, et al. Acute traumatic rupture of the thoracic aorta treated with endoluminal stent grafts. *J Trauma* 2002;52(6):1173–1177.

62. Ouriel K. Peripheral arterial disease. *Lancet* 2001;358: 1257–1264.

63. Thrombolysis in the management of lower limb peripheral arterial occlusion: A concensus document. Working Party on Thrombolysis in the Management of Limb Ischemia. *Am J Cardiol* 1998;81:207–218.

64. Giordano JM. Surgical treatment of Takayasu's disease. *Cleve Clin J Med* 2002;69(Suppl 2):S146–S148.

65. Dieter RS, Chu WW, Pancanowski JP, et al. The significance of lower extremity peripheral vascular disease. *Clin Cardiol* 2002;25:3–10.

38

Cardiac Toxicology

James Edward Weber

HIGH YIELD FACTS

- A multitude of drugs intended for a variety of treatment indications, in addition to drug-drug interactions, can have adverse effects on the cardiovascular system.
- Abnormal cardiac function results from alteration of adequate systemic vascular resistance, cardiac pump function, or conduction.
- Initial management includes general supportive care, preventing ongoing exposure, preventing further gastrointestinal absorption, and enhancing excretion.
- Advanced therapeutic measures depend on the toxin, and frequently include the use of specific medical therapy (antidotes, antibodies), or mechanical therapy (hemodialysis, intraaortic balloon counterpulsation [IABC], cardiopulmonary bypass [CPB]) when indicated.

INTRODUCTION

Ingestions of substances, whether therapeutic medications or toxic materials, frequently exhibit deleterious effects on the cardiovascular system. Regardless of the culprit substance, maintenance of adequate oxygen delivery and tissue perfusion depends on preservation of three key components: (1) adequate systemic vascular resistance, (2) cardiac contractility, and (3) integrity of the cardiac rhythm. Correspondingly, the cardiotoxic effects of drugs may be clinically manifested by the development of (1) hypotension or hypertension, (2) congestive heart failure or pulmonary edema, or (3) conduction abnormalities or arrhythmias.

Prompt recognition of these specific cardiovascular abnormalities by the emergency physician is essential in determining the particular class or type of drug responsible as well as administration of potentially life-saving treatment.

Hemodynamic Abnormalities

The majority of medications or toxins that affect blood pressure do so by modification of the normal chemical interaction at the postganglionic sympathetic neurons. The interaction between these nerve endings and the receptors on blood vessels determines vascular tonicity and blood pressure.

Norepinephrine (NE) is synthesized and stored in presynaptic vesicles in the nerve ending. With sympathetic stimulation, NE is released into the synapse, and subsequently one of three actions occurs: (1) NE may be metabolized by catechol-*o*-methyltransferase (COMT) or monoamine oxidase (MAO), (2) may be actively pumped back into the neuron, or (3) may bind to receptor sites on the postsynaptic blood vessel. NE binding to alpha-receptors on the blood vessels cause vasoconstriction; conversely, catecholamines that bind to beta-receptors cause vasodilatation, which clinically results in a decrease in blood pressure.

Drug-Induced Hypertension

The majority of drugs or toxins that cause an increase in blood pressure are mediated by alpha-receptors. Their mechanism of action typically falls into one of four categories: (1) stimulating release of NE storage granules, (2) decreasing uptake of NE into presynaptic cleft, (3) decreasing the degradation of NE, or (4) directly interacting with alpha-receptors. Those drugs which increase NE release or decrease uptake are termed "indirect acting" agents. Although physical examination alone will infrequently establish the culprit drug in any toxic ingestion, nearly all drugs that may cause hypertension as one of their symptoms fall into the category of sympathomimetic, tricyclic antidepressant (TCA), or beta-receptor agonists (Table 38-1).

Drug-Induced Hemodynamic Instability

A large number of drugs are capable of inducing hypotension and or hemodynamic instability (Table 38-2). Certain classes of agents exert their hypotensive effects as a consequence of surpassing their intended therapeutic effects. Drug-induced hypotension can occur directly or indirectly, as a result of coexisting hypoxia, anaphylaxis, hypovolemia, or arrhythmias. Identification of the culpable agent often requires the incorporation of a detailed history, physical examination (including the identification of specific toxidromic features), and laboratory studies.

Table 38-1. Classes of Drugs and Toxins that may Induce Hypertension

Alpha-Mediated Effects
Direct alpha-adrenergic agonists
Indirect alpha-adrenergic agonists
Combined direct and indirect alpha-adrenergic agonists

Non-Alpha-Mediated Effects
Stimulants of RAAS
Beta-adrenergic receptor agents
    Nonselective
    Predominantly beta-2 selective
Cholinomimetics
Nicotine
Renal toxins (secondary effect)
Steroids
Thromboxane (via angiotensin II)
Vasopressin

Source: Modified from Hessler, R.A. *Goldfrank's Toxicologic Emergencies*, 7th ed. McGraw-Hill, New York, 2002, p. 320.

Congestive Heart Failure

The second type of medication-induced cardiotoxic effect is congestive heart failure or pulmonary edema. Pulmonary edema can be further subdivided into (1) cardiogenic or (2) noncardiogenic. Cardiogenic pulmonary edema occurs as a result of the medication's direct effects on cardiac contractility, thus impairing cardiac output resulting in volume

Table 38-2. Drug Classes or Toxins that may Cause Hypotension

Antihypertensives
Adrenergic antagonists
ACE inhibitors
Centrally acting alpha-2-antagonists
Peripherally acting alpha-1-antagonists
Ganglionic blocking agents
Vasodilators
Antianginals
Antidepressants
Antiparkinson agents
Diuretics
CNS depressants
Antipsychotics
Toxins causing volume depletion

Source: Modified from Hessler, R.A. *Goldfrank's Toxicologic Emergencies*, 7th ed. McGraw-Hill, New York, 2002, p. 323.

overload. Numerous drugs can exert depressant effects on cardiac contractility, either by acute or chronic exposure. Noncardiogenic pulmonary edema (NCPE) is defined as increased intraalveolar fluid in the lungs with preserved cardiac output. Although several mechanisms for NCPE have been proposed, no single etiology has been ascertained. Hypoventilation, hypoxia, and direct capillary epithelial toxins have been proposed. NCPE has been reported with drugs such as solvents, salicylates, stimulants, opioids, nonsteroidal anti-inflammatory drug (NSAIDs), and cocaine.

Drug-Induced Conduction Abnormalities

The etiology of cardiac conduction abnormalities or arrhythmias that affect myocardial cellular function occur either directly, or indirectly via the CNS. With the exception of specific agents known to precipitate conduction abnormalities (e.g., calcium-channel blockers [CCB] and antiarrhythmics), the underlying mechanism is usually unknown. Regardless of the underlying mechanism, arrhythmias result from electrophysiologic disturbances of electrolyte channels, which inadvertently affect the normal myocardial cell action potential.

Cardiac arrhythmias are can be produced by the disruption of any of three different mechanisms: (1) automaticity, (2) reentry, and (3) triggering. Catecholamines and digoxin are examples of drugs that cause myocardial pacemaker cells to spontaneously depolarize more rapidly, thus increasing automaticity. Reentry phenomena occurs when an early impulse (atrial or ventricular premature beat) triggers an impulse after a branch point is no longer refractory to stimulation, thus resulting in retrograde conduction. Reentry mechanisms are responsible for most of the proarrhythmic effects of antiarrhythmic agents. Triggered arrhythmias occur after the depolarization period, during the resting phase of the action potential. Additionally, some drugs exert their cardiotoxic effects by propagation of electrical impulses through the conduction system. The result includes first, second, or third degree (complete) heart block. When conduction is delayed through the right or left bundle branches, the result may be widening of the QRS complex or prolongation of the QT interval.

General Therapeutic Strategies
Drug-Induced Hypertensive Emergencies

Regardless of the mechanism, drug-induced hypertensive emergencies are often transient, and once NE depletion (*washout*) occurs, hypotension may actually ensue. Therefore, aggressive therapy to treat overdoses such TCA or cocaine is usually unnecessary. However, if the blood pressure remains severely elevated, or if the patients displays evidence of end-organ dysfunction, therapy with a short-acting intravenous agent should be used in small initial doses, and with careful monitoring. Short-acting benzodiazepines, such as lorazepam, are first-line therapy.[1] In patients with drug-induced hypertensive emergencies refractory to benzodiazepines, short-acting antihypertensive agents such as sodium nitroprusside should be considered as a second-line agent. Labetalol, a nonselective beta-2-blocker and alpha-blocker, has demonstrated efficacy for hypertensive emergencies associated with sympathomimetic poisoning and is considered a third-line agent. However, labetalol should be used in carefully titrated doses because of its predominantly beta-blocking properties. Propranolol is contraindicated because it blocks only beta-2-receptors, leaving unopposed alpha-adrenergic stimulation and actually worsening hypertension.[2]

Drug-Induced Hemodynamic Instability

Agents used to optimize cardiac output and blood pressure in cardiogenic shock and arrest states are discussed in detail, see page 35. The first step in managing toxic patients with hemodynamic abnormalities is to aggressively support the vital signs. Intravenous fluids should be administered, and restricted only by the presence of congestive heart failure. Crystalloid administration should precede administration of vasopressor or inotropic agents. If the exact cardiotoxic agent responsible for hypotension is identified, other pharmacologic strategies may be more effective.

Drug-Induced Pulmonary Edema

In general, early aggressive intervention is warranted with drug-induced pulmonary edema. Initial management of drug-induced pulmonary edema mimics that of pulmonary edema caused by a pure cardiac source. Efforts should be directed at reducing preload and afterload, while increasing cardiac output. Management considerations should include supplemental oxygen, or alternatively, noninvasive or endotracheal intubation when appropriate. Simultaneously, patients should receive aggressive hemodynamic support. After initial stabilization, a pulmonary artery catheter (Swan-Ganz) may be useful for distinguishing cardiac versus NCPE, and assist in guiding therapy in critically ill patients. Although irreversible structural disease may be present, cardiotoxic patients with pulmonary edema frequently have a reversible process. No specific antidotes exist for drug-induced pulmonary edema.

Drug-Induced Arrhythmias

In general, the generation of cardiac arrhythmias are rarely attributable to a specific drug. Treatment should be directed at reversing the precise conduction abnormality present. Advanced cardiac life support (ACLS) protocols should be followed for drug-induced arrhythmias and conduction abnormalities. In the presence of hypotension, chest pain, or congestive heart failure, tachyarrhythmias should be treated with electrical cardioversion. In the absence of hemodynamic compromise, appropriate selection of an antiarrhythmic agent may be useful in terminating the event. Specific therapy directed at the culpable toxin should be administered if available. The treatment of drug-induced tachyarrhythmias initially depends on the hemodynamic status of the patient. In patients with supraventricular arrhythmias who are hemodynamically stabile, careful observation and monitoring, along with enhanced drug elimination, is the safest strategy. The presence of a wide QRS complex should be presumed to be ventricular tachycardia until proven otherwise.

The initial treatment of drug-induced bradycardia initially includes atropine. Internal pacing is the definitive treatment for patients who fail to respond to atropine therapy, or in the presence of hypotension, myocardial ischemia, or congestive heart failure.

Pathophysiology and Management of Specific Agents

Recognition and treatment of hemodynamic abnormalities is often required prior to identification of the drug or toxin responsible. Initial clinical measures should always include the prevention of continuous exposure and further gastrointestinal absorption by using activated charcoal and application of enhanced elimination techniques. Additional interventions vary depending on the drug or toxin, and frequently include the use of specific medical therapy or mechanical intervention (Table 38-3).

Beta-Blocker Toxicity

Beta-adrenergic blocking agents decrease cardiac contractility and heart rate, with a consequential decrease in cardiac output and blood pressure. Beta-1-receptors increase the force and rate of myocardial contraction and atrioventricular (AV) node conduction velocity. Blockade of beta-receptors results in decreased production of intracellular cyclic adenosine monophosphate (cAMP) with the resultant cardiovascular effects due to suppression of

Table 38-3. Cardiac Toxicity Therapies

Treatment	VP	Atro	AD	CaCl	Ins	HCO3	VD	AR	HD	CP	IABC	CPB
Beta-blocker	+*	+†	+‡		(−)§				+¶	+a	+b	+b
CCB	+*	+†		+c	(−)§						+b	+b
Opiate			+d									
TCA	+*				+e			+e				+b
Cocaine							+f	+e				
Digoxin		+†	+g	(−)	+h	+h		+i		+a		

Abbreviations: VP = vasopressors, Atro = atropine, AD = antidote, CaCl = calcium chloride, Ins = insulin, HCO3 = sodium bicarbonate, VD = vasodilators, AR = antiarrhythmic, HD = hemodialysis, CP = cardiac pacing, IABC = intraaortic balloon counterpulsation, CPB = cardiopulmonary bypass, Dob = dobutamine, DA = dopamine, NE = norepinephrine, EPI = epinephrine, PE = phenylephrine, NTG = nitroglycerin, BNZ = benzodiazepines, VD = volume of distribution.

*Dob, DA, NE, and EPI may be effective at ↑doses. For TCA OD, alpha-agonists NE or PE preferred.
†Atro 0.5 mg IV repeated q 5 min prn.
‡Initial dose of glucagon is 2–5 mg IV, followed by a dose of 10 mg if needed. Clinical endpoint is improvement in BP rather than increase in HR.
§Insulin-euglycemia or pump therapy not yet recommended.
¶May be effective for beta-blockers with small VD.
a CP considered; capture may be difficult. Not necessary for digoxin toxicity if Fab available.
b May be lifesaving for shock refractory to medical therapy.
c CaCl 1–3 mg slow IV push, in absence of digoxin toxicity.
d Initial naloxone dose 2 mg IV. Synthetic opiate OD may require higher doses.
e HCO3 1–2 me/kg IV to alkalinize blood pH to 7.50–7.55. If refractory arrhythmias persist, lidocaine should be considered.
f NTG and BNZ first line for chest pain. Phentolamine is second-line agent if refractory.
g Digoxin-specific Fab given 10–20 vials empirically. Quick estimate for adults: #vials = (digoxin serum level × Pt wt (kg))/100.
h Should be given with D_{50} and exchange resins for hyperkalemia if Fab not immediately available.
i For digoxin-induced VT or VF, phenytoin up to 1000 mg IV (50 mg/min max rate) or lidocaine 1 mg/kg IV bolus followed by 1–4 mg/min infusion.

circulating catecholamines. Beta-blockers, therefore, reduce heart rate, blood pressure, myocardial contractility, and myocardial oxygen consumption. Significant toxicity manifests as bradycardia, AV block, and/or hypotension. The clinical toxicity manifestations of a specific beta-blocker vary with lipid solubility, oral availability, metabolism, membrane-stabilizing activity, and intrinsic sympathomimetic activity.[3] The negative inotropicity of beta-blockers contributes more to the occurrence of hypotension than rate-related decreases in cardiac output; and bradycardia may not be present in otherwise symptomatic patients.[4]

The initial treatment for beta-blocker-induced hypotension and bradycardia consists of atropine and intravenous crystalloid. The response to atropine is often incomplete, thus necessitating additional therapy. Glucagon is considered by many to be the antidote of choice, despite inconsistent success rates.[5] The inotropic effects of glucagon are qualitatively similar to those of catecholamine agents but are not mediated by the beta-

receptors. As a result, glucagon can work in patients undergoing beta-blockade therapy, whereas catecholamines cannot gain access to the receptors. Hypotension and bradycardia caused by beta-blocker poisoning may respond more predictably to glucagon than to catecholamine therapy.

In general, the initial dose of glucagon is 2–5 mg intravenously, followed by a dose of 10 mg if needed. An upper limit dose has not been established. There are reports of benefit from calcium chloride with beta-blocker toxicity.[6,7] However, for drug-induced shock from other than for CCB overdose, this is not recommended due to limited data.[8] Adrenergic support with dobutamine, dopamine, NE, and epinephrine may be useful in some patients, but they may require higher than usual doses to be effective. Recently intravenous insulin, with sufficient glucose to maintain euglycemia, has been found to produce excellent results in experimental models of beta-blocker overdose.[9] Although the mechanism is undefined, the benefit is probably related to improved energy handling by the myocytes, and the result is enhanced inotropism. Although animal studies are promising, recommendations for the use of insulin-euglycemia or insulin pump therapy have been withheld until comparative human data are available.

Mechanical strategies are worth consideration in refractory cases. Charcoal hemoperfusion and dialysis may be appropriate for beta-blocking agents such as atenolol, nadolol, and acebutolol, which have a high level of urinary excretion and a small volume of distribution. External pacemakers may be employed, but capture or acceleration may be difficult. The use of circulatory assist devices such as IABC or emergency CPB may be lifesaving in patients with drug-induced shock refractory to maximal medical therapy.[10,11]

Calcium-Channel Blocker Toxicity

The cardiovascular effects of CCB overdose are due to peripheral vasodilation, decreased chronotropic and inotropic properties, and impairment of cardiac conduction. CCB overdose also results in suppression of insulin release from the pancreas and decreased free fatty acid utilization by the myocardium, thus further depressing cardiac contractility. Therefore, CCB overdose may cause profound hypotension and bradycardia, often accompanied by various degrees of AV heart block.

Although CCB and beta-blocker agents are often classified together, subtle differences in presentation are noteworthy. For example, patients with CCB poisoning more often remain conscious despite profound vital sign abnormalities. Conversely, the opposite is true of patients who have taken an overdose of beta-blockers. Whether this difference occurs because calcium-channel blockers promote neuronal stability by inhibiting the influx of calcium or because most beta-blockers are highly lipophilic is not known. In general, overdose by short-acting agents is characterized by rapid progression to cardiac arrest. Overdose by extended release formulations result in delayed onset of arrhythmias, shock, and sudden cardiac collapse.

For patients in CCB-induced shock, catecholamine type vasopressors are considered first-line drug therapy. In patients with CCB-induced shock refractory to conventional catecholamine vasopressor therapy, calcium chloride infusions, at a dose of 1–3 g slow IV push, are recommended.[8] Additional calcium infusions, either bolus or drip, are warranted in patients who demonstrate a beneficial hemodynamic response to initial calcium therapy. While high-dose calcium chloride (4–6 g) may overcome some of the adverse effects of CCBs, it rarely restores normal cardiovascular status. In addition, calcium should

be administered only after digoxin toxicity has been excluded. Although calcium infusions may be beneficial in other types of drug-induced shock, it currently is only recommended for CCB-induced shock because of limited supportive data.[8] Glucagon has been reported to be beneficial in patients unresponsive to calcium,[12,13] Insulin-glucose infusions resulted in hemodynamic improvement in a case series of five CCB poisoned patients. However, the incremental benefit of insulin-glucose therapy was confounded by the use of other additional therapies.[14] Finally, CCBs are highly protein bound, therefore, dialysis is not useful for enhancing elimination. IABC or CPB may be considered for hypotensive patients unresponsive to medical interventions.[15]

Opiates

Opiate overdose may cause CNS-mediated hypotension. CNS sedation results in decreased sympathetic stimulation to the heart and peripheral vasculature, and may result in a subsequent decrease in heart rate and contractility, as well as peripheral vasodilatation and subsequent hypotension. Local effects on peripheral vasculature further increase venous capacitance, which is of mild benefit in congestive heart failure. However, this property further augments the hypotensive effect of opiates. The vagotonic effects of opiates block reflex sympathetic cardiac heart rate stimulation that occur as a result of hypotension, thus bradycardia may ensue. Lastly, certain agents also have a direct myocardial depressant effect, which may further augment hypotension.

In cases of suspected opiate overdose, assisted ventilation and reversal with naloxone should be administered. Naloxone therapy need not be withheld until assisted ventilation has started. Naloxone can be administered intravenously, intramuscularly, sublingually, or via endotracheal tube. Providers should be aware that the effects of naloxone do not last as long as those of heroin (45–70 min vs. 4–5 hours).[11] Higher doses of naloxone may be required to reverse the effects of the more potent synthetic opioids, such as propoxyphene, codeine, methadone, hydrocodone, oxycodone, and fentanyl. If initial doses of naloxone restores adequate respiration, but further therapy is needed, repeat boluses or continuous infusion can be used. The typical infusion dose is one-half to two-thirds of the initial dose that reversed the initial respiratory depression. Nalmephine, a long-acting opioid antagonist, can be used to treat overdoses, but may result in prolonged withdrawal symptoms.[16] Most physicians recommend admission of any patient who requires a second dose of naloxone, or who fails a 6-hour observation period in the ED. Because of the risk of NCPE, some authorities recommend admission of heroin overdose patients who present with significant respiratory depression. However, this complication is usually evident within minutes of patient arrival. Thus, the patient who is asymptomatic following heroin overdose, and has not demonstrated recrudescent toxicity during a 6-hour period of observation, may be discharged safely.

Cyclic Antidepressants

Medications with alpha-adrenergic blocking properties, such as TCA, phenothiazines, or alpha-1-receptor blocking agents, may induce hypotension. The additional effects of TCAs are numerous, and are related to the multitude of their pharmacologic actions. TCAs inhibit the reuptake of NE, serotonin, and to a lesser extent, dopamine. The subsequent sympathomimetic effects are thought to contribute to the development of cardiac arrhythmias. Inhibition of fast Na^+ channels leads to delayed depolarization, and culminates in depression of myocardial contractility, AV blocks, hypotension, wide QRS complex, and cardiac ectopy.

Sodium bicarbonate is the drug of choice for treating ventricular dysrhythmias and/or hypotension due to TCA toxicity.[11] The goal is to achieve a systemic pH of 7.50–7.55. However, the optimum pH is best determined by clinical endpoints, such as narrowing of the QRS complex, or cessation of the arrhythmia. Hypotension, refractory to volume expansion, is best treated with a pure alpha-agonist such as NE or phenylephrine, rather than dopamine.[17] For arrhythmias resistant to sodium bicarbonate therapy, lidocaine is the antiarrhythmic agent of choice. Procainamide is contraindicated for the treatment of TCA-induced arrhythmias, because its class Ia antiarrhythmic properties would be expected to worsen TCA-induced cardiac toxicity.[11] Forced diuresis, hemodialysis, and charcoal hemoperfusion are ineffective in TCA overdoses. The use of CPB in TCA overdose has been successful in animal models, and may be considered in cases of shock refractory to medical therapy.[9]

Cocaine

Cardiovascular complications of cocaine use include hypertension, arrhythmias, myocardial ischemia or infarction, and less commonly, aortic dissection.[18] Chest pain is the most frequently reported cardiac consequence of cocaine abuse, with acute myocardial infarction (AMI)

occurring in 6% of such cases.[19] Numerous factors have been implicated in the pathophysiology of cocaine-associated myocardial ischemia, including coronary artery vasoconstriction,[20] platelet aggregation,[21,22] in situ thrombus formation,[23,24] and premature atherosclerosis.[25,26] However, the relative contributions of individual pathophysiologic mechanisms have not been widely investigated and are poorly understood. A recent angiographic study supports that patients with cocaine-induced AMI have microvascular flow impairment similar to AMI in the absence of cocaine, with both demonstrating significant impairment in epicardial and microvascular flow compared to normal patients.[27]

Chest pain of ischemic origin typically responds to a combination of nitroglycerin and/or benzodiazepines.[28,29] The administration of aspirin is indicated, because of the effect of cocaine on increased platelet aggregation and thrombosis.[30] For refractory chest pain, phentolamine, a potent alpha-adrenergic antagonist may be considered. Severe, sustained hypertension may be treated with other vasodilators such as nitroprusside. The use of beta-adrenergic receptor blockers is a topic of continuous debate. Nonselective beta-blockers (propranolol) are contraindicated in patients with cocaine acute coronary syndrome (ACS).[11] Disagreement exists over the role of selective beta-1 (esmolol) and mixed (labetalol) adrenergic receptor blockers in cocaine-induced ACS. Esmolol and metoprolol will not aggravate hypertension, but may induce hypotension. Although labetalol has been reported to be effective in isolated cases, it has predominant beta effects and is nonselective. According to consensus guidelines, the use of beta-receptor antagonists for cocaine ACS are neither recommended nor contraindicated at this time.[11] Thrombolysis for cocaine-induced AMI may be considered when other interventions have failed and invasive reperfusion strategies are not available. Thrombolytic agents are contraindicated in the presence of cocaine-induced hypertensive emergencies. For cocaine-induced ventricular tachycardia or fibrillation, sodium bicarbonate and lidocaine are considered first-line drug therapies in hemodynamically stable patients.[11] The use of beta-receptor blockers in patients with cocaine-associated ventricular tachycardia is contraindicated.

Digoxin and Cardiac Glycosides

Cardiac glycosides and specifically digoxin, inhibit the active transport of Na^+ and K^+ across cell membranes by binding to a specific site on the Na^+K^+ ATPase. These glycosides increase inotropicity due to an increase of cytosolic Ca^{2+} during systole. During repolarization and relaxation, calcium is pumped back into the sarcoplasmic reticulum by a Ca^{2+} ATPase and is removed intracelluarly by a Na^+Ca^{2+} and a sarcolemmal Ca^{2+} ATPase. Excessive increases in digoxin levels result in an excess of intracellular Ca^{2+}, which results in a transient late depolarization that may be accompanied by additional ectopy. Therefore, digitalis toxicity may simulate almost every known type of dysrhythmia. Although no dysrhythmia is diagnostic of digitalis toxicity, AV junctional block of varying degrees, along with increased ventricular automaticity, are the most common manifestations, occurring in 30–40% of such patients.[31] Hyperkalemia is the most problematic electrolyte disturbance in *acute* digitalis toxicity, and occurs primarily due to inhibition of the Na^+K^+ATPase pump. Elevated serum potassium levels with digitalis intoxication cause further depolarization of myocardial conduction tissue, particularly the AV node, leading to an exacerbation of conduction delays. Thus, hyperkalemia is prognostically more important than initial ECG changes or the serum digoxin concentration.[32] Hypokalemia occurs more commonly with chronic digitalis use, and is most likely secondary to kaliuresis induced by concomitant loop diuretic use in patients with congestive heart failure.

The therapeutic range of digoxin is 0.5–2.0 ng/mL. However, serum levels must be interpreted with consideration of concurrent medication use and metabolic abnormalities, and should not be the sole determinant of toxicity. Patients with life-threatening digitalis toxicity should receive digoxin-specific antibody fragments. Indications for antibody administration include severe ventricular dysrhythmias, symptomatic bradydysrhythmias unresponsive to atropine, a serum potassium concentration of ≥5 meq/L with suspected digoxin toxicity, or a serum digoxin concentration of ≥15 ng/mL at any time or ≥10 ng/mL at steady state. In circumstances where digoxin-specific antibody therapy is not immediately available, the drugs of choice for ventricular dysrhythmias include phenytoin and lidocaine. These agents are useful because they mitigate enhanced automaticity without significantly slowing conduction throughout the AV node. Class IA antidysrhythmic agents may worsen AV-nodal block and are therefore contraindicated.

Digitalis toxic patients with supraventricular bradyarrhythmias should receive atropine despite inconsistent success rates. Beta-adrenergic receptor antagonists may further depress nodal activity. Isoproterenol may exacerbate ventricular ectopy in digitalis toxic patients, and should be avoided. External or transvenous pacemakers have limited utility and early use of digoxin-specific Fab should be administered as first-line therapy.[33]

Electrolyte disturbances, particularly hypokalemia, hypercalcemia, and hypomagnesemia can exacerbate digitalis-induced arrhythmias. The use of calcium chloride, known to be beneficial in nondigitalis toxic patients, can lead to fatal outcomes if used in digitalis toxic patients, because intracellular hypercalcemia already exists. Intravenous insulin, dextrose, sodium bicarbonate, and oral cation exchange resins should be administered to lower the serum potassium if digoxin-specific Fab is not immediately available for severe hyperkalemia.

SUMMARY

A large number of drugs and toxins have the potential to interact with the heart or vascular system to cause hypertension or hypotension, congestive heart failure, or rhythm disturbances. These abnormalities may occur individually, or in combination, and may suggest a particular class of drugs or toxin. Recognition and treatment of hemodynamic abnormalities is often required prior to identification of the culprit substance. Initial clinical measures include the prevention of continuous exposure and further gastrointestinal absorption, and enhanced elimination. Additional measures will vary depending on the drug or toxin, and frequently include the use of specific medical therapy or mechanical intervention.

REFERENCE

1. Advanced Challenges in Resuscitation: ECC Guidelines. *Circulation* 2000;I-223:102.
2. Ramoska E, Sacchetti AD. Propranolol-induced hypertension in treatment of cocaine intoxication. *Ann Emerg Med* 1985;14:1112.
3. Love JN, Howell JM, Litovitz TL, et al. Acute beta-blocker overdose: Factors associated with the development of cardiovascular morbidity. *J Toxicol Clin Toxicol* 1996;34:273.
4. Love JN, Enlow B, Howell JM, et al. Electrocardiographic changes associated with (Beta)-blocker toxicity. *Ann Emerg Med* 2002;40:603.
5. Taubolet P, Cariou A, Berdeaux A, et al. Pathophysiology and management of self-poisoning with beta-blockers. *J Toxicol Clin Toxicol* 1993;31:531.
6. Brimacombe JR, Scully M, Swainston R. Propanolol overdose: A dramatic response to calcium chloride. *Med J Aust* 1991;155:267.
7. Pertoldi F, D'Orlando L, Mercante WP. Electromechanical dissociation 48 hours after atenolol overdose: Usefulness of calcium chloride. *Ann Emerg Med* 1998;31:777.
8. Albertson TE, Dawson A, deLatorre F, et al. TOX-ACLS: Toxicologic oriented advanced cardiac life support. *Ann Emerg Med* 2001;37:S78.

9. Kerns W, Schroeder D, Williams C, et al. Insulin improves survival in a canine model of acute beta-blocker toxicity. *Ann Emerg Med* 1997;29:748.

10. Grossman JI, Furman S. Intra-aortic balloon augmentation during drug-induced myocardial depression. *Surgery* 1971;70:304.

11. Albertson TE, Dawson A, deLatorre F, et al. TOX-ACLS: Toxicologic oriented advanced cardiac life support. *Ann Emerg Med* 2001;37:S78.

12. Papadopoulos J, O'Neill MG. Use of glucagon infusion in the management of massive nifedipine overdose. *J Emerg Med* 2000;18:453.

13. Mahr NC, Valdes A, Lamas G. Use of glucagons for acute intravenous diltiazem toxicity. *Am J Cardiol* 1997;79:1570.

14. Yuan TH, Kerns WP, Tomaszewski CA, et al. Insulin-glucose as adjunctive therapy for severe calcium channel antagonist poisoning. *J Toxicol Clin Toxicol* 1999;37:463.

15. Holzer M, Sterz F, Schoerkhuber W, et al. Successful resuscitation of a verapamil-intoxicated patient with percutaneous cardiopulmonary bypass. *Crit Care Med* 1999;27:2818.

16. Kaplan JL, Marx JA, Calabro JJ, et al. Double-blind, randomized study of nalmefene and naloxone in emergency department patients with suspected narcotic overdose. *Ann Emerg Med* 1999;34:42.

17. Tran TP, Panacek EA, Rhee KJ, et al. Response to dopamine vs norepinephrine in tricyclic antidepressandt-induced hypotension. *Acad Emerg Med* 1997;4:864.

18. Larkin GL, Graeber GM, Hollingsed MJ. Experimental amitryptiline poisoning: Treatment of severe cardiovascular toxicity with cardiopulmonary bypass. *Ann Emerg Med* 1994;23:480.

19. Lange RA, Hillis LD. Medical progress: Cardiovascular complications of cocaine use. *N Engl J Med* 2001;345:351.

20. Weber JE, Chudnofsky CR, Boczar M, et al. Cocaine associated chest pain: How common is myocardial infarction? *Acad Emerg Med* 2000;7:873.

21. Lange RA, Cigarroa RG, Yancy CW, et al. Cocaine-induced coronary artery vasoconstriction. *N Eng J Med* 1989;321:1557.

22. Togna G, Tempesta E, Togna AR, et al. Platelet responsiveness and biosynthesis of thromboxane and prostacyclin in response to in vitro cocaine treatment. *Haemostasis* 1985;15:110.

23. Rezkalla SH, Mazza JJ, Kloner RA, et al. Effects of cocaine on human platelets in health subjects. *Am J Cardiol* 1993;72:243.

24. Zimmerman FH, Gustafson GM, Kemp HG. Recurrent myocardial infarction associated with cocaine abuse in a young man with normal coronary arteries: Evidence for coronary artery spasm culminating in thrombus. *J Am Coll Cardiol* 1987;9:964.

25. Stenberg RG, Winniford MD, Hillis LD, et al. Simultaneous acute thrombosis of two major coronary arteries following intravenous cocaine use. *Arch Pathol Lab Med* 1989;113:521.

26. Mittleman RE, Wetli CV. Cocaine and sudden "natural" death. *J Forensic Sci* 1987;32:11.

27. Dressler FA, Malekzadeh S, Roberts WC. Quantitative analysis of amounts of coronary arterial narrowing in cocaine addicts. *Am J Cardiol* 1990;65:303.

28. Weber JE, Hollander JE, Murphy, et al. Quantitative comparison of coronary artery flow and myocardial perfusion in patients with acute myocardial infarction in the presence and absence of recent cocaine use. *J Thromb Thrombolysis* 2002;14:239.

29. Baumann BM, Perrone J, Hornig SE, et al. Randomized, double-blind placebo-controlled trial of diazepam, nitroglycerin, or both for treatment of patients with potential cocaine-associated acute coronary syndromes. *Acad Emerg Med* 2002;7:878.

30. Honderick T, Williams D, Seaberg D, et al. A prospective, randomized, controlled trial of benzodiazepines and nitroglycerin or nitroglycerin alone on the treatment of cocaine associated with acute coronary syndromes. *Am J Emerg Med* 2003;21:39.

31. Heesch CM, Wilhelm CR, Restich J, et al. Cocaine activates platelets and increases the formation of circulating platelet containing microaggregates in humans. *Heart* 2003;83:688.

32. Mahdyoon H, Battilana G, Rosman H, et al. The evolving pattern of digoxin intoxication. Observations art a large urban hospital from 1980–1988. *Am Heart J* 1990;120:1189.

33. Bismuth C, Gaultier M Conso F, et al. Hyperkalemia in acute digitalis poisoning: Prognostic significance and therapeutic implications. *Clin Toxicol* 1979;6:153.

34. Taboulet P, Baud FJ, Bismuth C, et al. Acute digitalis intoxication: Is pacing still appropriate? *J Toxicol Clin Toxicol* 1999;31:261.

39

Hypertensive Emergencies

Brian S. Oliver
Kenneth C. Jackimczyk
Raymond E. Jackson

HIGH YIELD FACTS

- Treat the patient, not the blood pressure.
- Initiate treatment with titratable intravenous agents that have a rapid onset and a short duration of action.
- Treat with the concept of autoregulation in mind.
- Reduce the mean arterial pressure (MAP) 10–25% within 1 hour in patients with acute end-organ dysfunction.

INTRODUCTION

What is a Hypertensive Emergency?

Hypertension, defined as a blood pressure persistently greater than 140/90 millimeters of mercury (mmHg),[1] is a common chronic medical condition affecting 50 million Americans and as many as 1 billion people worldwide. Essential hypertension can be successfully treated by a variety of long-term medicines and lifestyle modifications. Patients who remain compliant and proactive with a medication regimen have less than a 1% risk of developing a hypertensive emergency, defined as an inappropriately elevated blood pressure that threatens the function of vital organs and requires immediate therapy. Examples include severely elevated blood pressure with any of the following clinical entities: worsening renal failure, myocardial ischemia, encephalopathy, aortic dissection, pulmonary edema, or hemorrhagic stroke.

Since hypertensive emergencies are relatively rare, they are difficult to study in isolation from other serious illnesses. Additionally, most of the medical literature on hypertensive emergencies focuses on immediate blood pressure reduction as the measured outcome rather than on improvement of end-organ function or mortality.[2]

Because of the paucity of evidence supporting any single treatment regimen there is a wide variability in practice among clinicians. In this chapter, we discuss the principles used for recognition and treatment of hypertensive emergencies.

Hypertensive "Urgencies"

Many authors use the term hypertensive urgency in reference to a marked elevation in blood pressure without end-organ damage or dysfunction. This is not a useful classification since there are not data demonstrating that these patients benefit from urgent treatment. Many hypertensive patients have diastolic pressures that chronically run above 110 mmHg with no evidence of acute end-organ damage. Rapid lowering of blood pressure in these patients can result in significant morbidity and mortality and should be abandoned as a routine emergency department practice. Evidence suggests these patients should be started on an oral antihypertensive, such as diuretic or angiotensin converting enzyme (ACE) inhibitor, and scheduled for close follow-up.[1,3]

GENERAL PRINCIPLES

Treat the Patient, Not the Pressure

The definition of a hypertensive emergency does not include a specific level of diastolic or systolic pressure, although systolic blood pressures (SBP) above 180 mmHg and diastolic blood pressures (DBP) above 110 mmHg are generally referred to as a "severe" elevation.[1] The patient's measured pressure should never supercede the clinical presentation, because the outcome of any severe hypertensive episode depends on many factors including age, comorbid disease, the rapidity of the blood pressure elevation, treatment compliance, and the presence of previous end-organ disease.[4] As an example, the approach and treatment for two patients with pressures of 240/140 mmHg may vary depending on their presentation. An asymptomatic patient requires evaluation for evidence of end-organ dysfunction followed by initiation of medical therapy, education, and close followup. A second patient with the identical blood pressure who is in acute pulmonary edema would require rapid initiation of intravenous therapy and admission to a critical care unit.

As a general principle, once the physician recognizes the presence of an emergent hypertensive condition, the MAP should be reduced by 10–25% within 1 hour. Regardless of what the blood pressure cuff reads, resolution of the patient's symptoms is the primary indication that adequate blood pressure reduction has been achieved. Many adverse events can be avoided if the goals of treatment remain clinical improvement rather than physician comfort with the pressure displayed on a monitor. Treating the patient and not the pressure is the key concept.

Autoregulation

The cornerstone of the pathophysiology of hypertensive emergencies is autoregulation. Autoregulation is the concept that organs keep their blood flow constant over a wide range of MAP. The MAP is defined with the following formula:

$$MAP = \frac{systolicBP + (2 \times diastolicBP)}{3}$$

Tissue perfusion and blood flow in the cerebrovascular system, coronary arteries, and renal vasculature are all controlled by autoregulation. Normotensive patients exhibit autoregulation over a range in the MAP of 60–130 mmHg. Vascular beds of the heart, brain, and kidneys respond to chronically elevated blood pressure by shifting the autoregulatory curve to the right, or to higher pressures (see Fig. 39-1). For example, a man with long-standing poorly controlled hypertension may maintain an average MAP of 140–150 mmHg rather than 90 mmHg. His autoregulatory curve will have reset itself at higher

pressure (see Fig. 39-1). Points B and C represent the range of autoregulation on his "new" curve. Any MAP less than point C or greater than point B will lead to a failure of autoregulation and subsequently to abnormal perfusion. This chronically hypertensive patient can be harmed by lowering his pressures to the normotensive range (below point C) where blood flow deceases dramatically with decreasing pressure resulting in organ ischemia. The goal in hypertensive emergencies is not to achieve normotension, but to reestablish an organ's normal, adequate blood flow. At point B the MAP would still be considered hypertensive, but the patient maintains blood flow on the flat part of the autoregulatory curve.[5] Hypertensive emergencies usually occur at a MAP about 25% above the patient's normal, represented by point A. This MAP will cause increased blood flow and vascular damage due to a loss of autoregulation.

From a physiologic standpoint, an autoregulatory shift occurs when chronically elevated blood pressure causes intimal and medial myocyte proliferation in medium and small arteries. This myocyte hypertrophy allows stronger vasoconstriction but inhibits vasodilation. Vessels can maintain constant blood flow over a higher range of blood pressures, but the autoregulatory curve has been shifted to a higher pressure and hypoperfusion occurs at the middle and low ends of normotension.[6,7]

It is important to note that effective antihypertensive therapy reverses the vessel damage done by chronic

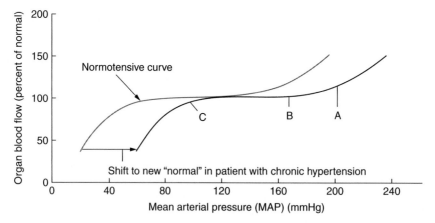

Fig. 39-1. Autoregulation. The grey curve above, labeled normotensive, shows the normal relationship between blood pressure and blood flow in the cerebral, coronary, and renal vasculature. The black curve applies to a patient with long-standing or suboptimal therapy for hypertension. See the text for a discussion of points A, B, and C. For reference, the MAP correlates to blood pressure through the equation (systolic BP + 2 × diastolic BP)/3. (Source: Adapted from Lycette CA, Doberstein C, Rodts GE, et al. *Neurosurgical Critical Care, Current Critical Care Diagnosis & Treatment*, 2nd ed. New York: McGraw-Hill, 2003, Fig. 31-3.)

hypertension, and averts the shift in the autoregulation curve to higher pressures. This is a strong argument for preventative medicine with regard to hypertension.[8]

Initial Examination

All patients with severe elevations in blood pressure require a thorough clinical evaluation. A focused history should be done with attention to symptoms suspicious for end-organ damage. The history should include details about previous therapy for hypertension, how successful the treatment was, and the severity of previous blood pressure elevations. Any previous history of target organ dysfunction is also important. Other historical features, such as the use of recreational drugs or monoamine oxidase inhibitors may be important, as these historical facts could alter the response to treatment.[9]

The blood pressure should be measured at least twice on two separate occasions and averaged, as this may eliminate spurious abnormal blood pressure readings. Blood pressure readings in both arms with a pulse or pressure differential may lead the clinician to suspect aortic dissection.[10] The remaining physical examination should focus on the hallmarks of severe hypertension. An ophthalmologic examination should be performed. The presence of retinal hemorrhages and/or papilledema confirm the diagnosis of a hypertensive emergency. The cardiac examination should focus on signs of heart failure such as abnormal heart or lung sounds, peripheral edema, and jugular venous distention. A complete neurologic examination is necessary and should include a mental status examination, visual fields, and a search for any focal sensory or motor deficits.

The laboratory assessment of a patient with an extremely elevated blood pressure should, at a minimum, include tests of renal and cardiac function. An electrocardiogram, chest x-ray, complete blood count, electrolytes, blood urea nitrogen, creatinine, and urinalysis should be done.[11,3] Any symptomatic patient requires further studies focused on the specific complaint. Simultaneously, the patient should begin receiving therapy consistent with the severity of symptoms.

Treatment Principles

A hypertensive emergency requires treatment in a monitored setting. The general goal is a 10–25% decrease in the MAP over 1 hour. An exception applies for two clinical entities; first, a patient with aortic dissection needs rapid blood pressure lowering to the lowest clinically tolerated blood pressure. Second, cerebrovascular emergencies require judicial titration of blood pressure, because rapid decreases will compromise cerebral blood flow due to impaired cerebral autoregulation.

All patients with hypertensive emergencies should be observed by the treating physician for clinical improvement or deterioration, especially when cerebral, cardiac, or renal ischemia is suspected. Close observation is also required in elderly patients and those with comorbid conditions, since they have a higher likelihood of poor tolerance to therapy.[12]

Pharmacotherapy

The ideal treatment for hypertensive emergencies is a titratable intravenous medication with a rapid onset, a short duration of action, and no side effects.[2] Hypotension is a potential side effect of any blood pressure-lowering medication and the best way to avoid clinical deterioration due to hypotension is by using a drug whose effects are easily terminated. Table 39-1 summarizes the key facts about the most common parenteral medications used in acute blood pressure reduction.

Intravenous sodium nitroprusside has been the mainstay for treatment of hypertensive emergencies. It is widely used and efficacious, but requires invasive monitoring and is light sensitive, which requires shielding, usually with aluminum foil. It has the added problem of releasing cyanide as a toxic metabolite, especially when the drug is used for periods longer than 24–48 hours or in patients with preexisting renal disease or hepatic failure. Nitroprusside is also known to raise intracranial pressure and should be used with care in focal neurologic processes and head injuries.[2]

Esmolol is an ultra short-acting beta-blocker available in intravenous form and is used widely for hypertensive emergencies. It may also be used in combination with nitroprusside for aortic dissections and other conditions where reflex tachycardia may be a problem. Esmolol requires a bolus dose to reach steady state. Beta-blockers must be used with caution if concurrent cocaine use is suspected due to the potential for unopposed alpha-adrenergic effects.

Enalaprilat is the only parenteral ACE inhibitor available in the United States. It is relatively short acting, but takes 30 min to reach maximum effect. An oral form is also available, so transition to oral maintenance therapy is facilitated. The degree of blood pressure reduction is somewhat unpredictable and depends on pretreatment renin level, but it has proven to be safe and effective. It may be particularly useful in patients where a high renin level is suspected, such as renal vasculitis and adrenergic crises including cocaine or methamphetamine intoxication.[13]

Table 39-1. Parenteral Medications for Treatment of Hypertensive Emergencies

Drug	Mechanism of Action	Initial Dose (IV)	Onset	Duration	Contrain-dications	Main use	Caution	Adverse Effects
Sodium nitro-prusside	Smooth muscle dilator	0.05 μg/kg/min	Seconds	1–2 min	Hepatic dysfunction	Combo with esmolol in aortic dis-section	Coronary steal, increases ICP, light sensitive, worsens azotemia	Thiocyanate and cyanide Toxicity, nausea, vomiting
Fenoldopam	Dopamine agonist	0.1 μg/kg/min	2–4 min	10 min	None	Any, renal	Worsens glaucoma	Tachycardia, headache, flu
Nitroglycerin	Direct vasodilator	5–10 μg/min	2–5 min	3–5 min	Space occupying lesion in CNS	Cardiac chest pain	Space occupying CNS lesion	Headache, tolerance
Enalaprilat	ACE inhibitor	0.675–1.25 mg push	15–30 min	6 h	Renal artery stenosis	Heart failure, high renin	Hypovolemia	Hypotension, renal failure angioedema
Labetalol	Alpha- and beta-blockade	20–80 mg push Repeat q 10 min	5–10	4–8 h	Asthma, COPD	Pregnancy-induced hypertension	Heart failure	Vomiting, Heart block, dizzy bronchocon-striction
Esmolol	Beta-blocker	250–500 μg/kg first min, then 50 μg/kg/min	1–2 min	10–20 min	Asthma, COPD	Aortic Dissection, Cardiac Ischemia	Adrenergic crises, meth, cocaine	Hypotension, nausea, brady bronchocon-striction
Phentolamine	Alpha-blocker	5 mg	1–2 min	15–30 min	Cardiac ischemia except when cocaine induced	Adrenergic crises, clonidine withdrawal	Proarrhythmic	Hypotension, reflex tachycardia
Hydralazine	Arteriolar dilator	10–20 mg	10 min	6 h	Cardiac ischemia, aortic dissection	Pregnancy-induced hypertension	Raises ICP, and changes cerebral blood flow distribution	Increases cate-cholamines, reflex tachycardia
Nicardipine	Calcium-channel blocker	2 mg push then 4 mg/h	15–30 min	40 min	Aortic stenosis	Subarachnoid hemorrhage	Caution with cardiac ischemia, heart failure, or beta-blocker	Headache, tachycardia

Source: Modified with permission from Judith Tintinalli, et al. *Emergency Medicine: A Comprehensive Study Guide*, 6th ed. New York: McGraw-Hill, 2004.

An emerging alternative to sodium nitroprusside is fenoldopam. It has been proven safe and effective at lowering blood pressure in dose-dependent fashion with minimal negative side effects.[14] Fenoldopam is a dopamine agonist with activity in the enteric, coronary, cerebral, splanchnic, and renal vasculature. It increases creatinine clearance, and promotes natriuresis and is especially useful in chronic hypertensives with preexisting renal disease.[15,16]

Nicardipine is a longer-acting, water-soluble dihydropyridine calcium-channel blocker. It is useful in the setting of subarachnoid hemorrhage to decrease cerebral vasospasm. It should be avoided in acute heart failure and cardiac ischemia.

Nitroglycerin (NTG) lowers systemic vascular resistance and blood pressure in a dose-dependent fashion. It decreases preload more than afterload and is most useful in cardiac ischemia with hypertension.

Phentolamine is an alpha-adrenergic blocker used in the therapy of pheochromocytoma. It has a predictable and dramatic effect on blood pressure. As an alpha-blocker it is also useful in the therapy of cocaine, methamphetamine, or other adrenergic hypertensive emergencies. It will reduce systolic pressure more than diastolic and causes significant reflex tachycardia.[5]

Poor compliance with or withdrawal from oral antihypertensive medications is often the inciting event for hypertensive emergencies. If so, reinstitution of the previous oral medication may provide safe and effective therapy, provided the clinical picture allows sufficient time for the drug to take effect. Clonidine may be particularly useful when the patient has recently quit using clonidine and has rebound hypertension.[5]

Otherwise, oral agents should be avoided until after the emergent illness has been stabilized. Oral nifedipine has been used in the past for treatment of severe pressure elevations. This method of therapy has been strongly condemned in both the adult and pediatric literature because of multiple poor outcomes due to precipitous drops in blood pressure.[17] Both oral hydralazine and oral labetalol may be used in gestational hypertension. Both are discussed later in this chapter. Hydralazine should be avoided in nonpregnant hypertensive emergencies as it has an unpredictable rate of metabolism, which can lead to excessive hypotension.[2]

Selection of pharmacotherapy in hypertensive emergencies is difficult because there is both a lack of good outcomes-based literature and a variety of opinions among experts in the field. Most authors support the use of nitroprusside as a first-line agent, due to its predictability and short duration of action. Growing support exists, however, for the primary use of fenoldopam or enalaprilat as first-line agents. There are also many illness with specific therapies discussed in the following sections and in Table 39-1.

The literature does not provide definitive evidence to support any one treatment over others. The Cochrane library has a position paper and evidence-based review forthcoming on the treatment of hypertensive emergencies. However, the treatment of hypertensive emergencies will likely remain a matter of controversy until more outcomes-based data are gathered and published.[18]

HYPERTENSIVE CARDIAC EMERGENCIES

Chest Pain

Patients frequently present to the emergency department with chest pain. An extreme elevation of blood pressure does not alter the differential diagnosis for a patient with chest pain; in fact, some degree of hypertension is normal in the setting of acute coronary syndrome (ACS) due to high adrenergic tone. Extreme hypertension with chest pain should raise the suspicion of aortic dissection or cardiac ischemia.

Acute Coronary Syndrome

When ischemic chest pain is accompanied by extreme elevations in blood pressure the progression to myocardial damage may be accelerated. The patient who has an acute myocardial infarction or unstable angina and an elevation of blood pressure has increased the myocardial work, which adds to the imbalance between oxygen supply and demand. Any increase in the MAP directly increases afterload, increasing oxygen demand potentially decreasing coronary blood flow. Any patient with severely elevated blood pressure should routinely be evaluated for acute ischemic injury. If an ACS is recognized in a patient with elevated blood pressure, treatment aimed at judiciously lowering the blood pressure should begin immediately.

The blood pressure can be effectively lowered using treatment modalities which also treat ACS. Intravenous NTG not only dilates coronary arteries, but also acutely reduces systemic vascular resistance. The initial NTG dose of 5–10 μg/min can be titrated rapidly and stabilized once chest pain relief occurs. If there are no contraindications, an intravenous beta-blocker, such as metoprolol or esmolol should be used to further decrease the myocardial oxygen demand. A coronary steal syndrome has been described in patients on sodium nitroprusside with a fixed coronary lesion. Therefore, it is not the agent of choice in patients with markedly elevated pressures and acute coronary ischemia.[6] Treating an elevated blood pressure should never delay definitive reperfusion therapy.

Aortic Dissection

Acute dissection of the thoracic aorta requires prompt and thoughtful intervention. Hypertension is the etiology for aortic dissection in more than 90% of patients. Inflammatory disorders account for the bulk of nonhypertensive dissections. Aortic arch dissections and aneurysms carry an immediate mortality of 1–2% per hour and require emergent surgical therapy regardless of the medical therapy employed. Distal dissections are far less lethal carrying a 1-month mortality of 10%. The surgical indications for distal dissections are less clear as the surgical mortality approaches 35% and medical therapy may be employed.[19]

Proximal and distal dissections present with identical symptoms, including an abrupt onset of severe chest, back, or abdominal pain. The dissecting segment may involve the carotid or coronary arteries, leading to signs of acute cerebral or cardiac infarction. Any neurologic deficit in the presence of chest pain requires an evaluation for aortic dissection. A chest radiograph may reveal apical capping and a widened mediastinum, but a chest CT or angiography is required for definitive diagnosis. No diagnostic study should delay definitive treatment of the blood pressure.

Medical therapy in the dissecting patient is aimed at stabilization and resuscitation. Treatment is aimed at not only controlling the blood pressure but also reducing the shear forces generated by vigorous systolic contractions. These shear forces can extend the dissection by separating the layers of the arterial wall. The goal of immediate therapy is to attain the lowest tolerated blood pressure where there are no signs or symptoms of cardiac, cerebral, or renal dysfunction.

A combination of esmolol and sodium nitroprusside effectively reduces both blood pressure and shear forces in most patients with dissection.[20] The dose of esmolol is 250–500 μg/kg in the first minute and then 50 μg/kg/min titrated for heart rate greater than 60. Sodium nitroprusside is initiated at 0.5 mg/kg/min and can be rapidly titrated to the desired blood pressure. It should start after esmolol to avoid reflex tachycardia.[12] Conversion to an oral antihypertensive agent and oral beta-blocker should begin early so that the side effects of thiocyanate and cyanide toxicity can be avoided. An alternative choice for treatment of aortic dissection is intravenous labetalol. It has a mixed alpha- and beta-blocker effect and decreases the blood pressure and shear forces. Labetalol is given as a 20-mg intravenous push, and the dose can be repeated, or doubled, every 10 min. It has a longer duration of action, so dosing must be carefully monitored. If the patient will be receiving emergent surgery, a shorter-acting agent may be preferable.

Acute Pulmonary Edema

Acute pulmonary edema may occur with left ventricular failure induced by high blood pressure. Treatment of acute pulmonary edema hinges on the presence or absence of cardiac ischemia. If cardiac ischemia is suspected, NTG and morphine should be used initially. If there is no evidence of cardiac ischemia, enalaprilat, with its renin inhibition, is an excellent choice for therapy.

If respiratory failure is imminent, triple therapy with nitroprusside, NTG and enalaprilat will effectively reduce the blood pressure and may avert intubation. Close blood pressure monitoring is needed so that the NTG and nitroprusside can be safely titrated down once the enalaprilat begins to take effect. An intravenous diuretic should also be given immediately unless there are clinical signs of hypovolemia. Beta-blocking agents should generally be avoided in the patient with acute congestive heart failure.

ACUTE NEUROLOGIC HYPERTENSIVE EMERGENCIES

Altered Mental Status

Hypertensive encephalopathy is a rare, but devastating complication of acute hypertension, defined as an alteration in mental status along with signs and symptoms of significantly elevated blood pressure. These signs and symptoms may include severe headache, nausea and vomiting, as well as altered mental status ranging from lethargy or confusion to coma. Symptoms may progress over hours and can lead to coma and death. Seizures can also be the presenting symptom. Headache alone in the presence of a significantly elevated blood pressure does not constitute a hypertensive emergency.

Initial findings on physical examination may include decreased strength, changes in visual acuity, and ophthalmologic changes such as papilledema and alternating areas of arteriolar constriction and dilation.[8] A CT scan of the head is necessary to rule out intracerebral hemorrhage or structural CNS lesions. The CT scan should not delay therapy in an encephalopathic patient.

Encephalopathy is a result of a loss of autoregulation leading to hyperperfusion. This hyperperfusion causes damage to the endothelium and clotting eventually occurs within the cerebral vessels. Ultimately, a drastic decrease in blood flow will result, worsening the encephalopathy. The loss of autoregulation makes the patient exquisitely vulnerable to cerebral hypoperfusion with an overly aggressive reduction in blood pressure, so the clinician must be judicious in the choice of blood pressure lowering agents.

The treatment goal in hypertensive encephalopathy is to lower the MAP so that the cerebral blood flow returns to normal. A decrease of 10–15% of the MAP in 30–60 min may result in symptomatic relief and return that patient to the flat part of their autoregulatory curve. (See Fig. 39-1) More rapid lowering of the blood pressure is contraindicated, as it can lead to hypoperfusion. Hypoperfusion is a particular concern in the elderly and those with long standing hypertension.[2]

Because of their rapid onset and short duration of action, both sodium nitroprusside and intravenous fenoldopam are good choices for initial therapy in the patient with hypertensive encephalopathy. Care should be used with any long-acting agents since decreased cerebral blood flow can occur with overzealous treatment. After the initial MAP is reduced by 10–15%, the pressure can be further lowered into an acceptable range over the next 48 hours.

Acute Stroke Syndromes

It may be difficult to sort out the cause-and-effect relationship between hypertension and CNS dysfunction in the patient with an acute stroke syndrome. The stroke or hemorrhage may be the etiology of the pressure elevation (Cushing's effect), or the hypertension may be the cause of the stroke. Because other forms of CNS dysfunction (thrombotic stroke, intracranial hemorrhage, and subarachnoid hemorrhage) are more common than hypertensive encepthalopathy, they must be excluded in the patient with CNS findings and hypertension. Diagnostic testing should generally precede treatment, unless there are obvious signs of organ damage outside the CNS due to the elevated pressure.

Pretreatment diagnostic testing is necessary because, a loss of autoregulation in tissue near an intracranial injury causes tissue blood flow to be directly pressure dependent, so viable tissue at the margins surrounding the injured area may be sensitive to small reductions of pressure. Aggressive antihypertensive treatment in stroke patients may promote ischemic injury by decreasing blood flow to these watershed areas.

A recent evidence-based review found a lack of outcome-based evidence to support lowering the blood pressure in the setting of an acute stroke.[21] Therapy to lower an elevated blood pressure should only be attempted in a patient with a stroke when there is clear evidence of hypertensive target organ damage outside the CNS. In this setting, a controlled reduction of the MAP by 10% may be attempted. The best agent for this is fenoldopam at 0.01 µg/kg/min, because of its short duration of action and minimal CNS side effects. Although small doses of intravenous labetalol may also be effective. If a fibrinolytic agent is considered, the blood pressure must be controlled following the published guideline of reducing the pressure below 185/110 mmHg prior to thrombolysis.[22]

Patients with intracerebral hemorrhage who also have a substantially increased blood pressure are at an increased risk of rebleeding. There is no evidence, however, that lowering the initial blood pressure decreases the number of repeat hemorrhages.[23] Despite a lack of evidence, it is common clinical practice to treat the blood pressure in patients with intracerebral hemorrhage. Commonly used endpoints for blood pressure control are a systolic BP of 170–220 mmHg and diastolic BP 105–120 mmHg.[11] A short-acting agent such as fenoldopam may be used.

If no discernable cause for the CNS dysfunction can be determined, and the role of an elevated blood pressure is uncertain, the blood pressure should be reduced. Severe elevation of pressure (BP > 220/120 mmHg) requires titrating the mean blood pressure downward 10–15%, while closely monitoring the patient's response. The clinician should accomplish this in a controlled, gradual manner with agents that are short acting and fully reversible.

ACUTE RENAL INJURY

Acute renal pathology can be the cause or the result of acute hypertension. However, deterioration of renal function in the face of an elevated pressure is considered a hypertensive emergency. Renal blood flow follows the same principles of autoregulation as do the brain and heart.[24]

Severely elevated blood pressure with proteinuria, along with elevation of the BUN and creatinine are diagnostic of a hypertensive emergency. Fenoldopam, which increases creatinine clearance, is emerging as the best choice in hypertensive emergencies associated with acute renal insufficiency. Sodium nitroprusside and labetalol are also reasonable choices for immediate treatment. Cyanide toxicity, however, can occur more quickly with fulminate renal failure.[25] ACE inhibitors can worsen renal failure and should be avoided.

Patients with renal insufficiency associated with a hypertensive emergency should have their blood pressure slowly and carefully lowered. Marked decreases in blood pressure can worsen renal failure, so a 10–25% decrease

---

in the MAP in 1–2 hours is a reasonable goal, with further reduction in pressure over the next 24–48 hours. Diuretics may be appropriate in obvious fluid overload but should be used with caution, as they will worsen renal failure in a hypovolemic patient.[8]

HYPERTENSIVE EMERGENCIES IN CHILDREN

Hypertensive emergencies are exceedingly rare in children. Children manifest these emergencies in ways similar to adults. Headache tends to be a prominent symptom and should not be ignored in this age group. Mental status changes are a late and ominous finding in children with hypertensive encephalopathy. Other symptoms and signs include altered visual acuity, proteinuria, and papilledema.[26]

Marked elevation of blood pressure in children is usually the result of renal disease. Also in the differential diagnosis is drug ingestion, coarctation, neuro-endocrine tumors, and intracranial pathology. Pharmacologic therapy in children is similar to adults. Nicardipine and nitroprusside are widely used but there is no strong evidence supporting any particular treatment regimen. Due to its unpredictable effect, nifedipine should be avoided.[27]

GESTATIONAL HYPERTENSION

Gestational hypertension is defined as an elevated blood pressure greater than 140/90 mmHg after 20 weeks' gestation. Preeclampsia is gestational hypertension plus proteinuria, and may include other symptoms and signs

such as hyperreflexia, confusion, headache, and epigastric pain. Eclampsia includes the above symptoms plus seizures. See Table 39-2 for the definitions of the mild and severe forms of gestational hypertension, preeclampsia, and eclampsia. Severe preeclampsia and eclampsia are hypertensive emergencies. They occur most commonly in primagravidas and in multigravidas over the age of 35, especially those with a prior history of renal or hypertensive disease. Gestational hypertension, preeclampsia, and eclampsia are not seen before 20 weeks except with gestational trophoblastic disease and in women with preexisting renal or hypertensive diseases. Patients with gestational hypertension may be discharged with close follow-up. Those with preeclampsia should be seen by an obstetrician in the hospital but do not always require admission. Anyone with severe preeclampsia or eclampsia requires admission to the hospital for testing and immediate therapy.[28]

During preeclampsia and eclampsia, uterine blood flow decreases, necessitating monitoring of fetal heart tones. Laboratory tests should include a complete blood count, liver function panel, and electrolytes, plus a urinalysis. These labs will help discern the severity of disease as well as revealing a variant of preeclampsia called the HELLP (**h**ypertension, **e**levated **l**iver enzymes, and **l**ow **p**latelets) syndrome.

The initial emergency treatment is to lower the blood pressure into the normal range with magnesium sulfate and labetalol. Magnesium sulfate has both antihypertensive and antiepileptic properties. It is given as a 4-g intravenous bolus, followed by a 1–2 g/hour infusion. Therapeutic levels are 6–8 meq/L. Excessive magnesium

Table 39-2. Criteria for Gestational Hypertension, Preeclampsia, and Eclampsia[*]

Gestational hypertension	BP >140/90 mmHg on two occasions at least 6 h apart.
Severe gestational hypertension	BP >160/110 mmHg for longer than 6 h.
Preeclampsia	Gestational hypertension (>140/90 mmHg) and mild proteinuria of 300 mg to 5 g may have mild symptoms of right upper quadrant pain with nausea or vomiting, thrombocytopenia (>100,00), and abnormal liver enzymes.
Severe preeclampsia	Requires one or more of the following: Severe gestational hypertension (>160/110 mmHg) with mild proteinuria, or gestational hypertension (>140/90 mmHg) plus severe proteinuria of >5 g/day or gestational hypertension and severe multiorgan involvement with right upper quadrant pain, elevated LFTs, oliguria, pulmonary edema, thrombocytopenia (<100,000), altered mental status, or visual changes.
Eclampsia	Preeclampsia or severe preeclampsia with seizures or coma.

[*]All criteria require a gestational age greater than 20 weeks.
Source: Modified with permission from Judith Tintinalli, et al. *Emergency Medicine: A Comprehensive Study Guide*, 6th ed. New York: McGraw-Hill, 2004.

sulfate administration can lead to loss of reflexes (>8 meq/L), hypotension, and eventual respiratory arrest (>12 meq/L). Thus, reflexes must be monitored at least every 2 hours, and when they disappear, the infusion must be stopped. Labetalol is safe and efficacious and is often used with magnesium for blood pressure lowering. Hydralazine 10–20 mg IV may also be given. Sodium nitroprusside can be used, but the infusion should not be prolonged and thiocyanate levels must be monitored. The definitive treatment is delivery of the fetus.[29] Postpartum preeclampsia and eclampsia can develop up to 2 weeks postpartum and may be treated as above.

Diuretics are contraindicated in gestational hypertension or preeclampsia, as this is a volume-contracted state, despite the presence of peripheral edema. Often the treatment of these patients requires stabilization for transport to a hospital with high-risk labor and delivery capabilities.

SUMMARY

Though rare, hypertension-induced organ failure requires prompt and thoughtful action. Key principles include: (1) treat the patient not the blood pressure; (2) treat with a short-acting agent with few side effects; (3) treat with autoregulation in mind; and(4) initially have the goal of a 10–25% reduction in MAP in the first hour. Remember the hypertensive emergencies where blood pressure control is required outside of the above guidelines, which are aortic dissection, and hemorrhagic or embolic stroke.

REFERENCES

1. Joint National Committee on Prevention, Detection and treatment of High Blood Pressure (JNC VII): *The Seventh Report of the Joint Committee on Prevention, Detection, Evaluation and Treatment of High Blood Pressure*, Washington DC:U.S. Dept. of Health and Human Services, 2004.
2. Cherney D, Straus S. Management of patients with hypertensive urgencies and emergencies: A systematic review of the literature. *J Gen Intern Med* 2002;17:937–945.
3. Varon J, Marik P. The diagnosis and management of hypertensive crises. *Chest* 2000;118:214–227.
4. Shayne PH, Pitts SR. Severely increased blood pressure in the emergency department. *Ann Emerg Med* 2003;41:513–529.
5. Elliot WJ. Hypertensive emergencies. *Crit Care Clin* 2001;17(2):435–451.
6. Tietjen CS, Hurn PD, Ulatowski JA, et al. Treatment modalities for hypertensive patients with intracranial pathology: Options and risks. *Crit Care Med* 1996; 24(2):311–322.
7. Wu MM, Chanmugan A. Hypertension. In: Tintinalli J, Stapczynski JS, Kelen GD (eds.), *Emergency Medicine, A Comprehensive Study Guide*, 6th ed. New York: McGraw-Hill, 394–403.
8. Straandgard S, MacKenzie ET, Jones JV, et al. Studies on the cerebral circulation of the baboon in acutely induced hypertension. *Stroke* 1977;7:287–290.
9. Vaughan CJ, Delanty N. Hypertensive emergencies. *Lancet* 2001;356:411–417.
10. Rodgers KG, Jones JB. Back pain. In: John A Marx, Robeg S Hockberger, Ron M Walls, et al. (eds.), *Rosen's Emergency Medicine, Concepts and Clinical Practice*, 5th ed. Philadelphia, PA: Mosby, 2002:233–241.
11. Peters H, Clarke M. The utility of laboratory data in the evaluation of the asymptomatic hypertensive patient (abstract). *Ann Emerg Med* 2002;40(4):S48.
12. Parmele KT, McDonald AJ. Hypertension. In: Harwood-Nuss A, Wolfson AB (eds.), *The Clinical Practice of Emergency Medicine*, 3rd ed. Philadelphia, PA: Lippincott Williams & Wilkins, 2001:720–725.
13. Blumenfeld JD, Laragh JH. Management of hypertensive crises: The scientific basis for treatment decisions. *Am J Hypertension* 2001;14:1154–1167.
14. Panacek EA, Bednarczyk EM, Dunbar LM, et al. Randmoized, prospective trial of fenoldapam versus sodium nitroprusside in the treatment of acute severe hypertension. *Acad Emerg Med* 1995;2:959–965.
15. Shusterman NH, Elliot WJ, White WB. Fenoldapam but not nitroprusside, improves renal function in severely hypertensive patients with impaired renal function. *Am J Med* 1993;95:161–168.
16. Tumlin JA, Dunbar LM, Oparil S, et al. Fenoldapam, a dopamine agonist, for hypertensive emergency: A multicenter randomized trial. *Acad Emerg Med* 2000;7:653–662.
17. Leonard MB, Kasner SE, Feldman HI, et al. Adverse neurologic events associated with rebound hypertension after using short acting nifedipine in childhood hypertension. *Pediatr Emerg Care* 2001;17(6):435–437.
18. Perez M. Cochrane Hypertension Group, personal communication, 2004.
19. Nienaber CA, Eagle KA. Aortic dissection: New frontiers in diagnosis and management. Part I. From etiology to diagnostic strategies. *Circulation* 2003;108(5):628–635.
20. Nienaber CA, Eagle KA. Aortic dissection: New frontiers in diagnosis and management. Part II. Therapeutic management and follow up. *Circulation* 2003;108(6):772–778.
21. Bath P, et al. The Cochrane Stroke Group, Interventions for deliberately altering blood pressure in acute stroke. *Coch Database Syst Rev* 2001;3 (Abstract).
22. Smith S, Johnston C, Easton JD. Cerebrovascular diseases. In: Kasper D, Fauci A, Longo D, et al. (eds.), *Harrison's Principles of Internal Medicine*, 16th ed. 2005, Chap. 349.
23. Willmot M, Leonardi-Bee J, Bath PM. High blood pressure in acute stroke and subsequent outcome: A systematic review. *Hypertension* 2004;43(1):18–24.

24. Persson PB. Renal blood flow autoregulation in blood pressure control. *Curr Opin Nephrol Hypoertens* 2002; 11(1):67–72.

25. Freiderich JA, Butterworth JF. Sodium nitroprusside: Twenty years and counting. *Anesth Analg* 1995;81(1):152–162.

26. Murphy C. Hypertensive emergencies, advances and updates in cardiovascular emergencies. *Emerg Med Clin North Am* 1995;13(4):973–1007.

27. Groshong T. Hypertensive crisis in children. *Pediatr Ann* 1996;25(6):368–376.

28. Sibai BM. Diagnosis and management of gestational hypertension and preeclampsia. *Ob Gyn* 2003;102(1):181–192.

29. Montan S. Drugs used in hypertensive diseases in pregnancy. *Curr Opin Obstet Gynecol* 2004;16(2):111–115.

PART VI

PEDIATRIC CARDIOLOGY

40

A Diagnostic and Management Approach to the Pediatric Patient with Heart Disease

Sharon E. Mace

INTRODUCTION

Congenital heart disease occurs in about 1% of term live births[1] and 2% of premature infants[2] (excluding premature infants with patent ductus arteriosus, which occurs in 31% of premature infants <1500 g).[3] This incidence does not include bicuspid aortic valves (found in 2–3% of adults)[4] or mitral valve prolapse. Congenital heart disease is still the number one cause of death in children with congenital malformations.[2,5]

Patients with congenital heart disease may present at any age, from newborn to adulthood. Because of the postnatal changes occurring with the transitional circulation, a neonate with congenital heart disease may have no signs or symptoms in the newborn nursery (and be undiagnosed), only to return symptomatic within days to weeks. The average length of stay (LOS) for neonates after delivery has dramatically decreased in the last few decades,[6] while the rate of neonatal visits to emergency departments has increased.[7] According to one study, the LOS for mothers and infants status post an uncomplicated vaginal delivery was <24 hours in over 50%.[8] The likelihood exists (and may be increasing in view of the decreased neonatal LOS)[6–8] that these undiagnosed

HIGH YIELD FACTS

- Patients with pediatric heart disease are a large and growing population that the emergency physician is likely to encounter. Since the longevity of this population has markedly increased, these patients may present at any age with a diverse spectrum of clinical presentations.

- Any pediatric patient presenting with chest pain, syncope, hypertension, congestive heart failure (CHF), cyanosis, respiratory distress, or shock should have pediatric heart disease in the differential diagnosis.

- Infants with ductal-dependent lesions usually present in the first few days or weeks of life with the abrupt onset of cardiogenic shock. In addition to the usual ABCs, treatment with a prostaglandin E_1 (PGE_1) infusion may be considered.

- A PGE_1 infusion will keep the ductus arteriosus open. The dose is a bolus of 0.1 µg/kg followed by an infusion at 0.1 µg/kg/min.

- In infants, CHF occurring in the first few weeks to months of life is most commonly from left-to-right shunt lesions, and may present with signs/symptoms different from adults/older children.

- Common complications in patients who are status post cardiac surgery for congenital heart disease include dysrhythmias, residual or recurrent lesions, shunt dysfunction, acute/chronic neurologic events, and even sudden death.

- Emergency treatment for tetralogy of Fallot (Tet) spells includes positioning, oxygen, morphine, and a bolus of normal saline. If there is no response to these first-line measures, additional therapy may involve bicarbonate, beta-adrenergic blockade (propranolol), and phenylephrine.

infants will be seen in the emergency department, often with a variety of nonspecific complaints.

In addition, with the progress in pediatric cardiology/cardiovascular surgery over the past few decades,[9–15] the number of pediatric congenital heart disease patients surviving to adolescence and adulthood has grown exponentially.[16,17] The incidence of adults with congenital heart disease (corrected or uncorrected) is increasing at approximately 5% per year.[16]

In the United States alone, there are about one million adults with congenital heart disease (this number does not include infants, children, and adolescents with pediatric heart disease). In developed countries, it is estimated there are as many adult patients with congenital heart disease as there are children and adolescents with congenital heart disease.[17]

All these factors make it likely that the emergency physician will encounter patients of all ages with congenital heart disease; some of whom will have known diagnosed congenital heart disease while others are undiagnosed, or even misdiagnosed.[18]

The clinical presentation of infants and children with congenital heart disease is quite variable, ranging from asymptomatic patients with a heart murmur, to stable symptomatic patients with chest pain, syncope, or hypertension; and critically ill infants in extremis with cyanosis, respiratory distress, CHF, and/or cardiogenic shock (Table 40-1). Because of the varied age-related differences in presentation, and the complexity of pediatric heart disease, such patients can be a diagnostic challenge. Furthermore, some of these patients may need life-saving interventions.

It is not unusual for patients with congenital heart disease to be unrecognized or misdiagnosed. Ten percent of infants with congenital heart disease who died in the first year of life, and 25% of those who died in the first week of life, did not have the diagnosis made before death.[8] The most common misdiagnoses are a respiratory illness: such as pneumonia or a viral upper respiratory illness, and feeding problems. Indeed it can be difficult or impossible, in a patient with known cardiac disease, to distinguish between an exacerbation of their underlying heart disease and a new illness, especially respiratory disease. Some clinical findings may be identical in patients with respiratory disease and patients with heart failure, for example, tachypnea and rales.

Patients with a chief complaint of chest pain, syncope, hypertension, respiratory distress, cyanosis, CHF, and shock should have congenital heart disease in the differential diagnosis. However, patients with congenital heart disease may present with signs and symptoms seemingly unrelated to heart disease (Table 40-1). For example, the infant seen with a chief complaint of "poor feeding" may not have an underlying gastrointestinal disorder but instead may be easily fatigued during routine feedings because of heart failure.[18] Sweating during feeding, stopping in the middle of a feeding, or taking a prolonged time to feed may signify fatigue and dyspnea from CHF.

What clues can the clinician obtain in order to answer the question: Does this patient have pediatric heart disease and if yes, what should the management/treatment be? The history, physical examination, and some simple tests can assist in making the diagnosis and determining initial therapy.

HISTORY

The history of poor growth or failure to thrive (FTT) can occur with pediatric heart disease because of greater oxygen consumption and increased work of breathing. This results in a higher expenditure of calories because of inadequate tissue perfusion and a lesser availability of cellular substrate.[18] There is also a higher incidence and increased severity of respiratory infections, especially respiratory syncytial virus (RSV), in patients with cardiovascular malformations.[19] Feeding difficulties may be due to dyspnea during feeding, caused by increased pulmonary venous pressure. Fussiness, irritability, tachypnea, and

Table 40-1. Presenting Signs/Symptoms in Patients with Pediatric Heart Disease

- Murmur
- Failure to thrive (poor weight gain)
- Poor growth
- Difficulty feeding
- Difficulty breathing (respiratory distress/respiratory failure)
- Infections: pneumonia, sepsis
- Respiratory symptoms: tachypnea, rales, wheezing (cardiac asthma), hemoptysis, cyanosis, cough, clubbing, dyspnea
- Exercise intolerance
- Palpitations/dysrhythmias
- Apnea
- Fever (infections/inflammatory endocarditis, pericarditis, myocarditis)
- Dysrhythmias
- Chest pain
- Syncope
- Hypertension
- Cyanosis (*Blue Baby*)
- Congestive heart failure
- Shock (circulatory collapse)

excessive perspiration can be the pediatric manifestation of exertional dyspnea. Hemoptysis is unusual in pediatric patients but can occur with pulmonary congestion.

The prenatal and birth history may provide clues to the presence of congenital heart disease. A maternal history of acute illness especially during the first trimester may be associated with various syndromes (e.g., TORCH) that have congenital heart disease as a part of the complex. TORCH represents the following congenital infections that frequently have associated congenital cardiovascular malformation: toxoplasmosis, "other" infections, rubella, cytomegalovirus, and herpes.

Infants of diabetic mothers have a nearly three times higher occurrence of congenital heart disease than in the general population.[18] Maternal diabetes, especially when poorly controlled, is associated with a hypertrophic obstructive cardiomyopathy in newborns.[20] Maternal collagen vascular disease (e.g., systemic lupus erythematosus) also has been associated with complete heart block in newborns, due to placental transfer of maternal antibodies to the conduction tissue.

Maternal ingestion of drugs/toxins can have a teratogenic effect. Fetal alcohol syndrome, caused by excessive maternal alcohol ingestion, is associated with increased incidence of ventricular septal defect (VSD). Medications associated with a higher incidence of cardiac malformations are phenytoin, lithium (with Ebstein's anomaly), and thalidomide. The perinatal history may be helpful in differentiating noncardiac respiratory disease (e.g., meconium aspiration or asphyxia) from cardiac causes of respiratory distress and/or cyanosis.

PHYSICAL EXAMINATION

The general appearance is important. Is the child/infant critically ill, in need of immediate resuscitation, suffering from respiratory distress, or resting comfortably? The vital signs are essential. A fever suggests an infection. Hypothermia can occur with infection/sepsis, poor perfusion, or environmental exposure. Marked tachycardia can occur with paroxysmal supraventricular tachycardia. Sinus tachycardia in a pediatric congenital heart disease patient can be a neurohumoral response from increased adrenergic tone and catecholamine release secondary to poor cardiac output (CO). However, tachycardia can also be a nonspecific response to various stresses from infection to pain. Bradycardia may be due to a complete heart block, which may be congenital or a postoperative complication of cardiac surgery. Bradycardia, in the context of sepsis, is an ominous sign.

Respiratory findings of tachypnea, wheezing, rales, cyanosis, clubbing, and cough can be found in patients with pulmonary disease or with pulmonary congestion from heart failure. Tachypnea is present with CHF or low CO/shock. A low pulse oxygen saturation occurs with impaired CO, cyanotic congenital heart disease, or respiratory disease. However, administering 100% supplemental oxygen will significantly increase the oxygen saturation in a patient with respiratory disease, and to a lesser degree in those with poor myocardial function and a low CO, but will usually have a negligible effect in patients with cyanotic congenital heart disease. This is the basis for the hyperoxia test (see below).[21]

The blood pressure (BP) in the arms and legs should be measured. Differences in BP between the arms and legs suggest coarctation of the aorta or an interruption of the aortic arch. A significant heart murmur generally indicates a cardiac etiology for cyanosis or respiratory distress. However, some of the serious cyanotic heart defects may not have a murmur initially (such as transposition of the great vessels), or may have only a nondescript systolic murmur, as with a single ventricle. Furthermore, when there is poor CO/low flow state, a murmur may not be present. Later when cardiac flow and output improve, a murmur may be heard.

Heart sounds may suggest a cardiac basis for the patient's symptomatology. A single S_2 occurs in pulmonary atresia and truncus arteriosus. A wide fixed split S_2 is typical of an atrial septal defect (ASD). A gallop rhythm, with a prominent S_3, occurs with decreased ventricular compliance and increased resistance to ventricular filling, and suggests cardiac failure and myocardial dysfunction. A fourth heart sound is uncommon in children, but is associated with cardiomyopathy, hypertension (systemic or pulmonic), and severe semilunar valve stenosis. A systolic ejection click occurs with dilatation of the aorta, or pulmonary trunk, and is always abnormal after the first day of life. Inspection of the precordium may reveal a precordial bulge, indicating cardiac enlargement. Palpation of the precordium may also detect a thrill or an abnormal cardiac impulse.

The abdomen should be examined. Hepatomegaly may occur with right-sided heart failure. The peripheral pulses should be palpated in all four extremities. Differences between the upper and lower extremities, or between the arms, occur with aortic coarctation or an aortic arch abnormality. The quality of the pulses can suggest various disorders. For example, weak thready pulses indicates low CO, and bounding pulses with a wide pulse pressure occurs with a patent ductus arteriosus or aortic valve insufficiency.

The extremities should be examined for signs of cyanosis, clubbing, or edema. In infants and children, peripheral edema is an uncommon manifestation of heart failure. Cool pale moist extremities, from catecholamine-induced peripheral vasoconstriction, may be a clue to decreased CO. The skin examination may disclose an ashen grey color in a child with metabolic acidosis and poor peripheral perfusion/shock, a bluish hue in cyanotic congenital heart disease or respiratory disease, or the pink plethoric appearance of a patient with heart failure.

The infant/child should be examined for the abnormal facies or stigmata, any syndromes/chromosomal abnormalities, and for noncardiac disorders. Although the cause of most congenital heart disease is unknown, certain cardiac defects are associated with various chromosomal abnormalities and syndromes including trisomy 21, Turner syndrome, and the DiGeorge syndrome. The term "CATCH 22" describes the major features of these syndromes: cardiac defects, abnormal facies, thymic aplasia, cleft palate, and hypocalcemia.

Certain noncardiac disorders may have a cardiac component. For example, specific types of muscular dystrophy may have myocardial involvement, in addition to the peripheral muscle abnormalities. Cardiac involvement can cause myocardial dysfunction and/or dysrhythmias. Rheumatologic disorders, such as lupus erythematous, may be associated with pericarditis or myocarditis. In addition to the characteristic rash and arthralgias, patients with Lyme disease may have AV-nodal block and/or myopericarditis.

Ancillary Studies

A few simple noninvasive tests are essential in the evaluation of the pediatric heart disease patient. These include the ECG and a chest roentgenogram. The neonatal ECG reflects the physiologic and hemodynamic changes that occur in the transition from the fetal circulation to the postnatal circulation. In the near-term fetus, pulmonary vascular resistance (PVR) and systemic vascular resistance are about equal; therefore, the work of the right ventricle (RV) and the left ventricle (LV) are similar (RV work is about 1.3 times LV work) which causes a nearly equal RV mass and LV mass.[22,23] Thus, in the first few days of life the ECG shows a rightward axis and a right-sided predominance. With postnatal changes, systemic vascular resistance increases while the PVR decreases, leading to a thinning of the right ventricular wall.[22,23] Therefore, in the first week of life, there is a "physiologic" right ventricular hypertrophy,[22,23] with gradual progression to the "normal" adult ECG pattern of LV predominance, by about 3–4 years of age.

The chest roentgenogram is useful in detecting cardiomegaly, assessing pulmonary vascularity, and may reveal a characteristic pattern suggestive of specific cardiac defects, (e.g., the "snowman" appearance with total anomalous pulmonary venous return [TAPVR], see page 513; the "egg on a string" of transposition of the great arteries [TGA], see page 511; or the "boot shaped" heart of a tetralogy of Fallot [TOF], see page 505). The chest roentgenogram is also essential in ruling out other causes of respiratory distress or cyanosis, such as pneumonia or pneumothorax.

The "hyperoxia" test is the response in PaO_2 to administration of 100% supplemental oxygen.[21] This test has been used to differentiate cyanotic congenital heart disease from other causes of cyanosis. In patients with respiratory disease such as pneumonia, breathing 100% oxygen for 20 min will significantly increase the PaO_2 by overcoming the ventilation perfusion mismatch. An intracardiac shunt can generally be eliminated from consideration if the PaO_2 increases by >150 mmHg after 100% FiO_2. In patients with neurologic disease causing hypoventilation, assisted ventilation will also lead to a normal PaO_2. In general, patients with cyanotic congenital heart disease will not significantly increase their PaO_2 with 100% FiO_2 administration, unlike patients with pulmonary disease, low CO, shock, sepsis, or hypoventilation.

The echocardiogram has become the diagnostic test of choice for confirming congenital heart disease. In many patients, this simple, painless, noninvasive test has supplanted cardiac catheterization. Cardiac catheterization may still be needed in some patients who have complicated cardiac anatomy that needs further definition prior to surgery, when pulmonary hypertension may be present, and for therapeutic procedures such as a balloon atrial septostomy or interventional balloon valvuloplasty.

Occasionally, other studies ranging from exercise testing, CT scan, MRI scan, and laboratory tests (hematocrit in polycythemic patients, blood cultures in endocarditis, various strep titers/tests in rheumatic fever, rheumatologic studies for possible lupus myopericarditis etc.) will be useful in the diagnosis of the pediatric patient with heart disease.

Approach to the Patient with Pediatric Heart Disease

There are many different cardiovascular malformations. The common ones and their incidence[2,24–29] are given in Table 40-2. For the clinician, an approach based on clinical manifestations is useful. Based on presentation, patients will be seen with a pathologic murmur (but may be asymptomatic) chest pain, syncope, hypertension, palpitations/dysrhythmia, cyanosis, heart failure, and cardiogenic shock. Asymptomatic patients with a pathologic murmur,

Table 40-2. Common Congenital Heart Defects and their Relative Incidence[*]

Congenital Cardiac Defect	Fyler	Hoffman	Kramer	Mitchell	Campbell	Hoffman
Ventricular septal defect	16.6	31.3	28.1	29.5	30.5	32.4
Atrial septal defect (secundum)	3.1	6.1	8.0	7.4	9.8	7.5
Patent ductus arteriosus	6.5	5.5	6.2	8.3	9.7	7.1
Coarctation of aorta	6.5	5.5	7.6	5.0	6.8	5.0
Tetralogy of Fallot	9.4	3.7	10.4	3.9	5.8	5.2
Pulmonic valve stenosis	3.5	13.5	7.7	8.6	6.9	7.0
Aortic valve stenosis	3.3	3.7	5.8	3.8	6.1	4.0
d-Transposition of great arteries	11.2	3.7	6.3	2.6	4.2	4.5
Hypoplastic left ventricle	7.9	0.6	—	3.1	—	2.9
Hypoplastic right ventricle	6.0	0.6	—	2.4	—	2.3
Truncus arteriosus	1.5	2.5	—	1.7	4.2	1.4
Total anomalous pulmonary venous return	2.6	0.6	—	0.7	—	1.0
Tricuspid atresia	1.6	0.6	—	0.9	2.2	—
Other	12.1	17.8	14.8	18.5	—	11.4
Endocardial cushion defect	5.3	3.7	5.1	3.6	—	3.8
Double outlet right ventricle	2.8	0.6	—	—	—	1.2
Single ventricle	—	—	—	—	—	—

[*]The first authors are listed (references 24–29).

and stable patients with chest pain, syncope, or hypertension, may represent congenital heart disease. Emergency department assessment may include an electrocardiogram and chest roentgenogram and occasionally an echocardiogram in addition to a thorough history and physical examination and appropriate referral.

The remaining symptomatic patients with congenital heart disease can be grouped into three categories: cyanosis, heart failure, and/or cardiogenic shock. Patients may belong to more than one category such as heart failure and cyanosis.

The Pediatric Patient with Cyanosis

Cyanosis is a bluish color of the skin and mucous membranes caused by an increased quantity of reduced hemoglobin (deoxyhemoglobin) or hemoglobin derivatives in the capillaries. Generally, cyanosis is detectable if the arterial saturation is ≤85%, although in some individuals it may not be detectable until an arterial saturation ≤75%, especially if they are dark skinned. Cyanosis is usually looked for in the tongue, the lips, nail beds, earlobes, and conjunctiva. Central cyanosis must be distinguished from acrocyanosis. Acrocyanosis is isolated transient peripheral cyanosis that occurs in normal infants/children who do not have heart disease. Cyanosis suggests hypoxia, although the absence of cyanosis does not rule out tissue hypoxia. Tissue hypoxia can be present without cyanosis. However, when cyanosis is present, clinical investigation is warranted.

The differential diagnosis of cyanosis/hypoxia is extensive. Pulmonary disease is the most common cause, although other etiologies from shock to anatomic abnormalities, airway obstruction, hypoventilation, methemoglobinemia, and congenital heart disease should be considered.[30,31] The specific etiology is somewhat affected by the age of the patient. In the neonate, common respiratory etiologies for respiratory distress or cyanosis are persistent fetal circulation, meconium aspiration, respiratory distress syndrome, extrinsic compression (as from a pneumothorax or congenital diaphragmatic hernia), congenital respiratory tract defects (e.g., tracheomalacia, choanal atresia, laryngeal web, laryngeal cysts), and infection (pneumonia and sepsis). Sepsis and shock are two important causes of cyanosis that are in the differential diagnosis of cyanosis at any age. Hypoventilation, whether from central nervous system (CNS) abnormalities, spinal cord/spinal nerve disease, or peripheral neuromuscular problems (from peripheral nerve lesions) can lead to cyanosis.

Cyanosis in patients with congenital heart disease can be explained by either inadequate pulmonary blood flow, "mixing lesions" or if a significant amount of deoxygenated blood is pumped via the systemic circulation to the body (and usually a significant amount of oxygenated blood returns to the lungs) (Table 40-3). Two common situations that demonstrate inadequate pulmonary blood flow with a right-to-left shunt are hypercyanotic spells and Eisenmenger syndrome. Specific cyanotic congenital heart defects are categorized into two groups by the presence of either a decreased or increased pulmonary blood flow on chest x-ray (see Chap. 42 on congenital heart disease).

HYPERCYANOTIC (TET) SPELLS: DIAGNOSIS AND MANAGEMENT

Patients with TOF may have Tet or hypercyanotic spells.[1] Hypercyanotic spells are life threatening. Patients with Tet spells have severe dyspnea, tachypnea, worsening cyanosis, labored breathing, and often syncope. Tet spells are precipitated by exertion, whether from feeding, crying, exercise, straining at stool, and so on. Tet spells may last for a few minutes to hours. They can lead to seizures, stroke, or even death.

Table 40-3. Cyanotic Congenital Heart Defects

Decreased pulmonary blood flow
  Impaired inflow into right ventricle
    Hypoplastic right heart
    Severe tricuspid stenosis/atresia
    Ebstein's anomaly
  Impaired inflow into pulmonary artery
    Tetralogy of Fallot (with severe pulmonic stenosis)
    Tricuspid insufficiency secondary to myocardial ischemia/infarction
    Pulmonary atresia
    Severe pulmonic stenosis
    Double outlet right ventricle with pulmonic stenosis
    Transposition of the great vessels with ventricular septal defect and pulmonic stenosis
Increased (or normal) pulmonary blood flow
    Truncus arteriosus
    Single ventricle
    Total anomalous pulmonary venous return

The pathophysiology of Tet spells is increased ventricular outflow tract obstruction causing an increased right-to-left shunt across the VSD, increased hypoxia, metabolic acidosis, and hypercarbia. The acidosis and hypoxia produce a further drop in systemic vascular resistance that only serves to increase the shunt, in addition to stimulating the CNS centers of respiration leading to hyperpnea.

Emergency treatment for a Tet spell includes positioning by placing the infant in a knee chest position (this increases venous return, and increases systemic vascular resistance which decreases the right-to-left shunt across the VSD), giving oxygen (decreases the hypoxia), morphine sulfate (0.2 mg/kg/dose IM, or SQ), and a bolus of normal saline 10 mL/kg (to increase preload). With a severe Tet spell and no response to the initial measures, additional pharmacologic therapy is indicated. To counteract the metabolic acidosis, sodium bicarbonate IV (1 meq/kg) is administered. Beta-adrenergic blockage is accomplished by propranolol IV (0.1 mg/kg up to a maximum of 0.2 mg/kg) or esmolol IV (0.5–1.0 mg/kg), followed by a continuous infusion to decrease hypercontractility of the RV outflow tract. Lastly, phenylephrine, an alpha-agonist, is used to increase systemic vascular resistance (dose 10 µg/kg IV bolus then maintenance drip at 2–5 µg/kg/min).

Therapy for a Tet spell is administered in a stepwise fashion. Usually, the first-line management: positioning, oxygen administration, morphine, and calming the infant/child will abort the Tet spell.

Eisenmenger Syndrome

Congenital heart disease patients with a large unrestricted left-to-right shunt (for example, a VSD) have an increased volume overload with increased blood flow going to the lungs. If corrective surgery is not done, pulmonary hypertension will eventually develop. When the pulmonary hypertension becomes severe, the shunt direction reverses to become right to left, with resultant cyanosis. The change in direction of shunt flow usually takes place by adolescence or early adulthood.

In addition to cyanosis, signs and symptoms of Eisenmenger syndrome include fatigue, dyspnea on exertion, hemoptysis, and palpitations from atrial arrhythmias (secondary to atrial enlargement).

Polycythemia occurs to compensate for the chronic hypoxia. Unfortunately, the hyperviscosity accompanying the polycythemia can cause complications. These include dizziness, paresthesias, headache, visual changes, or a cerebrovascular accident. A brain abscess can occur from a right-to-left shunt of an infected embolus.

With the onset of the right-to-left shunt, the murmur usually disappears, and the P_2 is loud because of the pulmonary hypertension. Right ventricular hypertrophy is present on the ECG and there is decreased pulmonary vascularity (*pruned pattern*) on the chest radiograph.

Management of patients with Eisenmenger syndrome is to avoid actions that aggravate the hyperviscosity/cyanosis such as dehydration, high altitude, strenuous activity, vasodilators, and pregnancy. Such actions may increase morbidity and mortality.

Congestive Heart Failure in Infants and Children

Congestive heart failure is a physiologic condition in which the CO is unable to meet the metabolic demands of the tissues. CO is a function of the stroke volume (SV) and heart rate (HR), where $CO = SV \times HR$. SV depends on preload (filling volume), afterload (the resistance to the ejection of blood by the ventricles or systemic vascular resistance), and contractility.

Although the physiologic principles of heart failure are similar in adults and pediatric patients; the etiology, signs/symptoms, and management may differ (Tables 40-4 to 40-6) In infants/children, a common etiology of increased preload is left-to-right shunts as with an ASD, VSD, or patent ductus arteriosus. Outlet obstructions, in addition to systemic hypertension, are causes of increased afterload. Examples of left-sided outlet obstruction in infants/children are coarctation of the aorta, critical aortic stenosis, and hypertrophic obstructive cardiomyopathy (HOCM). There are many causes of impaired contractility. Myocarditis/cardiomyopathy are causes of poor myocardial function. Dysrhythmias may decrease CO by insufficient filling time during diastole (as with tachycardias) or by impaired CO (occurring with bradycardia). In adults, the most common causes of CHF are: ischemia (coronary artery disease), hypertension, and calcified valvular disease. In pediatrics, the most common cause of CHF is congenital heart disease (Table 40-4).

The clinical presentation of CHF in infants and children can be subtle, differs somewhat from adults, and is easily misdiagnosed as other disorders (e.g., sepsis, pneumonia) (Table 40-5). Heart failure symptoms/signs that are similar in adults and children include difficulty breathing, dyspnea (shortness of breath if able to verbalize), limited exercise tolerance (dyspnea on exertion, stops to rest while playing), diaphoresis, tachycardia, tachypnea, wheezing, rales, and cyanosis (hypoxia). However, symptoms such as peripheral edema, jugular venous distention, and anasarca

Table 40-4. Causes of Congestive Heart Failure in Pediatric Patients

---

- Infectious: myocarditis from viruses (especially enteroviruses), bacteria (diphtheria, tuberculosis, hemophilus), parasites (Chagas disease), fungus, rickettsia (myocarditis can also be idiopathic)
- Rheumatologic/connective tissue disorders: acute rheumatic fever, Kawasaki syndrome, Lyme disease, systemic lupus erythematosus
- Drugs/toxins: cocaine, chemotherapy (Adriamycin), cardiac drugs (digoxin, beta-blockers, calcium-channel blockers)
- Neuromuscular: muscular dystrophy (some forms affect peripheral muscle and heart muscle)
- Tumors: primary or metastatic cancers to the myocardium, endocardium, or pericardium
- Metabolic: electrolyte abnormalities (Na, K, Ca, Mg)
- Endocrine: thyroid disorders
- Trauma: cardiac tamponade, myocardial contusion
- Pericardial disease/pericarditis: infections, uremia, rheumatologic diseases, tumors
- Myocardial infarction/ischemia: can occur in pediatrics—from anomalous coronary arteries, or vasculitis (Kawasaki syndrome, periarteritis nodosum, and so on)
- Heart rate:
  Tachycardias: decreased diastolic filling
  Bradycardias: impaired output
- Preload
  Cardiac: left-to-right shunts: ventricular septal defect, atrial septal defect, patent ductus arteriosus, arteriovenous fistula, atrioventricular canal defects
  Hematologic: severe anemia
  Excess volume: iatrogenic: excessive fluid administration (neonates/infants are especially vulnerable)
  Renal failure
- Afterload
  Systemic hypertension (left-sided failure), pulmonary hypertension (right-sided failure)
  Outflow tract obstruction: coarctation of aorta, critical aortic stenosis, hypertrophic obstructive cardiomyopathy

---

occur infrequently with pediatric heart failure. Other non-specific symptoms occur in infants/children with CHF: feeding difficulties, irritability, and FTT (Table 40-5).

Poor growth occurs because the infant/child with CHF is struggling to meet the body's basic metabolic demands and extra oxygen consumption/work needed for growth. Feeding requires an additional expenditure of energy/work, which the failing heart has difficulty providing. The result is feeding intolerance, manifested by diaphoresis during feeding (a classic symptom of CHF in infants), prolonged time to feed, stopping in the middle of feeds, or "spitting up."

Respiratory symptoms are very common in the infant/child with CHF, and range from "chest congestion," wheezing, cough, cyanosis, hemoptysis (from pulmonary congestion or edema), to respiratory distress/failure. Frequent or recurrent respiratory infections are a typical presentation of pediatric patients with volume overload. A clue that the presentation may be CHF is the absence of

fever and rhinorrhea. Consider cardiac disease in an afebrile pediatric patient with tachypnea and tachycardia. One caveat to remember, however, is that the onset of a new infection can lead to cardiac decompensation in a patient with heart disease because of their limited cardiac reserve.

With CHF, the BP may be elevated initially because of increased sympathetic activity and adrenergic tone (a compensatory mechanism for CHF) and low, later in the course of the disease, because of poor myocardial contractility and inability to compensate.

Rales or wheezing (*cardiac asthma*) can occur from pulmonary venous congestion (left-sided heart failure). Hepatomegaly, peripheral edema, and anasarca may indicate an increased right-sided filling pressure from right heart failure.

The cardiovascular examination can be instrumental in differentiating heart disease from primary respiratory problems. Inspection and palpation of the precordium may reveal a hyperdynamic heart with an increased

Table 40-5. Manifestations of Congestive Heart Failure in Infancy/Children

Symptoms
- Poor feeding (especially sweaty with feeding or stops in middle of feeding, or prolonged time to feed)
- Irritability
- Failure to thrive
- Poor weight gain
- Frequent respiratory infections
- Squatting (with TOF to decrease left-to-right shunt)

Signs
- Tachycardia, tachypnea, diaphoresis
- Wheezing, rales, cough, and respiratory distress
- Hyperactive precordium
- Increased ventricular impulse
- Shift of PMI
- Ventricular lift, heave
- Thrill
- Gallop rhythm
- Hepatomegaly
- Splenomegaly
- Peripheral edema: uncommon, late sign
- Jugular venous distention: uncommon, late sign
- Anasarca: uncommon, late sign
- Shock: delayed capillary fill, decreased thready pulses, hypotension, sweaty

and/or displaced point of maximal impulse (PMI), and a ventricular lift, are findings consistent with CHF.

The chest radiograph demonstrates cardiomegaly with CHF, increased pulmonary vascularity with left-sided CHF, and possibly a clue to the specific congenital cardiac lesion. The ECG may detect hypertrophy, ST-T-wave changes, Q waves, and dysrhythmias. The echocardiogram will determine the ejection fraction (EF) and usually the specific underlying abnormality. Cardiac catheterization may be necessary in some patients for diagnosis and/or therapeutic interventions.[9–12,14,15]

The typical age when infants with significant left-to-right shunts are seen with CHF manifestations is about 6 weeks. This corresponds to the postnatal gradual decline in PVR. Soon after birth, the initially high PVR prevents significant left-to-right shunting. With the decreasing PVR, the amount of left-to-right shunt increases.

Management of the pediatric CHF patient includes general supportive care, pharmacologic therapy, and specific therapy depending on the underlying etiology (Table 40-6).

Cardiogenic Shock: Ductal-Dependent Lesions

Congenital heart disease patients whose blood flow (systemic or pulmonary) is maintained through a patent ductus arteriosus will become symptomatic, with acute heart failure and circulatory collapse/cardiogenic shock when the ductus closes (Table 40-7). This generally occurs in the first week of life. The infant may have had no obvious clinical manifestations of congenital heart disease in the newborn nursery or in the first few days at home, but can present later in acute shock/circulatory failure.

Consider the possibility of a ductal-dependent congenital heart defect in any neonate in the first few weeks of life with circulatory collapse. Associated findings may be with severe metabolic acidosis, low BP/shock, poor peripheral perfusion (delayed capillary fill), ashen grey color, tachypnea, respiratory distress, cyanosis, and/or CHF. Life-saving therapy is an infusion of PGE_1. This is done to maintain patency of the ductus arteriosus until definitive treatment of the specific cardiac lesion can be done in the operating room or by interventional cardiac catheterization.

A PGE_1 infusion will keep the ductus arteriosus open. The dose is a bolus of 0.1 µg/kg followed by an infusion at 0.1 µg/kg/min. Attention to the ABCs is especially important since the side effects of PGE_1, which are dose dependent, include apnea, hypotension, bradycardia, seizures, and tremors. An immediate consultation with the pediatric cardiologist is warranted when a PGE_1 infusion is being considered and such infants should be admitted to the neonatal or pediatric intensive care unit.

The differential diagnosis of circulatory collapse/shock in critically ill infants is extensive and ranges from sepsis to child abuse (shaken baby syndrome), but congenital heart disease should be a consideration.

Cardiogenic Shock

Cardiogenic shock in the pediatric patient may result from dysrhythmias, left ventricular outflow tract obstruction (congenital as with severe coarctation/severe aortic stenosis, HOCM, cardiomyopathy from toxins/drugs, following cardiac surgery, and in the late stages of septic shock). Management of the pediatric patient in shock involves the ABCs to perfuse the tissues/cells with oxygenated blood. Specific therapy is outlined in Table 40-6.

Complications Occurring in Patients with Pediatric Cardiovascular Disease

Although there have been major advances in the treatment of patients with pediatric cardiovascular disease,[9–15]

Table 40-6. Management of the Pediatric Patient with Congestive Heart Failure and/or Shock

General supportive care
- Positioning (heads up position decreases work of breathing)
- NPO with IVF (decreases risk of aspiration if tachypneic, decreases work of feeding)
- Antipyretics for fever (elevated temperature increases oxygen consumption)
- Restrict fluids unless dehydrated or in shock or otherwise in need of volume replacement
- Check electrolytes (diuretics less effective with low K, Mg, cardiac contractility improved) correct abnormalities
- Treat underlying infections
- Sedation: morphine
- Supplemental oxygen
- If severe respiratory distress/severe hypoxia/respiratory failure from CHF/or pulmonary edema, may need ventilatory support: BVM, BiPAP, intubation with PEEP

Pharmacologic treatment
- Diuretics: furosemide, bumetanide, spironolactone
- Digoxin: improves contractility (may precipitate arrhythmias in certain patients—use with caution)
- Inotropes: dopamine, dobutamine
- Pressors: epinephrine, norepinephrine, isoproterenol
- Afterload reduction: angiotension converting enzyme (ACE) inhibitor (use with caution in patients with renal insufficiency and right-to-left shunts)
- Vasodilators: sodium nitroprusside
- Heart rate control:
  Tachycardia: adenosine, beta-blockers, calcium-channel blockers
  Bradycardias: atropine, epinephrine, pacing

Mechanical (if severe/critical)
- ECMO
- Balloon pump

Specific therapy
- Cardiac tamponade: pericardiocentesis
- Supraventricular tachycardia: Valsalva maneuvers, adenosine (verapamil contraindicated in infants/young children)
- Bradycardia: pacing
- Infective endocarditis: antibiotics
- Kawasaki syndrome: IVIG, high-dose aspirin
- Acute rheumatic fever: antibiotic to treat group B streptococci
- Tet spell: keep child calm/comfortable, knee-chest position, oxygen, morphine, bolus 10 cc/kg NS, propranolol, phenylephrine
- Severe anemias: transfusion with packed RBCs
- Cardiothoracic surgery to relieve obstruction, repair nonfunctioning valve etc.

complications can occur (Table 40-8). The complications can be grouped on the basis of likelihood of need for future reintervention.[32]

Patients who have "true complete repair" have surgery that restores normal cardiac anatomy and function. These patients usually lead a "normal" life without a need for further surgery. Patients with a secundum ASD, or a simple VSD, or a patent ductus arteriosus are in this category.

Patients with "anatomic repairs with residual lesions" will have relief of their symptoms, but have abnormal physiology and remaining anatomic defects. Patients' status post valve repair/valvulotomy, repair of TOF, or status post atrioventricular canal defect repair fit into this group. They will often need reoperation.

Patients whose surgery necessitates use of prosthetic materials, such as conduits, prosthetic valves, or baffles, will need reoperation to replace the prosthetic device because of growth of the patient and degeneration of the prosthetic material. Patients with truncus arteriosus, or pulmonary atresia with a VSD, fall into this category.

Table 40-7. Ductal-Dependent Congenital Heart Lesions

Systemic blood flow depends on the ductus arteriosus (blood flows right-to-left through the ductus from the pulmonary artery to the aorta)

> Interrupted aortic arch
> Severe coarctation of the aorta
> Critical aortic stenosis
> Hypoplastic left heart syndrome
> Mitral atresia with intact ventricular septum
> Severe mitral stenosis with an intact ventricular septum

Pulmonary blood flow depends on the ductus arteriosus (blood flow left-to-right through the ductus of the aorta to the pulmonary artery)

> Tetralogy of Fallot with severe pulmonic stenosis
> Critical pulmonic stenosis
> Hypoplastic right heart syndrome
> Tricuspid atresia with intact ventricular septum
> Pulmonary atresia with intact ventricular septum

Note: This is not an all-inclusive list but gives some common lesions.

"Physiologic" repairs correct the abnormal physiology but not the abnormal anatomy. Therefore, these patients will undoubtedly experience complications needing future medical and/or surgical management. Patients with transposition of the great vessels who have undergone an atrial switch operation (e.g., Mustard or Senning procedure) are an example of a "physiologic" repair.

In addition to the need for future reoperation,[32–34] there are other difficulties that occur in the pediatric heart disease population.[35] Arrhythmias may be the most common problem.[34–40] Arrhythmias may occur in the immediate postoperative period, or months to years later. They can be diverse, from sick sinus syndrome to ventricular tachycardia and may lead to syncope or sudden death.[34,35,41,42] The cause of the dysrhythmia may be from the underlying defect (as with Ebstein's anomaly), the surgical repair, medications, or electrolyte abnormalities. A pacemaker or automatic internal cardiac defibrillator (AICD) may be necessary, or a surgical catheter ablation procedure. The complaint of syncope, chest pain, or palpitations, in the pediatric heart disease patient, should be concerning as a warning for sudden death. Nonspecific symptoms such as irritability in infants may also be a harbinger for sudden death.[42]

Problems with the prosthetic material (conduit, baffle, prosthetic valve, or the surgical shunt) can occur. The

Table 40-8. Complications of Pediatric Heart Disease

- Electrolyte disturbances (from medications)
- Arrhythmias
- Chest pain
- Anticoagulation: inadequate → thrombosis, over anticoagulated → bleeding
- Syncope
- Sudden death
- Myocardial dysfunction → heart failure
- Myocardial fibrosis (from chronic hypoxia)
- Endocarditis
- Poor growth
- Increased susceptibility to respiratory illnesses including respiratory syncytial virus
- Problems with prosthetic materials
- Cerebral emboli (in right-to-left shunt)
- Cerebral abscess (in right-to-left shunt)
- Cerebrovascular accident
- Air embolus (in right-to-left shunt)*
- Residual lesion at surgical site
- Recurrent lesion at surgical site
- Rupture/leakage at the surgical site
- Need for "redo" because of patient growth
- Shunt dysfunction, shunt "clots" off
- Neurologic events: acute/chronic: seizures, stroke, neurodevelopmental abnormalities
- Psychosocial conditions: developmental problems
- Complications of heart transplantation: graft vs. host disease; complications of immunosuppression

Immediate postoperative period:
- Myocardial dysfunction → heart failure
- Pleural effusion
- Pericardial effusion
- Pulmonary emboli
- Wound infections
- Postperfusion syndrome

*Requires extra precaution when placing a line in a patient to avoid iatrogenic air emboli.

prosthetic material (e.g., conduit or baffle) may leak or be torn, loosen (sutures may be dislodged, dehiscence may occur), become displaced, restenose, be compressed (externally or internally by restenosis), obstruct,[34] be considered a "technical failure," or need a "bailout" procedure.[33]

There can be dysfunction of the surgical shunt. When a shunt is placed to increase blood flow, there is usually a continuous murmur heard over the shunt, and there is relief of the cyanosis. When the shunt narrows (as with obstruction from thrombosis), cyanosis increases (oxygen saturation falls) and the usual shunt murmur decreases or disappears. Management of shunt dysfunction involves supportive measures, including 100% O_2, and transfer to a tertiary center with pediatric cardiology/cardiothoracic surgery capability. Surgical shunt replacement, or definitive surgical repair, is usually necessary. Thrombolytics are not recommended in the ED, although they have been used in a few cases.

Pulmonary hypertensive crisis can occur in patients with increased pulmonary artery pressure. Typically, this occurs in patients with a large VSD. During any procedure, or if the patient is in pain, pulmonary vasospasm can occur. This results in a right-to-left shunt across the VSD as occurs with a Tet spell. The symptoms and complications are similar to that of the Tet spell: cyanosis, lethargy, even seizures, and death. Therapy to be instituted is 100% O_2 to cause pulmonary vasodilatation, alkalinization with intravenous bicarbonate, and analgesic/anxiolytic agents.

Ventricular dysfunction and heart failure[34,35,43] may occur from volume or pressure overload, chronic cyanosis (leading to myocardial fibrosis), complications of the surgical repair (prolonged bypass), and so on. Such myocardial dysfunction can lead to heart failure and its related complications including death.

Hypercyanotic (Tet) spells, Eisenmenger syndrome, residual pulmonary hypertension/pulmonary vascular disease, and endocarditis are all potential problems. Emboli and thrombosis can occur.[44] Patients on anticoagulant therapy can have bleeding problems/hemorrhage.

Reintervention to correct any residual or recurrent lesions or for other complications may need to be done on an emergent basis.[33–35] For example, if valvular insufficiency suddenly worsens causing heart failure, or cardiogenic shock.

Myocardial infarction and ruptured aneurysm/pseudoaneurysm are other cardiac causes of morbidity and mortality.[34,42,43] Patients with chronic hypoxemia, from cyanotic congenital heart disease, often have a "compensatory" polycythemia, which may need therapeutic phlebotomy. The high blood viscosity from the polycythemia can lead to cerebrovascular injury. A sudden drop in hematocrit in such polycythemic patients may precipitate failure or cause other problems.

Complications related to therapy, both surgical and medical, are not uncommon. In the immediate postoperative period wound infections, deep vein thrombosis, pulmonary emboli, and pleural effusions are potential problems. Toxicity from medications whether from antiarrhythmics, digoxin, or diuretics, can also occur. Dehydration and electrolyte abnormalities can quickly result from illnesses accompanied by vomiting/diarrhea.

Infants and children with heart disease have an increased susceptibility to respiratory infections especially RSV infections.[19] The added stress from an infection and/or fever may be a precipitant for heart failure or worsening cyanosis in such patients.

Cerebral emboli/thrombosis and abscess can be a significant cause of morbidity and mortality in patients with congenital heart disease.[35,44] When obtaining vascular access, especially in patients with right-to-left shunts, the health care worker should take precautions to avoid an air emboli. Neurologic events, both acute and chronic, ranging from seizures to strokes can occur.[35,44,45]

Poor growth, developmental delay, and neurodevelopmental abnormalities have been reported in patients with congenital cardiovascular disease.[46,47] The mechanisms of CNS injury are multifactorial and complex. Some of the factors are presence of multiple congenital anomalies, preoperative hemodynamic instability with possible hypoxic-ischemic brain injury, intraoperative events (e.g., effects of cardiopulmonary bypass), chronic low normal blood flow, chronic hypoxia, chronic polycythemia, and the risk of emboli/thrombosis.

In addition to the advances in palliative/corrective cardiac surgery and transcatheter procedures, cardiac transplantation is an option for some patients with congenital cardiovascular defects or those with acquired heart disease.[48]

REFERENCES

1. Hoffman JIE, Christianson R. Congenital heart disease in a cohort of 19,502 births with long-term follow-up. *Am J Cardiol* 1978;42:641–647.
2. Bernstein D. Epidemiology and genetic basis of congenital heart disease. In: Behrman RE, Kliegman RM, Jenson HB (eds.), *Nelson Textbook of Pediatrics*, 17th ed. Philadelphia, PA: W.B. Saunders, 2004:1499–1502.
3. The Vermont Oxford Trials Network: Very low birth weight outcomes for 1990. *Pediatrics* 1993;91:540–545.
4. Subramanian R, Olson LJ, Edwards WD. Surgical pathology of pure aortic stenosis: A study of 374 cases. *Mayo Clin Proc* 1984;59:683–690.
5. Rosenthal G. Prevalence of congenital heart disease. In: Garson A Jr, Bricker JT, Fisher DJ, et al. (eds.), *The Science and Practice of Pediatric Cardiology*. Baltimore, MD: Williams & Wilkins, 1998:1083–1106.
6. Margolis HM. A critical review of studies of newborn discharge timing. *Clin Pediatr* 1995;34(12):626–634.
7. Sacchetti AD, Gerardi M, Sawchuk P, et al. Boomerang babies: Emergency department utilization by early discharge neonates. *Pediatr Emerg Care* 1997;13(6):365–368.
8. Kuehl KS, Loffredo CA, Ferencz C. Failure to diagnose congenital heart disease in infancy. *Pediatrics* 1999; 103(4):743–747.

9. Balmer C, Beghetti M, Fasnacht M, et al. Balloon aortic valvuloplasty in paediatric patients: Progressive aortic regurgitation is common. *Heart* 2004;90(1):77–81.

10. Mendelsohn AM, Shim D. Inroads in transcatheter therapy for congenital heart disease. *J Pediatr* 1998;133(3):324–333.

11. Grech ED. Non-coronary percutaneous intervention. *Br Med J* 2003;327:97–100.

12. Budts W, Gewillig M, VandeWerf F. Left-to-right shunting in common congenital heart defects: Which patients are eligible for percutaneous interventions? *Acta Cardiologica* 2003;58(3):199–205.

13. Rosenkranz ER. Caring for the former pediatric cardiac surgery patient. *Pediatr Clin North Am* 1998;45(4):907–941.

14. Rao PS, Gupta ML, Balaji S. Recent advances in pediatric cardiology-electrophysiology, transcatheter and surgical advances. *Indian J Pediatr* 2003;70(7):557–564.

15. Tworetsky W, Marshall AC. Balloon valvuloplasty for congenital heart disease in the fetus. *Clin Perinatol* 2003; 30(3):541–550.

16. Moodie DS. Adult congenital heart disease. *Curr Opin Cardiol* 1994;9:137–142.

17. Webb GD. Advances in adult congenital heart disease. *Cardiol Clin* 2002;20(3):Xi–Xii.

18. Moller JH. Clinical history and physical examination. In: Moller JH, Hoffman HIE (eds.), *Pediatric Cardiovascular Medicine*, Churchill-Livingston, Philadelphia, 2000:97–110.

19. Respiratory syncytial virus. In: Pickering LK, Baker CJ, Overturf GD, et al. (eds.), *Red Book 2003 Report of the Committee on Infectious Diseases*. Elk Grove Village, IL: American Academy of Pediatrics, 2003:523–528.

20. Mace SE, Hirschfield SS, Riggs T, et al. Echocardiographic abnormalities in infants of diabetic mothers. *J Pediatr* 1979;95(6):1013–1019.

21. Bernstein D. Cyanotic congenital heart disease: Evaluation of the critically ill neonate with cyanosis and respiratory distress. In: Behrman RE, Kliegman RM, Jenson HB (eds.), *Textbook of Pediatrics*, 17th ed. Philadelphia, PA: W.B. Saunders, 2004:1523–1524.

22. Bernstein D. The fetal-to-neonatal circulatory transition. In: Behrman RE, Kliegman RM, Jenson HB (eds.), *Textbook of Pediatrics*, 17th ed. Philadelphia, PA: W.B. Saunders, 2004:1479–1481.

23. Brook MM, Heymann MA, Teitel DF. The heart. In: Klaus MH, Fanaroff AA (eds.), *Care of the High-Risk Neonate*, 5th ed. Philadelphia, PA: W.B. Saunders, 2001:393–424.

24. Fyler DC, Buckley LP, Hellenbrand WE. Report of the New England Regional Infant Cardiac Program. *Pediatrics* 1980;65(2):375–461.

25. Hoffman JIE, Christianson R. Congenital heart disease in a cohort of 19,502 births with long-term follow-up. *Am J Cardiol* 1978;42:641–647.

26. Kramer HH, Majewski F, Trampisch HJ. Malformation patterns in children with congenital heart disease. *Am J Dis Child* 1987;141:789–795.

27. Mitchell SC, Korones SB, Berendes HW. Congenital heart disease in 56,109 births. *Circulation* 1971;KLIII:323–332.

28. Campbell M. Incidence of cardiac malformations at birth and later and neonatal mortality. *Br Heart J* 1973;35: 189–200.

29. Hoffman JIE. Congenital heart disease: Incidence and recurrence. In: Rudolph CD, Rudolph AM, Hostetter MK, et al. (eds.), *Rudolph's Pediatrics*, 21st ed. New York: McGraw-Hill, 2003:1780–1782.

30. Mace SE. The pediatric patient with acute respiratory failure: Clinical diagnosis and pathophysiology. *Pediatric Emerg Med Reports* 2001;6(3):21–32.

31. Mace SE. Dyspnea. In: Mahadevan SV (ed.), *Clinical Emergency Medicine: A Guide for the Practitioner in the Emergency Department*. Cambridge, UK: Cambridge University Press, 2004.

32. Friedli B, Faidutti B, Oberhansli L, et al. Late results of surgery for congenital heart defect. *Helv Chir Acta* 1990;57:533–543.

33. Monro JL, Alexiou C, Salmon AP, et al. Re-operations and survival after primary repair of congenital heart defects in children. *J Thorac Cardiovas Surg* 2003;126(2): 511–520.

34. Dearani JA, Danielson GK, Puga FJ, et al. Late follow-up of 1095 patients undergoing operation for complex congenital heart disease utilizing pulmonary ventricle to pulmonary artery conduits. *Ann Thorac Surg* 2003;75(2):399–411.

35. Kaemmerer H, Fratz S, Bauer U, et al. Emergency hospital admissions and three-year survival of adults with and without cardiovascular surgery for congenital cardiac disease. *J Thorac Cardiovasc Surg* 2003;126(4):1048–1052.

36. Mavroudis C, Deal BJ, Backer CL. Arrhythmia surgery in association with complex congenital heart repairs excluding patients with Fontan conversion. *Semin Thorac Cardiovasc Surg Pediatr Card Surg Annu* 2003;6:33–50.

37. Ashburn DA, Harris L, Downnar EH, et al. Electrophysiologic surgery in patients with congenital heart disease. *Semin Thorac Cardiovasc Surg Pediatr Card Surg Annu* 2003;6: 51–58.

38. Deal BJ, Mavroudis C, Baker CL. Beyond Fontan conversion: Surgical therapy of arrhythmias including patients with associated complex congenital heart disease. *Ann Thorac Surg* 2003;76(2):542–553.

39. Greason KL, Dearani JA, Theodoro DA, et al. Surgical management of atrial tachyarrhythmias associated with congenital cardiac anomalies: Mayo Clinic Experience. *Semin Thorac Cardiovasc Surg Pediatr Card Surg Annu* 2003;6: 59–71.

40. Mavroudis C, Backer CL, Kohr LM, et al. Bidirectional Glenn shunt in association with congenital heart repairs: The 1 1/2 ventricular repair. *Ann Thorac Surg* 1999;68: 976–982.

41. Nollert CD, Dabritz SH, Schmoeckel M, et al. Risk factors for sudden death after repair of tetralogy of Fallot. *Ann Thorac Surg* 2003;76(6):1901–1905.

42. Fenton KN, Siewers RD, Rebovich B, et al. Interim mortality infants with systemic-to-pulmonary artery shunts. *Ann Thorac Surg* 2003;76:152–157.

43. Reddy WV, McElhinney DB, Sagrado T, et al. Results of 102 cases of complete repair of congenital heart defects in patients weighing 700 to 2500 grams. *J Thorac Cardiovasc Surg* 1999;117(2):324–331.

44. Dees E, Lin H, Cotto RB, et al. Outcome of pre-term infants with congenital heart disease. *J Pediatr* 2000;137(5):653–659.

45. Clancy RR, McGaurn SA, Wernovsky G, et al. Risk of seizures in survivors of newborn heart surgery using deep hypothermic circulatory arrest. *Pediatrics* 2003;111(3):592–601.

46. Ikle L, Hale K, Fashaw L, et al. Developmental outcome of patients with hypoplastic left heart syndrome treated with heart transplantation. *J Pediatr* 2003;142(1):20–25.

47. Wernovsky G, Newburger J. Neurologic and developmental morbidity in children with complex congenital heart disease. *J Pediatr* 2003;142(1):6–8.

48. Michielon G, Parisi F, Squitieri C, et al. Orthotopic heart transplantation alternative for high-risk Fontan candidates. *Circulation* 2003;108(Suppl II):II-140–II-149.

41

Pediatric Acquired Heart Disease

Sharon E. Mace

HIGH YIELD FACTS

- There is no diagnostic test for Kawasaki disease. The diagnosis is based on clinical criteria: fever plus any four of conjunctival injection, oropharyngeal involvement, cervical lymphadenopathy, peripheral extremity changes, and a rash.

- Cardiac involvement leads to the development of coronary artery aneurysms in 20–25% of untreated Kawasaki disease.

- Patients with Kawasaki disease should be hospitalized for cardiac evaluation and treated with intravenous immune globulin (IVIG), and high-dose aspirin. Treatment with IVIG prevents the coronary abnormalities.

- Acute rheumatic fever (ARF) is an inflammatory disease affecting the heart, joints, brain, blood vessels, and subcutaneous tissue resulting from a prior streptococcal pharyngitis.

- The diagnosis of ARF is based on the Jones criteria. ARF can be prevented by antistreptococcal antibiotic therapy.

- Bacterial endocarditis should be considered in any at-risk patient with fever, a new or changing murmur, and elevated acute phase reactants.

- Fever and nonspecific complaints (malaise, myalgias, and arthralgias) may be the only clinical findings of bacterial endocarditis.

- Syncope in pediatric patients is a common complaint, usually benign, but can be due to a serious life-threatening cardiac disease.

- A thorough history and physical examination along with an ECG can help distinguish the benign from significant life-threatening cardiac disease as a cause of syncope or chest pain in pediatric patients.

KAWASAKI DISEASE

Kawasaki disease is the number one cause of acquired heart disease in children in the developed world and the United States.[1–3] Furthermore, its frequency worldwide is on the rise.[2–5] Kawasaki disease was named "mucocutaneous lymph node syndrome" because of the striking involvement of the mucous membranes, skin, and lymph nodes in affected children. The Japanese physician, Kawasaki, first described the disorder in 1967.[6] Kawasaki disease is probably the same disorder described previously as infantile periarteritis nodosa.[7] The disorder occurs throughout the world and has been found in all ethnic groups although there is a predilection for the Asian population, especially the Japanese.[8]

Kawasaki syndrome is an acute febrile, exanthematous multisystem vasculitis affecting primarily pediatric patients. Ninety five percent of all patients are less than 10 years old.[9,10] The peak age of occurrence in the United States is 18–24 months, 50% of patients are <2 years old, and 80% of patients are <5 years old.[9,10]

Since there is no diagnostic test for Kawasaki syndrome, the diagnosis is based on clinical findings. The diagnostic criteria are fever lasting for at least 5 days, not be explained by another disease process, plus four of the following:

(a) Bilateral bulbar conjunctival injection without exudates

(b) Oropharyngeal involvement (dry cracked lips, strawberry tongue, erythematous pharynx)

(c) Acute nonsuppurative cervical lymphadenopathy (one or more nodes >1.5 cm)

(d) Peripheral extremity changes (indurated hands/feet with erythematous palms/soles, periunguinal desquamation)

(e) generalized polymorphous erythematous rash[11,12]

One important caveat to remember is the diagnosis can be made and treatment started if fever and ≥4 other criteria are met even if the fever has been present less than the "requisite" 5 days' duration.[13]

The acute phase begins with the abrupt onset of a high fever. The fever is usually >104°F, unresponsive to antibiotics and the usual antipyretics, and lasts 1–2 weeks if untreated. The hallmark of the bilateral bulbar conjunctival injection, which occurs in about 90% of patients, is a lack of discharge. The strawberry tongue is similar to that occurring with streptococcal infections. The lymph nodes are nonsuppurative, usually large and nontender. The rash is generalized and can take almost any appearance: morbilliform, maculopapular, scarlatiniform, or erythema multiforme but not vesicular.

Several days after the onset of the fever; pain, swelling, and edema of the hands and feet occur. This is followed by cutaneous desquamation during the second to third weeks primarily involving the tips of the fingers/toes, the palms, and the soles of the feet.

The most important system involvement is cardiac since about 20–25% of untreated patients will develop coronary artery aneurysms, generally occurring between weeks 1 and 4 after disease onset.[14] Less commonly, pericarditis, myocarditis, and/or endocarditis can occur.[14]

Other clinical manifestations that may be present are gastrointestinal (abdominal pain, vomiting, diarrhea, gall bladder hydrops, hepatosplenomegaly), genitourinary (sterile pyuria), musculoskeletal (transient arthralgias/arthritis), neurologic (aseptic meningitis), pulmonary (pneumonia on chest roentgenogram), typmpanitis, and irritability in infants.[14]

Kawasaki syndrome has four phases: acute (febrile), subacute, recovery (convalescent), and chronic. The acute (febrile) phase, days 1–11, is when classic diagnostic clinical signs are present.[1] Key findings during the subacute phase, days 11–21, are desquamation, thrombocytosis, and resolution of fever.[1] During the recovery phase, days 21–60, most clinical signs resolve, and the acute phase reactants become normal.[1] Long-term cardiac sequelae can occur during the chronic phase and involve coronary occlusive disease, aneurysmal rupture, cardiac small vessel disease, and perhaps even early coronary atherosclerosis.[15–18]

Atypical or incomplete Kawasaki disease is diagnosed when patients have a fever and less than four of the other criteria.[19] Incomplete Kawasaki syndrome occurs most often in infants (age <12 months) who are more susceptible to the development of coronary artery aneurysms and in whom clinical findings may be subtle making the diagnosis more difficult.[20] Persistent fever in an infant may be the only sign of Kawasaki disease. Echocardiography can be invaluable in making the diagnosis in cases of atypical Kawasaki syndrome.

There is no pathognomic test for Kawasaki disease. Typical findings on the complete blood count are leukocytosis, with a left shift (increased neutrophils), normochromic normocytic anemia, and thrombocytosis (after the first week of acute illness). Markedly elevated phase reactants (erythrocyte sedimentation rate, C-reactive protein), a two- to threefold rise in liver function tests, and sterile pyuria from urethritis, are usually present. Important clues to the diagnosis are the negative tests for rheumatologic disorders (e.g., anti-nuclear antibody (ANA), rheumatoid factor) and for acute infections (blood, urine, cerebrospinal fluid, throat cultures). ECG changes, found in about one-third of patients, include prolonged PR interval, left ventricular hypertrophy, non-specific ST-T abnormalities, abnormal Q waves, and ventricular dysrhythmias. An infiltrate or cardiomegaly may be noted on the chest radiograph. Echocardiography should be done to detect coronary artery abnormalities, pericardial effusions, or impaired myocardial contractility. The incidence of death is <0.01%, usually in the first 6 weeks from myocardial infarction (the most common cause), rupture of an aneurysm, or myocarditis.[14]

Risk factors for coronary artery abnormalities are age <1 year, male gender, Asian ethnicity, prolonged fever >16 days, ECG abnormalities, markedly increased sedimentation rate (>101 mm/hour), an elevated white blood cell count (>30,000/mm^3), high percent neutrophils (>68%), low hematocrit (<32.5), and low serum albumin (<3 g/L).[21,22]

The differential diagnosis includes rheumatologic disorders (such as juvenile rheumatoid arthritis), other vasculitis (e.g., polyarteritis nodosa), Stevens-Johnson syndrome, and acute infections. Infections may be bacterial (scarlet fever, sepsis, toxic shock syndrome), viral (rubella, Epstein-Barr virus, adenovirus), or rickettsial (Rocky-Mountain spotted fever).[1,8,11]

Ultimately, the etiology of Kawasaki disease is unknown, but an immune response to an infectious agent is most likely.[13] A recent theory postulates that a bacterial toxin (either staphylococci or hemolytic streptococci) colonizes the gastrointestinal tract in a genetically susceptible individual, which stimulates a superantigen response by the body.[8,12,13,23]

Anti-inflammatory therapy should be given as soon as the diagnosis is made or suspected. Early gamma-globulin administration prevents coronary abnormalities and leads to faster symptom resolution, usually within 24–48 hours.[14,24] The treatment of choice is high-dose IVIG as a single dose of 2 g/kg over 10–12 hours. The single dose is more effective than divided doses.[25] High-dose aspirin is also given during the acute phase, both for its antithrombotic and anti-inflammatory effects, in a dose of 80–100 mg/kg/day in four divided doses.[14,26,27] In patients failing the initial therapy of IVIG and aspirin, a repeat dose of IVIG at 2 g/kg can be given.[28] There has been much controversy regarding the use of corticosteroids. Currently steroids are not recommended routinely but are used in some patients (such as those patients refractory to standard IVIG therapy or with life-threatening complications of Kawasaki disease).[26–29] An early study found a greater incidence of coronary artery aneurysms in patients treated with prednisolone.[30] However, recent studies using corticosteroids have shown a benefit.[31,32]

An echocardiogram is warranted early in the acute phase (in the first week) and toward the end of the recovery phase (6–8 weeks after symptom onset) to evaluate for carditis.[14]

Coronary arteriography also demonstrates the coronary artery abnormalities but is infrequently needed. In patients without coronary abnormalities, full recovery can be expected and even children with cardiac involvement do well, although long-term cardiac complications can occur.[15–17]

ACUTE RHEUMATIC FEVER

Rheumatic fever is the most common cause of acquired heart disease in children and young adults throughout the world.[33] Even though the occurrence of rheumatic fever has shown a dramatic decrease over the past few decades in developed countries, including the United States and Western Europe,[34] its incidence is still high in the United States because of a resurgence in certain areas.[35–38]

ARF is a diffuse inflammatory disease of the connective tissue; mainly the heart, joints, brain, blood vessels, and subcutaneous tissues. It is a delayed nonsuppurative sequelae of an upper respiratory tract infection with group A beta-hemolytic streptococci. Because, the risk of rheumatic fever can be nearly eradicated by appropriate antibiotic therapy of group A beta-hemolytic streptococcal pharyngitis,[39] it is critical to diagnose it in order to eliminate or minimize future significant heart disease.

Failure to treat a group A beta-hemolytic streptococcal pharyngitis is a prerequisite for the subsequent development of ARF. The pathogenesis involves a pharyngitis caused by rheumatogenic strains of group A beta-hemolytic streptococci in a susceptible host. This is followed by an immune reaction, associated with certain HLA-DR alleles, which causes inflammation in various tissues/organs, notably the heart, joints, brain, blood vessels, and connective tissue. The latent period between the acute streptococcal infection and rheumatic fever is a mean of 18 days (range 7–35 days), and for Sydenham's chorea from 2 to 6 months.[40]

There is no pathognomonic test for ARF. The diagnosis is based on the modified Jones criteria,[34,41] requiring two major, or one major and two minor criteria, plus supporting evidence of antecedent group A streptococcal infection. The major Jones criteria are arthritis, carditis, chorea, erythema marginatum, and subcutaneous nodules. The minor criteria are arthralgias, fever, elevated acute phase reactants (erythrocyte sedimentation rate or C-reactive protein), and prolonged PR interval on ECG.[34] Evidence of a previous group A streptococcal infection can be confirmed by a positive throat culture or rapid streptococcal antigen test, an elevated or rising streptococcal antibody titer, or recent scarlet fever.[34]

About 2–3 weeks after a streptococcal infection, the clinical manifestations begin. These are usually an initial arthritis, followed by carditis.[42] Arthritis, the most common

major manifestation, is typically migratory, affecting the large joints. The pain, redness, heat, and swelling of the inflamed joint(s) quickly resolves with salicylates.

Signs of myocarditis are a resting tachycardia in an afebrile patient, heart block (especially a prolonged PR interval), cardiomegaly, and heart failure. A new murmur, especially mitral insufficiency, heralds the onset of endocarditis (valvular inflammation). The most frequently encountered lesions of rheumatic carditis are rheumatic valvulitis, especially mitral and/or aortic insufficiency, and heralds the onset of endocarditis. Heart failure can be due to severe valvular disease or myocarditis. Pericarditis, possibly detected by the presence of a friction rub, signifies pancarditis, which has a high mortality.

Other symptoms of rheumatic fever include Sydenham's chorea (St. Vitus' dance). This is characterized by involuntary purposeless uncoordinated choreiform movements of the extremities. Clumsiness with fine motor tasks, emotional lability, crying, fidgeting, and poor writing are other manifestations. Erythema marginatum is an irregular serpiginous erythematous macular rash, varying in size/shape, and often evanescent. Subcutaneous nodules are nontender, freely movable, about 1-cm diameter nodules on the extensor tendons of extremities.

Hospitalization may be necessary for patients with ARF in order to establish the diagnosis, evaluate the heart, and initiate treatment. A course of antibiotic therapy with penicillin or erythromycin is recommended, in order to eliminate the streptococci, even if the throat culture and rapid streptococcal tests are negative. High-dose aspirin will treat the carditis and arthritis. A recent study found that naproxen (15–20 mg/kg, divided to bid) was an acceptable alternative to aspirin for the treatment of ARF.[43] The use of corticosteroids is controversial, often reserved for use with severe carditis or chorea, and without proven benefit.[44] Intravenous immunoglobin is also not recommended.[44] Long-term follow-up of patients with ARF is needed for endocarditis prophylaxis, monitoring for reoccurrence, and treatment of cardiac complications including heart failure.

Appropriate antimicrobial therapy is effective in the prevention of rheumatic fever.[39] A recent report suggests that intramuscular penicillin is more effective than oral penicillin and more frequent injections are also more efficacious in the prevention of rheumatic fever.[45,46]

INFECTIVE ENDOCARDITIS

Infective endocarditis is a microbial infection of the heart's endothelial (endocardial) surface. Endocarditis can affect prosthetic or native heart valves, septal defects, the mural endocardium, and intracardiac/intravascular devices, such as intracardiac patches or baffles, surgically constructed shunts, and central venous catheters.

The incidence of endocarditis has increased in the past few decades and will probably continue to do so in the future.[47–52] There are many reasons for this, and include advances in treatment of congenital heart disease, increased number of cardiac surgeries, greater use of prosthetic materials, increased use of indwelling catheters, expanded use of neonatal/pediatric intensive care units and medical technology, increase in number of immunocompromised patients, neonatal and/or pediatric intensive care unit graduates, and growing rates of intravenous drug abuse. Individuals with the greatest risk for endocarditis are those with congenital or acquired valvular heart disease, and those with prosthetic materials in the cardiovascular system.

Bacteremia can colonize an area of endothelium damaged by abnormal blood flow hemodynamics. There are many portals of entry for bacteria, and include dental caries, genitourinary or gastrointestinal or airway procedures, skin infections, indwelling catheters/devices, intravenous drug abuse, and body piercing/tatooing.[53–58] The vast majority of endocarditis is due to bacteria, although fungi, rickettsiae, or viruses can be the cause. The most common microorganisms are *Streptococcus viridans* and *Staphylococcus aureus*.[47–53] Other less frequent microorganisms are the HACEK group (*Hemophilus, Actinobacillus, Cardiobacterium, Eikenella, Kingella*), other streptococci/enterococci, coagulase-negative staphylococcus, gram-negative bacilli, and fungi.[47–50,59,60] Enterococci, fungi, and HACEK organisms are frequently found in newborns and immunocompromised patients.[59,60] Fungal endocarditis has been reported in drug abusers, and hospitalized infants with indwelling central venous catheters.[54,55,61]

Signs and symptoms generally begin within 2 weeks of the bacterial seeding, and are often nonspecific, mild, and easily overlooked.[62,63] Fever is the most frequent manifestation.[47–51,60] Nonspecific complaints of malaise, myalgia, or arthralgias are common. A new or changing murmur occurs only about half the time. Less common signs are splenomegaly, neurologic changes, peripheral emboli, petechiae, and congestive heart failure. The classic findings of Roth spots, splinter hemorrhages, Janeway lesions, and Osler nodes are rare. The physician should have a high index of suspicion for endocarditis in any patient with congenital or acquired heart disease who has a fever or any of the above signs/symptoms.

The clinical manifestations of endocarditis occur as a result of (1) the immunologic response to the vegetation, including fever, myalgias, and arthralgias, (2) peripheral emboli causing neurologic symptoms, hematuria, splinter hemorrhages, etc, and (3) impaired heart function by direct local effect of the infection resulting in cardiac valve dysfunction (most commonly, insufficiency).

Laboratory findings commonly found with endocarditis include elevated acute phase reactants (sedimentation rate, C-reactive protein), anemia, hematuria, and a positive rheumatoid factor.

A positive blood culture with endocarditis is found about 90% of the time.[66] A positive blood culture in an infant/child with heart disease does not automatically mean endocarditis is present, although the possibility must be considered. Conversely, in a patient with heart disease who has risk factors for endocarditis, blood cultures should be obtained. Culture negative endocarditis occurs,[66–68] and may be due to recent antibiotic therapy or fastidious organisms that are difficult to grow in culture. The incidence of true culture negative endocarditis in patients who have not received antibiotics is probably less than 5%.[69] In the future, the use of polymerase chain reaction (PCR) may aid in the identification of the infecting organism, when blood cultures are negative.[67,68,70]

Echocardiography can be a diagnostic adjunct; however, the detection rate for endocarditis in pediatric patients is about 60–86%.[64,65] The failure rate is probably higher for infants/children with complex congenital heart disease because their anatomy/shunts are more difficult to visualize on the echocardiogram.

Patients with a fever, typical signs/symptoms of endocarditis, and a positive blood culture, are not a diagnostic challenge. Others may lack classic findings, especially those with acute onset, right-sided endocarditis, infants, and neonates. Criteria for the diagnosis of infective endocarditis (von Reyn, Duke, Beth Israel) use various parameters (clinical, pathologic, microbiologic, echocardiographic), and may be helpful in such cases.[71–73] However, the validity of such criteria for infants and children has not been fully established.[74–76]

Once the responsible organism is known, specific antibiotic therapy can be started. In some, appropriate broad-spectrum coverage may be instituted after blood cultures and specialist consultation are obtained.

Surgery to remove the vegetation, or replace the infected valve, may need to be done in some patients if there is persistent bacteremia, myocardial abscess, severe valve failure, recurrent emboli, or arrhythmias unresponsive to usual therapy. Before antibiotics, endocarditis was uniformly fatal. Even with today's therapeutic advances, the mortality rate is still 6–14%. Therefore, prevention is critical. A synopsis of the American Heart Association guidelines regarding the prevention of bacterial endocarditis is given in Tables 41-1 to 41-3.[77,78]

Table 41-1. Common Procedures for Which Antibiotic Prophylaxis is Recommended

- Dental: extractions, root canal, implants, periodontal procedures, cleaning (if bleeding is anticipated) initial placement of orthodontic bands
- Respiratory: rigid bronchoscopy, flexible bronchoscopy with biopsy, surgical procedures: tonsillectomy, adenoidectomy
- Gastrointestinal: esophageal dilatation, variceal sclerotherapy, endoscopic retrograde cholangiography, biliary tract surgery, surgery involving the intestinal mucosa
- Genitourinary: cytoscopy, urethral dilatation

SYNCOPE IN THE PEDIATRIC PATIENT

Syncope is an abrupt brief transient loss of consciousness with loss of postural tone, which resolves spontaneously. It is a frequent complaint in patients of all ages, and is responsible for 3% of emergency department (ED) visits.[79] Syncope accounts for 2% of pediatric ED visits[80] and 1% of pediatric hospital admissions.[81] In adults, syncope accounts for 1–6% of inpatient admissions.[82–84] The incidence of syncope varies with age. It is infrequent in preschool age children (<5 years of age), while up to half (15–50%) of adolescents have had one or more syncopal episodes.[81,85–87]

Although there are many causes of syncope,[88–91] the final common pathway involves decreased cerebral blood flow (with decreased oxygen and glucose) delivered to the reticular activating system in the brainstem or both cerebral hemispheres. Generally, decreased cardiac output results in inadequate cerebral perfusion and syncope results.

It is crucial to recognize the cardiovascular causes of syncope because cardiovascular syncope may be a harbinger for sudden death. Pediatric heart disease patients have an increased risk of dysrhythmias and sudden death. In pediatric patients, the most common cause of dysrhythmias leading to syncope is congenital heart disease.[92] Especially vulnerable to sudden death from dysrhythmias

are patients with Eisenmenger syndrome (see page 469), and those who have had cardiac surgery for congenital cardiac defects.[93] Sudden death in patients with a structurally "normal" heart has been associated with the long QT syndrome, bradyarrhythmias (e.g., sick sinus syndrome, complete heart block), Wolf-Parkinson White syndrome (WPW), the Brugada syndrome, and ventricular tachycardias. There are many diverse causes for these dysrhythmias, which may be inherited or acquired. Some of these causes include medications, toxins, electrolyte abnormalities, myocarditis/cardiomyopathies, myocardial ischemia, a history of cardiac surgery (with damage to the heart conducting system), infections (such as diphtheria, Chagas disease), rheumatologic disorders (Lyme disease, systemic lupus erythematosus), and neuromuscular disorders (muscular dystrophy, Kearns-Sayre disease, and other generalized disorders affecting the myocardium).

Any cardiac disorder causing obstruction to blood flow can also lead to syncope and sudden death. Cardiac syncope can occur with aortic stenosis, coarctation of the aorta, hypertrophic obstructive cardiomyopathy (HOCM), pulmonic stenosis, cardiac tumors (such as an atrial myxoma), primary pulmonary hypertension, Eisenmenger syndrome, and pericarditis (with tamponade). The number one cause of sudden death in young athletes is HOCM.

Myocardial disease, whether from myocarditis, ischemia, other disorders damaging the myocardium (tumors,

Table 41-2. Common Procedures for Which Antibiotic Prophylaxis is not Recommended

- Dental: orthodontic appliance removal or adjustment, local anesthetic injections, fluoride treatments, oral radiographs
- Respiratory: intubation, flexible bronchoscopy without biopsy, tympanostomy, tube placement/removal
- Gastrointestinal: endoscopy without biopsy
- Genitourinary: urinary catheterization, circumcision
- Gynecologic: cesarean section, vaginal delivery
- Cardiac: cardiac catheterization with/without device placement, transesophageal echocardiography
- Other: skin biopsy

Table 41-3. Cardiac Conditions for Which Prophylaxis is/is not Recommended

A. Endocarditis prophylaxis recommended high-risk category
- Cyanotic congenital heart disease: e.g., tetralogy of Fallot, transposition, truncus, total anomalous pulmonary venous return, tricuspid valve abnormalities
- Surgically constructed systemic—pulmonary shunts or conduits
- Prosthetic cardiac valves
- Previous bacterial endocarditis

B. Endocarditis prophylaxis recommended moderate-risk category
- Most other cardiac congenital cardiac malformations (other than in A or C)
- Acquired valve dysfunction (rheumatic heart disease)
- Hypertrophic cardiomyopathy
- Mitral valve prolapse (with valvular regurgitation or thickened leaflets)

C. Endocarditis prophylaxis not recommended negligible risk category
- Cardiac pacemakers, implanted defibrillators
- Isolated secundum atrial septal defect
- Surgical repair without residual done after 6 months of age for ASD, VSD, or PDA
- Previous Kawasaki disease without valvular dysfunction
- Innocent (physiologic) murmurs

Source: Adapted from the American Heart Association Recommendations (References 77, 78).

connective tissue diseases, and so on), can cause cardiac syncope. Vascular causes of syncope range from aortic dissection to subclavian steal and thoracic outlet syndrome.

Although cardiac syncope is not the most common etiology of pediatric syncope (vasovagal syncope is the most frequent etiology),[81,91] because it is a high-risk cause, an ECG is probably indicated in any ED patient (pediatric or adult) with syncope.

Clues to the possibility that the patient may have cardiac syncope and is at high risk for sudden death are a history of congenital or acquired heart disease, status post cardiac surgery, family history of sudden death or arrhythmias (such as WPW), abnormal cardiac examination (nonphysiologic murmur, abnormal heart sounds, thrill, abnormal

pulses/blood pressure), associated cardiac symptoms such as chest pain dyspnea on exertion, palpitations, fast or slow pulse/heartbeat, and systemic diseases that can affect the heart, including rheumatologic diseases, and vasculitis.

CHEST PAIN IN THE PEDIATRIC PATIENT

Pediatric chest pain is very common.[94] It is usually benign, most often musculoskeletal or idiopathic, but can be from serious life-threatening disease.[95–99] The incidence of "idiopathic" chest pain may be overestimated. Several studies have found a high incidence of exercise-induced asthma or gastroesophageal disease (especially reflux) when pediatric patients underwent further evaluation.[100,101] The history, physical examination, and occasionally ancillary studies (e.g., ECG and chest radiograph) are instrumental in differentiating benign from serious causes of pediatric chest pain.

Risk factors from a possible life-threatening etiology for the chest pain are previous cardiac surgery, known congenital or acquired heart disease, chest pain with exercise, chest pain with associated symptoms (including syncope or dyspnea), and chest pain associated with signs of heart disease, or with systemic disorders that may have a cardiac component.

Factors suggesting a cardiac etiology are drug/use (including illegal drugs such as cocaine, glue sniffing, or steroids), toxins, or a positive family history of familial hyperlipidemia, sudden death, arrhythmias, WPW, or long QT syndrome. Associated cardiovascular symptoms may suggest a cardiac etiology, and include dyspnea on exertion, orthopnea, palpitations, irregular or slow or fast heart beat, syncope/near syncope.

Other diagnoses may affect the myocardium, and should be considered. For example, the child with a fever and rash or joint pain may have chest pain from a vasculitis (e.g. polyarteritis nodosa, Wegener's granulomatosis, Takayasu's arteritis, or hypersensitivity vasculitis), or a rheumatologic disease such as juvenile rheumatoid arthritis, systemic lupus, erythematosus, or Lyme disease.

The cardiovascular examination is important in the evaluation of the pediatric patient with chest pain and should include inspection, palpation, and auscultation. Any cardiac abnormalities from a heave, thrill, increased/displaced point of maximal impulse (PMI), a single S_2 (as with truncus arteriosus), a fixed widely split S_2 (as with an atrial septal defect), or an S_3 or S_4 (implying valvular disease), suggest cardiac pathology as a cause of the chest pain. A pericardial rub signifies pericarditis and a pathologic murmur may indicate congenital or acquired heart disease. The pulses in all four extremities are important parts of the physical examination, and may reveal the wide bounding pulses of a patent ductus arteriosus or aortic insufficiency, or discrepancies suggesting coarctation. Likewise, the blood pressure may disclose previously unrecognized hypertension or coarctation of the aorta.

The general physical examination may reveal the abnormal facies or stigmata of an underlying syndrome (e.g., Marfan disease, Ehlers Danlos syndrome, Turner syndrome, or Down syndrome) that has a high association with congenital cardiac defects. The remainder of the physical examination may uncover a collagen vascular disease, neuromuscular disorder, vasculitis, or systemic infection that has a cardiac component.

Cardiac causes of chest pain in pediatric patients may be from an acute coronary syndrome (as in Kawasaki disease, premature atherosclerosis, or from an anomalous coronary artery), valvular disease (significant aortic or pulmonic stenosis), severe hypertension (systemic or pulmonic), outflow tract obstruction (typically HOCM), pericarditis, or myocardial disease (cardiomyopathy, myocarditis, infiltrating diseases of myocardium).

A thorough history/physical examination and appropriate ancillary studies (typically an ECG and chest radiograph, occasionally other studies) will help differentiate the benign from life-threatening causes of chest pain. The ECG is a simple noninvasive, inexpensive test that can be extremely valuable. A chest radiograph may also be useful.

REFERENCES

1. Rowley A, Shulman ST. Kawasaki's disease. In: Behrman RE, Kliegman RM, Jenson HB (eds), *Nelson Textbook of Pediatrics*, 17th ed. Philadelphia, PA: W.B. Saunders, 2004:823–826.
2. Harden A, Alves B, Sheikh A. Rising incidence of Kawasaki disease in England: Analysis of hospital admission data. *Br Med J* 2002;324:424–425.
3. Yanagawa H, Nakamura Y, Yashiro M, et al. Incidence survey of Kawasaki disease in 1997 and 1998 in Japan. *Pediatrics* 2001;107:E33.
4. McCrindle BW, Lobo L, Nagpal S, et al. The epidemiology of Kawasaki disease in Ontario and Canada. *Pediatr Res* 2002;53(1):159 (abstract #8).
5. Chang RKR. Hospitalizations for Kawasaki disease among children in the United States, 1988–1997. *Pediatrics* 2002;109(6):e87 (abstract).
6. Kawasaki T. Pediatric acute febrile mucocutaneous lymph node syndrome with characteristic desquamation of fingers and toes: My clinical observation of 50 cases [in Japanese]. *Jpn J Allergol* 1967;16:178–222. Translation by H Shike, C Shimizu, JC Burns [online 2002]. Available at: http//www.pidj.com/
7. Landing BH, Larson EJ. Are infantile periarteritis nodosa with coronary artery involvement and fatal mucocutaneous lymph node syndrome the same: Comparison of 20 patients from North America with patients from Hawaii and Japan. *Pediatrics* 1977;59:651–662.
8. Barron KS. Kawasaki disease etiology, pathogenesis, and treatment. *Cleve Clin J Med* 2002;69(Suppl 2):S1169–S1178.
9. Holman RC, Curns AT, Belay ED, et al. Kawasaki syndrome hospitalizations in the United States, 1997 and 2000. *Pediatrics* 2003;112(3):495–501.
10. Belay ED, Holman RC, Maddox RA, et al. Kawasaki syndrome hospitalizations and associated costs in the United States. *Public Health Rep* 2003;118:464–469.
11. Rowley AH, Shulman ST. Kawasaki syndrome. *Pediatr Clin North Am* 1999;46(2):313–329.
12. Meissner HC, Leung DKM. Kawasaki syndrome: Where are the answers. *Pediatrics* 2003;672–676.
13. Newburger JW, Taubert KA, Shulman ST, et al. Summary and abstracts of the seventh international Kawasaki Disease symposium. *Pediatr Res* 2003;53(1):153–157.
14. Pickering LK, Baker CJ, Overturf GD, et al. Kawasaki syndrome. *Red Book: 2003 Report of the Committee on Infectious Diseases*, 26th ed. Elk Grove Village, IL: American Academy of Pediatrics, 2003:392–395.
15. Kato H, Koike S, Yamamoto M, et al. Coronary aneurysms in infants and young children with acute febrile mucocutaneous lymph node syndrome. *J Pediatr* 1975;86:892–898.
16. Kato H, Akagi T, Sugimura T, et al. Kawasaki disease. *Coron Artery Dis* 1995;6:194–206.
17. Hirata S, Nakamura Y, Matsumoto K, et al. Long-term consequences of Kawasaki disease among first-year junior high school students. *Arch Pediatr Adolesc Med* 2002;156:77–80.
18. Dajani AS, Taubert KA, Takahashi M, et al. Guidelines for long-term management of patients with Kawasaki disease. Report from the Committee on Rheumatic Fever, Endocarditis, and Kawasaki disease. Council on Cardiovascular Disease in the young, American Heart Association. *Circulation* 1994;89:916–922.
19. Rowley AH. Incomplete (atypical) Kawasaki disease. *Pediatr Infect Dis J* 2002;21:563–566.
20. Ganizi J, Miron D, Spiegel R, et al. Kawasaki Disease in very young infants: High prevalence of atypical presentation and coronary arteritis. *Clin Pediatrics* 2003;42:263–267.
21. Zhang T, Yanagawa H, Oki I, et al. Factors relating to the cardiac sequelae of Kawasaki disease one month after initial onset. *Acta Paediatr* 2002;91:517–520.
22. Honkanen VEA, McCrindle BW, Laxer RM, et al. Clinical relevance of the risk factors for coronary artery inflammation in Kawasaki disease. *Pediatr Cardiol* 2003;24:122–126.
23. Leung DYM, Meissner HC, Shulman ST, et al. Prevalence of superantigen-secreting bacteria in patients with Kawasaki disease. *J Pediatrics* 2002;140(6):742–746.

24. Tse SML, Silverman ED, McCrindle BW, et al. Early treatment with intravenous immunoglobulin in patients with Kawasaki disease. *J Pediatr* 2002;140:450–455.

25. Newburger JW, Takahashi M, Beiser AS, et al. A single intravenous infusion in the treatment of acute Kawasaki syndrome. *N Engl J Med* 1991;324:1633–1639.

26. Brogan PA, Bose A, Burgner D, et al. Kawasaki disease: An evidence-based approach to diagnosis, treatment, and proposals for future research. *Arch Dis Child* 2002; 86:286–290.

27. Lang B, Duffy CM. Controversies in the management of Kawasaki disease. *Best Pract Res Clin Rheumatol* 2002; 16(3):427–442.

28. Shulman ST. Is there a role for corticosteroids in Kawasaki disease? *J Pediatr* 2003;142:601–603.

29. Dale RC, Saleem MA, Daw S, et al. Treatment of severe complicated Kawasaki disease with oral prednisolone and aspirin. *J Pediatr* 2000;137:723–726.

30. Kato H, Koike S, Yokoyama T. Kawasaki disease: Effect of treatment on coronary artery involvement. *Pediatrics* 1979;63:175–179.

31. Sundel RP, Baker AL, Fulton DR, et al. Corticosteroids in the initial treatment of Kawasaki disease. *J Pediatr* 2003; 142:611–616.

32. Okada Y, Shinohara M, Kobayashi T, et al. Effect of corticosteroids in addition to intravenous gamma globulin therapy on serum cytokine levels in the acute phase of Kawasaki disease in children. *J Pediatr* 2003;143: 363–367.

33. Aboub EM. Acute rheumatic fever. In: Allen HD, Clark EB, Gutgesell HP, Driscoll DJ (eds.),*Moss and Adams Heart Disease in Infants, Children, and Adolescents*, 6th ed. Philadelphia, PA: Lippincott Williams & Wilkins, 2001: 1226–1241.

34. Guidelines for the diagnosis of rheumatic fever. Jones Criteria, 1992 update. Special Writing Group of the Committee on Rheumatic Fever, Endocarditis, and Kawasaki Disease of the Council on Cardiovascular Disease in the Young of the American Heart Association. *JAMA* 1992;268(15):2069–2073.

35. Veasy LG, Wiedmeier SE, Orsmond GS, et al. Resurgence of acute rheumatic fever in the intermountain area of the United States. *N Engl J Med* 1987;316:421–427.

36. Kaplan EL, Johnson DR, Cleary PP. Group A streptococcal serotypes isolated from patients and sibling contacts during the resurgence of rheumatic fever in theUnited States in the mid-1980's. *J Infect Dis* 1989;159:101.

37. Kavey RE, Kaplan EL. Resurgence of acute rheumatic fever. *Pediatrics* 1989;84:585–586.

38. Kaplan EL, Hill HR. Return of rheumatic fever: Consequence, implications, and needs. *J Pediatr* 1987;111(2):244–246.

39. Pickering LK, Baker CJ, Overturf GD, et al. Group A streptococcal infections. *Red Book: 2003 Report of the Committee on Infectious Diseases*. Elk Grove Village, IL: American Academy of Pediatrics, 2003:573–584.

40. El-Said GM, El-Refall MM, Sorour KA, et al. Rheumatic fever and rheumatic heart disease. In: Garson A Jr, Bricker JT, Fisher DJ, Neish SR (eds.), *The Science and Practice of Pediatric Cardiology*, 2nd ed. Baltimore, MD: Lippincott Williams & Wilkins, 1998:1691–1724.

41. Ferrieri P. Proceedings of the Jones Criteria Workshop. *Circulation* 2002;106:2521–2523.

42. Tani LY, Veasy LG, Minich LL, et al. Rheumatic fever in children younger than 5 years: Is the presentation difference? *Pediatrics* 1993;112(5):1065–1068.

43. Hashkes PJ, Tauber T, Somekh E, et al. Naproxen as an alternative to aspirin for the treatment of arthritis of rheumatic fever: A randomized trial. *J Pediatr* 2003;143(3): 399–401.

44. Cilliers AM, Manyemba J, Saloojee H. Anti-inflammatory treatment for carditis in acute rheumatic fever. *Coch Database Syst Rev* 2003;(2):CD003176.

45. Manyemba J, Mayosi BM. Penicillin for secondary prevention of rheumatic fever. *Coch Database Syst Rev* 2002; (3):CD002227.

46. Manyemba J, Mayosi BM. Intramuscular penicillin is more effective than oral penicillin in secondary prevention of rheumatic fever—a systemic review. *SAMJ* 2003; 93(3):212–218.

47. Saiman L, Prince A, Gersony WM. Pediatric infective endocarditis in the modern era. *J Pediatr* 1993;122: 847–853.

48. Ashkenazi S, Levy O, Blieden L. Trends of childhood infective endocarditis in Israel with emphasis on children under 2 years of age. *Pediatr Cardiol* 1997;18:419–424.

49. Awadallah SM, Kavey RE, Byrum CH, et al. The changing pattern of infective endocarditis in childhood. *Am J Cardiol* 1991;68:90–94.

50. Mylonakis E, Calderwood SB. Infective endocarditis in adults. *N Engl J Med* 2001;345:1318–1330.

51. Van Hare GF, Ben-Shachar G, Liebman J, et al. Infective endocarditis in infants and children during the past 10 years: A decade of change. *Am Heart J* 1984;107:1235–1240.

52. Johnson DH, Rosenthal A, Nadas AS. A forty-year review of bacterial endocarditis in infancy and childhood. *Circulation* 1975;51:581–588.

53. Ako J, Ikari Y, Hatori M, et al. Changing spectrum of infective endocarditis: Review of 194 episodes over 20 years. *Circulation* 2003;67(1):3–7.

54. Brown PD, Levine DP. Infective endocarditis in the injection drug user. *Infect Dis Clin North Am* 2002;16(3):645–665, viii-ix.

55. Wilson LE, Thomas DL, Astemborski J, et al. Prospective study of infective endocarditis among injection drug users. *J Infect Dis* 2002;185(12):1761–1766.

56. Satchithananda DK, Walsh J, Schofield PM. Bacterial endocarditis following repeated tattooing. *Heart* 2001; 851(1):11–12.

57. Friedel JM, Stehlik J, Desai M, et al. Infective endocarditis after oral body piercing. *Cardiol Rev* 2003;11(5):252–255.

58. Weinberg JB, Blackwood RA. Case report of Staphylococcus aureus endocarditis after navel piercing. *Pediatr Infect Dis J* 2003;22(1):94–96.

59. Pearlman SA, Higgins S, Eppes S, et al. Infectious endocarditis in the premature neonate. *Clin Pediatr* 1998; 37(12):741–746.

60. Feder HM, Roberts JC, Salazar JC, et al. HACEK endocarditis in infants and children: Two cases and a literature review. *Pediatr Infect Dis J* 2003;22:557–562.

61. Mayayo E, Moralejo J, Camps J, et al. Fungal endocarditis in premature infants: Case report and review. *Clin Infect Dis* 1996;22(2):366–368.

62. Ferrieri P, Fewitz MH, Gerber MA, et al. Unique features of infective endocarditis in childhood. *Pediatrics* 2002; 109(5):931–943.

63. Opie GF, Fraser SH, Drew JH, et al. Bacterial endocarditis in neonatal intensive care. *J Paediatr Child Health* 1999; 35(6):545–548.

64. Bitar FF, Jawdi RA, Dbaibo GS, et al. Paediatric infective endocarditis: 19-year experience at a tertiary care hospital in a developing country. *Acta Paediatrica* 2000;89(4): 427–430.

65. Humpl T, McCrindle BW, Smallhorn JF. The relative roles of transthoracic compared with transesophageal echocardiography in children with suspected infective endocarditis studies. *J Am Coll Cardiol* 2003;41(11):2068–2071.

66. Werner AS, Cobbs CG, Kaye D, et al. Studies on the bacteremia of bacterial endocarditis. *JAMA* 1967;202:199–203.

67. Lamas CC, Eykyn SJ. Blood culture negative endocarditis: An analysis of 63 cases presenting over 25 years. *Heart* 2003;89:258–262.

68. Werner M, Anderson R, Olaison L, et al. A clinical study of culture-negative endocarditis. *Medicine* 2003;82(4): 263–273.

69. Bayer AS, Bolger A, Taubert KA, et al. Diagnosis and management of infective endocarditis and its complications. *Circulation* 1998:2936–2948.

70. Gauduchon V, Chalabreysse L, Etienne J, et al. Molecular diagnosis of infective endocarditis by PCR amplification and direct sequencing of DNA from valve tissue. *J Clin Microbiol* 2003:763–766.

71. Von Reyn CF, Levy BS, Arbeit RD, et al. Infective endocarditis: An analysis based on strict case definitions. *Ann Intern Med* 1981;94:505–518.

72. Durack DT, Lukes AS, Bright DK. New criteria for diagnosis of infective endocarditis: Utilization of specific echocardiographic findings. Duke Endocarditis Service. *Am J Med* 1994;96:200–209.

73. Li JS, Sexton DJ, Mick N, et al. Proposed modifications to the Duke criteria for the diagnosis of infective endocarditis. *Clin Infect Dis* 2000;30:633–638.

74. Stockheim JA, Chadwich EG, Kessler S, et al. Are the Duke criteria superior to the Beth Israel criteria for the diagnosis of infective endocarditis in children? *Clin Infect Dis* 1998;27:1451–1456.

75. Michelfelder EC, Ochsner JE, Khoury P, et al. Does assessment of pretest probability of disease improve the utility of echography in suspected endocarditis in children? *J Pediatr* 2003;142:263–267.

76. Del Pont JM, De Cicco LT, Vartalitis C, et al. Infective endocarditis: Clinical analyses and evaluation of two diagnostic criteria. *Pediatr Infect Dis J* 1995;14(12):1079–1086.

77. Dajani AS, Taubert KA, Wilson W, et al. Prevention of bacterial endocarditis. Recommendations by the American Heart Association. *Circulation* 1997;96(1):358–366.

78. Dajani AS, Taubert KA, Wilson W, et al. Prevention of bacterial endocarditis. Recommendations by the American Heart Association. *JAMA* 1997;277(22):1794–1801.

79. Day SC, Cook EF, Funkestein H, et al. Evaluation and outcome of emergency room patients with transient loss of consciousness. *Am J Med* 1982;73:15–23.

80. Owens TR. Sudden cardiac death: Is your patient at risk? *J Resp Dis* 1998;19:384–396.

81. Pratt JL, Fleisher GR. Syncope in children and adolescents. *Pediatr Emerg Care* 1989;5:80–82.

82. Kapoor WN, Karpf M, Wieand S, et al. A prospective evaluation and follow-up of patients with syncope. *N Engl J Med* 1983;309:197–204.

83. Martin GJ, Adams SL, Maritno HG, et al. Prospective evaluation of syncope. *Ann Emerg Med* 1984;13:499–504.

84. Gendelman HE, Linzer M, Gabelman M, et al. Syncope in a general hospital patient population. *NY State J Med* 1983;83:1161–1165.

85. Murdoch BD. Loss of consciousness in healthy South African men. *S Afr Med* 1980;57:771–774.

86. Williams RL, Allen BD. Loss of consciousness: Incidence, causes and electroencephalographic findings. *Aerospace Med* 1962;33:545–551.

87. Dermksian G, Lamb LE. Syncope in a population of healthy young adults. *JAMA* 1958;168:1200–1207.

88. Driscoll DJ, Jacobsen SJ, Porter CJ, et al. Syncope in children and adolescents: A population based study of incidence and outcome. *Circulation* 1996;94:1–54.

89. Mace SE. In: Harwood-Nuss AL (ed.), *Pediatric Syncope. The Clinical Practice of Emergency Medicine*, 4th ed. Philadelphia, PA: Lippincott Williams & Wilkins, 2004.

90. Ozme S, Alshan D, Valaz K, et al. Causes of syncope in children: A prospective study. *Int J Cardiol* 1993;40:111–114.

91. McHarg ML, Shinnar S, Rascoff H. et al. Syncope in childhood. *Pediatr Cardiol* 1997;18:367–371.

92. Klitzner TS. Sudden cardiac death in children. *Circulation* 1990;82:629–632.

93. Berger S, Dhala A, Friedberg DZ. Sudden cardiac death in infants, children, and adolescents. *Pediatr Clin North Am* 1999;46:221–234.

94. Kocis KC. Chest pain in pediatrics. *Pediatr Clin North Am* 1999;46(2):189–203.

95. Rowe BH, Dulberg CS, Peterson RG, et al. Characteristics of children presenting with chest pain to a pediatric emergency department. *Can Med Assoc J* 1990;143(5):388–394.

96. Selbst SM, Ruddy RM, Clark BJ, et al. Pediatric chest pain: A prospective study. *Pediatrics* 1988;82(3):319–323.

97. Selbst SM, Ruddy R, Clark BJ. Chest pain in children. Followup of patients previously reported. *Clin Pediatr* 1990;29(7):374–377.

98. Zavaras-Angelidou KA, Weinhouse E, Nelson DB. Review of 180 episodes of chest pain in 134 children. *Pediatr Emerg Care* 1992;8:189–192.

99. Fyfe DA, Moodie DS. Chest pain in pediatric patients presenting to a cardiac clinic. *Clin Pediatr* 1984;23:321–324.

100. Wiens L, Sabath R, Ewing L, et al. Chest pain in otherwise healthy children and adolescents is frequently cause by exercise induced asthma. *Pediatrics* 1992;90(3):350–353.

101. Sabri MR, Ghavanini AA, Haghighat M, et al. Chest pain in children and adolescents: Epigastric tenderness as a guide to reduce unnecessary work-up. *Pediatr Cardiol* 2003;24(1):3–5.

42

Pediatric Congenital Heart Disease
Acyanotic Congenital Heart Defects

Sharon E. Mace

HIGH YIELD FACTS

- The three main presentations of symptomatic patients with congenital heart disease are cyanosis, congestive heart failure, and shock.

- Left-to-right (L → R) shunt lesions are a common cause of heart failure in pediatric patients. The most common L → R shunts are ventricular septal defect (VSD), atrial septal defect (ASD), and a patent ductus arteriosus (PDA).

- Infants with acyanotic congenital heart disease may present in shock, needing emergent resuscitation including the ABCs and often a prostaglandin E_1 (PGE_1) infusion. Such lesions include the hypoplastic left heart syndrome, severe coarctation of the aorta, and critical aortic stenosis.

- Interference with the complex embryologic development of the heart results in specific congenital cardiac defects. Three structures: the ductus venous (DV), the ductus arteriosus (DA), and the foramen ovale (FO) are responsible for the fetal pattern of blood flow. After birth, the DA and the FO can be critical for survival of infants with various congenital heart defects.

ANATOMY, PHYSIOLOGY, AND EMBRYOLOGY

In order to understand the various congenital cardiac defects, a review of the fetal circulation, the changes occurring after birth (*transitional* circulation), the neonatal circulation, and cardiac embryology is necessary.

FETAL CIRCULATION

In the adult and the child, the pulmonary and systemic circulations are arranged in series (Fig. 42-1). Deoxygenated blood returns to the right side of heart via the inferior vena cava (IVC) and superior vena cava (SVC) into the right atrium (RA), enters the right ventricle (RV) where the deoxygenated blood is ejected to the pulmonary circulation. The oxygenated blood returns from the lungs and is pumped by the left side of heart to the systemic circulation.

This is compared with the more complex fetal circulation which is in parallel (Fig. 42-2). In the fetus, the placenta performs the functions of the lung for gas and metabolite exchange, and has responsibility for oxygenation of desaturated blood. Three structures: the DV, FO, and the DA are essential in creating a different pattern of blood flow in the fetus[1-3] (Figs. 42-3 and 42-4).

Oxygenated blood in the fetus comes from the placenta via the umbilical vein (UV). Umbilical venous blood is split almost equally into two parts with about half the blood going directly into the IVC via the ductus venosum (DV) while the other 50% goes through the left half of the liver entering the hepatic microcirculation then into the left hepatic vein before entering the IVC. Blood in the thoracic IVC contains blood from three sources: venous return from the fetus' lower body, the DV, and the hepatic veins. Blood from these three sources enters the thoracic IVC, but does not mix completely, with a preferential flow or "streaming" of blood into various cardiac chambers. The more highly oxygenated blood from the DV and left hepatic vein flows preferentially across the FO into the left atrium (LA) then the left ventricle (LV) and into the ascending aorta (AA_O) to supply the upper part of the fetus' body especially the cerebral and myocardial circulation. The desaturated blood from the venous circulation from the fetus' upper body including the head/neck/myocardium returns to the SVC. SVC blood and desaturated blood from the lower part of the fetus' body in the IVC streams preferentially into the RA, then into the RV and into the main pulmonary trunk where the majority of blood (~87.5%) passes through the DA into the descending aorta (DA_O) and then to the placenta to become oxygenated. Only about 12.5% of the RV output goes to lungs and then returns (still desaturated) to the LA where it combines with the oxygenated blood coming through the FO from the IVC via the DV and the left hepatic veins.[4] Left atrial blood passes into the LV to then be ejected into the AA_O supplying the upper part of the fetus with oxygenated blood. (See Table 42-1.)

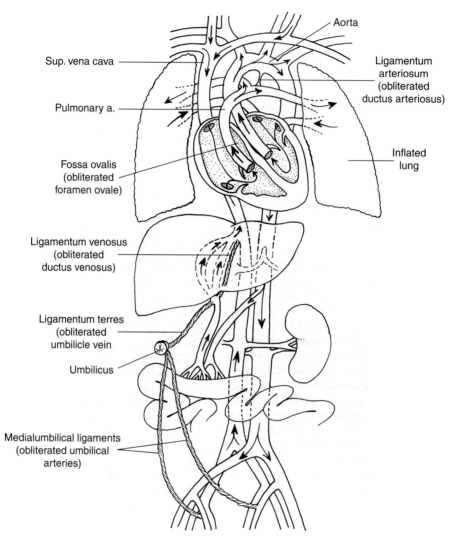

Aorta

Sup. vena cava

Pulmonary a.

Ligamentum
arteriosum
(obliterated
ductus arteriosus)

Fossa ovalis
(obliterated
foramen ovale)

Inflated
lung

Ligamentum venosus
(obliterated
ductus venosus)

Ligamentum terres
(obliterated
umbilicle vein

Umbilicus

Medialumbilical ligaments
(obliterated umbilical
arteries)

Fig. 42-1. Postnatal circulation. (Source: Adapted from Cochard LR. *Netter's Atlas of Human Embryology*. Teterboro, NJ: ICON Learning Systems, 2002:105.)

POSTNATAL CHANGES: THE TRANSITIONAL CIRCULATION

At birth, the first breath ushers in many changes. A major (≈10-fold) increase in pulmonary blood flow occurs with the onset of breathing.[4] With the advent of ventilation, intraalveolar fluid is replaced by air and the oxygen concentration increases. These changes coupled with the release of vasodilators such as bradykinin and prostaglandins results in a decrease in pulmonary vascular resistance (PVR).

There is an initial marked drop in PVR due to relaxation of the resistance vessels. This is followed by a further gradual decline in PVR over the following 2–6 weeks of life. During this time, the pulmonary arterioles transition from the fetal type containing much smooth muscle in

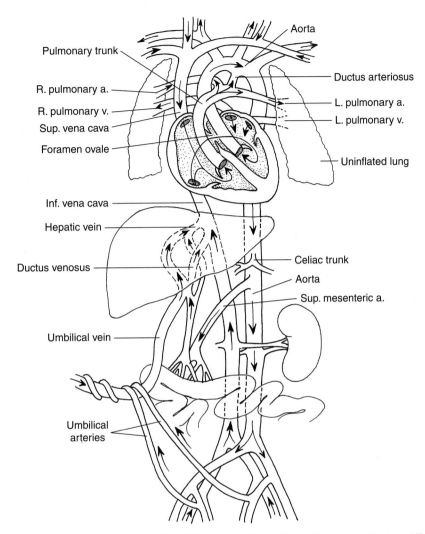

Fig. 42-2. Fetal circulation. (Source: Adapted from Cochard LR. *Netter's Atlas of Human Embryology*. Teterboro, NJ: ICON Learning Systems, 2002:104.)

the medial layer of the arterioles to the adult type with a minimal amount of smooth muscle in the media. The "physiologic anemia" normally occurring in the first few months of life results in a decreasing hematocrit. The decreasing viscosity of blood from the declining hematocrit causes a further drop in PVR.

In summary, four components cause the postnatal decline in PVR: (1) the increased oxygen concentration occurring with lung inflation, (2) replacement of lung fluid with air, (3) structural changes in the pulmonary resistance vessels (with decreased muscle in the medial layer), and (4) the decreased blood viscosity.

Closure of the Ductus Arteriosus

Like the pulmonary vessels, the DA contains smooth muscle in its medial layer. Prostaglandins are responsible for keeping the DA in a relaxed state and thus, patent.

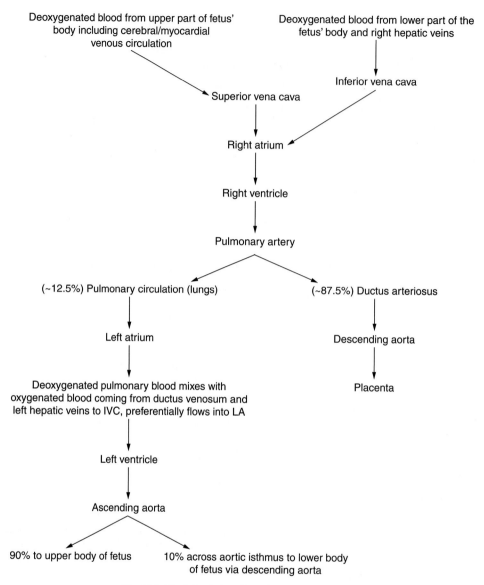

Fig. 42-3. Fetal circulation: flow of deoxygenated blood.

After birth, serum prostaglandin levels drop precipitously due to loss of supply from the placenta and to metabolism of any remaining prostaglandin by the pulmonary circulation. Postnatally, active constriction of the DA occurs due to: (1) increased local oxygen concentration, (2) the pulmonary release of vasoconstrictive mediators, and (3) to the loss of the vasodilating effect of the prostaglandins.

In term infants, functional closure of the DA usually occurs within the first 12 hours. Permanent closure via thrombosis, fibrosis, and intimal proliferation takes several weeks. Factors, such as hypoxia and/or acidosis, allow the DA to remain patent or to reopen.

This is of critical importance since a prostaglandin infusion to keep the DA patent can be life saving in certain infants with congenital heart disease.

A large percent of premature infants, especially very low birth weight (<1250 g) infants, have a PDA. The presence of a PDA in such preterm infants often complicates their

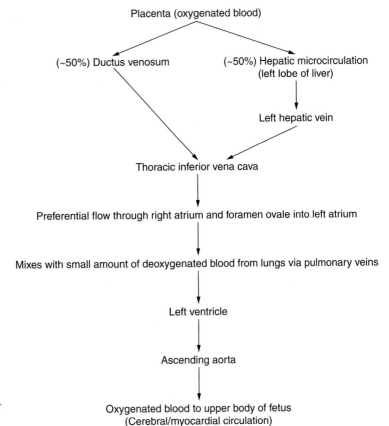

Fig. 42-4. Fetal circulation: flow of oxygenated blood.

clinical course and worsens their respiratory distress syndrome. In this case, management may include closure of the PDA with indomethacin, an inhibitor of prostaglandin synthesis.

Closure of the Foramen Ovale

Postnatal alterations in the pattern of blood flow occur with the removal of the placenta.[1-3] There is a sharp decrease in blood flow through the IVC to the atria, a tremendous increase in pulmonary blood flow, and a change in the pressure relationships in the LA and RA. In the fetus, RA pressure is greater than LA pressure so blood from the DV and the left hepatic vein flows from the RA through the FO into the LA. Postnatally, LA pressure forces closure of the valve-like flap of the FO. However, anatomic closure may be incomplete with a probe patent FO lasting for years even into adulthood. This is important since shunts through the FO may occur with certain types of congenital heart disease.

EMBRYOLOGY

In the embryo, the first recognizable cardiac precursors are a group of cells located on both sides of the embryo's central axis.[1] These two groups of cells form into paired cardiac tubes, which fuse in the midline to form the primitive heart tube[1-3] (Fig. 42-5). Myoblasts migrate into the area and surround the primitive heart tube. The myoblasts are muscle-forming cells which will become the myocardium.[3]

The primitive heart tube, formed during the first gestational month, has four parts in series: sinus venosus, primitive atria, primitive ventricle, and the bulbus cordis (Fig. 42-3). The inferior aspect of the bulbus cordis will become the RV. The superior segment of the bulbus cordis is the conotruncus. The conotruncus consists of the conus cordis and the truncus arteriosus. The truncus arteriosus will divide into the outflow of both ventricles (the aorta and pulmonary trunk).[3] Blood flows into the sinus venosus then the primitive atria, next into the primitive ventricle, then into the bulbus cordis and exits through the conotruncus.

Table 42-1. Differences in Fetal Circulation from the Mature Circulation in the Child or the Adult

	Fetus	**Child and Adult**
Oxygenated blood	From placenta via UV (50% of UV blood enters hepatic circulation, 50% via DV) which both join IVC	From lungs
Deoxygenated blood	Via DA to DA$_O$, then to UA to placenta to become oxygenated	IVC, SVC to RA to RV to PA to lungs to become oxygenated
SVC blood flow	SVC blood in RA → preferentially through TV into RV → PA (same as adult)	SVC blood in RA → through TV into RV through PV into PA
IVC	Left hepatic vein + DV (oxygenated blood) to IVC to RA → preferentially through FO → LA → through mitral valve → LV → AA$_O$ → fetal upper body	IVC to RA to RV
Right ventricular outflow	≈12.5% to lungs 87.5% bypasses lungs, goes to PA through DA to DA$_O$ to lower part of fetal body then returns via UA to placenta	≈100% to lungs to become oxygenated
Flow through DA	From PA through DA to DA$_O$	DA is obliterated, remnant is ligamentum arteriosum
RV output	1.3 times greater than LV output	RV output = LV output
Amount of work	RV does greater volume of work than LV	LV does greater work because of higher systemic pressure
"Dominant" ventricle	RV (ejects ~2/3 CVO), LV (ejects ~1/3 CVO)	LV
Thicker ventricle	RV	LV
Circuit	Parallel	Series
Pulmonary vessels	Vasoconstricted	—
Pulmonary vascular resistance	Increased	—

Abbreviations: SVC: superior vena cava, IVC: inferior vena cava, DV: ductus venosum, UV: umbilical vein, UA: umbilical artery, DA$_O$: descending aorta, RA: right atrium, RV: right ventricle, LA: left atrium, LV: left ventricle, AA$_O$: ascending aorta, TV: tricuspid valve, MV: mitral valve, AV: aortic valve, DA: ductus arteriosus, FO: foramen ovale, CVO: combined ventricular output.

This heart tube then evolves during the second gestational month into a heart with two parallel systems each composed of an atrium, ventricle, and great artery.

As early as 21–22 days, the embryonic heart begins to contract demonstrating the phases of the cardiac cycle akin to that in the adult heart.[2–3] Segments of the embryonic heart tube that become part of the mature heart are listed in Table 42-2.

Cardiac Looping

Formation of the heart tube is followed by cardiac looping and cardiac septation. At about 23 days, the heart tube begins cardiac looping: the process of bending ventrally and toward the right. Looping (d-loop) results in the future LV being relocated leftward and the primitive atria

relocated superiorly and posteriorly, and the bulbus cordis relocated to the right and anteriorly.[2] The future RV is positioned rightward in continuity with the truncus arteriosus (the Ao and PA in the mature heart). Cardiac looping is an early embryonic appearance of the right-left asymmetry present in the mature heart. When abnormal cardiac looping occurs in the developing fetus, there is a high probability of major congenital cardiac defects.

When an l-loop occurs, the heart loops to the left instead of the right. The result is a reversal of the normal positions of the ventricles in the chest, placing the morphologic RV on the left and the morphologic LV on the right. Situs inversus is when the l-loop reversal of the normal positions of the ventricles occurs with reversal of the left-right axis in all other organs. Patients with situs inversus may have otherwise "normal" cardiac

Table 42-2. Comparison of Primitive Cardiac Tube Structure with the Mature Heart Structure

Primitive Cardiac Tube Structure	Mature Heart Structure
Sinus venosus	Part of the right atrium (right auricle)
Primitive atrium	Parts of right and left atria
Primitive ventricle	Most of LV
Bulbus cordis	Most of RV
Conotruncus	
Conus cordis	Outflow region of RV, LV
Truncus arteriosus	Aorta and pulmonary artery

development. But when l-loop occurs with normal situs of all other organs except the heart, "isolated dextrocardia," serious congenital heart defects are the rule. When the process of cardiac looping is abnormal, congenital cardiac defects such as double outlet right ventricle (DORV) and double inlet left ventricle (DILV) occur. In DORV, both the Ao and the PA arise from the RV. In DILV, both the oxygenated left atrial blood and the deoxygenated right atrial blood enter the LV. When cardiac looping occurs, the proximal and distal ends of the primitive cardiac tube are fixed and differential growth causes the heart tube to bend rightward. Then the bulboventricular part of the tube doubles over on itself, causing the right and left ventricle to lie side by side.

Cardiac Septation

Cardiac looping is followed by cardiac septation (Fig. 42-6). When normal cardiac looping is finished, the heart's external form resembles a mature heart with the various components of the heart now in proper position and alignment, while the internal appearance is that of a tubular organ with numerous ridges that resemble primitive chambers. There is now a common atrium (which will be divided into the left and right atrium). The common atrium is connected to the primitive ventricle (which will become the future LV) by the atrioventricular (AV) canal. The bulboventricular foramen connects the primitive ventricle with the bulbus cordis (which is the future RV). The distal segment of the bulbus cordis becomes the conus, an outlet

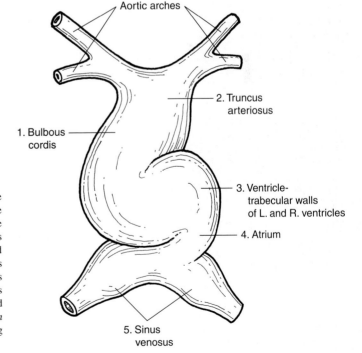

Aortic arches

1. Bulbous cordis

2. Truncus arteriosus

3. Ventricle-trabecular walls of L. and R. ventricles

4. Atrium

5. Sinus venosus

Fig. 42-5. Primitive heart tube. Key: 1. The superior segment of the bulbous cordis (the conotruncus consists of the conus cordis and the trucus arteriorsus). 2. Truncus arteriosus divides into the outflow of both ventricle (aorta and pulmonary artery). 3. Primitive ventricle becomes part of left ventricle. 4. Primitive atrium becomes parts of right and left atria. 5. Sinus venosus becomes part of right auricle. (Source: Adapted from Cochard LR. *Netter's Atlas of Human Embryology.* Teterboro, NJ: ICON Learning Systems, 2002:103.)

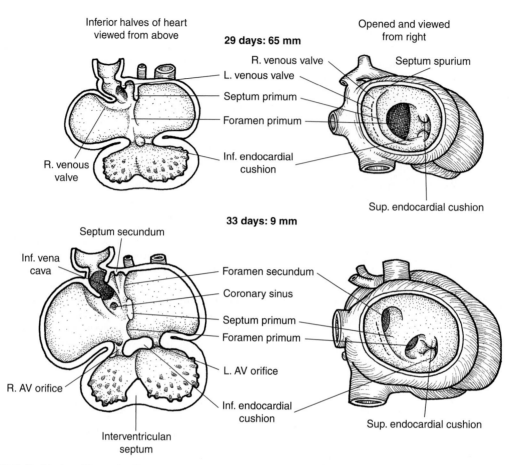

Inferior halves of heart
viewed from above
29 days: 65 mm
Opened and viewed
from right

R. venous valve
L. venous valve
Septum primum
Foramen primum
Inf. endocardial cushion
R. venous valve
Septum spurium
Sup. endocardial cushion

33 days: 9 mm
Septum secundum
Inf. vena cava
Foramen secundum
Coronary sinus
Septum primum
Foramen primum
L. AV orifice
R. AV orifice
Inf. endocardial cushion
Interventriculan septum
Sup. endocardial cushion

Fig. 42-6. Partitioning of heart tube. (Source: Adapted from Cochard LR. *Netter's Atlas of Human Embryology.* Teterborg, NJ: ICON Learning Systems, 2002:98.)

segment, which goes into the truncus arteriosus. Ingrowth of various masses of tissues will result in the formation of the four-chambered heart.

Septation of the Atria and Atrial Septal Defects

Septation of the common atria into the right and left atria occurs by growth of two parallel septa (septum primum and septum secundum) coming down from the roof of the atria and by a small part of the endocardial cushion tissue just above the AV valves. As septum primum grows downward toward the AV canal, an interatrial opening, the ostium primum occurs. Numerous perforations located in the upper part of septum primum occur and then combine to form a single opening, the ostium secundum. The

importance of these two interatrial openings is to allow the right to left flow of the oxygenated blood in the fetus from the placenta (via the DV and left hepatic vein to the IVC) into the LA, then the LV, out the AA_O to supply oxygenated blood to the upper body of the fetus. When the ostium primum closes (forming part of the atrial septum), the ostium secundum remains open in the fetus allowing the right-to-left interatrial flow. The thin septal primum tissue abuts against the thicker septum secundum and the centrally located fossa ovalis to form the one-way valve of the FO. This allows for the preferential flow of blood from the RA to the LA in the fetus. After birth, the changes in pressure close the FO.

Thus, there are several types of ASDs: primum defects, secundum (FO), or sinus venosus defects. Atrial secundum defects are in the region of the fossa ovalis. Atrial secundum defects are caused by a lack of tissue needed to close the FO. This can be caused by excessive resorption of the septum primum and/or by an abnormally large FO. Primum defects are related to endocardial cushion defects. Failure of fusion of the endocardial cushions and AV septum leads to the primum defect. Sinus venosum defects are due to an incomplete absorption of the sinus venosum into the RA and/or abnormal development of septum secundum. Sinus venosum ASDs (subcaval ASD) are located just below the entrance of the SVC into the RA.

Septation of the Ventricles, Endocardial Cushion Defects, and Ventricular Septal Defects

The ventricular septum is formed by the fusion of three embryologically different parts: muscular, inlet, and outlet septa. The muscular septum, which makes up the majority of the ventricular septum, originates from an outgrowth of tissue where the primitive ventricle (future LV) and bulbus cordis (future RV) join. Muscular VSDs are when there is a deficiency of this extension of muscular tissue. There is a conotruncal septum which separates the aorta and pulmonary artery. Downward growth of this conotruncal septum results in closure of the outlet ventricular septum. Failure of closure of the ventricular septum in this region results in a supracristal VSD, so named because the VSD is located above the crista, a conspicuous band of muscle in the RV. Inlet VSDs are a type of endocardial cushion defect.

Perimembranous VSD, the most common type of VSD, occurs in the area where all three of these components (e.g., muscular, outlet, and inlet sections) meet. Thus, missing of any or all of these three parts from the ventricular septum can result in a perimembranous VSD.

Endocardial Cushion Defects

The atria are connected to the primitive ventricle (future LV) by the AV canal. The function of endocardial cushions is to septate the inlet to the ventricles, which is known as the AV canal. There are four protrusions of tissue around the edge of the AV canal. These outgrowths of tissue are the endocardial cushions. Their purpose is to help septate the heart into four chambers. The endocardial cushions meet and fuse to form the septum intermedium, which also meets the septum primum. In addition to their key role in septation of the AV canal into right and left AV canals, the endocardial cushions also act as primitive heart valves. Thus, growth of the endocardial cushions separates the AV canal into tricuspid and mitral channels in addition to forming the inferior part of the atrial septum and the inlet section of the ventricular septum.

Abnormal development in this area can lead to numerous congenital heart defects. The most serious congenital heart defect is a complete AV canal with a large continuous ASD and VSD, missing AV valvular tissue, and one common AV valve overlying the ventricular septum. A less severe defect is an ostium primum defect. This consists of a large opening in the inferior part of the atrial septum; a VSD located below the AV valves and a displaced mitral valve. Various other endocardial cushion defects can occur, ranging from a VSD in the area of the inlet to a cleft in the mitral valve.

The Conotruncus and Defects of the Great Vessels

The most distal part of the primitive cardiac tube, the conotruncus, develops into the aorta and pulmonary outflow tracts. There are four steps in the transition of the conotruncus into the Ao and PA. They are: (1) growth of the conotruncal cushions, (2) neural crest cells migrating into the conotruncus, (3) resorption of the subaortic conus, and (4) leftward migration of the conotruncus. Interference in any of these processes results in various congenital heart defects.

The endocardial cushions grow and fuse, thereby separating the conus into the right and left ventricular outflow tracts and the truncus into the aortic and pulmonic valves. Migration of neural crest cells into the growing conotruncal septum is mandatory for normal development, although their exact role is not known. The congenital heart defect, truncus arteriosus, occurs when there is a failure of septation of the conotruncus. With truncus arteriosus, there is a single truncal valve instead of two semilunar (e.g., aortic and pulmonic) valves, and one common aortic and pulmonary trunk instead of a separate Ao and PA.

Early in development, the conotruncus is located over the bulbus cordis (future RV). The aortic section of the conotruncus migrates leftward to position the Ao over the LV. Muscle from the left part of the conus must be resorbed in order to allow for the leftward movement of the aortic part of the conotruncus. When there is failure of resorption of the subaortic conus, this leftward migration cannot occur so a DORV occurs. With DORV, both the PA and the Ao arise from the RV. When the subpulmonic conus, instead of the subaortic conus resorbs, the pulmonary outflow tract moves leftward causing a d-transposition of the great arteries. The Ao arises from the RV and the PA from the LV in d-transposition of the great vessels. Normal resorption of the subaortic conus followed by inadequate partial migration results in tetralogy of Fallot, characterized by a dextroposed overriding Ao, pulmonic stenosis, and a VSD.

Pulmonary Veins

The primitive lung buds arise as an out-pocketing of the foregut. Initially the venous drainage of the lung beds is by the splanchnic plexus via the umbilicovitteline and cardinal veins. The common pulmonary veins (PV) develop as a small outgrowth from the posterior aspect of the LA. Simultaneously as the umbilicovittelne and cardinal veins are resorbed, the common PV enlarges. The common PV is merged into the LA, allowing direct flow into the LA. Abnormal development of the common PV or failure to join with the splanchnic plexus causes total anomalous venous return with persistence of the primary venous connection.

Cor triatriatum is a type of abnormal pulmonary venous development in which the common PV is inadequately connected into the LA causing the formation of a constricting membrane between the common PV and the LA.

ACYANOTIC CONGENITAL HEART DISEASE: CONGENITAL HEART LESIONS THAT PRESENT WITH CONGESTIVE HEART FAILURE

Left-to-Right Shunt Lesions

Left-to-right shunts occur when blood in the left-sided cardiac chambers (LA or LV) or great vessel (Ao) is diverted to the right-sided cardiac chambers (RA or RV) or great vessel (PA). Since the blood in the left side of the heart is fully oxygenated, cyanosis does not occur. However, the volume of blood flow to the lungs is increased since all of the systemic venous return plus some oxygenated blood diverted from the left side of the heart flows into the lungs.

Under normal conditions, the volume of blood going to the lungs (Q_p = pulmonary blood flow) is equal to the volume of blood going to body (Q_s = systemic blood flow). Thus, the ratio $Q_p/Q_s = 1$. In general, a small shunt indicates a $Q_p/Q_s \leq 1.5$, a moderate shunt is a Q_p/Q_s of $1.5 - 2/0$, and with a large shunt $Q_p/Q_s > 2.0$. Thus, with a left-to-right shunt one or more right-sided chambers/structures suffers from volume overload and may also have a pressure overload depending on the size of the left-to-right shunt, the location, and the pulmonary vascular resistance (PVR). For example, with a small restrictive VSD (Q_p/Q_s <1.5), there is increased blood flow in the RV, PA, and to the lungs from the "normal" desaturated blood returning to the RA from the vena cava plus the oxygenated blood directed across the VSD from the LV to the RV. Pressure in the RV and PA are normal or mildly elevated. With a large VSD, there is a greater increase in blood flow in the RV, PA, and lungs than with the small VSD, and pressures

in the RV and PA are markedly elevated and equal to the LV pressure.

There are four main congenital cardiac shunt lesions: VSD, ASD, PDA, and endocardial cushion defects.

Ventricular Septal Defect

Ventricular septal defect is the most common congenital heart lesion, comprising about one-third of all congenital cardiac malformation.[5] Defects may be found in any location of the ventricular septum. There are four types of VSD: (1) perimembranous (membranous, infracristal)—most common type, (2) supracristal (infundibular, conal, subpulmonary, outlet)—located above a band of muscle, the crista supraventricularis, in the right ventricular outflow tract, just below the pulmonic valve, (3) muscular VSD—in the muscular part of the ventricular septum, and (4) inlet VSD—septal defects located just below the tricuspid valve (posterior inferior to the perimembranous defect) (Fig. 42-7).

The clinical manifestations depend on the amount of left-to-right shunt going from the LV to RV. The amount of flow and the physical findings are a function of the size of the VSD, the type/location of the VSD, and the downstream PVR as compared to the systemic vascular resistance (SVR).

A cardiac murmur may be the only manifestation of a small- or moderate-sized VSD. With a large VSD, in the newborn period, the amount of left-to-right shunt through the VSD is limited by the increased PVR. Over the next 4–6 weeks, with the usual postnatal decline in PVR, the amount of shunt increases and heart failure/pulmonary edema occurs, typically, at about 1 month of age.

The physical findings for a small VSD may only be a holosystolic murmur (heard best at lower left sternal border if a muscular VSD, and at the upper left sternal border if a supracristal or membranous VSD), and often a palpable precordial thrill. The precordial impulse, S_1, and S_2 are normal as is the ECG and chest roentgenogram.

Physical examination findings with moderate to large VSDs include: increased right ventricular impulse at the lower left sternal border, increased laterally displaced left ventricular impulse, palpable precordial thrill, loud P_2, holosystolic murmur along left sternal border, and a gallop rhythm (middiastolic murmur from flow through the mitral valve). Occasionally, patients with a supracristal VSD have associated aortic insufficiency with presenting signs and symptoms of the aortic insufficiency. Left ventricular hypertrophy is found on the ECG with moderate VSDs because of the left ventricular volume overload. With large VSDs, left or right ventricular hypertrophy is present on the ECG. Echocardiography can confirm the diagnosis of

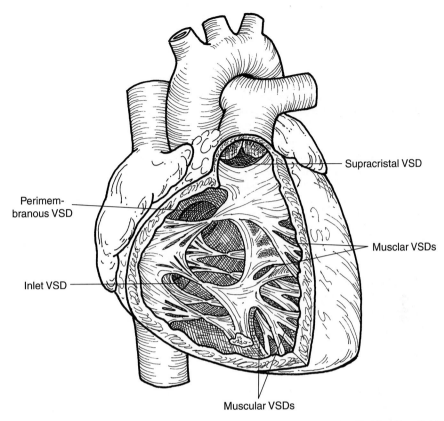

Fig. 42-7. Ventricular septal defect. (Source: Adapted from Emmanouilides G, Riemenschneider T, Allen H, et al. *Moss and Adams Heart Disease in Infants, Children and Adolescents*. Baltimore, MD: Williams & Wilkins, 1995:726.)

a VSD. Cardiac catheterization is generally reserved for those with possible pulmonary vascular disease to determine if they are a surgical candidate. The standard treatment of heart failure and pulmonary edema is indicated in those patients with the moderate to large VSDs who are symptomatic.

The size of the VSD is a major determinant of the prognosis and management. A significant percent of small VSDs will close spontaneously, usually within the first year of life and surgical repair is not recommended for small VSDs. Patients with large VSDs especially those with pulmonary hypertension should be closed electively, usually between 6 and 12 months of age, in order to prevent the development of pulmonary vascular disease.[6] Children with moderate-sized VSDs who have cardiomegaly and ECG evidence of ventricular hypertrophy should also be closed. Surgical closure, often with a patch, has been the method of VSD closure.[7] Transcatheter closure of selected perimembranous and muscular VSDs using various devices

(amplatzer ventricular septal occluder, Rashkind umbrella device, or a detachable coil) is gaining acceptance.[8–10] This has the advantage of avoiding cardiopulmonary bypass which is required for surgical patch closure. The main complications, embolization of the device or valvular insufficiency, have occurred in a few patients.[8,9] Endocarditis prophylaxis is required for all patients with VSDs irregardless of the size.[11]

Patent Ductus Arteriosus

The DA is normally patent in the fetus but should close within the first few days of life.[1–4] A PDA is fairly common accounting for about 10% of all congenital cardiac malformations excluding premature infants in whom the incidence of PDA is extremely high[12,13] (Fig. 42-8). A PDA is present in 80% of infants with a birthweight <1200 g, and 45% of those with a birthweight <1750 g,[6] while another study found a 31% incidence of

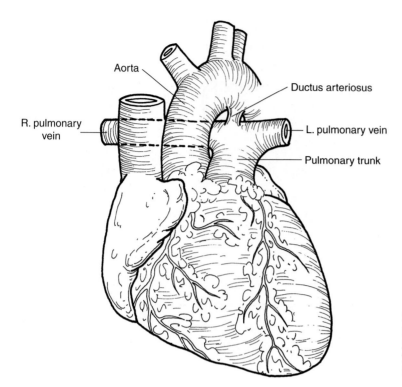

Aorta

Ductus arteriosus

R. pulmonary vein

L. pulmonary vein

Pulmonary trunk

Fig. 42-8. Patent ductus arteriosus. (Source: Adapted from Cochard LR. *Netter's Atlas of Human Embryology.* Teterboro, NJ: ICON Learning Systems, 2002:110.)

PDA in infants weighing 501–1500 g.[13] Closure of a PDA is required in 70% of preterm infants delivered before 28 weeks' gestation.[14] A PDA should be suspected in a premature infant with respiratory distress syndrome whose clinical course worsens.[15]

The most common presentation of a PDA in term infants and children is a continuous "machinery" type murmur heart best at the left infraclavicular area with "bounding" peripheral pulses from the wide pulse pressure caused by "runoff" (flow) from the Ao to the PA during diastole. In premature and newborn infants the murmur often is only heard in systole.

Patients with a small PDA are asymptomatic with a normal ECG and a normal chest roentgenogram. Patients with a large PDA may develop heart failure, have left or combined ventricular hypertrophy on ECG, and cardiomegaly with increased pulmonary vascularity on the chest roentgenogram. Echocardiography is used to diagnose a PDA.

There are many potential complications associated with a PDA in addition to the heart failure and pulmonary vascular disease occurring with a large PDA. These complications include endocarditis, calcification of the ductus, and aneurysms of the ductus. These complications can occur even with a small PDA.[16] Therefore, closure of a PDA is recommended in all PDAs whether they are symptomatic or not.[16] The risk of endocarditis is greater than the risk of closure. Closure can be achieved by several techniques: (1) pharmacologic using indomethacin IV[17] (successful in many preterm infants, not used in term infants or children), (2) transcatheter devices (placement of coils[18,19] or various occluder devices[20–23]), and (3) surgery (ligation and division of the PDA). Management also includes therapy for heart failure/pulmonary edema when present, and endocarditis prophylaxis until the ductus is closed.

Atrioventricular Canal Defects (Endocardial Cushion Defect) (AV Septal Defect)

Atrioventricular canal defects, about 5% of all congenital heart lesions, occur when there is defective development of the endocardial cushion (Fig. 42-9). There is a deficiency or absence of septal tissue just above and below the normal level of the AV valves, in the area generally occupied by the AV septum. Such lesions may be incomplete or complete. With a complete AV canal the inferior part of the atrial septum and part of the ventricular septum are missing and

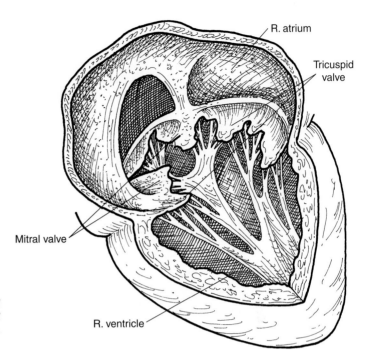

R. atrium

Tricuspid valve

Mitral valve

R. ventricle

Fig. 42-9. Complete AV septal defect. (Source: Adapted from Emmanouilides G, Riemenschneider T, Allen H, et al. *Moss and Adams Heart Disease in Infants, Children and Adolescents.* Baltimore, MD: William & Wilkins, 1995:710.)

there is one large common AV valve instead of two distinct AV (e.g., mitral and tricuspid) valves. Thus, the whole center part of the heart is absent. This defect is frequent in patients with Down syndrome. Incomplete (partial) AV canal defects include ostium primum ASD, common atrium, cleft mitral valve, and AV septal defects.

With a complete AV canal defect, there is left-to-right shunting at both the atrial and ventricular levels and sometimes, shunting of blood from the LV to the RA due to the missing AV septum. The valvular insufficiency further adds to the volume load on the ventricle(s). Pulmonary hypertension and the rapid onset of elevated PVR are characteristic, and will lead to Eisenmenger syndrome (see page 469).

Typically, heart failure and frequent respiratory infections occur in infants with complete AV septal defects. In addition to signs of heart failure and failure to thrive, physical examination reveals cardiomegaly often with a systolic thrill at the lower left sternal border, a precordial bulge/lift, a normal or accentuated S_1, widely split S_2 if there is torrential pulmonary blood flow, a low pitched mid-diastolic rumbling murmur at the lower left sternal border, a pulmonary systolic ejection murmur from the increased pulmonary blood flow, and a mitral insufficiency (MI) murmur at the apex.

The ECG has characteristic findings with a complete AV canal: left axis deviation, superior frontal axis, Q waves in leads I and AVL (counterclockwise frontal plane loop) and ventricular (combined or isolated right) hypertrophy, incomplete right bundle branch block (RSR complex in V_1). Marked cardiomegaly with prominence of all four cardiac chambers, enlargement of the pulmonary artery, and increased pulmonary vascularity is present on the chest roentgenogram. Echocardiography establishes the diagnosis, although cardiac catheterization is performed for preoperative surgical evaluation and to determine if pulmonary vascular disease is present. The presence of valvular disease in addition to a VSD increases the complexity of surgical repair compared with a simple VSD.[24]

Atrial Septal Defects

Atrial septal defects, about 10% of congenital cardiac malformations,[12] can occur in any location on the atrial septum. (Fig. 42-10). There are three common types of ASD: secundum, primum, sinus venosum, and rarely the atrial septum is almost totally absent creating essentially one large atrium.

The ostium secundum ASD, the most common type of ASD, is located in the area of the fossa ovalis (Fig. 42-11).

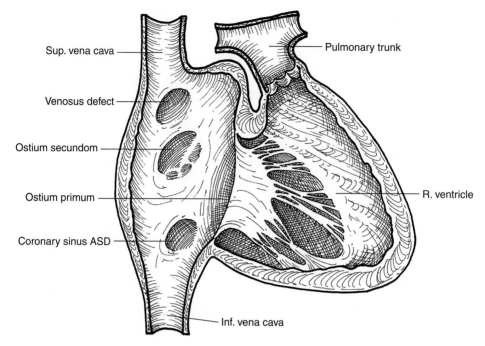

Fig. 42-10. Atrial septal defects. (Source: Adapted from Emmanouilides G, Riemenschneider T, Allen H, et al. *Moss and Adams Heart Disease in Infants, Children and Adolescents.* Baltimore, MD: Williams & Wilkins, 1995:688.)

It is the consequence of inadequate formation of the septum secundum and/or increased reabsorption of the septum primum. Sinus venosus ASDs are found in the posterior superior portion of the atrial septum and are frequently accompanied by partial anomalous drainage of the right upper PV (Fig. 42-12). The sinus venosus ASD is caused by misalignment of the right PV to either the SVC or IVC followed by resorption of the surface between the PV(s) and the vena cava.

An ostium primum defect is considered a type of partial AV canal defect. The inferior part of the AV septum is missing. There is usually an associated AV valve insufficiency (most often the mitral valve, infrequently the tricuspid valve). The shunt from the LA to the RA across the ASD is usually moderate to large.

Most often, patients with an ASD are asymptomatic and are discovered because of a heart murmur. Often these ASD murmurs are not recognized until the patient is about 3–5 years of age. Although heart failure and poor growth can occur in patients with an ASD, this is the exception occurring in <10% of ASD patients. However, if there is another associated lesion, then congestive heart failure,

and failure to thrive are more likely with symptom onset in infancy or in the first few years of life.

The classic findings in ASD patients are: increased RV impulse along lower left sternal border, normal S_1, wide fixed split of S_2, systolic ejection murmur along left sternal border (from increased flow through the pulmonic valve). When a moderate to large ASD is present, a mid-diastolic rumble at either the left or right lower sternal border is also heard and signifies increased blood flow across the tricuspid valve. ECG findings depend on the size and type of ASD. If there is a small left-to-right shunt with a secundum or sinus venosus ASD, the ECG can be normal, although an RSR' may be present in the right precordial leads which can also be found in normal children/infants. Moderate to large shunts are denoted by right atrial hypertrophy, right ventricular hypertrophy, and right axis deviation.

Patients with an ostium primum defect may be asymptomatic, while other patients with large left-to-right shunts and severe mitral insufficiency have fatigue, decreased exercise tolerance, and frequent respiratory infections. Typical cardiac findings are: wide fixed split

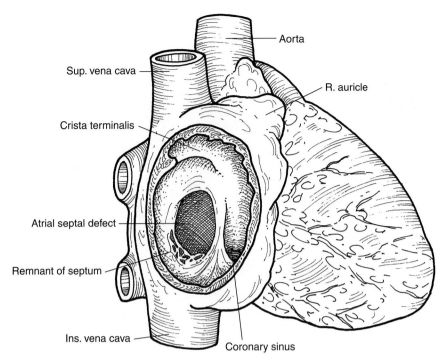

Fig. 42-11. Ostium secundum defect. (Source: Adapted from Cochard LR. *Netter's Atlas of Human Embryology.* Teterboro, NJ: ICON Learning Systems, 2002:108.)

S_2 (hallmark of all types of ASD), a normal or prominent S_1, a pulmonary systolic ejection murmur, often a pulmonic click, a middiastolic rumbling murmur at the lower left or right sternal border, and if mitral insufficiency is present (which is usually the case) the apical harsh murmur of mitral insufficiency.

The ECG demonstrates right ventricular hypertrophy and right atrial hypertrophy. With an ostium primum defect, there is left axis deviation and an initial counter-clockwise frontal plane loop (Q waves in I, and AVL), while other types of ASD have right axis deviation. First-degree heart block and incomplete right bundle branch block are common. A normal chest radiograph is found when the shunt is small, while cardiomegaly and increased pulmonary vascularity occur with larger shunts. Echocardiography is employed for definitive diagnosis. Closure of an uncomplicated ASD is generally done around 2–4 years of age. Surgery by patch closure or direct suture is done to close ASDs. In the future as improvements in transcatheter devices for closing ASDs occur, such transcatheter devices will be increasingly

employed for closure of uncomplicated ASDs.[25,26] Endocarditis prophylaxis is given except for secundum ASDs.[11]

Long-term complications occurring in untreated ASDs are: right atrial enlargement, right ventricular enlargement/hypertrophy and fibrosis, heart failure, arrhythmias, paradoxical embolization, and pulmonary vascular disease.[6]

CONGENITAL HEART LESIONS THAT PRESENT WITH CARDIOGENIC SHOCK

Hypoplastic Left Heart Syndrome

Hypoplastic left heart refers to various congenital heart defects that have in common underdevelopment or hypoplasia of the left side of the heart and/or of the AA_O. The hypoplastic left heart syndrome includes hypoplasia of the AA_O, severe coarctation of the aorta, aortic valve atresia or severe stenosis, and mitral valve atresia or severe stenosis. The common physiology includes a RV that maintains both the pulmonic and systemic

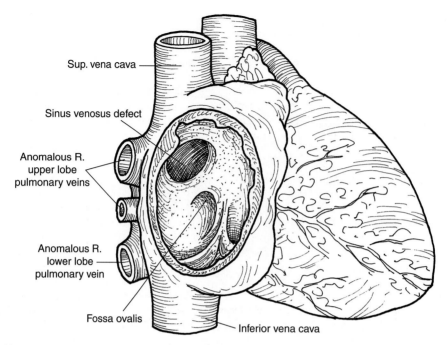

Fig. 42-12. Sinus venosus defect. (Source: Adapted from Cochard LR. *Netter's Atlas Human Embryology*. Teterboro, NJ: ICON Learning Systems, 2002:108.)

circulations, and an atretic or a small nonfunctional LV. The hypoplastic left heart syndrome is an example of a total mixing lesion since saturated pulmonary venous blood is shunted across a patent FO or an ASD into the RA where it combines with the desaturated blood returning from the body via the vena cava. If the ventricular septum is intact, the entire right ventricular output enters the PA. Blood flow to the body is via the DA to the descending Ao also with retrograde filling of the ascending Ao and coronary arteries.

The cardinal features of the hypoplastic left heart syndrome are hypoperfusion or even shock and cyanosis. Depending on the size of the interatrial communication either pulmonary overcirculation if a nonrestrictive ASD, or pulmonary venous hypertension if a tiny restrictive FO, can occur.

Closure of the DA soon after birth leads to shock with signs of hypoperfusion, weak or absent peripheral pulses, hypotension, delayed capillary fill, and mottling of the skin with a typical grayish blue skin color. Cardiomegaly with a right ventricular parasternal lift and a systolic murmur are present. The chest roentgenogram findings are cardiomegaly with increased pulmonary vascularity. The ECG typically shows atrial hypertrophy. The echocardiogram

shows the hypoplasia of the left side of the heart thus confirming the diagnosis.

Therapy consists of correction of metabolic abnormalities from acidosis to hypoglycemia, prevention of hypothermia, and PGE_1 infusion, which maintains systemic blood flow by keeping the DA open. Management for the hypoplastic left heart syndrome involves the Norwood procedure or orthotopic heart transplantation.[27,28] A recent modification of the Norwood procedure (see page 516) using a RV to PA conduit instead of a modified Blalock-Taussig shunt may further improve outcome/survival for these patients.[29,30]

Coarctation of the Aorta

Coarctation of the Ao is a narrowing of the Ao, typically located just beyond the origin of the left subclavian artery. It accounts for about 5–8% of all congenital cardiac malformations. It may be an isolated finding or part of a syndrome (e.g., Turner syndrome).

The clinical presentations of coarctation of the Ao vary greatly and are determined by the severity of the obstruction, the patient's age, and whether other accompanying defects are present. Coarctation of the Ao can manifest acutely with life-threatening cardiogenic shock in neonates or after early infancy in a less acute fashion.

In infants with critical or severe coarctation of the Ao, a PDA provides for systemic blood flow from right to left, from the PA across the DA to the Ao below the point of constriction. As the DA begins to close, the infant develops signs and symptoms of heart failure then cardiogenic shock. Differences in the pulses and blood pressures between the extremities and differential cyanosis between the right arm (receives blood flow from before the constricted portion of the aorta) and the legs (receives blood flow from the DA after the narrowed part of the aorta) are clues to the diagnosis. However, since these neonates are critically ill, in shock with poor peripheral perfusion, any differences in the pulses may be difficult to appreciate. A murmur is generally not present because of the low cardiac output. In addition to the ABCs, a PGE_1 infusion may stabilize the patient until corrective surgery can be done.

The clinical manifestations after early infancy are variable and less severe. Most patients are symptom free when a murmur or elevated blood pressure is detected. Physical examination reveals discrepancies in the blood pressure and pulses between the extremities, a delay in the femoral pulse compared to the brachial pulse, and a murmur. The murmur is best heard in the left infraclavicular area, the axilla, and posteriorly over the left chest medial to the scapula, all areas concordant with the auscultory regions of the thoracic Ao. The murmur peaks in late systole and may extend into early diastole. Occasionally, a continuous murmur from collateral blood vessels can also be ausculted. The ECG may show left ventricular hypertrophy or be normal. The heart size and pulmonary vascularity are generally normal on the chest radiograph but rib notching due to rib erosion by collateral vessels is often present in children of school age or older (≥ 6 years of age). Echocardiography and more recently MRI have been used to diagnose the lesion. Management has been surgical repair[31,32] or percutaneous balloon angioplasty to dilate the constricted aortic segment.[33,34]

Critical Aortic Stenosis

As with coarctation of the Ao, aortic stenosis may present as a critically ill infant in heart failure and/or cardiogenic shock, or at a later age (after 1 year of age) with less acute and less severe manifestations. Again, a typical murmur of aortic stenosis may not be present because of the low cardiac output. The management of the hemody-

namically unstable neonate with critical aortic stenosis is identical to that for critical coarctation of the Ao and hypoplastic left heart syndrome. Maintain the patient with the ABCs and a PGE_1 infusion until the patient can get definitive therapy in the operating room[35,36] or the cardiac catheterization laboratory.[37] With critical aortic stenosis, either surgical valvulotomy or percutaneous balloon valvotomy during cardiac catheterization can be done to relieve the stenosis.

Up to 10–15% of patients with congenital aortic stenosis present by 12 months of age. They are seen with the signs and symptoms of heart failure or are in cardiogenic shock. After 1 year of age, the clinical manifestations of aortic stenosis are less acute. Some patients may be asymptomatic and are evaluated for a murmur, while older children may have symptoms of fatigue, dyspnea on exertion, syncope, and chest pain. The classic systolic ejection murmur heard best at the cardiac base and radiating to the carotids is present in children over 1 year of age. Other physical examination findings may include a palpable systolic thrill, a palpable left ventricular lift, and an opening click if the stenosis is valvular. With mild stenosis, the ECG is normal, but with moderate to severe stenosis left ventricular hypertrophy is present. The chest radiograph often shows poststenotic dilatation of the AA_O. If there is severe stenosis, left ventricular enlargement, left atrial enlargement, and pulmonary vascular congestion is apparent on the chest roentgenogram. Otherwise the heart size and vascularity are within normal limits. Patients with aortic stenosis need endocarditis prophylaxis and should be followed since the gradient across the valve often increases.

REFERENCES

1. Moore KL, Persaud TVN. The cardiovascular system. In: *Before We Are Born-Essentials of Embryology and Birth Defects.* Philadelphia, PA: W.B. Saunders, 2003:264–304.
2. Larsen WJ, Sherman LS, Potter SS, et al. Development of the heart. In: *Human Embryology.* New York: Churchill Livingstone, 2001:157–193.
3. Moore KL, Persaud TVN, Sheota K. The cardiovascular system. In: *Color Atlas of Clinical Embryology.* Philadelphia, PA: W.B. Saunders, 2000:198–215.
4. Brook MM, Heymann MA, Teitel DF. The heart. In: Klaus MH, Fanaroff AA (eds.), *Care of the High-Risk Neonate,* 5th ed. Philadelphia, PA: W.B. Saunders, 2001:393–424.
5. Hoffman JIE. Congenital heart disease: Incidence and recurrence. In: Rudolph CD, Rudolph AM, Hostetter MK, et al. (eds.), *Rudolph's Pediatrics,* 21st ed. New York: McGraw-Hill, 2004:1780–1782.

6. Driscoll DJ. Left to right shunt lesions. *Pediatr Clin North Am* 1999;46(2):355–368.

7. Bol-Raap G, Weerheim J, Kappetein AP, et al. Follow-up after surgical closure of congenital ventricular septal defect. *Eur J Cardiothorac Surg* 2003;24(4):511–515.

8. Arora R, Trehan V, Kumar A, et al. Transcatheter closure of congenital ventricular septal defects: Experience with various devices. *J Intervent Cardiol* 2003;16(1):83–91.

9. Thanopoulos BD, Karanassios E, Tsaousis G, et al. Catheter closure of congenital/acquired muscular VSDs and perimembranous VSDs using the Amplatzer devices. *J Intervent Cardiol* 2003;16(5):399–407.

10. Bass JL, Kalra GS, Arora R, et al. Initial human experience with the Amplatzer perimembranous ventricular septal occluder device. *Catheter Cardiovasc Interv* 2003;58(2):238–245.

11. Dajani As, Taubert KA, Wilson W, et al. Prevention of bacterial endocarditis. Recommendations by the American Heart Association. *Circulation* 1997;96(1):358–366.

12. Campbell M. Incidence of cardiac malformations at birth and later and neonatal mortality. *Br Heart J* 1973;35:189–200.

13. The Vermont-Oxford Trials Network: Very low birthweight outcomes for 1990. *Pediatrics* 1993;91:540–545.

14. Clyman RI. Ibuprofen and patent ductus arteriosus. *N Engl J Med* 2000;343(10):728–730.

15. Brooks MM, Heymann MA, Teitel DF. The heart. In: Klaus MH, Fanaroff AA (eds.), *Care of the High-Risk Neonate*, 5th ed. Philadelphia, PA: W.B. Saunders, 2001:393–424.

16. Brickner ME, Hillis LD, Lange RA. Congenital heart disease in adults. *N Engl J Med* 2000;342(4):256–263.

17. Van Overmeire B, Smets K, Lecoutere D, et al. A comparison of ibuprofen and indomethacin for closure of patent ductus arteriosus. *N Engl J Med* 2000;343(10):674–681.

18. Hijazi ZM, Geggel RL. Transcatheter closure of large patent ductus arteriosus (>or = to 4 mm) with multiple Gianturco coils: Immediate and mid-term results. *Heart* 1996;76(6):536–540.

19. Uzun O, Hancock S, Parsons J, et al. Transcatheter occlusion of the arterial duct with Cook detachable coils: Early experience. *Heart* 1996;76(3):269–273.

20. Thanopoulos BD, Tsaousis GS, Djukic M, et al. Transcatheter closure of high pulmonary artery pressure persistent ductus arteriosus with the Amplatzer muscular ventricular septal defect occluder. *Heart* 2002;87(3):269–273.

21. Berdis F, Moore JW. Balloon occlusion delivery technique for closure of patent ductus arteriosus. *Am Heart J* 1997;133(5):601–604.

22. Jaeggi ET, Fasnacht M, Arbenz U, et al. Transcatheter occlusion of the patent ductus arteriosus with a single device technique: Comparison the Cook detachable coil and the Rashkind umbrella device. *Int J Cardiol* 2001;79(1):71–76.

23. Rao PS, Kim SH, Choi JY, et al. Follow-up results of transvenous occlusion of patent ductus arteriosus with the buttoned device. *J Am Coll Cardiol* 1999;33(3):820–826.

24. Atrioventricular septal defect. In: Kouchoukos NT, Blackstone EJ, Doty DB, et al. (eds.), *Kirklin/Barratt-Boyes Cardiac Surgery*, Churchill Livingstone, Philadelphia, 2003:801–849.

25. Staniloae CS, El-Khally Z, Ibrahim R, et al. Percutaneous closure of secundum atrial septal defect in adults a single center experience with the amplatzer septal occluder. *J Invasive Cardiol* 2003;15(7):393–397.

26. Mills NL, King TD. Late follow-up of nonoperative closure of secundum atrial septal defects using the King-Mills double umbrella device. *Am J Cardiol* 2003;92(3):353–355.

27. Chang RKR, Chen AY, Klitzner TS. Clinical management of infants with hypoplastic left heart syndrome in the United States, 1988–1997. *Pediatrics* 2002;110(2):292–298.

28. Gutgesell HP, Massaro TA. Management of hypoplastic left heart syndrome in a consortium of university hospitals. *Am J Cardiol* 1995;76:809–811.

29. Pizarro C, Malec E, Maher KO, et al. Right ventricle to pulmonary artery conduit improves outcome after stage 1 Norwood for hypoplastic left heart syndrome. *Circulation* 2003;108(10 Suppl II):II-155–II-160.

30. Maher KO, Pizzaro C, Gidding SS, et al. Hemodynamic profile after the Norwood procedure with right ventricle to pulmonary artery conduit. *Circulation* 2003;108(7):782–784.

31. Walhout RJ, Lekkerkerker JC, Oron GH, et al. Comparison of polytetrafluoroethylene patch aortoplasty and end-to-end anastomosis for coarctation of aorta. *J Thorac Cardiovasc Surg* 2003;126(2):521–528.

32. Manganas C, Illiopoulos J, Chard RB, et al. Reoperation and coarctation of the aorta: The need for lifelong surveillance. *Ann Thorac Surg* 2001;72(4):1222–1224.

33. Rao PS, Jureidini SB, Balfour IC, et al. Severe aortic coarctation in infants less than 3 months: Successful palliation by balloon angioplasty. *J Invasive Cardiol* 2003;15(4):202–208.

34. Hernandez-Gonzales M, Solorio S, Conde-Carmona I, et al. Intraluminal aortoplasty vs. surgical aortic resection in congenital aortic coarctation. A clinical random study in pediatric patients. *Arch Med Res* 2003;34(4):305–310.

35. Brown JW, Ruzmetov M, Vijay P, et al. Surgery for aortic stenosis in children: A 40-year experience. *Ann Thorac Surg* 2003;76:1398–1411.

36. Thomson JDR. Management of valvular aortic stenosis in children. *Heart* 2004;90(1):5–6.

37. Reich O, Tax P, Marek J, et al. Long-term results of percutaneous balloon valvoplasty of congenital aortic stenosis: Independent predictors of outcome. *Heart* 2004;90(1):70–76.

43

Pediatric Congenital Heart Disease
Cyanotic Heart Defects

Sharon E. Mace

HIGH YIELD FACTS

- The three main presentations of symptomatic patients with congenital heart disease are: cyanosis, congestive heart failure, and shock.

- Cyanotic heart lesions are categorized by those that have decreased pulmonary blood flow (such as tetralogy of Fallot [TOF]) or increased pulmonary blood flow (such as truncus arteriosus).

- Infants with cyanotic congenital heart disease may present in shock, needing emergent resuscitation including the ABCs and often a prostaglandin E_1 (PGE_1) infusion. Such lesions include the TOF, pulmonary atresia, critical pulmonic stenosis (PS), and transposition of the great arteries (TGA).

- Common causes of cyanotic congenital heart disease are the "five Ts": tetralogy of Fallot, TGA, truncus arteriosus, tricuspid valve abnormalities, and total anomalous pulmonary venous return (TAPVR).

- Use of IV prostaglandin can be life saving in infants with ductus arteriosus dependent lesions. Such infants may present with cyanosis and/or cardiogenic shock.

SPECIFIC CONGENITAL HEART DEFECTS

There are numerous classifications of congenital heart disease, often based on physiology. Such classifications include: (1) whether cyanosis is present or absent, (2) whether pulmonary blood flow is increased, decreased, or normal, (3) type of anatomic defect: shunt, obstruction, transposition, or complex lesions, (4) whether congestive heart failure (or shock) is present or absent, and (5) with or without persistent fetal circulation.

Specific Cyanotic Congenital Heart Defects

The "five Ts" are a common listing of five common causes of cyanotic congenital heart disease that begin with the letter T. They are tetralogy of Fallot, transposition of the great arteries, truncus arteriosus, tricuspid atresia, and total anomalous venous return. Tricuspid atresia has been recently revised to "tricuspid valve abnormalities" (TVA).[1] Cyanotic congenital heart lesions included in TVA are tricuspid atresia, tricuspid valve stenosis, hypoplastic right ventricle syndrome, and tricuspid valve displacement (*Ebstein's anomaly*).

CYANOTIC CONGENITAL HEART DEFECTS WITH DECREASED PULMONARY BLOOD FLOW
Tetralogy of Fallot

Tetralogy of Fallot involves a dextroposed overriding aorta, obstruction of the right ventricular outflow tract (RVOT) (e.g., some form/degree(s) of pulmonic stenosis (PS), a ventricular septal defect (VSD), and resultant right ventricular hypertrophy (Fig. 43-1). The TOF has an additional atrial septal defect (ASD). TOF is the most common cause of cyanotic congenital heart disease after infancy.[2]

The obstruction at the RVOT leads to a right-to-left shunt across the VSD. In the left ventricle (LV), the deoxygenated shunted blood mixes with oxygenated blood from the LA, and the mixed somewhat desaturated blood is pumped to the systemic circulation resulting in cyanosis.

The history may reveal poor growth, and exercise intolerance relieved by squatting. Typical findings on physical examination are a holosystolic VSD murmur at the left 3rd intercostal space (ICS), a systolic diamond-shaped PS murmur at the left second ICS, and an abnormal second heart sound (single S_2 or split with a soft P_2). The chest roentgenogram reveals decreased pulmonary vascularity, an enlarged right ventricle (RV), and a boot-shaped heart with a concavity in the left heart border in the region generally occupied by the pulmonary artery (PA). The ECG shows right axis deviation and right ventricular hypertrophy. A right-sided aortic arch occurs in ~25% of TOF patients.

The clinical presentation of patients with TOF is variable.[3] Infants with severe right ventricular outflow obstruction present as a critically ill cyanotic neonate with no murmur, decreased arterial oxygen saturation,

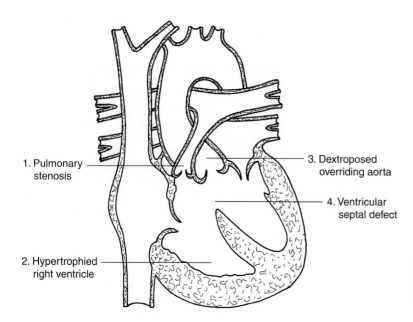

1. Pulmonary stenosis

2. Hypertrophied right ventricle

3. Dextroposed overriding aorta

4. Ventricular septal defect

Fig. 43-1. Tetralogy of Fallot. (Source: Adapted from Larson WJ. *Essentials of Human Embryology*. New York: Churchill-Livingstone, 1998:120.)

and dependence on a patent ductus arteriosus (PDA) for blood flow to the lungs. Intravenous PGE$_1$ in addition to the usual ABCs is essential therapy to stabilize the infant until cardiothoracic surgery can be done.[4]

Another presentation is that of a patient who is not cyanotic as a neonate but becomes symptomatic later in the first year of life. As the infant grows, there is increasing hypertrophy of the right ventricular infundibulum causing worsening PS with an increasing right-to-left shunt. These patients become symptomatic later in the first year of life with cyanosis and dyspnea on exertion. Infants and toddlers will play for a brief period then sit or lie down. In order to relieve the dyspnea from physical activity, children will assume a squatting position. Especially during the first 2 years of life "paroxysmal hypercyanotic attacks" or "Tet" spells can occur.

Patients with mild right ventricular outflow obstruction, the "pink Tet," may be seen with heart failure due to the large left-to-right shunt.

Previously, a systemic artery to PA anastomosis to increase pulmonary blood flow was performed followed by later repair with patch closure of the VSD and opening of the RVOT obstruction.[5–7] The Waterson, Potts, and Blalock-Taussig shunts (see page 516) were used in the past with the modified Blalock-Taussig shunt used more recently.[4] Currently, complete repair is often done at the time of diagnosis[8] even in neonates since there were long-term complications associated with these shunts.[2] Complications

included pulmonary hypertension/pulmonary vascular disease, distortion of the PA branches, and LV volume overload.[2,9] Palliative shunts or balloon valvuloplasty are done in critically ill infants who are not candidates for complete repair if they have diminutive pulmonary arteries[2] or are very small premature infants[9] (although now surgery is being done even in premature infants).[10]

Hypoplastic Right Heart Syndrome

The hypoplastic right heart syndrome consists of various congenital heart defects, which have the common denominator of a small right ventricular cavity with hypertrophied walls.

Pulmonary Atresia with an Intact Ventricular Septum

Pulmonary atresia with an intact ventricular septum is one type of hypoplastic right heart syndrome. The pulmonary valve and RVOT are atretic. The only supply of blood flow to the lungs is via a PDA. Since there is no blood flow out of the RV, the right atrium (RA) pressure increases causing blood to shunt from the RA across the foramen ovale (FO) into the left atrium (LA) where it mixes with pulmonary venous blood and enters the LV. The LV is responsible for ejecting the combined left and right ventricular output.

As the ductus arteriosus (DA) closes in the first few hours or days of life, these neonates develop severe cyanosis and respiratory distress. The second heart sound is single and loud. Usually, there is no murmur although occasionally a continuous or systolic murmur from flow through the DA is present. The ECG reveals right atrial hypertrophy, left ventricular hypertrophy, and usually decreased right ventricular forces. The chest roentgenogram shows decreased pulmonary vascularity with a variable heart size. Without treatment these patients usually die within the first week of life.

The goal of ED management in addition to the usual ABCs is to maintain the patency of the ductus by an infusion of PGE_1. This will decrease the hypoxemia and acidosis allowing stabilization so interventional cardiac catheterization and surgery can be done. Palliative treatment usually includes an aortopulmonary shunt[11] to maintain adequate pulmonary blood flow often with a procedure to open the RVOT (e.g., pulmonary valvotomy) and/or an atrial septostomy.[4] The follow-up surgery varies depending on several factors including the RV/tricuspid valve size[4,12,13] and is either a "2 ventricle repair," a 1.5 ventricle repair,[14–16] or a one ventricle repair.[4,12,13] The 1.5 ventricle repair involves a cavopulmonary anastomosis with ASD closure so the inferior vena cava (IVC) flows to the RA, then RV and into the pulmonary arteries.[14–16] The one ventricle repair is a modified Fontan procedure with a RA to PA connection with an intraatrial tunnel.[4] Recently, percutaneous balloon valvotomy done during cardiac catheterization in selected patients has been effective in opening up the valve.[17]

Pulmonary Atresia with Ventricular Septal Defect

This congenital heart defect can be considered the most severe form of TOF in which the pulmonary valve is atretic and the RVOT is also atretic or hypoplastic. The clinical manifestation is similar to that of patients with severe TOF who present as cyanotic newborns dependent on ductal flow to the lungs. Again, PGE_1 is the pharmacologic drug of choice in addition to the usual supportive ABC measures.

Tricuspid Atresia

In tricuspid atresia, the tricuspid valve is atretic so there is no flow from the RA to the RV. The entire systemic venous return is shunted from the RA to the LA via the FO or an associated ASD. If there is no VSD, then there is a hypoplastic RV and an atretic PA. Pulmonary blood flow is ductal dependent. A PGE_1 infusion is mandatory in a cyanotic neonate with this congenital heart lesion.

If a VSD is present with tricuspid atresia, then the amount of pulmonary blood flow and the relative cyanosis is a function of (1) the size of VSD, and (2) if PS is present, and if so how severe is the PS. Infrequently, tricuspid atresia patients with a large VSD and no outflow obstruction have a high pulmonary blood flow and present with heart failure and mild cyanosis.

Patients with tricuspid atresia are usually cyanotic at birth. Unlike most other causes of cyanotic heart disease, such as TOF with an increased RV impulse and increased right ventricular forces on ECG, these patients have an increased LV impulse and left axis deviation and left ventricular hypertrophy on ECG. The chest roentgenogram usually demonstrates decreased pulmonary vascularity because of the PS-limiting pulmonary blood flow.

Management in severely cyanotic infants includes a PGE_1 infusion until surgery can be performed.

Patients with a small RV (or a small LV) whose hypoplastic ventricle is so small it cannot support a two ventricle circulation are considered a "single ventricle" physiology.[18] The goal of first stage palliation is to provide adequate balanced systemic (Q_s) and pulmonary blood flow (Q_p) ($Q_p \approx Q_s$), allow unobstructed atrial mixing of blood flow, and unobstructed systemic cardiac output. First stage palliation in single ventricle physiology (as with tricuspid atresia) is a systemic to pulmonary arterial shunt to increase pulmonary blood flow. The shunt is performed in the neonatal period. This is followed by a second stage palliation, usually done between 3 and 12 months of age. The second stage palliation forms a superior cavopulmonary connection in order to decrease the volume load on the single functional ventricle in order to avoid myocardial failure. This second stage palliative operation connects the superior vena cava (SVC) to the pulmonary arteries creating a bidirectional superior cavopulmonary shunt. Some institutions will do a "hemi-Fontan" surgery instead of a bidirectional superior cavopulmonary shunt for stage II.[19] Physiologically, the two procedures are similar. The hemi-Fontan creates a right atrial to right PA anastomosis in order to divert SVC flow to the pulmonary arteries.[19] The third stage, generally done between 1 and 5 years of age, is the Fontan operation. The Fontan procedure directs all inferior vena caval blood flow directly into the pulmonary circulation so that only pulmonary venous blood and coronary sinus blood returns to the common atrial chamber and single ventricle. The end result is a nearly complete separation of the systemic and pulmonary circulations. The Fontan procedure can be done using a lateral tunnel technique with placement of an intraatrial baffle or an extra conduit.[20,21] Surgical management is life saving for infants with tricuspid atresia (and other forms of single ventricle physiology), although early and late complications can occur and reoperation may be necessary.[22] Complications include occlusion of shunt by thrombosis (clotting off the baffle or conduit or shunt),[23] a "failing" Fontan circulation (with decreased exercise tolerance), AV valve regurgitation, cyanosis, arrhythmias, a protein losing enteropathy, myocardial dysfunction, thromboembolic complications, and hemodynamic abnormalities.[22,23]

Double Outlet Right Ventricle with Pulmonic Stenosis

With this lesion, the PA and the Ao both arise from the RV, and PS is present. The presentation and management are similar to TOF.

Ebstein's Anomaly

Ebstein's anomaly is a downward displacement of an abnormal tricuspid valve into the RV (Figs. 43-2 and 43-3). This lesion occurs when there is a failure of the normal separation of the tricuspid valve from the right ventricular

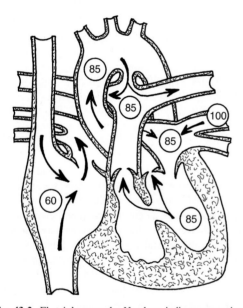

Fig. 43-2. Ebstein's anomaly. Numbers indicate approximate oxygen saturations. (Source: Adapted from Behrman RE, Kliegman RM, Jenson HB. *Nelson's Textbook of Pediatrics*. Philadelphia, PA: W.B. Saunders, 2004:1534.)

myocardium. The result is a RV separated into two parts by the abnormal tricuspid valve: a thin walled "atrialized" section contiguous with the right atrial cavity and a generally smaller section of normal myocardium. The RA is markedly enlarged because of tricuspid valve regurgitation. Effective right ventricular output is impaired because of the small poorly functioning RV. Right ventricular function and output may be so severely limited that there is "functional" pulmonary atresia. The increased volume of right atrial blood is shunted right to left through the FO into the LA.

The severity of the lesion and thus, the symptoms are quite variable. Newborns with severe Ebstein anomaly have marked cyanosis, massive cardiomegaly, and often die from hypoxemia and heart failure. Such infants are usually ductal dependent for pulmonary blood flow and require prostaglandin infusions until emergency cardio-thoracic surgery can be done.

Patients with milder forms of Ebstein's anomaly may present in adolescence or adulthood with symptoms/signs including fatigue, palpitations (from arrhythmias), and cyanosis. A holosystolic murmur from tricuspid regurgitation, a diastolic murmur at the lower left sternal border, and a gallop rhythm is typically present. The ECG reveals a right bundle branch block, atrial hypertrophy, and sometimes a Wolf-Parkinson-White syndrome. Older patients often have supraventricular dysrhythmias.

The preferred surgery for Ebstein's anomaly is tricuspid valve repair with closure of the associated ASD. The tricuspid valve may require replacement (in 20–30% of patients) because of severe deformity of the tricuspid valve.[24,25] Prior to corrective surgery, some patients had palliative surgery: bidirectional cavopulmonary shunts.[25] In neonates with severe Ebstein's anomaly some infants will undergo a Fontan procedure to create a univentricular heart because of a functional tricuspid and/or pulmonary atresia.[26]

Critical Pulmonic Stenosis

With critical PS there is such marked obstruction to blood flow through the severely narrowed pulmonic valve that pulmonary flow is decreased. The RV fills with blood which flows back into the RA through the tricuspid valve causing "functional tricuspid regurgitation." Blood is shunted through the FO from the RA to the LA, resulting in a mixing of deoxygenated venous blood with a negligible amount of oxygenated blood returning from the pulmonary veins. This blood flows into the LV and is ejected into the aorta resulting in systemic desaturation/hypoxia.

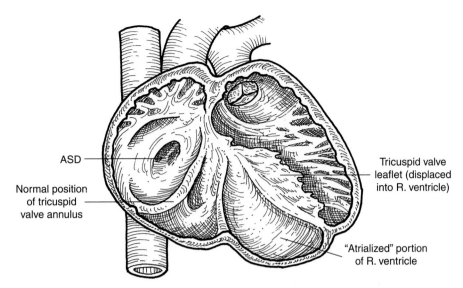

Fig. 43-3. Ebstein's anomaly. (Source: Adapted from Emmanouilides G, Riemenschneider T, Allen H, et al. *Moss and Adams Heart Disease in Infants, Children and Adolescents*. Baltimore, MD: Williams & Wilkins, 1995:919.)

The RA is markedly enlarged because of the tricuspid regurgitation while the left side of the heart has decreased filling and appears smaller. Physical examination reveals a tricuspid regurgitation murmur and usually right heart failure with marked hepatomegaly. The ECG shows right atrial hypertrophy. Decreased pulmonary blood flow and a prominence of the right heart border are seen on chest roentgenogram.

A PGE₁ infusion is crucial in maintaining pulmonary blood flow via the DA until the infant can be taken to the cardiac catheterization laboratory where balloon dilatation of the pulmonic valve is done or less frequently to surgery for a valvulotomy in order to open up the stenotic pulmonic valve.[27-29] Most patients will have some pulmonic regurgitation postprocedure and will require lifelong endocardial prophylaxis and follow-up.

CYANOTIC CONGENITAL HEART DISEASE WITH INCREASED PULMONARY BLOOD FLOW

Transposition of the Great Arteries

Transposition of the great arteries is a common congenital heart defect occurring in about 5% of all congenital heart disease. TGA is the most frequent diagnosis in critically ill neonates (age 0–30 days) with cardiac disease and is the most common cyanotic congenital heart defect in some series.[30]

In TGA, the Ao arises from the RV and the PA from the LV (Fig. 43-4). With the normal position of the great vessels the Ao is posterior and to the right of the PA. With d-TGA, the Ao is dextropositioned, located anterior and to the right of the PA.

Cyanosis occurs because desaturated blood from the body enters the RA then to the RV and then goes out the Ao to the body, while oxygenated pulmonary venous blood returns to the LA. Then it goes into the LV and PA only to return to the lungs. Without some mixing of blood via a FO and a patent DA, survival would not be possible. A VSD is present in approximately 50% of patients with TGA.

Isolated Transposition of the Great Arteries

Isolated TGA or simple TGA is a d-TGA with an intact ventricular septum. Postnatally when the DA starts to close, severe cyanosis occurs, since the small amount of blood shunting through the FO only provides a minimal amount of mixing of systemic and pulmonary blood.

The typical scenario of a patient with a simple TGA is a tachypneic neonate occurring within a few hours to days of birth. Without treatment, these infants will die from the severe prolonged hypoxemia and metabolic acidosis. The physical examination reveals cyanosis,

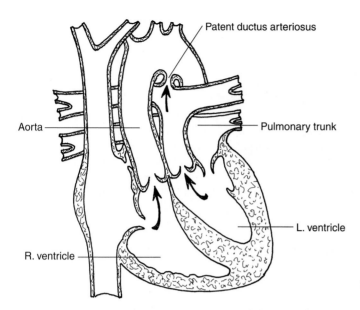

Patent ductus arteriosus

Aorta

Pulmonary trunk

L. ventricle

R. ventricle

Fig. 43-4. Transposition of the great arteries. (Source: Adapted from Larson WJ. *Essentials of Human Embryology*. New York: Churchill-Livingstone, 1998:120.)

tachypnea, a loud single S_2 (infrequently S_2 is split), and no murmur (rarely a soft systolic ejection murmur is present). The ECG demonstrates the usual neonatal right-sided dominance. The chest roentgenogram reveals increased or normal pulmonary blood flow, mild cardiomegaly, and a narrow mediastinum.

Management consists of the ABCs: correction of acidosis and any other abnormalities such as hypothermia and hypoglycemia, which will worsen the metabolic acidosis caused by the hypoxia and a stat PGE_1 infusion. Supplemental oxygen is given which will decrease PVR and increase pulmonary blood flow. Further therapy may include a Rashkind balloon atrial septostomy done during cardiac catheterization to enlarge the interatrial opening allowing for better mixing. Ideally, a successful Rashkind atrial septostomy will lead to a 35–50 mmHg increase in the arterial pO_2 and equal pressures in the right and left atria. Surgical therapy is the arterial switch (Jatene procedure) whereby the Ao and PA are incised and then reanastomosed to the correct position.

Surgical correction of an isolated TGA is by an atrial switch (Senning or Mustard) procedure or more recently an arterial switch (Jatene procedure), see page 516.[31,32] Atrial-level transposition of venous return (atrial switch) is accomplished in the Senning procedure by redesigning the RA and atrial septum or in the Mustard procedure by a pericardial baffle after excising the atrial septum.[32]

The atrial switch procedure redirects systemic venous blood through the mitral valve into the LV and out the PA while pulmonary venous blood is routed through the tricuspid valve into the RV and out the Ao. The atrial switch procedure results in a "physiologic" circulation with the RV functioning as the "systemic ventricle." The atrial switch surgery improved survival but was associated with complications. The complications were related to problems with the baffle (leakage, obstruction with increased venous pressure), RV (systemic) ventricle failure/dysfunction, and dysrhythmias (atrial arrhythmias especially atrial flutter, sinus node dysfunction, e.g., sick sinus syndrome), and sudden death.[32–38]

The arterial switch procedure has supplanted the atrial switch procedure whereby the Ao and PA are incised and then switched. The Ao is reanastomosed to the "neoaortic valve" (previously the pulmonic valve) arising from the LV. The PA is attached to the "neopulmonic valve" (formerly the aortic valve) arising from the RV. The great vessels are transected above the semilunar valves and coronary arteries so the coronary arteries need to be relocated to the neoaorta allowing for normal coronary circulation. The arterial switch procedure has better results than the atrial switch (Senning or Mustard) with less likelihood of reintervention, improved survival, and better functional class, although psychosocial disorders, particularly learning disorders are common.[31]

Transposition of the Great Arteries with Ventricular Septal Defect

For TGA with a small VSD, the clinical presentation and treatment is essentially the same as for TGA with an intact ventricular septum with the additional finding of a harsh systolic murmur at the lower left sternal border from the flow through the small restrictive VSD.

TGA with a large nonrestrictive VSD results in mixing of deoxygenated and oxygenated blood at the ventricular level such that cyanosis may not be as severe and heart failure symptomatology is the clinical presentation. Cyanosis may be mild, have a delayed onset, and a variable intensity. Cyanosis is usually identified during the first month of life although it may not be identified for several months.

Right ventricular prominence as with normal newborns is found on the ECG in neonates with TGA, but as the infant gets older right ventricular hypertrophy and right axis deviation are present. The chest roentgenogram findings are increased pulmonary vascularity, cardiomegaly, and a narrow superior mediastinum due to the anterior posterior position of the great vessel and thymic involution with an "egg on a string" appearance.

The diagnosis is usually made by echocardiography. Sometimes cardiac catheterization is performed and a Rashkind balloon atrial septostomy is done to decompress the LA even if there is sufficient mixing at the ventricular level. Surgical correction of TGA consists of the Jatene (arterial switch) procedure.[31,32] Previously an atrial switch (Senning or Mustard procedure) was performed.[31,32]

For patients with TGA, a VSD, and significant left ventricular outflow tract obstruction; a Rastelli procedure is done. The Rastelli operation results in an anatomic repair (LV to Ao, RV to PA) by closure of the origin of the pulmonary trunk from the LV, placement of an intracardiac baffle directing LV blood to the Ao, and a redirection of flow by a valved extracardiac conduit from RV to PA.[39,40] A recent report reviews the half-turned truncal switch operation for TGA with a VSD and PS.[41]

Uncorrected TGA with a VSD is usually fatal within the first year of life from heart failure, hypoxemia, and pulmonary vascular hypertension.

The clinical presentation of TGA with a VSD and PS is similar to TOF. The onset of symptoms depends on the severity of the PS. Cyanotic neonates should receive a PGE$_1$ infusion while cardiac catheterization and surgery are being arranged. A balloon atrial septostomy may be done during cardiac catheterization in order to increase atrial mixing and decompress the LA. Surgery is a stepwise approach: an aortopulmonary shunt to increase pulmonary blood flow in infancy, and a Rastelli operation or occasionally a Mustard operation done at a later date after the infant has experienced some growth.

"Congenitally Corrected" Transposition of the Great Arteries (ccTGA)

With ventricular inversion there is discordance of the atrioventricular relationships with the RA connected to the LV and the LA to the RV. ccTGA is characterized by ventricular inversion (RA to LV, LA to RV) and transposed great vessels (ventriculoarterial inversion—the Ao arises from the RV and the PA from LV). With L-TGA or levotransposition, the Ao arises to the left of the PA. The Ao and the PA usually lie side by side although occasionally the Ao may be anterior to the PA.

Thus, deoxygenated venous blood from the vena cava enters a normally positioned RA, goes through a bicuspid atrioventricular (mitral) valve into a morphologic LV located on the right side into the PA and into the lungs. Oxygenated pulmonary venous blood enters a normally positioned LA, goes through an atrioventricular (tricuspid) valve into a morphologic RV (but left-sided location) and then out a transposed Ao to the systemic circulation. Assuming there are no other cardiac defects, the hemodynamics would be adequate in this physiologically "corrected" circulation. Unfortunately, other abnormalities almost always exist and include VSD, PS, conduction defects, and Ebstein-like abnormalities of the left-sided tricuspid valve.

The clinical presentation of ccTGA varies depending on the other associated defects. Clues to the diagnosis on the chest radiograph include an abnormal position of the great vessels with a straight positioned ascending aorta comprising the upper left border of the heart. The ECG is generally abnormal; often with abnormal Q waves present in leads III, V, AVF, AVR and a missing Q wave in V$_6$.

Although echocardiography can suggest the diagnosis, cardiac catheterization is often done in order to map the conduction system so the bundle of His can be avoided during surgical repair of associated defects.

Recently, the "double switch" procedures have been advocated for surgical correction of ccTGA because of concerns regarding long-term use of the morphologic RV and tricuspid valve in the systemic circulation.[42–44] The "double switch" operations combines a Senning procedure plus an arterial switch procedure or a Senning and a Rastelli procedure. This has the advantage of using the morphologic LV and mitral valve in the systemic circulation.[42–44] The "double switch" operation: (1) connects the morphologic

LV with the Ao using an intraventricular baffle (which also closes the VSD), (2) connects the morphologic RV with the PA using an extracardiac conduit, and (3) performs an intraatrial transposition of venous return by a Senning or Mustard technique. Some institutions are using a bidirectional superior cavopulmonary anastomosis with a ccTGA physiologic repair[45] or with the "double switch" operation.[50] If there is severe pulmonic outflow tract obstruction, a valved extracardiac conduit is used to connect the left ventricle with the PA in a conventional repair of the ccTGA with a VSD and PS.[46,47]

Truncus Arteriosus

The pathophysiology of truncus arteriosus is a single arterial trunk overriding a VSD and receiving mixed blood from the left and right ventricles (Fig. 43-5). The single arterial trunk provides blood flow to the systemic, pulmonary, and coronary circulations. The solitary semilunar valve or "truncal" valve is abnormally formed. It has from two to six or seven cusps, and is generally regurgitant or stenotic. There are four subtypes of truncus arteriosus based on how the pulmonary arteries originate from the single arterial trunk. The large nonrestrictive VSD allows for total mixing of blood and results in equal RV and LV pressures.

In the first few hours or days of life when PVR is high, pulmonary blood flow is normal. With the drop in PVR in the first month of life, pulmonary blood flow increases and heart failure occurs. Cyanosis may be mild because of the increased pulmonary blood flow. If untreated, Eisenmenger syndrome develops.

The clinical presentation is a function of age and thus, PVR. In the first days of life when PVR is still increased, the clinical findings are mild cyanosis and a murmur. Later during infancy when PVR is decreased, there is tremendous pulmonary blood flow resulting in heart failure.

Clinical findings include a loud single second heart sound, a hyperdynamic precordium, a systolic ejection murmur at the mid left sternal border, usually with an early systolic ejection click and sometimes a thrill, an apical mid diastolic rumbling murmur from increased flow through the mitral valve, and if truncal insufficiency is present, a high pitched early diastolic murmur at the mid left sternal border.

Ventricular hypertrophy, either right, left, or combined, is present. Cardiomegaly from biventricular hypertrophy and increased pulmonary vascularity (after the first month of life) is present on the chest roentgenogram and a right aortic arch in 50% of patients. Echocardiography confirms the diagnosis and detects other associated defects such as an interrupted aortic arch.

In the past, palliative surgery with PA banding to decrease pulmonary blood flow was done. Now, surgery is usually done at about 6–8 weeks of age to decrease the

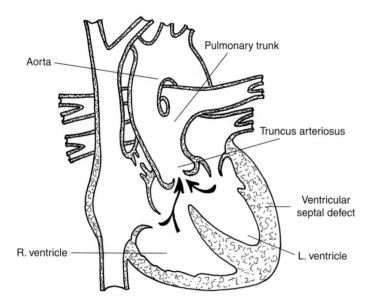

Fig. 43-5. Persistent truncus arteriosus. (Source: Adapted from Larson WE. *Essentials of Human Embryology*. New York: Churchill-Livingstone, 1998:126.)

likelihood of pulmonary vascular disease. The corrective surgery is patch closure of the VSD, and placement of a homograft conduit from the RV to the main PA.[48–50] With growth of the child, surgical revision(s) with replacement of the homograft will need to be done.[51–53] Insufficiency of the truncal valve is common and valve replacement is often necessary.[49,54]

Most untreated infants die within the first 2 years of life, although a few patients whose pulmonary blood flow is restricted by pulmonary vascular disease, may survive with Eisenmenger syndrome into early adulthood.

Total Anomalous Pulmonary Venous Return

Normally, the pulmonary veins return to the LA. With abnormal evolution of the pulmonary veins, either partial or complete anomalous pulmonary venous return can occur. Generally, partial venous return is an acyanotic congenital heart defect. With TAPVR, there is complete mixing of pulmonary venous and systemic venous return before or at the level of the RA, resulting in cyanosis (Fig. 43-6). The mixed blood in the RA follows two routes: either into the RV and then into the PA, or through a patent FO or an ASD into the LA.

With TAPVR, there is no direct route from the pulmonary veins into the LA. There are several alternative pathways either above or below the diaphragm or both. There are numerous sites where the anomalous pulmonary veins return: supracardiac (most common), cardiac, infracardiac, or mixed.[55,56] Pulmonary veins returning above the diaphragm may flow directly into the RA or into the coronary sinus (cardiac type), or via a "vertical vein" into the SVC (supracardiac type). Pulmonary veins draining below the diaphragm (infracardiac type) may enter a "descending vein" that joins a tributary of the IVC itself or even into the DV which closes shortly after birth. Severe obstruction can occur with anomalous pulmonary venous return above or below the diaphragm but is almost always present with infracardiac anomalous pulmonary venous return.

Signs and symptoms of TAPVR are determined by whether or not there is obstruction of pulmonary venous return. TAPVR with obstruction is a cardiothoracic surgical emergency since marked pulmonary congestion and pulmonary hypertension rapidly evolve leading to sudden deterioration. Furthermore, unlike most types of cyanotic congenital heart defects, PGE$_1$ infusion may not be helpful although it is usually given.

The clinical presentation depends on the degree of obstruction. Neonates with marked obstruction are critically ill with cyanosis, hepatomegaly, marked tachypnea, hemodynamic instability, and failure to respond to mechanical ventilation.[57] These neonates are often misdiagnosed with respiratory disease such as persistent pulmonary hypertension. They will have a rapid downhill course unless a prompt diagnosis is made and immediate surgery is done. Patients with mild to moderate obstruction and a large left-to-right shunt present with heart failure, mild cyanosis, PA hypertension, a gallop rhythm, and a systolic murmur at the left sternal border. The third group of patients do not have pulmonary venous obstruction or pulmonary hypertension and have mild cyanosis. This third group includes most of TAPVR patients with the cardiac type and about half the patients with the supracardiac type. With the cardiac type, pulmonary venous return goes to the coronary sinus or directly to the rRA. With the supracardiac type, pulmonary venous return is to the left or right SVC.

Patients with TAPVR must have a patent FO or an ASD in order for blood to reach the LA then the LV and the systemic circulation.

If there is no obstruction to pulmonary venous return then the manifestations of TAPVR are like that of an ASD with a right-to-left shunt. Unsaturated blood flows from the RA to the LA, and mixes with saturated blood returning from the pulmonary veins. The mixing causes blood that is not completely saturated to flow to the LV and out the Ao, which results in systemic cyanosis. Enlargement of the RA, RV, and PA occurs due to the increased venous return from both the systemic and pulmonary systems going to the RA.

On physical examination, a right ventricular impulse, a widely split S$_2$ with a loud P$_2$ component, and a systolic ejection murmur (from the increased pulmonary blood flow) at the mid/upper left sternal border are present.

Right atrial hypertrophy, a rightward QRS axis, and right ventricular hypertrophy is noted on ECG. The chest roentgenogram reveals cardiomegaly, increased pulmonary vascularity, and frequently a characteristic appearance: a snowman or figure of eight with supracardiac TAPVR, and marked pulmonary venous congestion with bilateral "fluffy" lung fields with infradiaphragmatic TAPVR. Dilatation of the vertical vein that enters the SVC and dilatation of the SVC causes the "snowman" appearance with supracardiac TAPVR. The appearance of the lungs with infradiaphragmatic TAPVR is from the obstruction of the pulmonary veins causing pulmonary venous congestion and may be confused with respiratory disease such as aspiration or pneumonia. Echocardiography is usually diagnostic. MRI and CT scan have also been used for diagnosing TAPVR. Occasionally, cardiac catheterization is done when there is very complicated pulmonary venous

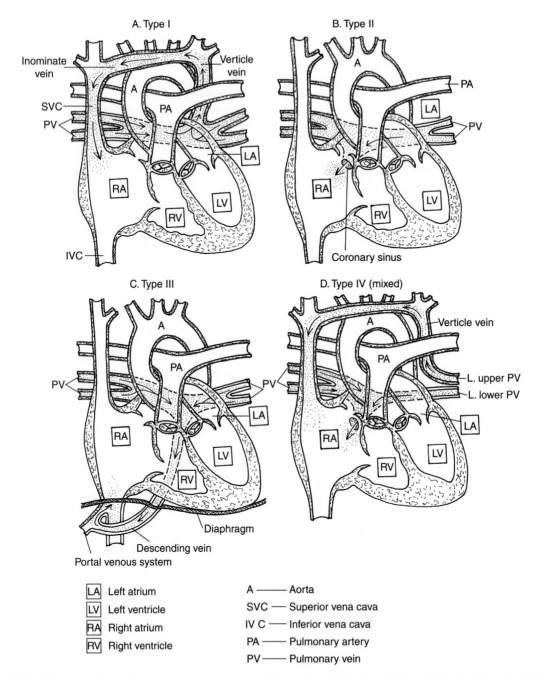

A. Type I

Inominate vein

Verticle vein

SVC

PV

A

PA

RA

LA

RV

LV

IVC

B. Type II

A

PA

LA

PV

RA

LV

RV

Coronary sinus

C. Type III

A

PA

PV

LA

RA

LV

RV

Diaphragm

Descending vein

Portal venous system

D. Type IV (mixed)

A

Verticle vein

PA

L. upper PV

L. lower PV

PV

RA

LA

LV

RV

LA	Left atrium
LV	Left ventricle
RA	Right atrium
RV	Right ventricle

A ——— Aorta
SVC — Superior vena cava
IV C — Inferior vena cava
PA ——— Pulmonary artery
PV ——— Pulmonary vein

Fig. 43-6. Total anomalous pulmonary venous return. (Source: Adapted from Pediatric cardiology. *Pediatr Clin North Am* 1999; 46(2):419.)

anatomy and if a Rashkind balloon atrial septostomy is needed to enlarge a restrictive FO or ASD.

Emergent corrective surgery is required for infradiaphragmatic TAPVR with obstruction. Treatment of pulmonary edema includes intubation with positive pressure ventilation and positive end-expiratory pressure (PEEP). Supplemental oxygen can be given but give as little as is needed, aiming for a desired systemic oxygenation saturation no greater than 90%. Higher oxygen saturations may cause further dilatation of the pulmonary vascular bed, which is already receiving torrential blood flow. If there is marked hypotension or shock, packed RBCs may be the fluid of choice (assuming polycythemia is not present).

Postoperative complications include pulmonary hypertension, arrhythmias, and pulmonary vein stenosis/obstruction (which may require reintervention, either reoperation or repeated balloon dilatation sometimes with a stent).[55,56,58–61]

Although there is some controversy over the use of a PGE_1 infusion with TAPVR, many still advocate its use.[62,63] The potential adverse effect is that the prostaglandin infusion, by keeping the DA patent, will increase pulmonary blood flow and worsen the pulmonary venous congestion. The potential benefits of a PGE_1 infusion are that it opens the DV which could decompress the obstructed infradiagramatic TAPVR. Thus, it may be appropriate to begin a PGE_1 infusion in any cyanotic neonate suspected of having congenital heart disease while awaiting definitive therapy.[62,63]

Single Ventricle (Double Inlet Ventricle, Univentricular)

Both atria (LA, RA) empty into one single ventricular chamber via one common atrioventricular valve or two separate atrioventricular valves with a single ventricle.[63] There is total mixing of the deoxygenated systemic venous return and the oxygenated pulmonary venous return in the single ventricular chamber. With single ventricle, also known as double inlet ventricle or univentricular heart, the morphology of the ventricular chamber may be that of a LV or RV or indeterminant. Both great vessels arise from the single ventricular chamber. The position of the Ao with respect to the PA may be posterior (which is normal) or malpositioned either anterior or side by side; and to the right or left. Pulmonary stenosis or atresia is a frequently associated lesion with single ventricle.

Clinical signs/symptoms and treatment depend on associated cardiac lesions. When pulmonic outflow obstruction is present, the presentation is like TOF with cyanosis without heart failure. In childhood findings include: dyspnea, fatigue, clubbing, polycythemia, cardiomegaly, a left parasternal lift, a systolic thrill, a loud single S_2, and a loud systolic ejection murmur.

Patients without pulmonary outflow obstruction have tremendously increased pulmonary blood flow. These patients present in infancy with mild to moderate cyanosis and heart failure. Symptoms including recurrent respiratory infections, failure to thrive, dyspnea, and tachypnea are common. Typical physical examination findings are cardiomegaly, a palpable left parasternal lift, a loud narrowly split S_2, a third heart sound, a mid-diastolic rumbling murmur from increased flow through the atrioventricular valve, and a mild nondescript systolic ejection murmur.

The ECG has variable findings: atrial hypertrophy is common, and right, left, or combined ventricular hypertrophy can occur (most often combined or right ventricular hypertrophy). The chest roentgenogram demonstrates cardiomegaly and increased pulmonary vascularity if there is no pulmonic outflow tract obstruction, or decreased pulmonary vascularity if PS is present. Echocardiography confirms the absence of a ventricular septum.

Without surgery, patients die in infancy from heart failure, or in adolescence/early adulthood from chronic hypoxia or pulmonary vascular disease (Eisenmenger syndrome). Surgical management depends on the associated defects. With severe PS, an aortopulmonary shunt is performed in order to provide adequate pulmonary blood flow. If pulmonary blood flow is torrential, PA banding is done to prevent pulmonary vascular disease and to manage the heart failure with a modified Fontan procedure (cavopulmonary isolation procedure) done at a later date. Because of the complications associated with the Fontan,[22,23,64–66] reintervention may be necessary[66] and other surgical options (septation into two ventricles[67] or PA division and shunt[68] or cardiac transplantation[69]) have been suggested.

SINGLE VENTRICLE PHYSIOLOGY

The term "single ventricle physiology" refers to any congenital cardiac defect in which there is no realistic possibility of surgically reconstructing a functional two ventricle heart.[18,70] Thus, other congenital heart lesions, such as tricuspid atresia, or pulmonary atresia with an intact ventricular septum, in addition to "single ventricle," are included in "single ventricle physiology." Surgical management for single ventricle physiology is generally based on a bidirectional Glenn shunt followed later by the Fontan operation and its variants.[18]

APPENDIX: PROCEDURES USED TO TREAT PATIENTS WITH CONGENITAL HEART DISEASE: CARDIAC CATHETERIZATION PROCEDURE

- Rashkind balloon atrial septostomy = catheter is directed across the FO from the RA into the LA, the catheter on the balloon is inflated then pulled back, thus tearing the atrial septum. The purpose is to increase the mixing of blood at the atrial level and/or to decompress the LA. A successful Rashkind procedure will increase the arterial pO_2 by 35–50 mmHg in an infant with cyanotic congenital heart disease (such as TGA).

SURGICAL PROCEDURES

Procedures to Decrease Pulmonary Blood Flow

- PA band (pulmonary trunk band)—a device (band) placed circumferentially around the PA which decreases pulmonary blood flow. The purpose is to prevent pulmonary hypertension with resultant pulmonary vascular disease.

Aortopulmonary Shunts to Increase Blood Flow

- Blalock-Taussig shunt = subclavian artery to ipsilateral PA anastomosis (e.g., right subclavian to right PA, or left subclavian to left PA).
- Glenn shunt = SVC to right PA anastomosis.
- Potts shunt = descending aorta to left PA.
- Waterston shunt = ascending aorta and right PA.
- Bidirectional superior cavopulmonary shunt = bidirectional Glenn shunt = palliative operation which diverts SVC blood from either one or both SVC to the right or left pulmonary arteries (palliative surgery for tricuspid atresia).

Surgery Repairs for Transposition of the Great Arteries

- Atrial switch operations provide "physiologic" repair by diverting systemic venous blood (deoxygenated) to the LA and pulmonary venous blood (oxygenated) to the RA via baffles constructed within the atria. Systemic venous deoxygenated blood reaches the morphologic LV and is pumped to the pulmonary circuit (e.g., PA to the lungs). Pulmonary (oxygenated) blood goes to the morphologic RV and is pumped to the systemic circuit (e.g., aorta (Ao)

and the body). The ventriculoatrial discordance remains. Postoperative result is: systemic venous deoxygenated blood → LA → LV → PA → lungs. Pulmonary venous (oxygenated) blood → RA → RV → Aorta → body.

- Mustard operation = atrial switch "physiologic" repair for TGA in which the atrial septum is excised and a pericardial patch is used to create the intraatrial baffle to direct blood flow from RA to LV and LA to RV.
- Senning operation = atrial switch "physiologic" repair for TGA in which incisions are made in the left atria and right atria, and an atrial septal flap is used to direct blood flow from RA to LV and LA to RV.
- Arterial switch operation (Jatene procedure) provides "anatomic" repair with blood flow from RV to PA and LV to Ao. The aorta and PA are incised and "switched" (reanastomosed) so the aorta arises from the LV and the PA from the RV. The coronary arteries are transplanted to the "neoaorta."

Surgery for Transposition of Great Arteries with Ventricular Septal Defect and Pulmonic Stenosis

- Rastelli operation = surgical repair with closure of VSD, and placement of an extracardiac RV to distal PA conduit attains physiologic and anatomic correction for TGA with VSD and PS (actually LVOT since the great vessels are transposed).

Surgery for Hypoplastic Left Heart

- Norwood procedure = three-stage reconstructive surgical palliation done for hypoplastic left heart. Ligation and transection of the distal main PA is followed by: (1) an anastomosis between the proximal main PA trunk and the ascending hypoplastic aorta (usually with a patch) creating a "neoaorta," (2) an aortic to PA anastomosis (with a Gore-Tex graft), (3) atrial septectomy to create large interatrial communication.

Surgery for "Single Ventricle" Physiology

- Fontan procedure = creation of a cavopulmonary tunnel or baffle that separates oxygenated from deoxygenated blood in the RA allowing blood from vena cava to flow directly into the pulmonary arteries, done for treatment "single ventricle physiology." The purpose is to separate the systemic and pulmonary venous blood, increase the systemic arterial saturation (decrease the cyanosis), and limit the work of the single ventricle to pumping a single cardiac output (to supply the systemic circulation).

- Hemi-Fontan procedure = creation of a right atrial to right PA anastomosis. The purpose is to divert superior vena caval flow to the pulmonary arteries.

REFERENCES

1. Waldman JD, Wernly JA. Cyanotic congenital heart disease with decreased pulmonary blood flow in children. *Pediatr Clin North Am* 1999;46(2):385–403.
2. Brickner ME, Hillis LD, Lange RA. Congenital heart disease in adults. *N Engl J Med* 2000;342(5):334–342.
3. Bernstein D. Tetralogy of Fallot. In: Behrman RE, Kliegman RM, Jenson HB (eds.), *Nelson Textbook of Pediatrics*, 17th ed. Philadelphia, PA: W.B. Saunders, 2004: 1524–1528.
4. Waldman JD, Wernly JA. Cyanotic congenital heart disease with decreased pulmonary blood flow in children. *Pediatr Clin North Am* 1999;46:385–403.
5. Gaynor JW, Spray TL. Congenital heart disease and anomalies of the great vessels. In: O'Neil JA Jr, Rowe MI, Grosfeld JL, et al. (eds.), *Pediatric Surgery*, 5th ed. St. Louis, MO: Mosby, 1998:1835–1848.
6. Duncan BW, Mee RB, Prieto LR, et al. Staged repair of tetralogy of Fallot with pulmonary atresia and major aortopulmonary collateral arteries. *J Thoracic Cardiovasc Surg* 2003;126(3):694–702.
7. Marshall AC, Love BA, Lang P, et al. Staged repair of tetralogy of Fallot and diminutive pulmonary arteries with a fenestrated ventricular septal defect patch. *J Thoracic Cardiovasc Surg* 2003;126(5):1427–1433.
8. Hennein HA, Mosca RS, Urcelay G, et al. Intermediate results after complete repair of tetralogy of Fallot in neonates. *J Thorac Cardiovasc Surg* 1995;109:332–344.
9. Therrien J, Marx GR, Gatzoulis MA. Late problems in tetralogy of Fallot recognition, management, and prevention. *Cardiol Clin* 2002;20:395–404.
10. Dees E, Lin H, Cotto RB, et al. Outcome of pre-term infants with congenital heart disease. *J Pediatr* 2000;137(5):653–659.
11. Pulmonary atresia and intact ventricular septum. In: Kourchoukos NT, Blackstone EH, Doty DB, et al. (eds.), *Kirklin/Barratt-Boyes Cardiac Surgery*, 3rd ed. Philadelphia, PA: Churchill-Livingstone, 2003:1095–1012.
12. Yoshimura N, Yamaguchi M, Ohashi H. et al. Pulmonary atresia with intact ventricular septum: Strategy based on right ventricular morphology. *J Thoracic Cardiovasc Surg* 2003;126(5):1417–1426.
13. Gupta A, Odim J, Levi D, et al. Staged repair of pulmonary atresia with ventricular septal defect and major aortopulmonary collateral arteries: Experience with 104 patients. *J Thoracic Cardiovasc Surg* 2003;126(6):1746–1752.
14. Kreutzer C, Mayorquim R de C, Kreutzer GOA, et al. Experience with one and a half ventricle repair. *J Thorac Cardiovasc Surg* 1999;117:662–668.
15. Numata S, Memura H, Yahihara T, et al. Long-term functional results of the one and one-half ventricular repair for the spectrum of patients with pulmonary atresia/stenosis with intact ventricular septum. *Eur J Cardiothorac Surg* 2003;24(4):516–520.
16. Miyaji K, Furuse A, Ohtsuka T, et al. Mid-term results of one and one-half ventricular repair in a patient with pulmonary atresia and intact ventricular septum. *Jpn Heart J* 1996;37(4):509–513.
17. Humpl T, Soderberg B, McCrindle BW, et al. Percutaneous balloon valvotomy in pulmonary atresia with intact ventricular septum: Impact on patient care. *Circulation* 2003; 108(7):826–832.
18. Tricuspid atresia and management of single-ventricle physiology. In: Kouchoukos NT, Blackstone EH, Doty DB, et al. (eds.), *Kirklin Barratt-Boyes Cardiac Surgery*. Philadelphia, PA: Churchill-Livingstone, 2003:1113–1176.
19. Jacobs ML, Pourmoghadam KK. The hemi-Fontan operation. *Semin Thorac Cardiovasc Surg* 2003;6:90–97.
20. Kumar SP, Rubinstein CS, Simsic JM, et al. Lateral tunnel versus extracardiac conduit Fontan procedure: A concurrent comparison. *Ann Thorac Surg* 2003;76:1389–1397.
21. Woods RK, Dyamenahalli U, Duncan BW, et al. Construction of extracardiac Fontan techniques: Pedicled pericardial tunnel versus conduit reconstruction. *J Thorac Cardiovasc Surg* 2003;125(3):465–471.
22. Petko M, Myung RJ, Wernovsky G, et al. Surgical reinterventions following the Fontan procedure. *Eur J Cardiothorac Surg* 2003;24:255–259.
23. Kammeraad J, Sreeram N. Acute thrombosis of an extracardiac Fontan conduit. *Heart* 2004;90(1):760.
24. Ebstein anomaly. In: Kouchoukos NT, Blackstone EH, Doty DB, et al. (eds.), *Kirklin/Barratt-Boyes Cardiac Surgery*, 3rd ed. Philadelphia, PA: Churchill-Livingstone, 2003: 1177–1199.
25. Chauvaud S, Berrebi A, d'Attellis N, et al. Ebstein's anomaly: Repair based on functional analysis. *Eur J Cardiothorac Surg* 2003;23(4):515–531.
26. VonSon JA, Falk V, Black MD, et al. Conversion of complex neonatal Ebstein's anomaly into functional tricuspid or pulmonary atresia. *Eur J Cardiothorac Surg* 1998;13:280–284.
27. Peterson C, Schilthuis JJ, Dodge-Khatami A, et al. Comparative long-term results of surgery versus balloon valvuloplasty for pulmonic valve stenosis in infants and children. *Ann Thoracic Surg* 2003;76(4):1078–1083.
28. Wang JK, Wu MH, Lee WL, et al. Balloon dilatation for critical pulmonic stenosis. *Int J Cardiol* 1999;69(1):27–32.
29. Hofbeck M, Singer H, Bukeitel G, et al. Balloon valvuloplasty of critical pulmonic valve stenosis in a premature neonate. *Pediatric Cardiol* 1999;20(2):147–149.
30. Fyler DC, Buckley LP, Hellenbrand WE. Report of the New England Regional Infant Cardiac Program. *Pediatrics* 1980;65(2):375–461.

31. Williams WG, McCrindle BW, Ashburn DA, et al. Outcomes of 829 neonates with complete transposition of the great arteries 12–17 years after repair. *Eur J Cardiothorac Surg* 2003;24(1):1–10.

32. Complete transposition of the great arteries. In: Kouchoukos NT, Blackstone EH, Doty DB, et al. (eds.), *Kirlin/Baratt-Boyes Cardiac Surgery*, 3rd ed. Philadelphia, PA: Churchill-Livingstone, 2003:1438–1508.

33. Hucin B, Voriskova M, Hruda J, et al. Late complications and quality of life after atrial correction of transposition of the great arteries in 12 to 18 year follow-up. *J Cardiovasc Surg* 2000;41:233–239.

34. Gelatt M, Hamilton RM, McCrindle BW, et al. Arrhythmia and mortality after the Mustard procedure: A 30-year single center experience. *J Am Coll Cardiol* 1997;29(1):194–201.

35. Wilson NJ, Clarkson PM, Barratt-Boyes BG, et al. Long-term outcome after the mustard repair for simple transposition of the great arteries. 28-year follow-up. *J Am Coll Cardiol* 1998;32(3):758–765.

36. Sagin-Saylam G, Somerville J. Palliative mustard operation for transposition of the great arteries: Late results after 15–20 years. *Heart* 1996;75(1):72–77.

37. Kirjavainen M, Happonen JM, Louhimo J. Late results of Senning operation. *J Thorac Cardiovasc Surg* 1999; 117(3):468–495.

38. Reddy V, Sharma S, Cobanoglu A. Atrial switch (Senning procedure) in the era of arterial switch operation: Current indications and results. *Eur J Cardiothorac Surg* 1996; 10(7):546–550.

39. Double outlet right ventricle. In: Kouchokos NT, Blackstone EH, Doty DB, et al. (eds.), *Kirlin/Baratt-Boyes Cardiac Surgery*, 3rd ed. Philadelphia, PA: Churchill-Livingstone, 2003:1509–1540.

40. Dearani JA, Danielson GK, Pua FJ, et al. Late results of the Rastelli operation for transportation of the great arteries. *Semin Thorac Cardiovasc Surg Annu* 2001;4:3–15.

41. Yamagishi M, Shuntok K, Matsushita T, et al. Half-turned truncal switch operation for complete transposition of the great arteries with ventricular septal defect and pulmonic stenosis. *J Thorac Cardiovasc Surg* 2003;125(4):966–968.

42. Devaney EJ, Charpie JR, Ohye RG, et al. Combined arterial switch and Senning operation for congenitally corrected transposition of the great arteries: Patient selection and immediate results. *J Thorac Cardiovasc Surg* 2003;125(3):500–507.

43. Duncan BW, Mee RBB, Mesia I, et al. Results of the double switch operation for congenitally corrected transposition of the great arteries. *Eur J Cardiothorac Surg* 2003;24:11–20.

44. Langley SM, Winlaw DS, Stumper O, et al. Midterm results after restoration of the morphologically left ventricle to the systemic circulation in patients with congenitally corrected transposition of the great arteries. *J Thorac Cardiovasc Surg* 2003;125(6):1229–1241.

45. Mavroudis C, Backer CL. Physiologic versus anatomic repair of congenitally corrected transposition of the great arteries. *Semin Thorac Cardiovasc Surg* 2003;6:16–26.

46. Congenitally corrected transposition of the great arteries and other forms of atrioventricular discordant connection. In: Kouchokos NT, Blackstone EH, Doty DB, et al. (eds.), *Kirlin/Baratt-Boyes Cardiac Surgery*, 3rd ed. Philadelphia, PA: Churchill-Livingstone, 2003:1549–1583.

47. Aeba R, Katogi T, Koizumi K, et al. Apico-pulmonary artery conduit repair of congenitally corrected transposition of the great arteries with ventricular septal defect and pulmonary outflow obstruction: A 10-year follow-up. *Ann Thorac Surg* 2003:1383–1388.

48. Dearani JA, Danielson GK, Puga FJ, et al. Late follow-up of 1095 patients undergoing operation for complex congenital heart disease utilizing pulmonary ventricle to pulmonary artery conduits. *Ann Thorac Surg* 2003;75(2):399–411.

49. Urban AE, Sinzobahamvya N, Brecher AM, et al. Truncus arteriosus: Ten-year experience with homograft repair in neonates and infants. *Ann Thorac Surg* 1998;66(6 Suppl): S183–S188.

50. Brizard CP, Cocrane A, Austin C, et al. Management strategy and long-term outcome for truncus arteriosus. *Eur J Cardiothorac Surg* 1997;11(4):687–695.

51. Heinemann MK, Hanley FH, Fenton KN, et al. Fate of small homograft conduits after early repair of truncus arteriosus. *Ann Thorac Surg* 1993;1409.

52. Elami A, Laks H, Pearl JM. Truncal valve repair: Initial experience with infants and children. *Ann Thorac Surg* 1994;57:397.

53. Rajasinghe HA, McElhinney DB, Reddy VM, et al. Long-term follow-up of truncus arteriosus repaired in infancy: A twenty-year experience. *J Thorac Cardiovasc Surg* 1997; 112(5):869–879.

54. Brown JW, Ruzmetov M, Okada Y, et al. Truncus arteriosus repair: Outcomes, risk factors, re-operation and management. *Eur J Cardiothorac Surg* 2001;20(3):221–227.

55. Hyde JA, Stumper O, Barth MJ, et al. Total anomalous pulmonary venous connection: Outcome of surgical correction and management of recurrent venous obstruction. *Eur J Cardiothorac Surg* 1999;15(6):735–740.

56. Choudhary SK, Bhan A, Sharma R, et al. Repair of total anomalous pulmonary venous connection in infancy: Experience from a developing country. *Ann Thorac Surg* 1999;68(1):155–159.

57. Fox RE, Crosson JE, Campbell AB. Radiological case of the mouth: Total anomalous pulmonary venous return. *Arch Pediatr Adolesc Med* 2001;155(2):193–194.

58. Bando K, Turrentine MW, Ensing GJ, et al. Surgical management of total anomalous pulmonary venous connection. Thirty-year trends. *Circulation* 1996;94(9 Suppl):II-12–II-16.

59. Ricci M, Elliott M, Cohen GA, et al. Management of pulmonary venous obstruction after correction of TAPVC: Risk factors for adverse outcomes. *Eur J Cardiothorac Surg* 2003;24(1):28–36.

60. Korbmacher B, Buttgen S, Schulte HD, et al. Long-term results after repair of total anomalous pulmonary venous connection. *Thorac Cardiovasc Surg* 2001;49(2):101–106.

61. Michel-Behnke I, Luedemann M, Hagel KJ, et al. Serial stent implantation to relieve in-stent stenosis in obstructed total anomalous pulmonary venous return. *Pediatr Cardiol* 2002;23(2):221–223.

62. Bullaboy CA, Johnson DH, Azar H, et al. Total anomalous pulmonary venous connection to portal system: A new therapeutic role for prostaglandin E_1? *Pediatr Cardiol* 1984; 5:115.

63. Grifka RG. Cyanotic congenital heart disease with increased pulmonary blood flow. *Pediatr Clin North Am* 1999; 46(2):405–425.

64. Marino BS. Outcomes after the Fontan procedure. *Curr Opin Pediatr* 2002;14(5):620–626.

65. Milanesi O, Stellin G, Colan SD, et al. Systolic and diastolic performance late after the Fontan procedure for a single ventricle and comparison of those undergoing operation at <12 months of age and at >12 months of age. *Am J Cardiol* 2002;89(3):276–280.

66. Petko M, Myung RJ, Wernovsky G, et al. Surgical reinterventions following the Fontan procedure. *Eur J Cardiothorac Surg* 2003;24(2):255–259.

67. Margossian RE, Solowiejczyk D, Bourloin F, et al. Septation of the single ventricle revisited. *J Thorac Cardiovasc Surg* 2002;124(3):442–447.

68. Bradley SM, Simsic JM, Atz AM, et al. The infant with single ventricle and excessive pulmonary blood flow: Results of a strategy of pulmonary division and shunt. *Ann Thorac Surg* 2002;74(3):805–810.

69. Michielon G, Parisi F, Squitieri C, et al. Orthotopic heart transplantation for congenital heart disease: An alternative for high-risk Fontan candidates? *Circulation* 2003;108(10) (Suppl II):II-140–II-149.

70. Schwartz SM, Dent CL, Musa NL, et al. Single-ventricle physiology. *Crit Care Clin* 2003;19:393–411.

INDEX

Page numbers followed by italic *f* or *t* denote figures or tables, respectively.

CK-MB. *See* Creatine kinase (CK)-MB
Clarithromycin, 404*t*
Clindamycin, 404*t*
Clopidogrel, 141–143, 154
Coagulation cascade, 74–75
Coarctation of the aorta, 502–503. *See also* Congenital heart disease
Cocaine, cardiac toxicity, 448*t*, 450
Colchicine, 424
Collagen vascular disorders, 252
Compression/decompression, active, 25
Compression/ventilation, simultaneous, 25
Computed tomography (CT)
 electron beam, for calcium scoring, 211–212
 in pericarditis, 422
Conduction defects. *See* Cardiac conduction blocks
Conduction systems. *See* Cardiac conduction system
Conduction time, prolonged, 220
Congenital heart disease
 anatomy and physiology
  ductus arteriosus closure, 489–490
  fetal circulation, 487, 489*f*, 490*f*, 491*f*, 492*t*
  foramen ovale closure, 490
  postnatal circulation, 487, 488*f*, 492*t*
  transitional circulation, 488–489
 atrial septal defects, 499–501, 500*f*, 501*f*, 502*f*
 atrioventricular canal defects, 498–499, 499*f*
 cardiac catheterization, 516
 cardiogenic shock in, 471, 472*t*, 501–503
 clinical presentation, 463, 464–465, 464*t*
 coarctation of the aorta, 502–503
 common defects, 467*t*
 complications, 471–474, 473*t*
 critical aortic stenosis, 503
 cyanosis in, 468–469, 468*t*
 diagnostic tests, 466
 double outlet right ventricle with pulmonic stenosis, 508
 ductal-dependent lesions, 471, 473*t*
 Ebstein's anomaly, 508, 508*f*, 509*f*
 Eisenmenger syndrome, 469
 embryology
  atrial septation, 494–495
  cardiac looping, 492–493
  cardiac septation, 493–494, 494*f*
  cardiac tube formation, 491–492, 493*f*, 493*t*

conotruncus and great vessels, 495
 endocardial cushion defects, 495
 pulmonary veins, 495
 ventricular septation, 495
heart failure in, 469–471, 470*t*, 471*t*, 472*t*, 496–501
high yield facts, 463, 487, 505
hypoplastic left heart syndrome, 501–502, 516
incidence, 463, 467*t*
left-to-right shunt lesions, 496
patent ductus arteriosus, 497–498, 498*f*
physical examination, 465–466
prenatal and birth history, 465
pulmonary atresia, 506–507
pulmonic stenosis, 508–509
single ventricle, 515, 516–517
surgical procedures, 516–517
tetralogy of Fallot, 468–469, 505–506, 506*f*
total anomalous pulmonary venous return, 513, 514*f*, 515
transposition of the great arteries, 509–512, 510*f*, 516
tricuspid atresia, 507–508
truncus arteriosus, 512–513, 512*f*
ventricular septal defect, 496–497, 497*f*, 516
Congestive heart failure. *See* Heart failure
Conotruncus, 495
Continuous positive airway pressure (CPAP), 333
Coronary angioplasty. *See* Percutaneous coronary intervention; Percutaneous transluminal coronary angioplasty
Coronary artery bypass graft (CABG)
 in acute myocardial infarction, 180, 180*t*
 in cardiogenic shock, 36, 37*f*
 trends in number performed, 64*f*
 in UA/NSTEMI, 178
Coronary artery disease. *See also* Acute coronary syndrome; Atherosclerosis; Cardiovascular disease
 demographics, 54–56
 economic issues
  cost of procedures, 63, 64*f*, 65*f*
  observation and admission protocols, 61–62, 62*t*, 63*f*
 historical perspective, 68–69
 prevalence, 53–54
 risk factors
  age, 54–55
  diabetes, 56–57

gender, 55–56, 55*f*
 hyperlipidemia, 57–58
 hypertension, 57
 physical inactivity, 58
 research, 59–60
 smoking, 57
Coronary calcium scoring, 211–212
Corrigan's pulse, 386
Corticosteroids
 mechanism of action and side effects, 352, 352*t*
 in pericarditis, 424
CPAP (continuous positive airway pressure), 333
C-reactive protein, 115
Creatine kinase (CK)-MB
 assays for, 111
 initial, 86–87, 87*t*
 multimarker strategy, 113
 pathophysiology, 110
 sensitivity and specificity, 112–113, 112*t*
 serial, 87*t*
 time changes in, 113–114, 114*t*
 timing of release, 110–111
CSM (carotid sinus massage), 241
C-type natriuretic peptide (CNP), 314, 315*f*
Cyanosis
 in congenital heart disease, 468–469, 468*t*, 505
 in Ebstein's anomaly, 508
 in single ventricle, 515
 in tetralogy of Fallot, 505–506
 in total anomalous pulmonary venous return, 513
 in transposition of the great arteries, 509, 511
 in tricuspid atresia, 507
 in truncus arteriosus, 512
Cyclosporin, 352, 352*t*

D
Defibrillation. *See also* Automated external defibrillator; Implantable cardioverter-defibrillator
 in cardiopulmonary resuscitation, 25
 early strategies
  controversies, 293–294
  first responder response, 292
  hospital-based, 294
  paramedic only response, 292
  public access, 292–293
 in presence of pacemaker, 283
 in ventricular fibrillation, 222